CRITICAL CARE ULTRASONOGRAPHY

NOTICE

Medicine is an ever-changing science. As new research and clinical experience broaden our knowledge, changes in treatment and drug therapy are required. The author and the publisher of this work have checked with sources believed to be reliable in their efforts to provide information that is complete and generally in accord with the standards accepted at the time of publication. However, in view of the possibility of human error or changes in medical sciences, neither the author nor the publisher nor any other party who has been involved in the preparation or publication of this work warrants that the information contained herein is in every respect accurate or complete, and they disclaim all responsibility for any errors or omissions or for the results obtained from use of the information contained in this work. Readers are encouraged to confirm the information contained herein with other sources. For example and in particular, readers are advised to check the product information sheet included in the package of each drug they plan to administer to be certain that the information contained in this work is accurate and that changes have not been made in the recommended dose or in the contraindications for administration. This recommendation is of particular importance in connection with new or infrequently used drugs.

CRITICAL CARE ULTRASONOGRAPHY

SECOND EDITION

Alexander B. Levitov, MD, FCCP, FCCM, RDCS
Professor of Medicine
Eastern Virginia Medical School
Department of Internal Medicine
Division of Pulmonary and Critical Care Medicine
Norfolk, Virginia

Paul H. Mayo, MD, FCCP
Division of Pulmonary, Critical Care, and Sleep Medicine
North Shore-Long Island Jewish Medical Center
New Hyde Park, New York
Hofstra North Shore-LIJ School of Medicine
Hempstead, New York

Anthony D. Slonim, MD, DrPH
Executive Vice President/Chief Medical Officer
Barnabas Health
West Orange, New Jersey
Professor, Medicine, Pediatrics, Community and Public Health
University of Medicine and Dentistry of New Jersey
New Jersey Medical School
Newark, New Jersey

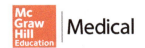

New York Chicago San Francisco Athens London Madrid Mexico City
Milan New Delhi Singapore Sydney Toronto

Critical Care Ultrasonography, Second Edition

Copyright © 2014 by McGraw-Hill Education. All rights reserved. Printed in China. Except as permitted under the United States Copyright Act of 1976, no part of this publication may be reproduced or distributed in any form or by any means, or stored in a database or retrieval system, without the prior written permission of the publisher.

1 2 3 4 5 6 7 8 9 0   CTP/CTP   19 18 17 16 15 14

ISBN 9781265833916
MHID 1265833915

This book was set in Berling by Aptara, Inc.
The editors were Brian Belval and Kim J. Davis.
The production supervisor was Catherine H. Saggese.
Cover photograph by Yonatan Y. Greenstein, MD
Project management was provided by Indu Jawwad of Aptara, Inc.

Library of Congress Cataloging-in-Publication Data

Critical care ultrasonography / [edited by] Alexander B. Levitov, Anthony D. Slonim, Paul H. Mayo. – Second edition.
  p. ; cm.
  Includes bibliographical references and index.
  ISBN 978-0-07-179351-3 (hardcover : alk. paper) – ISBN 0-07-179351-8 (hardcover : alk. paper)
  I. Levitov, Alexander, editor of compilation. II. Slonim, Anthony D., editor of compilation. III. Mayo, Paul H., editor of compilation.
  [DNLM: 1. Ultrasonography–methods. 2. Critical Care.   WN 208]
  RC78.7.U4
  616.07′543—dc23
                                              2013050216

McGraw-Hill Education books are available at special quantity discounts to use as premiums and sales promotions, or for use in corporate training programs. To contact a representative, please visit the Contact Us pages at www.mhprofessional.com.

To Irina and Alexandra for everything.
A.B.L.

To my wife Charlotte Malasky, MD, for all of her patience and support.
P.H.M.

To Terry, Michael, and Samantha . . . thanks for your love, support,
and devotion.
A.D.S.

CONTENTS

Contributors ix
Preface xiii
Acknowledgments xv

Section I: General Principles and Impact of Ultrasound Use in the ICU 1

1. Ultrasound in Critical Care Medicine: Improving Patient Care and Reducing Cost 3
   Nana E. Coleman
   Anthony D. Slonim

2. Physics of Sound, Ultrasound, and Doppler Effect and its Diagnostic Utility 9
   Alexander B. Levitov

3. Transducers, Image Formation, and Artifacts 23
   Alexander B. Levitov
   Joseph John

4. Training in Critical Care Ultrasonography 37
   Paul H. Mayo
   Alexander B. Levitov

5. Pediatric Critical Care: The Use of Bedside Ultrasonography 43
   William Tsai
   Shilpa Amara
   Anthony D. Slonim

Section II: Cardiac Sonography in the ICU . . . 55

6. Goal-directed Echocardiography in the ICU 57
   Seth Koenig
   Mangala Narasimhan
   Paul H. Mayo

7. Transthoracic Echocardiography: Image Acquisition 65
   Jose Cardenas-Garcia
   Paul H. Mayo

8. Transesophageal Echocardiography: Image Acquisition and Transducer Manipulation 77
   Viera Lakticova
   Paul H. Mayo

9. Echocardiographic Assessment of Left Ventricular Systolic and Diastolic Function 89
   Alexander B. Levitov
   Paul H. Mayo
   Louis Vastardis

10. Echocardiographic Evaluation of Preload Responsiveness 105
    Alexander B. Levitov
    Paul E. Marik

11. Echocardiographic Diagnosis and Monitoring of Right Ventricular Function 115
    Adolfo Kaplan
    Paul H. Mayo

12. Echocardiographic Diagnosis of Cardiac Tamponade 127
    Mikhail Litinski
    Keith Guevarra
    Anthony D. Slonim

13. Echocardiographic Diagnosis and Monitoring of Acute Myocardial Infarction and Associated Complications 135
    Rodney W. Savage

14. Echocardiographic Diagnosis of Cardiomyopathies 143
    Narinder P. Bhalla
    Marguerite Underwood
    Alexander B. Levitov

15. Echocardiographic Evaluation of Valve Function and Endocarditis 163
    Robert Arntfield
    Paul H. Mayo

16. Echocardiographic Evaluation of Cardiac Trauma 175
    Keith Guevarra
    Mikhail Litinski
    Anthony D. Slonim

Section III: Ultrasound Evaluation of the Neck, Trunk, and Extremities 183

17. Ultrasound Evaluation of the Neck and Upper Respiratory System 185
    Christian H. Butcher

18. Ultrasound Evaluation of the Pleura 197
    Lewis Eisen
    Peter Doelken
    Sahar Ahmad

19. Ultrasound Evaluation of the Lung 207
    Pierre Kory
    Paul H. Mayo

20. Ultrasound Evaluation of the Abdomen 219
    Sarah C. Shaves
    Heidi L. Frankel

21. Ultrasound Evaluation of the Renal System and the Bladder 235
    Yefim R. Sheynkin

22. Ultrasound Evaluation of the Pelvis 249
    Michael Blaivas

23. Ultrasound Evaluation of the Peripheral Vascular System 257
    James E. Foster, II
    Kevin Wiseman

Section IV: Ultrasound Guidance for Procedures 271

24. Ultrasound-Guided Transthoracic Procedures . . . 273
    Peter Doelken
    Paul H. Mayo

25. Ultrasound Guidance for Abdominal and Soft Tissue Procedures 285
    Sameh Aziz
    William J. Brunelli, Jr.
    James S. Cain

26. Peripheral and Central Neuraxial Blocks in Critical Care Medicine 297
    Santhanam Suresh

27. Ultrasound Guidance for Vascular Access 303
    Christian H. Butcher

28. Ocular Ultrasound 319
    David Evans

Appendix A: Glossary 327

Appendix B: Draft Ultrasound Reports By Body Region 335

Index 343

CONTRIBUTORS

▶ **Sahar Ahmad, MD**
Albert Einstein College of Medicine
Montefiore Medical Center
Division of Pulmonary Medicine
Bronx, New York

▶ **Shilpa Amara, PharmD**
Drug Information Specialist
Barnabas Health
South Plainfield, New Jersey

▶ **Robert Arntfield, MD, FRCPC, FCCP, FACEP, RDMS**
Assistant Professor
Director of Critical Care Ultrasound
Division of Critical Care and Division of Emergency Medicine
Department of Medicine
Western University
London, Ontario, Canada

▶ **Sameh Aziz, MD, FCCP, FACP**
Assistant Professor of Medicine
Pulmonary/Critical Care and Sleep Medicine
Assistant Professor of Medicine
Virginia Tech Carilion School of Medicine
Edward Via Virginia College of Osteopathic Medicine
Carilion Clinic
Roanoke, Virginia

▶ **Narinder P. Bhalla, MD**
River Region Cardiology Associates
Montgomery, Alabama

▶ **Michael Blaivas, MD, FACEP, FAIUM**
Professor of Medicine
University of South Carolina School of Medicine
Columbia, South Carolina

▶ **William J. Brunelli, Jr., MPAS, RDMS, RDCS, PA-C**
Radiology Associates of Roanoke, P.C.
Interventional Radiology
Lewis Gale Medical Center
Salem, Virginia

▶ **Christian H. Butcher, MD, FCCP**
Pulmonary and Critical Care Medicine
St Peter's Hospital Medical Group
Helena, Montana

▶ **James S. Cain, MD, FACP, FASN**
Clinical Assistant Professor of Medicine
Virginia Tech Carilion School of Medicine
Valley Nephrology Associates
Roanoke, Virginia

▶ **Jose Cardenas-Garcia, MD**
Division of Pulmonary, Critical Care, and Sleep Medicine
Long Island Jewish Medical Center
New Hyde Park, New York

▶ **Nana E. Coleman, MD, EdM**
Assistant Professor of Pediatrics
Weill Cornell Medical College
New York, New York

▶ **Peter Doelken, MD**
Associate Professor
Division of Pulmonary and Critical Care Medicine
Albany Medical College
Albany, New York

▶ **Lewis Eisen, MD**
Assistant Professor of Clinical Neurology
Associate Professor of Clinical Medicine
Division of Critical Care Medicine
Department of Medicine
Albert Einstein College of Medicine
Montefiore Medical Center
Bronx, New York

▶ **David Evans, MD, RDMS, RDCS, FACEP**
Medical Director of Ultrasound
Emergency Ultrasound Fellowship Director; Assistant Professor
Department of Emergency Medicine
Virginia Commonwealth University School of Medicine
Richmond, Virginia

▶ **James E. Foster, II, MD, FACS, RPVI**
Associate Professor, Department of Surgery
Virginia Tech Carilion School of Medicine
Medical Director, Non-Invasive Vascular Laboratory
Medical Director, Wound Care Center
Carilion Clinic
Roanoke, Virginia

▶ **Heidi L. Frankel, MD, FACS, FCCM**
Professor of Surgery
University of Southern California Keck School of Medicine
Director of Surgical Critical Care Services, Keck Hospital
Los Angeles, California

CONTRIBUTORS

▶ **Keith Guevarra, DO, FCCP**
Attending, Division of Pulmonary, Critical Care and Lung Transplant
Barnabas Health Lung Center
Newark Beth Israel Medical Center
Newark, New Jersey

▶ **Joseph John, PA-C, RVT**
Instructor
Department of Internal Medicine
Division of Critical Care Medicine
Eastern Virginia Medical School
Norfolk, Virginia

▶ **Adolfo Kaplan, MD**
Pulmonary and Sleep Center of the Valley
Weslaco, Texas

▶ **Seth Koenig, MD**
Division of Pulmonary, Critical Care, and Sleep Medicine
North Shore-Long Island Jewish Medical Center
New Hyde Park, New York
Hofstra North Shore-LIJ School of Medicine
Hempstead, New York

▶ **Pierre Kory, MD, MPA**
Program Director, Pulmonary and Critical Care Fellowship Program
Division of Pulmonary, Critical Care, and Sleep Medicine
Beth Israel Medical Center
New York, New York
Assistant Professor of Medicine
Albert Einstein College of Medicine
Bronx, New York

▶ **Viera Lakticova, MD**
Division of Pulmonary, Critical Care, and Sleep Medicine
North Shore-Long Island Jewish Medical Center
New Hyde Park, New York
Hofstra North Shore-LIJ School of Medicine
Hempstead, New York

▶ **Alexander B. Levitov, MD, FCCP, FCCM, RDCS**
Professor of Medicine
Eastern Virginia Medical School
Department of Internal Medicine
Division of Pulmonary and Critical Care Medicine
Norfolk, Virginia

▶ **Mikhail Litinski, MD**
Director, Division of Critical Care
Bayonne Medical Center
Bayonne, New Jersey

▶ **Paul E. Marik, MD**
Professor, Internal Medicine
Eastern Virginia Medical School
Norfolk, Virginia

▶ **Paul H. Mayo, MD, FCCP**
Division of Pulmonary, Critical Care, and Sleep Medicine
North Shore-Long Island Jewish Medical Center
New Hyde Park, New York
Hofstra North Shore-LIJ School of Medicine
Hempstead, New York

▶ **Mangala Narasimhan, DO**
Division of Pulmonary, Critical Care, and Sleep Medicine
North Shore-Long Island Jewish Medical Center
New Hyde Park, New York
Hofstra North Shore-LIJ School of Medicine
Hempstead, New York

▶ **Rodney W. Savage, MD, FACP, FACC, FSCAI**
Fellowship Director
VTC Interventional Cardiology Fellowship
Carilion Clinic
Roanoke, Virginia

▶ **Sarah C. Shaves, MD**
Assistant Professor, Radiology
Vice Chairman, Radiology Residency
Eastern Virginia Medical School
Norfolk, Virginia

▶ **Yefim R. Sheynkin, MD, FACS**
Associate Clinical Professor of Urology
SUNY at Stony Brook
Stony Brook, New York

▶ **Anthony D. Slonim, MD, DrPH**
Executive Vice President/Chief Medical Officer
Barnabas Health
West Orange, New Jersey
Professor, Medicine, Pediatrics, Community and Public Health
University of Medicine and Dentistry of New Jersey
New Jersey Medical School
Newark, New Jersey

▶ **Santhanam Suresh, MD**
Professor and Chair
Department of Pediatric Anesthesiology
Ann and Robert H. Lurie Children's Hospital of Chicago
Professor of Anesthesiology and Pediatrics
Northwestern University's Feinberg School of Medicine
Chicago, Illinois

▶ **William Tsai, MD**
Division of Critical Care Medicine
Levine Children's Hospital at Carolinas Medical Center
Charlotte, North Carolina

▶ **Marguerite Underwood, MSN, RN, RDCS**
Carilion Clinic Cardiology Services
Roanoke, Virginia

▶ **Louis Vastardis, RDCS**
Echocardiography
Sentara Heart Hospital
Norfolk, Virginia

▶ **Kevin Wiseman, BS, RVT**
Senior Vascular Technologist, Non-invasive Vascular Laboratory
Carilion Clinic
Roanoke, Virginia

PREFACE

In the interval of time since the first edition of this textbook was published, bedside ultrasonography, particularly for critically ill patients, has revolutionized the practice of critical care medicine and created a new standard of care for these vulnerable patients. As the use of bedside ultrasound has matured, there has been an explosion of scholarly work, pathways, protocols, and guidelines that support its routine use in everyday clinical care. In addition, fundamental training in bedside ultrasonography is now included in residency, fellowship, and postgraduate training for attending physicians.

Given these changes in the landscape, we are pleased to present the second edition of *Critical Care Ultrasonography*. While we have maintained the overall structure in this edition, we have been deliberate in incorporating feedback from readers and updates that keep pace with the evolution of the discipline. Further, because ultrasonography is a visual field, we have enhanced the visual aspects of content with additional figures and videos. We are hopeful that this book will continue to serve the spectrum of clinicians, from novice to expert, who are interested in a core textbook or a ready reference that helps to support clinical decision making.

Alexander B. Levitov, MD
Anthony D. Slonim, MD
Paul H. Mayo, MD

ACKNOWLEDGMENTS

We are indebted to many members of our team who helped us in updating and improving this textbook. First, we appreciate the effort of our authors who assisted us in assuring that state-of-the-art and evidence-based content were included in this edition of the book. Second, we appreciate the tireless efforts of our McGraw-Hill team, notably Brian Belval, Kim Davis, and James Shanahan. Finally, we are appreciative of those who supported us each day, including our colleagues and families, while we were busy trying to complete this volume.

SECTION I

General Principles and Impact of Ultrasound Use in the ICU

ULTRASOUND IN CRITICAL CARE MEDICINE: IMPROVING PATIENT CARE AND REDUCING COST

NANA E. COLEMAN & ANTHONY D. SLONIM

INTRODUCTION

More than a decade ago, the Institute of Medicine challenged medical care providers and systems to improve healthcare delivery across six essential areas: safety, effectiveness, efficiency, timeliness, equity, and patient-centeredness (Figure 1-1) in *Crossing the Quality Chiasm: A New Health System for the 21st Century*. Antecedent to the establishment of these goals, the same body recognized in *To Err is Human: Building a Safer Health System* that up to 100,000 patients in hospitals die needlessly each year from avoidable medical errors. Despite the extensive resources devoted by national and local governments, health systems, and individuals to improvements in patient safety and error reduction, disappointingly, studies demonstrate that since these seminal publications, *we have not achieved enough*. Medical errors continue to occur at an alarming rate; and as the definition of unacceptable hospital-based events broadens to include morbidities, such as hospital-acquired infections, pressure ulcers, and preventable delays in care, the disparity between the goals and reality of US health care is only more apparent.

Most recently, the paradigm for healthcare improvement has shifted to not only incorporate the impact of quality improvement on the individual patient, but on the population at large. With its focus on reducing the overall costs of care, optimizing the collective health of target populations, in addition to improving the individual patient care experience, the Institute for Healthcare Improvement's (IHI) "Triple Aim Initiative" seeks to unify strategies for patient safety and quality improvement within the context of a more integrated and collaborative care delivery model than previously witnessed (Figure 1-2). The IHI identified several principal elements to help guide achievement of these aims, including the reorganization of primary care services, an emphasis on population-based wellness goals, and the development of cost-reduction strategies. Finally, although the Triple Aim Initiative still prioritizes the six aims of improvement for the individual care experience as set forth in *Crossing the Quality Chiasm*, it goes further to integrate the concepts of better patient care, improved community health, and lower cost (Table 1-1).

As medical technologies and clinical practice evolve, it is imperative that they be considered in the framework of the patient experience, population health, and cost reduction (Figure 1-3) as defined by the Triple Aim Initiative. Only in so doing, can we, the consumers of health, be assured that our best interests remain at the forefront of such innovation. A striking example of one medical tool that has broad implications for each of these elements is bedside critical care ultrasonography. A rapid, noninvasive, high-yield radiographic modality, ultrasound is almost universally the gold standard diagnostic tool for the evaluation of obstetric and gynecologic abnormalities. Additionally, it has garnered widespread acceptance for guidance of regional anesthesia, invasive catheter placement, and as a first-line method of evaluating neonatal intracranial pathology. Given its unique features—portable, noninvasive, radiation-sparing, and dynamic—ultrasound is a desirable tool for optimizing the individual patient care experience, reducing healthcare costs, and improving population well-being. Particularly for critically ill populations for whom timely, minimal-risk, and high-yield diagnostics are essential, bedside ultrasound may be a transformative healthcare tool. In order to facilitate understanding of the value of critical care ultrasonography within the paradigm of the three aims, it is instructive to first overview the current practical application of ultrasound in the intensive care unit (ICU).

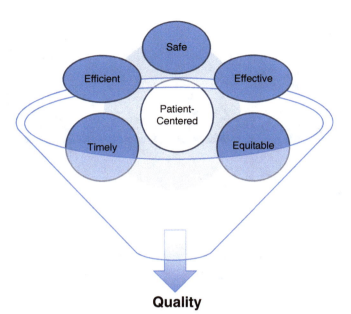

Figure 1-1 Institute of Medicine's six domains of quality improvement.

PRACTICAL APPLICATION OF ULTRASOUND IN THE ICU

Current literature suggests that the use of critical care ultrasound has enhanced technical proficiency among critical care providers; has improved procedural outcomes and in some instances, facilitated more timely diagnosis of medical problems than traditional radiographic methods. Furthermore, experiential reflection over time on the inherent advantages and pitfalls of bedside ultrasound has facilitated more judicious and efficacious application of this technology. Published guidelines now exist to define the ideal use of bedside ultrasound in various diagnostic and treatment algorithms. The enhanced safety profile of ultrasonography, in comparison to invasive or radiation-emitting techniques, has made it an attractive alternative across a broad range of clinical scenarios, including pulmonary, cardiac, and traumatic conditions.

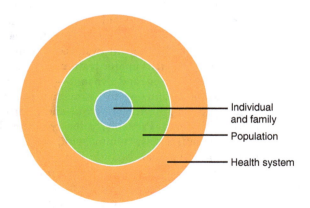

Figure 1-2 Schematic of the IHI Triple Aim Initiative. By improving the health of individuals and families, the overall wellness of a population improves and thus the costs to the system can be dramatically reduced.

TABLE 1-1
The Definitions of the Institute of Medicine Domains

Institute of Medicine Domain	Definition
Safety	To limit the unintentional harm associated with the delivery of health care
Effectiveness	To use evidence-based practice, the best scientific evidence, clinical expertise, and patient values to achieve the best outcomes for patients
Efficiency	To provide care that is done well and with limited waste
Equity	To provide care that is free from bias related to personal demographics, like gender, race, ethnicity, insurance status, or income
Timeliness	To provide care without unnecessary waits and to assure that patients have access to the care that they need
Patient centeredness	To provide care that reflects a focus on the patient's needs, including empathy, compassion, and respect

▶ Overview of Current Practice

Bedside chest ultrasound is now used almost routinely to assess pleural effusions at least as an adjunct to chest radiographs and in some cases for primary evaluation. It is also useful for the assessment of pneumothorax and with sufficient resolution, for evaluation of and differentiation between other alveolar or interstitial lung pathology. There presently exist hand-carried ultrasound devices used for intensive care patients that some now even advocate can be used as part of the daily, routine bedside evaluation of pulmonary disease. Given that thoracic ultrasound has both diagnostic and therapeutic benefits, it can serve to reduce the overall expenditures by use of a single study when appropriate. Recently, international guidelines were described to provide evidence-based consensus regarding the use of "point-of-care" lung ultrasound. Among the key statements was first, that chest ultrasonography more accurately assists in the diagnosis of pneumothorax than chest radiographs and secondarily that in pediatric patients, lung ultrasound is as accurate as chest radiography in diagnosing pneumonia. The consensus group further concluded that pulmonary ultrasonography is also valuable in monitoring aeration changes across the spectrum of parenchymal lung disease.

Although not as widespread as lung ultrasound, the role of "FADE" (Fast Assessment Diagnostic Echocardiography)

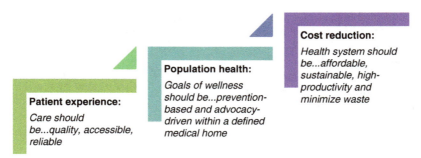

Figure 1-3 Key elements of quality in the triple aim model.

continues to grow in critical care medicine. Previously solely a procedural skill retained by cardiologists, intensivists and anesthesiologists both have begun to utilize rapid, focused echocardiography for the assessment of volume status, myocardial function, pericardial and valvular pathology, and hemodynamics. It is unlikely that bedside diagnostic echocardiograms can ever replace the sophistication of formal echocardiography; however, in acute situations, it may prove of benefit, especially when subspecialty expertise outside of the ICU is not imminently available. A specific inherent challenge of training noncardiologists to perform echocardiography is the variability in ascertaining procedural competence and maintenance of skill. Unlike cardiologists, who routinely perform this skill and thus have the ready opportunity to update and finesse their technical expertise, less frequent operators, such as intensivists, may rather place patients at risk if their diagnostic abilities are suboptimal. Moreover, unlike thoracic ultrasound for which there are fewer potential anatomical variants, subtle deviations from the normal in cardiac anatomy, particularly in children or after cardiac surgery, may distort the planes of view and thus, compromise diagnostic accuracy for the point-of-care ultrasonographer.

The utilization of focused assessment with sonography for trauma (termed "FAST") is broadly accepted and in many instances has become the standard of practice across emergency medicine and trauma departments, particularly in patients who are clinically unstable and for whom transfer to an area outside of the emergency department may result in greater morbidity, FAST is a useful tool for identifying the sequelae from blunt abdominal or thoracic injury in posttraumatic patients and guiding rapid intervention and therapy. Given the highly specific and moderately sensitive nature of this tool, it can help clinicians to stratify risk assessment and the need for follow-up care, especially in those patients who have borderline findings. Those educational studies which do exist claim that incorporation of focused ultrasound training in surgical and emergency medicine training programs is feasible with an acceptable level of competency attained by trainees.

Nowhere are these findings more relevant than in the case of neonates and children. Pediatric populations are especially vulnerable to procedural error and failure given their relatively small body habitus in comparison to adults; the frequent distortion of normal anatomical landmarks secondary to overlying vessels and their anatomical size; and their inability to readily cooperate with necessary positioning in the absence of substantive sedation and its associated risks. When critically ill, infants and children typically have lower thresholds for respiratory and hemodynamic collapse that may result from their primary disease process and are further exacerbated by the physiologic stress of painful procedures and the systemic effects of requisite sedation and analgesia. Additionally, while most parents will support and facilitate any intervention needed to help care for their sick child, even the most patient individuals are likely to become disheartened and unwilling when multiple procedural unsuccessful attempts are made. It is no wonder that ultrasound guidance for central vascular access in children has so quickly gained favor across most neonatal and pediatric critical care units.

▶ Challenges of Critical Care Ultrasound

Despite the clear benefit of intensive care ultrasound on patient care, provider quality, and system efficiency, the inherent risks associated with this emerging technology cannot be ignored. There are potential hazards associated with training highly skilled, yet undifferentiated practitioners in novel techniques. Although critical care physicians undergo years of training to become clinical subspecialists and possess extensive procedural expertise, adult learners are notoriously difficult to reeducate once they have moved from novice to master learners. New skills portend new technical, conceptual, and intellectual challenges that not all clinicians are willing to take the needed time to surmount. Additionally, maintenance of practical skill is difficult: first, when there are limited opportunities for skill mastery when one is outside of formal training, and second, when the motivation may be limited if in essence the existent practice "is not (thought to be) broken" in the first place.

As one can imagine, there is a learning curve for any new application or skill. Unfortunately, given the paramount consequences of misdiagnosis or clinical misadventures in critical care medicine, the margin of error is quite narrow. That being said, as practitioners seek to improve their ultrasound abilities, it is unclear how many patients may inadvertently suffer the undesirable consequences of time-delay, inaccurate or incomplete diagnosis, or direct injury all the while the learner hones his or her skills.

There exists also an inherent tension between those providers, who traditionally provided ultrasound services—radiologists, cardiologists, and sonographers, for example—and intensivists, who may try to mimic the same diagnostic or therapeutic outcomes; however, with far less training or expertise. One cannot ignore the potential *adverse* financial impact of this less costly, less invasive imaging modality on those who previously singularly provided these services. Arguably, equipping more providers to be able to perform this service can have clinical and even fiscal benefit for the larger health system; however, potentially at the expense of other sectors of the medical system.

▶ Provider Training and Education

Formal instruction in critical care ultrasound has taken various forms, from proprietary supplemental courses to the informal bedside "see one, do one, teach one" philosophy to high-fidelity simulation. In each of these formats, participants range from senior physicians to advanced practitioners and graduate medical trainees. What is typically common to the formal educational experience is a theoretical discussion surrounding ultrasound physics and technique, introduction to the direct application of ultrasound in the ICU, hands-on demonstration and/or experience with mannequins or observed media, and some form of certification or accreditation by the conclusion of the experience. Such courses are widely variable in academic and clinical rigor, the distribution of didactic versus practical experience, as well as in cost. In reality, the more pervasive approach to ultrasound education is through direct observation of (experienced) critical care operators with subsequent trial and error by the learning providers. Although the advantage of this method is that it provides real-life, real-time patient experience, the detriment lies in the inability to truly quantify competency and consistency among a range of providers.

▶ Summation

Clearly, the introduction of bedside ultrasound into critical care units has altered the manner in which intensive care is delivered. Most proponents of best practice would advocate the use of ultrasound guidance when available for vascular access and as a ready adjunct, if not primary tool for the diagnosis of certain critical conditions, including lung pathology, cardiac abnormalities, and traumatic injury. That being said, discrepancies exist between how ultrasound training and continuing education is provided in addition to the anticipated variance in provider proficiency and utilization of this tool. Naturally, further study of the benefits of intensive care ultrasound to the critically ill patient should consider factors, such as interprovider reliability, standardization of education for ultrasound training, and alternative uses of this technology to help facilitate better use of this tool in critical care practice.

BETTER CARE, HEALTH, AND COST: A NEW PARADIGM FOR CRITICAL CARE ULTRASOUND

Working to achieve the goals of quality and patient safety most recently outlined by the IHI requires both a working knowledge of the specified "triple aims," in addition to a broader awareness of how each and every medical intervention we incorporate into practice intersects with the path to better care, health, and cost. Having considered the scope of critical care ultrasonography in practical terms, we now focus our discourse on how this important technology can at once impact the patient care experience, overall wellness across patient populations, and cost effectiveness in the framework of these specific aims (Figure 1-4).

▶ Impact of Ultrasound on Patient Experience

Naturally, any clinical tool which results in timely and accurate diagnosis with minimal risk to the patient is attractive, if not utopian. Although not without its challenges, critical care ultrasound meets at least the minimal standard for such therapeutic goals. The ability for critically ill patients to remain in the ICU for radiographic evaluation as occurs with bedside ultrasound significantly decreases the morbidities associated with transporting seriously ill or unstable patients. Furthermore, because of its portability, in some institutions, ultrasound devices and technicians may be more readily accessible than traditional modalities, such as CT or MRI, when diagnostically appropriate. While it is known that there is some degree of interprovider variance with ultrasonography, the reliability of ultrasound can be significantly enhanced with standardized training and

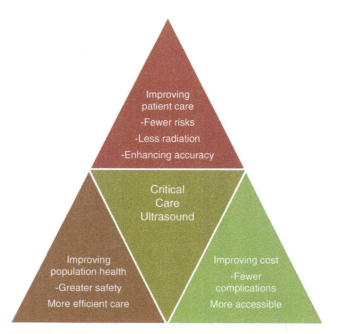

Figure 1-4 Critical care ultrasound and the triple aim.

opportunities for continued skill mastery. When applied precisely, ultrasound may decrease the time, discomfort, and risks associated with invasive patient procedures and thus serve to improve the patient care experience.

▶ Impact of Ultrasound on Population Health

The potential benefit of intensive care ultrasound on the individual patient is relatively clear; however, additional value of this technology exists to populations at large. When considered together, critically ill patients represent a high-risk, especially vulnerable group secondary to the pathophysiologic derangements that characterize their illnesses, their impaired ability to advocate effectively for their care, and the narrow therapeutic window, which underlies their care. For these individuals, the option of a clinically noninvasive, but diagnostically accurate tool, such as ultrasound, may result in fewer morbidities of their critical illness.

Pediatric patients represent another important sector of the population for whom recent literature would suggest that ultrasound has the potential to innovate current standards of medical practice in consideration of the serious intermediate and long-term risks associated with exposure to ionizing radiation in children. In light of the recent evidence that even moderate exposure to ionizing radiation can result in increased lifetime cancer risk and even impaired neuropsychological development in children, pediatric facilities are utilizing alternative means of radiographic imaging whenever possible for their patients. This trend and reevaluation of current practice standards is only certain to expand as more illnesses and conditions are linked to primary exposures in childhood.

Even for the general population, incorporation of bedside ultrasound into routine critical care practice has potential value. First, should any one of us or our loved ones unexpectedly require intensive care, would we not wish to benefit from those patient-specific advantages of ultrasound as outlined above if bedside ultrasound is the standard of care? Second, given its low-risk, high-yield safety profile, ultrasound could eventually replace other preventive health screening or surveillance modalities for certain conditions, especially as the technology and its specificity improves. Alternatively, it may also be used as an early screening tool to stratify higher risk patients, who may require more specific imaging, such that overall health resources may be more equitably and efficiently allocated among the population.

▶ Impact of Ultrasound on Cost Reduction

Health systems should be affordable and sustainable with high productivity and minimally wasteful. To affect these goals, each element of the health infrastructure must, therefore, in its own rite serve to exemplify these principles. The incorporation of ultrasound in the ICU engenders cost constraint and efficiency at the highest level. Taken together, the costs of training critical care personnel to use this technology, procuring the necessary equipment, and maintaining proficiency and skill among providers is far outweighed by the premiums exacted by complications of care. The use of ultrasound promotes safe practice in the true spirit of patient-centered care. By mitigating the unnecessary complications associated with invasive and blindly attempted procedures, ultrasound-based techniques both richly enhance the patient experience and effectively reduce the costs associated with medical errors.

Most health institutions will acknowledge that the availability of important radiologic studies is limited by cost, technical expertise, and resource availability grossly offset by demand. It is not uncommon for inpatients to wait days for follow-up imaging with MRI given the number of emergent or outpatient studies that are given priority. If ultrasound could be used instead for even a limited number of clinical conditions, the financial burdens of increased length of stay while awaiting tests, necessary overtime staffing to perform off-hour studies, and for complications associated with delays in diagnosis or treatment could be substantially reduced.

CONCLUSION

While we acknowledge that the road to quality improvement in health care is both laborious and at times painfully slow, it is clear that a paradigm, which emphasizes both the individual and shared benefits of a lower cost system, best embodies the frontier of safer medicine which patients and providers alike seek. In this chapter, we have considered the role of critical care ultrasound in the context of this "triple aim" of medical practice with the goal of achieving better care, better health, and better cost. This is a daunting, yet attainable mission, if only we maintain at the forefront of practice these unifying goals of care.

SUGGESTED READING

http://healthaffairs.org/blog/2012/03/09/the-toll-of-preventable-errors-how-many-dead-patients/. The Toll of Preventable Errors. Accessed January 31, 2013.

Institute of Medicine Committee on Quality of Health Care in America. Crossing the Quality Chasm: A New Health System for the 21st Century. Washington, DC: National Academies Press, 2001.

PHYSICS OF SOUND, ULTRASOUND, AND DOPPLER EFFECT AND ITS DIAGNOSTIC UTILITY

ALEXANDER B. LEVITOV

SOUND AND ULTRASOUND: ACOUSTIC PARAMETERS

All our lives we are surrounded by sounds. In fact, it is our ability to create and comprehend sounds in the form of speech that is integral to our human development. As physicians we assess heart sounds, breath sounds, and bowel sounds, but few will contemplate the nature of sound. Without understanding the physical properties of sound and their interactions with the surrounding medium, it is difficult to understand the images produced in clinical ultrasound. The critical care practitioner also often acts as a sonographer, whose responsibility is to operate the equipment, obtain images, distinguish between real structures and artifacts, and manipulate the transducer. Without a solid knowledge of basic sound principles, these tasks are virtually impossible.

A sound is a wave created by a moving (vibrating) object and comprises areas of increased (compressions) and decreased (rarefactions) densities. This wave moves through a medium with a fixed speed (propagation speed), transmitting its energy, while the vibrating matter of the medium returns to its original position with each cycle (see Chapter 2 in enclosed DVD). When the sound wave reaches an object, it is unable to penetrate, such as a wall; it may go around it (diffraction). This allows one to hear music around a corner. If the object is larger, such as a mountain, sound will bounce off (reflection) and return back to the source, creating a familiar phenomenon known as an echo. Echo was first described and named by the ancient Greeks.

Depending on the movement of the sound-generating object, the sound wave will acquire different characteristics known as acoustic parameters (Table 2-1). Some of those are related, while others are independent of each other. Though a sound wave is longitudinal with energy traveling in the same direction as the propagating wave, for the ease of representation it will be pictured as a transverse wave with energy distributed perpendicular to the direction of propagation like a wave on the surface of a pond (Figure 2-1).

▶ Frequency and Period

The time necessary for the sound wave to complete one cycle is known as its period. The cycle is complete when the sound source has produced one vibration and the matter in the medium has returned to its original resting position. The period is measured in units of time (Table 2-1). One can probably use the fractions of the year, but that would be rather inconvenient, so most of the time it is measured in milliseconds ([msec] 1 thousandth), microseconds ([μsec] 1 millionth of a second), or nanoseconds (1 billionth). For example, a guitar D string takes 2.5 msec to completely travel across the reference object, such as a guitar fret, from left to right and left again to where it started; the sound it has generated will have a period of 2.5 msec (Figure 2-2).

Related to the period is the frequency of the sound wave (Table 2-1). Frequency (f) is a number of cycles completed in 1 second. A standard measure of frequency is hertz (Hz), which was named for Heinrich Rudolf Hertz (1847–1894), the first person to transmit and receive radio waves. One Hz is one cycle per second. The same guitar string with the period lasting 2.5 msec will complete 400 periods in 1 second and therefore have a frequency of 400 Hz or 0.4 kilohertz (kHZ) (Figure 2-2). Frequency is the reciprocal of the period (Table 2-1). That is:

$$\text{Frequency} \times \text{period} = 1$$
$$f(\text{Hz}) = 1/\text{period}(\text{sec})$$
$$\text{period}(\text{sec}) = 1/f(\text{Hz})$$

- kHz: kilohertz, thousands of cycles per second with a period of milliseconds.

TABLE 2-1
Summary of Acoustic Parameters

Acoustic Parameter	Units	Determined by	Values in Diagnostic Ultrasound
Period	μs	Sound source	0.1–0.5 μs
Frequency	MHz	Sound source	2–10 MHz
Amplitude	dB	Sound source	—
Power	Watts	Sound source	—
Intensity	Watt/cm^2	Sound source	0.001–100 W/cm^2
Wavelengths	mm	Source and medium	0.1–0.6 mm
Propagation speed	m/s	Medium alone	1500–1600 m/s

- MHz: megahertz, millions of cycles per second with a period of microseconds.

Humans can hear sounds with frequencies ranging from 20 Hz to 20 kHz. Speech generates 100–220 Hz, and singing 50 Hz–1.5 kHz. The human ear is most sensitive to 3–4 kHz sounds. The sound in the range of human hearing is known as audible sound, or simply sound, with frequencies >20 kHz known as ultrasound and <20 Hz known as infrasound. Thus, a distinction between sound and ultrasound is really quite capricious if not entirely baseless. Many other animals have wider range of hearing. For example, the domestic cat can hear up to 50 kHz. Though an ultrasound wave is a sound wave in every respect, ultrasound waves (particularly in the MHz range) tend to travel in a straight line, and diffract less and reflect more off smaller objects than lower-frequency waves. Typical periods and frequencies for diagnostic ultrasound are 0.1–0.5 μsec and 2–10 MHz, respectively, and are determined by the ultrasound source known as a transducer, or a probe (Table 2-1). With frequencies, much greater than those of diagnostic ultrasound, ultrasound waves start to behave a lot like electromagnetic microwaves, but those frequencies are never reached in medical applications.

Most emitted and reflected sounds have a mixture of frequencies, with the lowest one being the so-called fundamental frequency, and its multiples are harmonic frequencies, or, simply, harmonics. These concepts are demonstrated by the movement of the guitar string (Figure 2-2).

AMPLITUDE, POWER, AND INTENSITY

As a sound wave propagates, the particles in the medium will move from the resting position. This creates areas of increased density and increased pressure on the surrounding area (compression). These changes in motion, pressure, and density will reach their peak and then subside with each vibration. The difference between a resting value of the parameter, such as density or pressure, and the peak one, during the period of

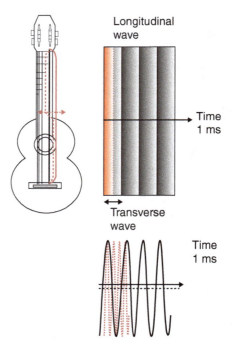

Figure 2-2 Guitar D string vibration is creating a longitudinal wave in fundamental (shades of gray) and first harmonic (shades of red) frequencies. The fundamental frequency longitudinal wave is represented below by a transverse wave of the same frequency. The red dotted wave is a first harmonic wave with half the period and twice the frequency of the fundamental wave. Fundamental period is 2.5 of a millisecond; fundamental frequency is 400 Hz (0.4 kilohertz [kHz]); first harmonic frequency is 0.8 kHz.

Nature of sound

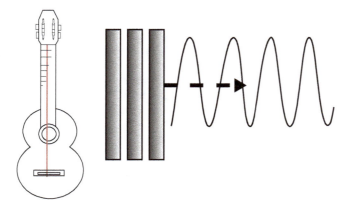

Figure 2-1 Guitar string vibration is creating a longitudinal wave. It is represented, however, as a transverse wave.

CHAPTER 2 PHYSICS OF SOUND, ULTRASOUND, AND DOPPLER EFFECT AND ITS DIAGNOSTIC UTILITY

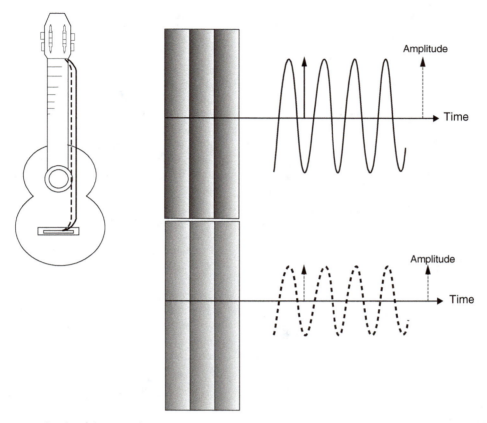

Figure 2-3 Different amplitude of the sound: —More medium displacement, higher amplitude; ---Less medium displacement, lower amplitude; Power = $k \times$ (amplitude)^2.

the sound wave, is referred to as amplitude. You can pluck the guitar string softly (with less amplitude), creating less motion (pressure, density), or vigorously (with more amplitude), but because the string has the same period and frequency, the sound would not change. Simply stated, amplitude is the loudness or volume of the sound whether one can hear the sound or not (Table 2-1). In ultrasound applications, it is often referred to as an output gain or acoustic power (Figure 2-3). Because amplitude is the difference or ratio between two values of the parameter with the same unit, it cannot be described in absolute units (Table 2-1). In other words, one can always produce a louder or softer sound. Therefore, a relative scale is used. The relative units of this scale are Bells. They are named for Graham Bell and are defined as 0.1 of the Bell or decibels (dB), which are the most commonly used units in acoustic measurements (Tables 2-1 and 2-2).

The scale is logarithmic, meaning that the number is described by how many multiples of 10 one needs to create it (Table 2-2). Thus, the logarithm of 100 is 2, of 1000 is 3, and of 1/100 is –2.

$$dB = 10 \times \log(A1/A2),$$ where $A1$ and $A2$ are the amplitudes of sounds being compared

More important, there are only two numbers to remember: 3 dB and 10 dB. Three decibels means 2-fold and 10 means 10-fold increase in the measured parameter, therefore –3 dB is 2 times less (one half) and –10 is 10 times less (0.1) than the original value. So if the parameter is pressure, then 3 dB sound will create twice the pressure on your eardrum (or be twice as loud) and 20 dB will be 100 times louder than the original one, while –3 dB will be only half that loud (Table 2-2).

It follows that power, or the amount of energy per second, delivered by the sound wave, is related to the amplitude and is in fact the amplitude squared (Table 2-1). When amplitude doubles, power increases fourfold.

$$\text{Power} = k \times (\text{amplitude})^2, \quad \text{where } k \text{ is a coefficient}$$

The unit of power is watt (joules/s), named for James Watt, the Scottish engineer. The power of the sound wave

TABLE 2-2	
Amplitude Ratios and Decibels	
Ratio of Sound 1/Sound 2	Decibels (dB)
1000:1	30
100:1	20
10:1	10
4:1	6
2:1	3
1:2	–3
1:10	–10

TABLE 2-3
Speed of Sound (Propagation Speed) in Different Tissues

Tissue	Speed of Sound (m/s)
Lung	300–1200
Fat	1450
"Soft tissue"	1540
Bone	2000–4000

distributed over the unit of surface is known as intensity (Table 2-1). Intensity is defined as the amount of energy per second delivered to the surface area of the medium. Intensity (measured in watt/cm^2) therefore will be directly proportional to power (amplitude) and inversely proportional to the area over which that power is applied. The same sound beam with the same power when applied to a smaller surface area will deliver more energy to that area and is said to be more intense. The typical intensity of the diagnostic ultrasound equipment is 0.001–100 watts/cm^2 (Table 2-1). In the case of diagnostic ultrasound, the "medium" is human tissue and the intensity will predict the bioeffect of the ultrasound (Tables 2-1 and 2-3). Those effects can be rather dramatic. One important example is ultrasonic lithotripsy, where the intensity of the ultrasound is used to decimate renal stones.

The speed of sound (propagation speed) is a fixed number and is related solely to the medium (Tables 2-1 and 2-3). This is a far-reaching statement and a unique feature of the physics of wave propagation. The speed of moving objects is an algebraic sum of the speed of the object and the observer. A couple of examples can help to demonstrate this point:

1. If a man is walking with the speed of 4 miles per hour (mph) down an escalator, which is moving at 3 mph relative to a stationary observer, he is moving at 7 mph.
2. If a police officer is chasing a getaway car and his car is moving at 110 mph, and the getaway car is moving at a 100 mph relative to that of the police officer, the speed of the chased car is −10 mph (the police officer is gaining on the getaway car).

It does not matter if the source of the sound or the observer is moving; the sound propagation speed remains the same (Table 2-1). A jet plane can fly faster than sound, but the roar of its engines will propagate at the same speed as if it were stationary on the ground; however, the frequency of the sound waves will change. If the sound is moving toward the observer, the period of the sound wave decreases and therefore the frequency increases (sound wave is compressed). If the sound is moving away, the opposite occurs (the wave is stretched). This is the so-called Doppler effect, which will be further discussed below, but for now remember: *nothing can change the speed of sound in a particular medium*; it is an established and fixed phenomenon.

Wavelength is the length of a single cycle and is measured in the units of length (Table 2-1 and Figure 2-4A). A picture of the wavelength is easy to confuse with that of the frequency; in fact, they will look exactly the same, but remember that here the axis is space, not time. Wavelength is determined by the frequency of the sound and the speed of sound in the medium (Table 2-1).

$$\text{Wavelength (mm)} = \text{speed of sound in the medium (mm/\mu sec)/frequency (MHz)}$$

Because the speed of sound in the medium is an intrinsic quality of the medium (Table 2-3), the wavelength in that medium will be inversely related to the frequency of the sound wave generated by the sound source (Table 2-1). In the same medium, the higher-frequency ultrasound therefore will generate a shorter wavelength. The longer the wavelength, the larger the size of the object the wave will need to encounter to be reflected. High-frequency ultrasound allows for reflection off smaller objects, which improves image quality (axial resolution) in the same medium (Figure 2-4B). In "soft tissue,"

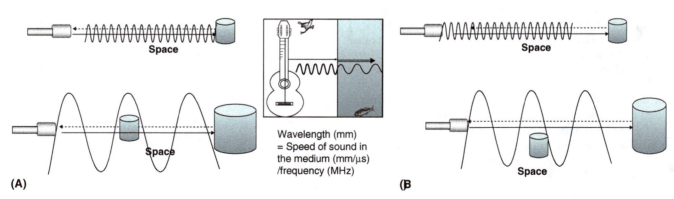

Figure 2-4 (A) Speed of sound in the medium is an intrinsic quality of the medium. As the speed of sound increases in the water, the wavelength becomes longer, while the frequency of the sound wave generated by the sound source does not change. In the same medium, higher-frequency ultrasound will create shorter wavelength. Shorter wavelength ultrasound produces better images by reflecting off smaller objects. Wavelength (mm) = Speed of sound in the medium (mm/μsec)/frequency (megahertz, MHz). (B) Shorter wavelength and higher-frequency ultrasound produce better images by reflecting off smaller objects. Because the speed of sound in the medium is an intrinsic quality of the medium, the wavelength in that medium will be inversely related to the frequency of the sound wave generated by the sound source.

CHAPTER 2 PHYSICS OF SOUND, ULTRASOUND, AND DOPPLER EFFECT AND ITS DIAGNOSTIC UTILITY

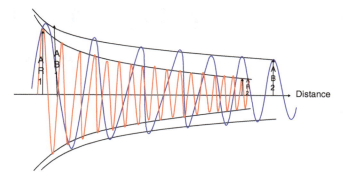

Figure 2-5 Both high-frequency red wave (R) and lower-frequency blue wave (B) attenuate (dampen) with distance. However, blue wave attenuates less. Ratio of initial amplitude A1 to final A2 illustrates the degree of attenuation and is measured in negative decibels (dB). AB1: AB2 > AR1: AR2.

TABLE 2-4

Relationship Between Elapsed Time and Distance to the Reflective Boundary in the "Soft Tissue"

Elapsed Time (μsec)	Depth of Reflective Boundary (cm)	Total Distance Traveled from the Source and Back (cm)
13*	1	2
26	2	4
52	4	8
130	10	20

*In "soft tissue," if the elapsed time is 13 μs the reflector is 1 cm deep.

sound with frequency of 1 MHz will have a wavelength of 1.54 mm, and 500 kHz a wavelength of 3.08 mm.

In "soft tissue": Wavelength (mm) = $1.54/f$ (MHz)

So in diagnostic ultrasound, the rule is: the higher the frequency, the shorter the wavelength, and the better the image. Useful values of wavelengths in diagnostic ultrasound are 0.1–0.08 mm.

INTERACTIONS OF ULTRASOUND AND MEDIUM

As the ultrasound wave travels through the medium, it releases some of its energy and reflects back to the source as an echo (Figure 2-6). The result is a dampening of the wave or reduction in its amplitude. This process is known as attenuation. Attenuation is dependent on the ultrasound frequency and the distance the ultrasound travels in the medium. Attenuation only affects the amplitude and the wave frequency or wave length. The greater the distance the ultrasound has to travel, the more attenuation will occur. To illustrate the relationship between frequency and attenuation, one just needs to rub one's hands together. The faster you do it (higher frequency), the hotter the hands will get, because more heat energy is released by friction. Attenuation is always measured in negative decibels, and in the soft tissues one MHz frequency signal will attenuate –0.5 dB per every centimeter it travels (Figure 2-5).

Attenuation = (–0.5 dB/cm/MHz) × travel distance (cm)

Heat generation will be discussed in the biological effects of the ultrasound, but reflection is important to image formation. It will also be discussed later in more detail, but some basics need to be addressed now.

When the sound wave strikes a boundary between two different tissue layers, some of the energy will proceed further, while the rest will return to the source of sound in the form of an echo. The timing and the energy of the echo signal will be related to the depth and the physical nature (acoustic impedance) of the boundary and will provide all the necessary information to create an image (Table 2-4 and Figure 2-6). The sound wave that is not

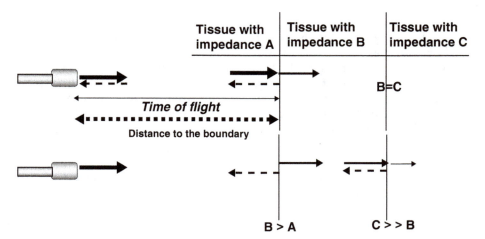

Figure 2-6 Normal incidence. If there is no difference in impedance between the two boundaries, no reflection will occur; the larger the difference, the greater the amount of ultrasound is reflected back to the source. Distance to the boundary can be calculated from the time it takes for the ultrasound to reach the boundary and return to the source (time of flight, elapsed time). In the soft tissues, distance to the boundary (mm) = elapsed time (μsec) × 0.77 mm/μsec.

TABLE 2-5
Comparison of High- and Low-Frequency Ultrasound Waves

	Image Depth	Attenuation	Image Quality	Axial Resolution	Lateral Resolution
Low frequency 2–5 MHz	Deep	Low	Lower	Lower (big number)	Lower (big number)
High frequency 5–10 MHz	Shallow	High	Higher	Higher (small number)	Higher (small number)

reflected will go on until the next tissue boundary is met. The same phenomenon will take place again until the signal is lost due to attenuation. Because energy is not created in the process, whatever is not reflected (or converted to heat and lost) will be transmitted. The amount of reflected ultrasound energy will depend on the physical properties of the boundary. Those properties can be summarized in a calculated number of acoustic impedance. Impedance is measured in units of Rayls (Z). The units are named for the physicist Robert John Strutt, 4th Baron Rayleigh.

Acoustic impedance (Rayls) = density (kg/m^3)
   × speed of sound (m/s)

Typical impedance of "soft tissues" is 1.25–1.75 Mrayls (1,250,000–1,750,000 Rayls).

The best reflection can be achieved when sound strikes a boundary between two layers with large differences in acoustic impedance at a 90° angle of incidence (normal incidence). If there is no difference in acoustic impedance between the two layers, no reflection will occur and no image can be formed (Figure 2-6). As a rule, at the boundary between two different "soft tissues" (i.e., fat/kidney) with similar impedance, only 1% of the sound is reflected in the form of echo and 99% is transmitted, while at soft tissues/bone interface roughly half of the sound is reflected back, and at tissue/air boundary, where the difference in impedance is the greatest, nearly all the energy is reflected (99%) and practically none is transmitted (Table 2-3). In this latter case, visualization of any structures below such boundary is impossible. The fine detail of the boundary (reflector) will only be reflected properly and visualized when the wavelength of the ultrasound is smaller than those details, thus the image will improve with an increase in ultrasound wave frequency (Tables 2-5 and 2-6). Regrettably, high-frequency waves also have high-attenuation rates and will not penetrate deeply into the tissues (Table 2-6).

That can be partially remedied by analyzing only returning echoes with frequencies that are multiples of the fundamental (emitted) one, the so-called tissue harmonics. For example, if the emitted sound wave has a frequency of 5 MHz, only echoes with frequency of 10 MHz are analyzed. Selecting those higher-frequency waves known as tissue harmonic imaging (THI) for image formation usually results in improved image quality.

When the two boundaries are separated by a distance much greater than the wavelength of the emitted ultrasound, they will appear separate on the image created by their respective echoes. However, as the boundaries get closer to each other, the timing interval between returning echoes becomes progressively shorter until finally they appear as a single object (Figure 2-7). The distance where two objects are perceived as two separate ones in the pass of the ultrasound wave (axial plane) is known as axial or longitudinal resolution. Resolution is measured in millimeters: the smaller the number, the better the image. The typical value of axial resolution for modern ultrasound equipment is about 0.1 mm (0.05–0.5 mm) (Figure 2-7).

For image formation, the ultrasound machine (system) always assumes that the reflective boundary is struck by the ultrasound at a 90° angle. However, in reality it is seldom the case and the result is that images become difficult to interpret. If the sound wave strikes the boundary at a non-90° incidence angle (oblique incidence), reflection may never reach the source of sound and image formation will be impossible (Figure 2-8). Moreover, ultrasound transmission and reflection with oblique incidence is difficult to describe mathematically, and if reflection does reach the sound source, ultrasound equipment will interpret it as if there has been normal incidence and may place the image in the wrong place, creating artifact. With normal incidence, the transmitted fraction of the sound wave will always follow the original direction of the beam. However, with the

TABLE 2-6
Factors Affecting Quality of the Ultrasound Image

Image Quality	Depth	Wave Frequency	Pulse	Focus
Better image	Shallow sample	High-frequency waves	Short SPL	Narrow focus
Worse image	Deep sample	Low-frequency waves	Long SPL	Wide focus

SPL = spatial pulse length.

CHAPTER 2   PHYSICS OF SOUND, ULTRASOUND, AND DOPPLER EFFECT AND ITS DIAGNOSTIC UTILITY

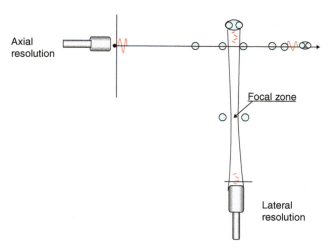

Figure 2-7 As two boundaries become closer in the pass of the ultrasound (axial plane), they will appear as one (limit of axial resolution). Two objects appearing as one in the plane perpendicular to the pass of the sound is a limit of lateral resolution. Axial resolution is always better (smaller number) than lateral resolution.

oblique incidence, if the speed of sound is different between the two layers of the boundary transmission, a bend, or refraction, will occur. Refraction is governed by Snell's law: sine of transmission angle/sine of incidence angle = speed of sound medium1/speed of sound medium^2 (Figure 2-8).

Ultrasound equipment assumes the same speed of sound in all tissues (1540 msec) and accordingly will not account

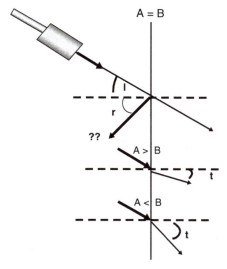

Figure 2-8 In oblique incidence, both transmission and reflection are unpredictable, except for the incidence angle I being equal to reflection angle r. If the speed of sound in both media is equal, transmission will follow the pass of the incident wave; otherwise refraction will occur. If the speed of sound in medium A is faster than in medium B, the transmission angle will be less than the incident angle. If the speed of sound in medium A is slower than in medium B, the transmission angle will be greater than the incidence angle (Snell's law). Sine t/Sine i = propagation speed B/A.

or compensate for refraction; therefore, refraction artifacts are common. To complicate things even further, once off the original pass, ultrasound might encounter unexpected reflective boundaries and take a "scenic" pass back to the transducer. None of these issues will be considered when the image is formed.

But if the sound is traveling in a straight line and strikes the reflector at 90° incidence, it is very easy to determine the reflector's depth. For this, one only needs to know the time needed for the echo to return to the sound source (transducer) and the speed of sound (Figure 2-6). Position (depth) of the reflective boundary can be calculated using the following formula:

Distance to the boundary (reflector) (mm)
= elapsed time (μsec) × 0.77 mm/μsec

WAVE INTERACTIONS

Besides interacting with the medium, the sound waves also interact with each other. As a longitudinal wave, the sound will transmit from the source in more or less concentric circles. An important analogy portrays this principle. One can sit behind a guitar player and still hear the music play. Due to wave interaction, however, when you sit in the front of the guitarist, the music is louder because of the ways in which the sound waves interact with each other. Two in-phase waves will sum creating a wave with higher amplitude (constructive interference), while waves in the counterphase will subtract, resulting in one with a lower amplitude (destructive interference) (Figure 2-9).

A bullhorn is designed to produce even more constructive interference creating a sound beam traveling in the direction it points. The waves in the center of the beam have the highest amplitude. Ultrasound waves emitted by the transducer diffract less, making beam formation even more precise. Wave interactions are described by Huygens' principle, which states that all constructive and destructive interferences within the beam will produce an hourglass-like final shape (Figure 2-9). The narrowest area (waist) of the beam is known as the focal point or focus. The beam with the narrowest focus will be able to distinguish two side-by-side objects as separate, while the beam with the broader focal point will fuse them into one image (Figure 2-6). This concept is known as lateral resolution. High-frequency sound waves have a narrower focal point and higher lateral resolution. Therefore, high-frequency ultrasound waves will improve both axial and lateral resolutions and are preferred for their ability to produce superior image quality, but can only be used for visualization of superficial structures due to high attenuation.

CONTINUOUS-WAVE AND PULSE ULTRASOUND

An ultrasound wave can be emitted continuously as a light from the headlight of the car or in pulses as a blinking turn signal. All imaging ultrasound waves are pulse waves, with

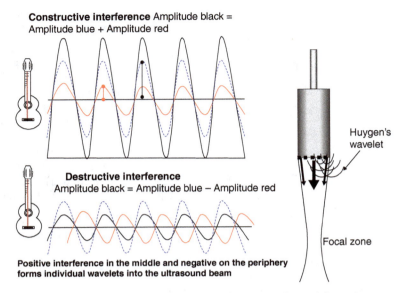

Figure 2-9 Interference and ultrasound beam formation. Positive interference in the middle and negative on the periphery form individual wavelets into the ultrasound beam.

an "on," or talking time, for producing a sound pulse and an "off" time for listening for the return echo signal. Imaging transducers serve as both transmitters and receivers.

The percentage of "on" time when the ultrasonic pulse is produced is known as the duty factor (Table 2-7). The usual duty factor in imaging ultrasound is 0.1–1%, so just as in a good human conversation, there is a lot of listening and very little talking. A duty factor of 100% means that continuous-wave, nonimaging (Doppler) ultrasound is used. The most familiar form of such a device is a "blackbox Doppler" used for finding a pulsatile artery. A duty factor of 0% means that the ultrasound machine is off. Several other terms need to be introduced in regard to the pulsatile nature of imaging ultrasound.

Pulse duration (PD) is the time during which the sound is emitted in each on/off phase. It is usually 0.5–3 μsec, with each pulse being a short wave composed of two to four cycles (Table 2-7 and Figure 2-10). Pulse repetition period (PRP) is the time of the entire on/off cycle (Table 2-7). Because the PD is fixed by the transducer, the only variable is an "off" or listening time. The deeper the imaging sample, the longer the time required for the echo pulse to return to the source, thus the longer the PRP necessary (Tables 2-4 and 2-7). Pulse repetition frequency (PRF) is a number of pulses emitted in 1 second (Table 2-7). PRF is measured in hertz and usually is 1–10 kHz in imaging ultrasound and will vary depending on the depth of the imaging sample. PRP and PRF are reciprocal numbers related in the following ways:

$$PRP\ (s) = 1/PRF\ (Hz)$$
$$PRF\ (Hz) = 1/PRP\ (s)$$

Note that though it is measured in the same units, PRF has no relationship to the frequency of the ultrasound wave produced during pulse generation that is measured in MHz.

Spatial pulse length (SPL) is the length of the pulse in space with a typical value of 0.1–1.0 mm (Table 2-7). Shorter pulses, just as shorter wavelengths of the pulse wave, reflect off the smaller objects. Shorter pulses produce better images by improving axial resolution.

Axial resolution can be described by the following relationship:

$$\text{Axial resolution} = SPL\ (mm)/2$$

TABLE 2-7
Summary of Pulsed-Wave Parameters

Parameter	Determined by	Units	Typical Value
Pulse duration	Ultrasound source alone	μs	0.5–3.0 μs
PRP	Source/changes with depth of image	msec	0.1–1.0 msec
SPL	Source and medium	mm	0.1–1.0 mm
PRF	Source/changes with depth of image	kHz	1–10 kHz
Duty factor	Source/changes with depth of image	%	0.1–1%

SPL = spatial pulse length; PRP = pulse repetition period; PRF = pulse repetition frequency.

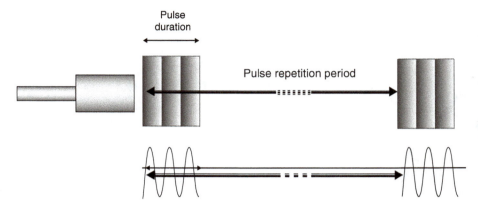

Figure 2-10 Pulse ultrasound. Pulse duration (PD) is the time during which the sound is emitted in each on/off cycle. It is usually 0.5–3 μsec and comprises two to four cycles. Pulse repetition period (PRP) is the time of the entire on/off cycle. Though difficult to depict graphically, PRP is usually 100–1000 times longer than PD. Duty factor = PD/PRP. Pulse repetition frequency (PRF) is the number of pulses emitted in 1 second. PRP (s) = 1/PRF (Hz), PRF (Hz) = 1/PRP (s). The deeper the image, the longer the PRP, the lower the PRF.

DOPPLER PHENOMENON AND ITS USE IN DIAGNOSTIC ULTRASOUND

First described by Christian Doppler, the Doppler phenomenon simply states that if the source of sound (transducer) and the object reflecting the sound (reflector) are moving in relationship to each other, the frequency of the reflected sound wave will change. If the reflector is moving toward the sound source, the sound waves will be compressed to a higher frequency (positive Doppler shift). If it is moving away from the sound source, the sound waves will be stretched to a lower frequency (negative Doppler shift) (Figure 2-11).

Subtracting the incident frequency from the frequency of the returning echo Doppler shift can be recorded, and because it falls into the audible range of 20 Hz–20 kHz, it can be heard by the operator. It is important to remember that the shift itself is riding "piggyback" on the inaudible original ultrasound wave usually measured in MHz. So if the reflector (such as blood or cardiac structures) is moving, the velocity and the direction of the movement can be calculated and imaged from the value of Doppler shifts using the equation below:

Reflector velocity
= (Doppler shift × propagation speed)/
2 × (incident f × cosine incidence angle)

Of those, the cosine of the incident angle is most important. The cosine of 90° angle is "0" and no reflector velocity can be measured. In fact, the closer the incidence angle to 0° or 180°, the closer the measured velocity to an actual one (Figure 2-11). This presents a problem if the image of the organ, such as a blood vessel, is to be obtained simultaneously with the blood flow velocity. The images are best at 90° incidences, but then no Doppler information can be

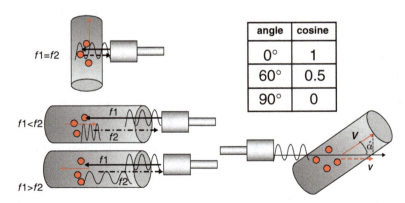

Figure 2-11 If the blood cell is moving toward the transducer, the frequency of the reflected signal will be higher than that of the emitted or incident one (positive Doppler shift). If the blood cell is moving away, the frequency of the returning signal will be lower than the incident frequency (negative Doppler shift). Doppler shift = f1 − f2. Doppler shift depends on the angle between the reflector (red blood cell) direction and the direction of the emitted sound wave. Doppler shift = 2× reflector speed × incident frequency × cos (angle ά)/propagation speed. With 90° angle there is no Doppler shift and the reflector velocity calculations are impossible. Velocity calculations are most accurate with 0° incident angle. f1 = incident frequency, f2 = reflected frequency, ά = incident angle.

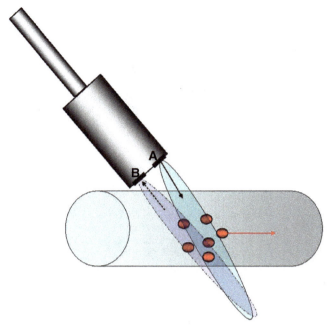

Figure 2-12 Continuous-wave Doppler. A is a transmitter element. B is a receiver element. The large area of overlap between the incident beam and the receiver beam results in an inability to assess where the sample is located. This is known as range ambiguity. Continuous wave can measure very high-flow velocities.

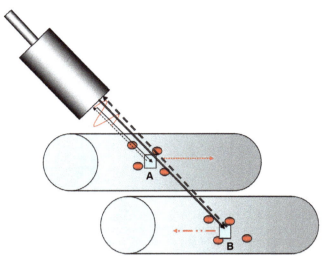

Figure 2-13 Pulsed-wave Doppler. The sample volume A is shallower and the position of the reflector (red blood cells) can be registered frequently. The sample volume B is deeper and the position of the reflector is sampled infrequently. Hence, the Nyquist limit = PRF/2 is exceeded and aliasing occurs.

obtained. So a compromise has to be reached between the image quality and the Doppler data. This compromise is achieved with a 60° incidence angle, which is often utilized in vascular studies.

The oldest, simplest, and perhaps most used Doppler modality is a continuous-wave Doppler (Tables 2-8 and 2-9). In this case, one part of the transducer constantly emits the incident ultrasound wave and the other constantly receives the returning wave. Processors subtract them and the resulting shift is heard by the operator. This is the construction of the "black box Doppler" found frequently in intensive care units (ICUs) and used by physicians and nurses when they are unable to palpate an arterial pulse (Figure 2-12). Continuous-wave Doppler is capable of detecting any flow velocity, but unable to tell where the sample is taken (Table 2-9). This "range ambiguity" results from large overlap between transmitted and received beams (Table 2-9).

When exact knowledge of the sample location is essential (i.e., stenotic aortic valve) pulsed-wave Doppler is used (Tables 2-8 and 2-9). Just as with the imaging pulsed ultrasound, the pulsed Doppler transducer serves both as a transmitter and a receiver. Echo signals from only one area, known as sample volume, are chosen for analysis, the rest are ignored (gating). This area is determined by the timing of the returned signal. This is known as range resolution (one knows exactly where the sample volume it taken) (Table 2-9). However, pulsed-wave Doppler has a fundamental problem. The transducer has to wait until the returned echo signal is received before the next incident pulse is transmitted (Table 2-8). Each pulse is a snapshot, and the rate of those snapshots decreases with increasing depth of the sample due to a longer time of flight (Figure 2-13).

Because the depth of the sample and PRP are directly related (see pulsed ultrasound parameters above), one can also say that the longer the PRP (the shorter the PRF), the lower the rate of Doppler snapshot(s) that record the position of the reflector. That results in aliasing (Table 2-9 and Figure 2-14).

Because of aliasing, with pulsed-wave Doppler measurements, high reflector velocities become inaccurate and the reflector may appear to be going in the direction opposite to the actual one (Table 2-8 and Figure 2-14). Aliasing is a sampling error, occurring when the sampling rate is too slow in comparison with the reflector velocity. The following example will illustrate this further.

TABLE 2-8
Continuous-Wave Versus Pulsed Doppler

Doppler Modality	Range Resolution	Aliasing	High Flow Velocity Detection
Continuous wave	No	No	Unlimited
Pulsed Doppler	Yes	Yes	Limited by Nyquist frequency

CHAPTER 2 PHYSICS OF SOUND, ULTRASOUND, AND DOPPLER EFFECT AND ITS DIAGNOSTIC UTILITY

TABLE 2-9
Comparison of Doppler Modalities

Doppler Modality	Pros	Cons
Continuous-wave Doppler	Identifies high flow velocity jets, no aliasing	Range ambiguity
Pulsed-wave Doppler	Range resolution (depicts location of the flow)	Aliasing with high flow velocities
Color flow Doppler	Direct two-dimensional flow information superimposed on anatomical images	Aliasing with high flow velocities

You are given snapshots of a unicyclist riding forward in a circus arena. You can see the position of the cyclist in the arena, but do not know if the cyclist's direction is going forward or backward. There is no timing mark on the snapshots and it takes him 5 minutes to complete the circle. If the snapshots are taken every minute, you will clearly see him moving forward. If sample snapshots are taken every 2.5 minutes, it is impossible to deduce if he is going backward or forward because he is only viewed on opposite sides of the arena. If the samples are taken every 4 minutes, you will have to conclude that the unicyclist is riding backward, because every sample snapshot will position him behind the previous one. He is still going forward, but low sampling frequency makes it appear otherwise. The same phenomenon explains why a plane propeller seems to be moving in the direction opposite to its true course. The eye's sampling ability is exceeded by the rate of rotation, similar to the way in which in old cowboy movies the wagon wheels seem to rotate in the opposite direction of their true trajectory because the film rate was too slow.

Doppler frequency at which aliasing will occur is known as a Nyquist limit and is equal to half of the PRF of the pulsed-wave Doppler (Table 2-8).

$$\text{Nyquist limit (kHz)} = \text{PRF}/2$$

So the deeper the sample volume, the lower the PRF, and therefore the lower the Nyquist frequency limit, the more aliasing is observed.

Doppler shift is also directly related to the transducer frequency. The higher-frequency probe will produce more Doppler shift and more aliasing. With the blood flow velocity of 2 msec, the high-frequency (7 MHz) probe will produce a Doppler shift of 3 kHz and a low-frequency (3.5 MHz) probe will only produce 1.5 kHz. If the Nyquist frequency limit is 2 kHz, the first transducer will show aliasing and the second will not (Figure 2-15).

Methods of controlling aliasing:

1. Use shallower sample volume = increase PRF
2. Decrease carrier ultrasound frequency
3. Change Doppler angle to 0°
4. Use continuous-wave Doppler

With pulsed Doppler, the Doppler frequency shift is very small (2300 times smaller) compared with the wave frequency of the pulse itself. This makes calculations from a single pulse difficult.

The problem can be partially solved by producing multiple ultrasound pulses (pulse packets or ensemble length) going in the same direction and interrogating the same sample volume. The Doppler shift of each pulse in the packet is measured separately, but then the packet is treated as a single pulse. This technique improves the accuracy of the velocity measurements and the sensitivity to low-flow states. Doppler shift is used to assess hemodynamic parameters such as stroke volume (SV) and to detect abnormal direction or velocity of blood flow in cardiac (echocardiography) and vascular ultrasound. Occasionally, it is also used in other modalities to detect movements of anatomical structures (e.g., pleura).

Doppler ultrasound has a number of important utilities. Normal blood flow is laminar, meaning that it is well organized, with the greatest flow velocity in the center and gradual decrease toward the vessel wall due to friction. At the level of the aorta, this bullet-like pattern represents blood ejection during systole. Doppler flow velocity will reflect it, describing different parts of the stream crossing the plane of Doppler interrogation over time. The integral of the flow velocity over time (velocity-time integral [VTI]) will enable the calculation of the vertical dimensions of the cross-section of the "bullet," while the aortic diameter (D) will allow the estimation at its base (cross-sectional area

8:1 Samples per rotation. Clockwise direction is obvious

2:1 Samples per rotation. Direction is obscure. Nyquist limit is reached

1:5 Samples per rotation. Red dot seems to move counterclockwise (aliasing has occurred)

Figure 2-14 Nyquist limit and aliasing.

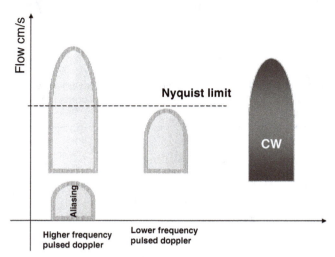

Figure 2-15 Eliminating aliasing. Aliasing can be eliminated by choosing the shallower sample (increased pulse repetition frequency, PRF), converting to continuous-wave Doppler, or choosing a lower-frequency pulsed-wave Doppler.

[CSA] = ($\pi \times \{D/2\}^2$). The product will provide the volume of the "bullet" and thus SV (Figure 2-16).

$$SV = VTI \times CSA$$

Those calculations are made by the equipment but are extremely dependent on the operator's ability to provide adequate Doppler data and proper measurement of the aortic diameter. As the blood flow reaches the area of the irregular lumen, predictable changes in flow velocity will take place at the site of the stenosis. The velocity will increase, reaching the highest velocity at the point of greatest narrowing (Figure 2-15). In the arterial bed there might be a loss of the pulsatile pattern, and in the venous bed a loss of phasic flow changes. At the exit point turbulent flow can develop. The pressure prior to stenosis (P_1) will increase and after the area of stenosis (P_2) will decrease, creating a pressure gradient. The predictable relationship between the flow velocity and pressure gradient was first described by Daniel Bernoulli. The Bernoulli principle states that as the speed of a moving fluid increases the pressure within the fluid decreases.

$$P_1 - P_2 = 4 \times (V_1^2 - V_2^2)$$

where P_1 is prestenotic pressure, P_2 poststenotic pressure, V_1 is prestenotic flow velocity, V_2 is poststenotic flow velocity.

The simplified Bernoulli equation will allow calculating the pressure gradient from maximal (peak) flow velocity by using the following formula:

$$\Delta P = 4 \times (P \text{ peak}^2)$$

where ΔP is pressure gradient and V is maximal flow velocity.

The Bernoulli equation is used extensively in cardiac echocardiography and vascular ultrasound. Usually, the pressure calculations are made by the equipment. However, it is important for the physician to know how those numbers are generated.

COLOR FLOW DOPPLER

Color flow Doppler is a multigated pulsed Doppler ultrasound technique, which means that multiple sample volumes are obtained and analyzed. Color flow Doppler is a pulsed modality and is therefore subject to aliasing and range resolution (Table 2-9). Multiple pulses in packets have different Doppler shifts that are averaged to provide mean or average flow velocities. Those flow velocities are measured not in one location, as with usual pulsed-wave Doppler or along the single line as with continuous wave, but on the two-dimensional grids and are usually combined with two-dimensional anatomical images (Table 2-9). The anatomical images are in black-and-white. Doppler information is provided in color, with negative Doppler shift (away from the transducer) usually depicted in the shades of blue and positive (toward the transducer) in the shades of red. Because it is not always presented in this way, a color map is provided to assist with identifying the direction and velocity of the flow. The upper part of the map shows flow toward the transducer and the lower part of the map shows flow away from it. The distance from the middle of the map bar is proportional to the flow velocity. In the upper part of the bar, the highest flow velocities are depicted on the top, and in the lower

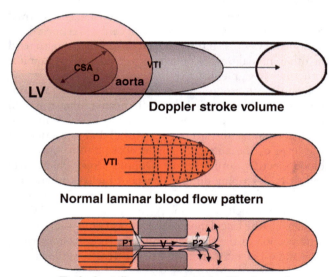

Figure 2-16 The normal laminar or parabolic blood flow pattern is bullet shaped with the highest flow velocity in the middle. Valvular or vascular stenosis is associated with an increase in pressure prior to the stenotic area, decreased pressure on exit, and increased flow velocity through the stenotic area. The pressure gradient is defined by the following relationship P1 – P2 = 4 × V² (simplified Bernoulli equation). The cross-sectional area of the vessel (i.e., aorta) CSA = $\pi \times \{D/2\}^2$. VTI × CSA will describe the volume of blood passing through the area during systole. For the proximal aorta, this will be stroke volume.

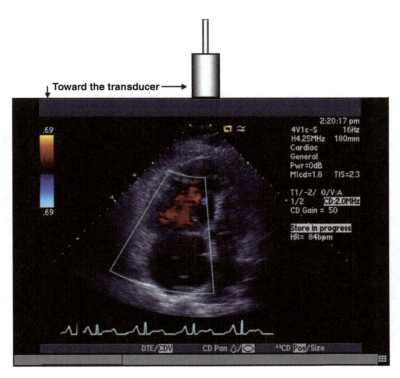

Figure 2-17 A colored map is provided for the colored Doppler of the right ventricle in this patient with pulmonary embolism.

part, on the bottom (Figure 2-17). As has been alluded to, the returning echoes will have different Doppler shift frequencies. When knowledge of individual frequencies is essential, spectral analysis is used. Digital techniques such as autocorrelation and fast Fourier transform (FFT) are performed by the computer chips and are of little interest to this book's intended audience. Additional information on the matter of spectral analysis of Doppler signals can be obtained from the list of suggested readings.

QUALITY ASSURANCE

Knowing the basic principles of imaging and Doppler ultrasound will enable the physician to participate in and understand the quality assurance program that will guarantee optimal images and prevent unnecessary downtime. In the ICU, problems ranging from inconvenience to adverse patient outcomes may be avoided with these approaches. Though the equipment manufacturer might provide support for maintaining the equipment in the form of a service contract, the ultimate responsibility for quality assurance rests with the operator. In the case of ICU ultrasonography, the operator is nearly always the physician. Routine quality assurance will also alleviate medical–legal problems that may arise from the use of the ultrasound equipment, particularly for invasive procedures.

Usually, imaging ultrasound equipment is tested on phantoms with standard physical characteristics (Figure 2-18). The most commonly used ones are the American Institute of Ultrasound in Medicine (AIUM) 100 mm test-object and tissue-equivalent phantoms. Both are commercially available. In these phantoms, the speed of sound is 1540 msec. Objects with different acoustic impedance are placed in different positions to assess the equipment's ability to visualize (resolution) and properly estimate their position (calibration) (Figure 2-18). The sensitivity of the machine is evaluated by its ability to detect objects in the far field. Axial resolution is evaluated by objects placed at a certain depth in the pass of the ultrasound beam and so is vertical calibration. Lateral resolution and horizontal calibration are checked by the objects placed perpendicular to the direction of the beam (Figure 2-18).

Mock cysts and tumors with different acoustic impedance are also placed in the tissue phantom to check the equipment's ability to detect their diameter and characteristics (Figure 2-18). Doppler phantoms usually utilize belts or strings moving at a standard speed to evaluate the system's ability to detect direction and velocity of the moving objects. More sophisticated Doppler testing phantoms pump echogenic (visible with the ultrasound) fluid into plastic pipes at known velocities.

BIOEFFECTS

Ultrasound images are produced by inducing tissue vibrations at ultrasonic frequency. There is little evidence to suggest that those vibrations have any biologic consequences. The same does not hold true for the ultrasound energy converted into heat. For instance, at the soft

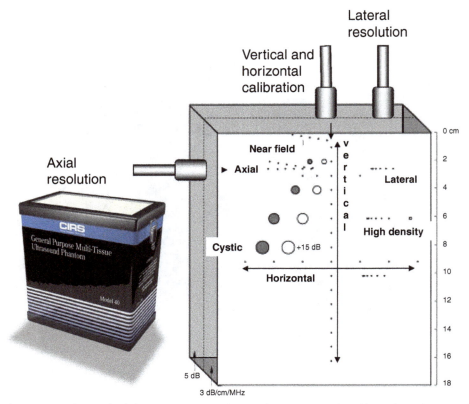

Figure 2-18 Tissue phantoms, with standard characteristics, can be used to assess axial and lateral resolution and calibration.

tissue–bone interface, roughly half of the sound is reflected back, but the remainder of the energy is absorbed by the bone, creating temperature elevation at this tissue–bone interface. This tissue heating is related to both the intensity and focus of the ultrasound beam. The more focused the ultrasound beam, the less the area of heat production, as the surrounding tissues dissipate thermal energy. This allowed the US Food and Drug Administration (FDA) and the AIUM to establish intensity limits: 100 mWatts/cm^2 for unfocused and 1000 mWatts/cm^2 (1 watt/cm^2) for focused ultrasound.

Aside from the thermal effects on the tissues, the other significant effect is called cavitation. Soft tissues contain microscopic areas of gas bubbles (gaseous nuclei) that can be heated by the ultrasound beam, resulting in their rapid expansion and ultimate bursting. This might create local mechanical stress and further tissue heating. Though little evidence for cavitation has been shown with diagnostic ultrasound, the possibility of tissue injury by that mechanism definitely exists.

This possibility prompted the AIUM in 1988 to issue a safety statement that is applicable even now to the use of diagnostic ultrasound, including its application in critical care medicine. As for ultrasound, the AIUM suggested that:

1. No study should be *performed* without valid reason.
2. No study should be *prolonged* without valid reason.
3. The minimal output power should be used to produce optimal images if the ultrasound machine allows control of output power. (*As low as reasonably achievable*, or ALARA principle.)

SUGGESTED READING

Edelman SK. *Understanding Ultrasound Physics*. 3rd ed. Huston, Tx: Esp Inc; 2004.
Hedrick WR, Hykes DL, Starchman DE. *Ultrasound Physics and Instrumentation*. 4th ed. St Louis, Mo: Elsevier Mosby; 2005.
Kremkau FW. *Diagnostic Ultrasound: Principles and Instruments*. 7th ed. St. Louis, Mo: Saunders Elsevier; 2006.
Miele FR. *Ultrasound Physics and Instrumentation*. 4th ed. Forney, Tx: Miele Enterpises; 2006.
Owen C, Zagzebski J. *Ultrasound Physics Review: A Q&A Review for the ARDMS Ultrasound Physics Exam*. Pasadena, CA: Davies Publishing Inc; 2008.

TRANSDUCERS, IMAGE FORMATION, AND ARTIFACTS

ALEXANDER B. LEVITOV & JOSEPH JOHN

Scan QR code or visit www.ccu2e.com for video in this chapter

TRANSDUCER STRUCTURE AND FUNCTION

Transducers are defined as devices converting one form of energy into another. In the case of ultrasound, electrical energy is converted into mechanical (acoustic) energy. The most familiar transducer is a telephone receiver, with an earpiece that converts electrical impulses into sound waves and a mouthpiece that converts sound energy into electricity. Imaging transducers combine both functions by emitting and receiving ultrasound pulses and converting them into electrical impulses for further processing. Nonimaging continuous-wave (CW) Doppler transducers, just like the telephone receiver, have two elements: one is constantly emitting sound and the other is receiving sound. Figure 3-1 shows the anatomy of the imaging transducer.

At the core of the ultrasound transducer (probe) is a sheet of piezoelectric material known as an active element, or simply the "crystal." It is usually made of lead zirconate titanate, or PZT. This material will create electricity when mechanically deformed (direct piezoelectric effect) and it itself deforms when electrical voltage is applied to its surface (reverse piezoelectric effect). The ability of some natural and man-made materials to create electricity when physically deformed was discovered by the brothers Pierre and Jacques Curie in 1880 and first used to produce ultrasound in sonar to track German U-boats during World War I in France in 1917. The piezoelectric effect of PZT irreversibly disappears as temperatures rise above 360°C (Curie point), making it impossible to sterilize ultrasound transducers with heat. The PZT crystal is one-half-wavelength thick (for the speed of sound in the active element itself). Connected to the PZT crystal is a wire that transmits electrical impulses from a pulse generator to the crystal during a pulse-generation phase, and away from it to the processor, during the "listening" phase, when an electrical impulse is generated in the PZT crystal by the returning echo. The listening phase is 10 times longer than the pulse duration, so the duty factor in imaging ultrasound transducers is 0.1–1% (see Chapter 2). The transducer can be also set to emit sounds of a so-called fundamental frequency, but receive echoes with frequencies that are multiples of the fundamental one. This tissue harmonic imaging is usually performed with returning frequencies that are twice (first harmonic) or even four times (second harmonic) higher than the fundamental one. Because the harmonic frequencies are generated in the tissues themselves, the image is resistant to certain artifacts and tends to be of a better quality. Behind the active element (PZT) is a backing or damping material. Just as a guitar string continues to produce sound after being struck once by the player, the electrical impulse, once it exits the PZT, will keep on ringing, producing longer pulse durations and spatial pulse lengths with deteriorating axial resolution. The backing material works like a guitarist's hand placed over the string, reducing the time that the PZT spends vibrating (ringing) after each electrical impulse and improving the image quality. The backing material is usually composed of tungsten-impregnated epoxy resin. CW Doppler transducers emit sound waves constantly and therefore do not require or contain any backing material (Figure 3-2).

In front of the PZT crystal is a matching layer that is a one-quarter wavelength thick. The difference in impedance results in an increase in reflection. The impedance of the matching layer is between that of the PZT crystal and the skin, in order to increase the transmission of the ultrasound from the active element into the tissues. To further reduce the impedance difference between PZT and skin, ultrasound gel is used. The impedance of the gel is less than that of the matching layer but more than that of the skin, making ultrasound transmission relatively smooth (Figure 3-1).

Wire, backing material, PZT crystal, and the matching layer are all housed in a case to protect them from the elements and to protect the patient and the operator from an

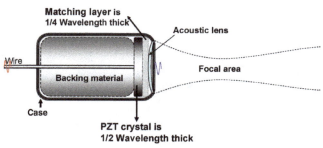

Figure 3-1 An imaging transducer both emits and receives signals. The PZT (piezoelectric) crystal converts electrical impulses from the wire into ultrasound and vice versa. A matching layer reduces internal reflections within the probe by gradually decreasing acoustic impedance. Backing material reduces the length of the pulse by preventing after-ringing dampening effect. Acoustic lenses improve focus. The case prevents electrical shock exposure for the patient and the operator.

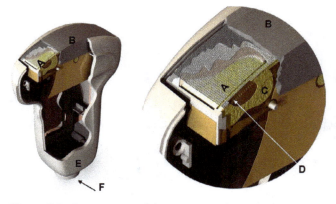

Figure 3-3 Components of the array transducer: A is PZT crystals, multiple crystals (active elements), can be activated separately; B is matching layer; C is backing material; D wires to each PZT element; E is a case; F cable all wires are still separated within the cable.

electrical shock (Figure 3-3). One should never attempt to use the transducer with a cracked housing or frayed wire.

Single-crystal transducers can produce several forms of imaging, of which only M-mode and two-dimensional (2D) (with mechanical scanning) are presently in use. A and B modes are only mentioned for their historical relevance (Figure 3-4). Both A-mode and B-mode will relate the strength of the signal to distance to the boundary where that signal is produced. This strength is either represented by the height (A-mode) or the brightness (B-mode) (Figure 3-4). B-mode of the single active element transducer will produce a series of dots arranged in a line. With multiple crystal or array transducers, each line produced by the single active element will coalesce with the one formed by its neighboring element to form a 2D image (see below). Because of this relationship, 2D images are sometimes called "B-mode," but this is technically incorrect. M-mode shows the position of the moving boundary over time, without reference to the signal's strength (Figures 3-4 and 3-5). M-mode is presently used in echocardiography and occasionally in noncardiac chest ultrasound for the diagnosis of pneumothorax, but 2D images are the primary mode used today. Two-dimensional imaging displays are used in all portable ultrasound machines available for intensive-care unit (ICU) use and in almost all diagnostic ultrasound equipment on the market.

Though 2D images can be produced by a single crystal transducer by mechanically moving the active element in a swinging motion across a scan plane (like moving a spotlight beam to see a deer in a night-time meadow), most of the modern transducers are composed of multiple active elements (Figures 3-3, 3-6, and 3-7). These so-called transducer arrays contain multiple PZT crystals with a separate wire attached to each element (Figures 3-3, 3-6, and 3-7). The electronic circuitry allows for each element to be activated separately in a specifically designed order. Arrays of active elements can be placed in a straight line (linear array), in an arc (convex or curved arrays), in concentric circles (annular arrays), or even in a checkerboard pattern (three-dimensional arrays) (Figures 3-3, 3-6, and 3-7). According to the sequence of element activation, transducers can also be divided into sequential arrays or phased arrays.

With sequential-array probes, groups of PZT crystals, usually arranged in linear or curved arrays, are fired in a sequence starting from one end to the other, 5–10 elements at a time, with each group firing immediately after its neighboring group. This is similar to a "wave" in a baseball stadium. When the activation sequence reaches the opposite end of the transducer, the process starts again. Linear sequential-array probes produce images only of the size of the transducer with a fixed focus, since each crystal in the array has its own focal zone and there is an inability to steer the beam. The image produced has a uniquely characteristic square shape (Figures 3-7 and 3-8). The linear-array probes are more common in vascular ultrasound. Convex sequential-array probes tend to be larger, with a fixed focus (for the same reason), but the image has a sector shape with a blunted top. Convex arrays have the

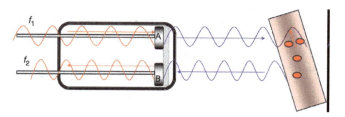

Figure 3-2 Continuous-wave Doppler transducer has two PZT crystals. One constantly emits and the other receives signals. Element A transmits continuous ultrasound waves with frequency f_1. Element B receives frequency f_2 ($f_1 - f_2$ = Doppler shift). Backing material is not necessary because continuous-wave signals require no dampening.

CHAPTER 3   TRANSDUCERS, IMAGE FORMATION, AND ARTIFACTS   25

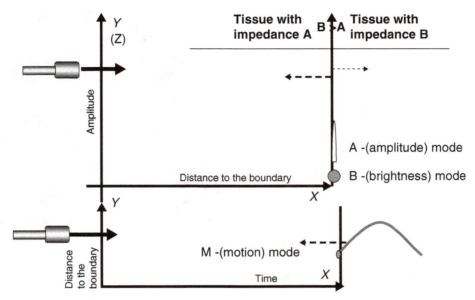

Figure 3-4 Display modes: A-mode displays amplitude of the signal and reflector depth; B-mode displays the same parameters, but the amplitude of the signal is represented by its brightness and not by the height; M-mode displays reflector depth over time.

advantage of a large near field and even larger far field and are used extensively in abdominal ultrasound, where large images are necessary (Figures 3-7 and 3-9).

Most transducers that critical care physicians will encounter will be linear, convex, or phased arrays. In phased-array probes, both beam steering and focusing is achieved electronically by sequencing the PZT crystal activation. Each active element is activated with an approximately 10-ns delay in a pattern created by a beam former in the ultrasound machine. Each PZT crystal in the array receives a signal in that predetermined pattern. There is also a similarly spaced delay in signal reception by the ultrasound machine. If the delay pattern is from the left to the right of the array, the beam is steered to the left. If the delay pattern is from right to left, the beam will be steered to the right. This will create the sweeping necessary to form 2D images without moving the active element (Figures 3-6 and 3-10).

The entire sweep from one side of the probe to the other will produce one imaging sector or frame. If the activation

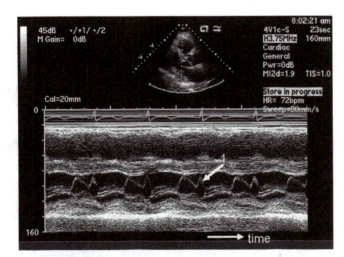

Figure 3-5 M-mode examination of the heart showing the position of different cardiac structures (intraventricular septum, mitral valve leaflets and inferior wall of left ventricle) plotted over time. Each 50 mm of the horizontal axis is 1 s. 1-Position of the anterior leaflet of the mitral valve at that time. Please note that brightness of the signal is of little relevance in an M-mode study.

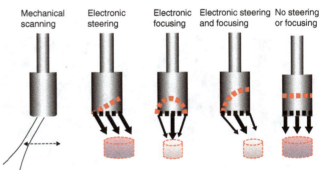

Figure 3-6 Mechanical scanning and phased-array probes offer a large acoustic footprint in the far field through a small window. They are common in cardiac ultrasound where the window is limited by intercostal spaces. In addition, phased-array probes offer electronic steering (sweeping) and focusing of the ultrasound beam. The operator is capable of selecting single or multiple focal points and the width of the sweep. A lack of moving parts also makes phased-array probes more reliable and durable.

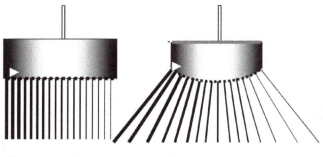

Figure 3-7 Two-dimensional imaging. Linear sequential arrays consist of multiple PZT crystals (elements) arranged in a line. Each one is connected to a separate wire. Elements are activated in groups from one end of the transducer to the other. A similar arrangement is present in a convex array, but the elements are arranged in a curve, giving this type of the transducer a wider view (larger footprint) in the far field. Elements in curved-array probe can be activated individually or in small groups.

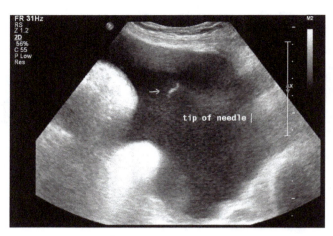

Figure 3-9 Image of the abdomen produced by the convex-array transducer. Notice a large acoustic footprint in both near and far field.

pattern is parabolic, the beam will be focused on a particular depth and the combination of patterns will produce both focusing and steering. Phased-array probes, regardless of how the active element patterns are arranged, are now the predominant probes used in echocardiography and are being used more frequently in vascular and general ultrasound.

The quality of the detail of the 2D image (spatial resolution) produced by an array probe depends on the number of separate ultrasound beams (lines) generated by the probe and the width of the sector necessary to produce the image. The line density, therefore, will depend on the number of the PZT crystals in the array probe and the sector width. To visualize the entire heart, for example, one will need a wider sector than the one necessary to visualize just the mitral valve. A cross section of the aorta will need a wider sector than a cross section of the carotid artery. The more lines per sector, the higher the line density, and the better the image quality and spatial resolution will be. Shallow images allow higher ultrasound frequency with better axial resolution per line and improved overall image quality (spatial resolution) (Figure 3-11 and Table 3-1). One complete sweep of either a mechanically or electronically steered beam will produce one frame of the 2D image. The sequence of the frames will create a video clip that can be observed or recorded by the operator. The number of frames per unit time is the temporal resolution of the exam. For continuous motion to be perceived as continuous, a minimal frame rate of 15 frames per second is necessary to provide a minimally acceptable temporal resolution. The more frames per second, the higher the temporal resolution. For a moving structure, like the heart, the higher the

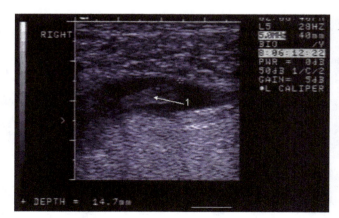

Figure 3-8 Vascular image (right common femoral vein) produced by linear sequential array transducer. Notice the image is square and is of the same size as a vessel. The solid-looking structure 1 in the middle of the vessel is a thrombus.

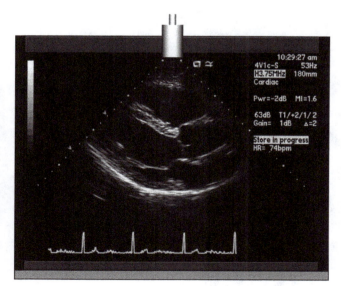

Figure 3-10 Echocardiographic image produced by the phased-array probe. Electronic steering enables the production of an image of the heart from a small acoustic window (intercostal space).

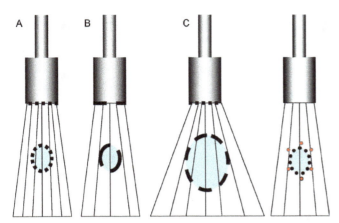

Figure 3-11 Probe A produces more ultrasound beams (lines) than probe B, with a resulting improvement in image quality (better spatial resolution). Probe C produces as many lines as probe A, but a wider sector decreases line density and degrades spatial resolution. Multifocusing requires more pulses per line and improves spatial resolution.

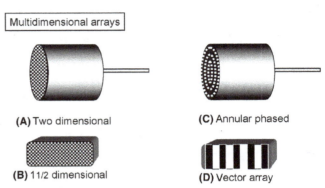

Figure 3-12 (**A**) Two-dimensional array is used to produce three-dimensional images. It has as many active elements in the vertical as in the horizontal plane. (**B**) One and one-half–dimensional array has more elements in the horizontal than vertical plane, makes a thin slice, and improves resolution in the vertical dimension. (**C**) In annular phased probe, PZT crystals are arranged in a concentric circular pattern and are activated from the innermost circle out. Each circle is focused on the particular depth (central shallower than outer ones), making it focused in all planes. Annular phased transducers are steered mechanically. (**D**) Vector arrays combine phased-array and sequential-array technology.

temporal resolution, the more real time is the image. The number of frames is limited by the time necessary to create a single frame. In any imaging, the previous pulse has to be received by the transducer and processed before the next one can be generated (Figure 3-11).

Temporal resolution is determined by the speed of sound in the medium and not controlled by the operator. The greater the distance the sound has to travel to deeper images, the longer the listening time of the transducer, the line density, and the amount of pulses necessary to create a frame (sector width and number of focal points) (Table 3-1).

In addition to commonly used imaging transducers, several specialty transducer types should be mentioned. Multidimensional transducers include 2D arrays used to create 3D ultrasound images (Figures 3-12 and 3-13) and one and one-half–dimensional arrays used to improve vertical components of the image by reducing beam width. Three-dimensional image capabilities are presently unavailable in portable ICU ultrasound equipment, but will undoubtedly become standard in the relatively near future. Annular phased arrays are automatically focused in multiple planes and are steered mechanically. These are used mostly in OB-GYN imaging. Vector arrays combine linear-, sequential-, and phased-array technologies in one transducer (Figure 3-12).

The construction of a pulsed Doppler transducer is very similar to that of a single-crystal imaging transducer, mentioned above. CW Doppler transducers emit ultrasound

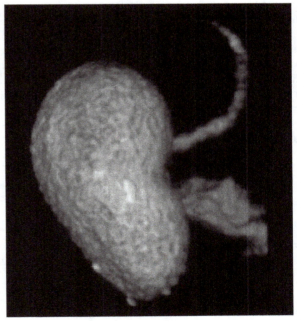

Figure 3-13 Three-dimensional ultrasound image of the kidney, produced using two-dimensional array.

TABLE 3-1
Factors Determining Spatial and Temporal Resolution of the 2D Image

Improved 2D Resolution	Depth	Sector Width	Line Density	Focusing
Spatial	Shallow	Narrow if the line density increases (zooming in)	High	Multiple
Temporal	Shallow	Narrow if the line density is unchanged	Low	Single

TABLE 3-2
Comparison of Different 2D Transducer Types

Transducer Type	Image Shape	Steering	Focusing
Mechanical	Sector	Mechanical	Fixed
Linear sequential array	Rectangle	None	Fixed
Linear phased array	Sector	Electronic	Electronic
Annular phased	Sector	Mechanical	Electronic
Convex sequential	Blunted sector	None	Fixed
Convex phased	Blunted sector	Electronic	Electronic
Vector	Flat top sector	Electronic	Electronic

waves continuously, just as their name implies, and therefore do not require any backing material (Figures 3-2 and 3-3). Different 2D transducer types are summarized in Table 3-2. Most modern transducers combine imaging and Doppler capabilities in a single probe.

IMAGE FORMATION

The formation of the ultrasound image requires proper flow of electrical impulses into the transducer and interpretation of direction, strength, frequency, and timing of the returning signal. The ultrasound machine or system makes all of that possible. Once an image is formed, it is displayed on a screen, usually in a digital format. In modern ultrasound systems, particularly portable ones that the ICU physician is likely to encounter, computer chips are increasingly used to simplify operation and optimize images (Figure 3-14). However, six common components are used in all ultrasound machines, irrespective of size or function, namely:

1. The master synchronizer organizes and times the flow of electrical signals within the system.
2. The pulser or beam former controls the firing pattern in the transducer and pulse amplitude, pulse-repetition frequency (PRF), and pulse-repetition period (PRP).
3. The transducer converts electrical signals received from the beam former into a sequence of ultrasound pulses and converts returning acoustic pulses into electrical impulses.
4. The receiver/processor contains the necessary elements for conversion of the returning electrical impulses into images (Table 3-3).
5. The display (screen, audio speakers, recording devices) presents data for interpretation and storage (usually in digital format).
6. Storage devices, also known as an archive, keep information more or less permanently for further review and to meet legal requirements.

Since the physician–sonographer will never come in contact with the master synchronizer, it is mentioned here, but will not be discussed further. Pulses or phased-array beam formers produce the sequence of electrical pulses that excite PZT crystals in the transducer. For the array transducer, separate electrical impulses are produced and timed separately for each PZT crystal. The voltage of those pulses may reach 500 volts, thus they present a real electrical hazard to the patient and the operator. *One should never use a transducer with a defective housing or frayed wire, no matter what the circumstances.* Traditionally, the amplitude of the output pulses (transducer output) was controlled by the operator, who could increase the amplitude of the electrical pulses in the pulser. In some larger echocardiography machines, this is still possible.

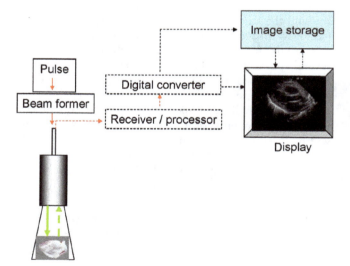

Figure 3-14 Basic components of the modern ultrasound system. The pulser generates electrical impulses organized by the beam former to electronically focus and steer (sweep) the ultrasound beam generated by the transducer. Active elements in the transducer convert electrical impulses into mechanical (acoustic) energy sent into the tissues. Incoming ultrasound echoes are converted into electrical impulses by the transducer and sent into the receiver/processor. The processor deciphers electrical information and an image is created. In modern systems, the image is displayed and stored in a digital format. Outgoing information is represented by solid arrows: red for electrical, green for ultrasound signals. Incoming information is represented by broken arrows.

CHAPTER 3 TRANSDUCERS, IMAGE FORMATION, AND ARTIFACTS

TABLE 3-3 Functions of the Receiver/Processor

Receiver Functions	Adjustable	Processing
Amplification	Yes	(Receiver gain) all signals are amplified and image becomes brighter when increased
Compensation	Yes	(TGC) deeper signals are amplified more
Compression	Yes	Gray-scale map is changed, dynamic range is decreased
Demodulation	No	Form and the direction of the signals are changed
Rejection	Yes	Only weak signals are rejected, strong are not affected

TGC, time-gain compensation.

High transducer output improves the signal-to-noise ratio and image quality. Presently, in almost all portable ultrasound systems, transducer output is set by the manufacturer and cannot be adjusted by the sonographer. The higher the amplitude of the electrical impulses and therefore the transducer output, the higher the potential to experience the adverse biological effects of ultrasound. Because manufacturers tend to improve image quality by setting the transducer output to the highest safe amplitude, it is incumbent upon the physician–sonographer not to prolong the examination unnecessarily.

A receiver/processor processes impulses received by the transducer and makes them suitable for the display (Table 3-3). The returning ultrasound and therefore electrical impulses are very weak and need to be amplified. The amplification, also known as receiver gain, is controlled by the operator and increases amplitude of all signals received by the transducer. In almost all imaging modalities, the amplitude (strength, volume) of the signal is presented on the screen as brightness. Increasing the receiver gain will increase the brightness of the entire image (Figure 3-15). After the signals have been amplified, signal compensation takes place. Compensation treats returning signals discriminately, depending on the depth of the image. Because the depth is derived from the time of flight, the control is known as time-gain compensation (TGC) or depth-gain compensation (DGC). Attenuation makes signals from greater depths (arriving later) disproportionately weaker compared with shallower (earlier arriving) echoes. Time-gain compensation amplifies returning signals to a greater degree if they have been received from the deeper parts of the image. Higher frequency traducers will produce quicker attenuating signals and require more TGC. Larger ultrasound systems usually have multiple controls increasing amplification of each depth separately, but in portable ICU equipment there may be only two TGC controls: shallow gain and deep gain, and the smoothness of the transitions is determined by the computer processing chips, which are often proprietary (Figure 3-16) (Video 3-1).

After compensation, signal compression takes place (Figure 3-17). Compression brings all signals within the brightness range visible to the human eye. Relative relationships between the signal amplitude continue to be the same (i.e., the highest are still the highest and the lowest are still the lowest), but the highest amplitude signals are

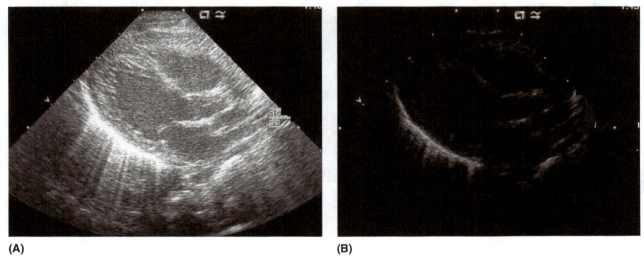

(A) (B)

Figure 3-15 Receiver gain controls the brightness of the entire screen. (**A**) Amplification settings that are too high; (**B**) settings that are too low. In either case, image quality is degraded.

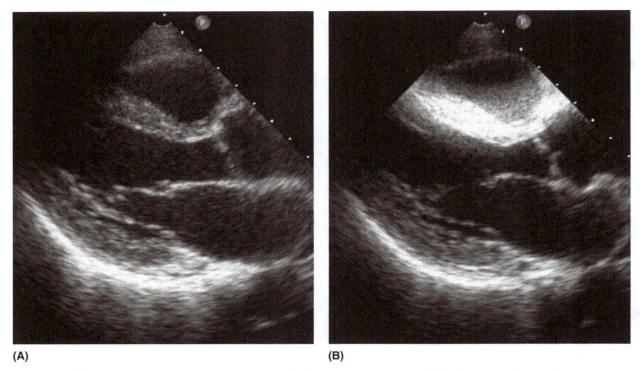

Figure 3-16 (**A**) Normal time gain compensation settings. (**B**) Overcompensation (too high of a gain) in the near field. Image quality is deteriorated (no fine details can be seen in the near field). Notice that both images are nearly identical in the far field. (Image courtesy of D. Adams, RDCS.)

reduced by an established number of decibels (dB) while the lowest amplitude signals are increased, so the difference between the highest and the lowest amplitude signals (dynamic range) is diminished. For example, if the original signal has a dynamic range of 100 dB and a compression of 30 dB takes place, the resulting dynamic range will be 70 dB. Visually, the dynamic range is represented by the gray scale of the image and is controlled either by the operator or set automatically by the processor, as in most portable systems. The wider the dynamic range (the less the compression), the more shades of gray represent the differences between the darkest and the brightest parts

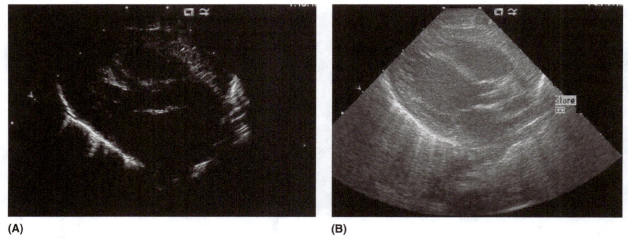

Figure 3-17 In most portable ultrasound systems compression is set automatically. In some, it is controlled by the operator, but in either case it sets the dynamic range of the image (the shades of gray representing the differences between the brightest and the darkest areas). In many ways, it is analogous to the contrast. (**A**) Image is overcompressed; it has narrow dynamic range with bistable (black and white) appearance, but also a high contrast. (**B**) Image is undercompressed; it has a wide dynamic range with multiple shades of gray, but the contrast is low. In either case, the image quality is degraded.

CHAPTER 3 TRANSDUCERS, IMAGE FORMATION, AND ARTIFACTS   31

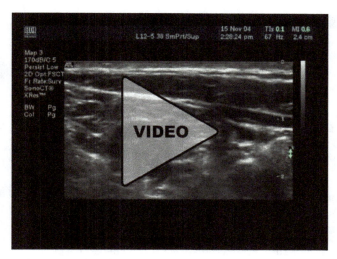

Video 3-1 Video of the cervical lymph node illustrating the use of overall gain and time gain compensation (TGC) controls. Note the side bar on the right side of the screen reflecting the amount of amplification applied to the signal (either overall or the echoes) returning from the specific depth (time of flight is used to determine the position of the boundary.). View at www.ccu2e.com

of the image and the lower is the contrast. The narrow dynamic range increases contrast, but makes images bistable (back and white), with lesser detail.

The vibration of the PZT crystal creates an alternating electrical current with positive and negative phases. Because ultrasound cannot identify negative electrical impulses, all negative voltages are converted to positive ones with the same amplitude (rectified). Then the signals are enveloped where all the changes in amplitude are evened out. Rectification and enveloping are collectively known as demodulation. Demodulation is performed by the processor in all systems and cannot be controlled by the operator (Figure 3-18).

After completion of demodulation, some low-level signals are rejected. Rejection does not affect high amplitude (bright) signals because they are usually meaningful to image formation. Low-amplitude signals can be rejected by the sonographer through the entire image if they do not appear meaningful and reduce image quality. Rejection can be fully or partially relegated to the computer chips in some portable ultrasound systems. Just as compression rejection increases the contrast, it narrows the dynamic range and results in some loss of the detail (Figure 3-17).

In modern ultrasound systems, processed signals are usually sent to a digital converter to be displayed in a digital format on the screen. Here again, computer chips are employed to improve the image. Digital images have the advantage of being virtually permanent, easy to disseminate, and allow, to some degree, the return to the original image format to do more analysis should new questions be raised. Digital archiving (a picture archiving and communication system, or PACS) can be entered easily at any time, after the images have been stored. The quality of the digital image is proportionate to the number of pixels available for the recording. At the present time, digital formats do not limit image quality. Throughout the ultrasound system the dynamic range is reduced from >100 dB in the transducer to 10–20 dB in the recorded images.

As one can see, the image generated by the ultrasound system is the result of complex processing. This makes this imaging modality the least intuitive of all, with the potential exception of nuclear medicine imaging. What complicates it even further is the fact that ultrasound imaging is based on a series of assumptions and the formation of the image requires multiple compromises (Tables 3-4 and 3-5). When the assumptions are faulty and compromises need to be made, image quality suffers and artifact production results. This by itself is neither bad nor good; in fact, some artifacts are an important part of the ultrasound diagnosis. However, it is important for the operator to be able to recognize which part of the image is real and which is not. The goal is not to achieve an "ideal image," reflecting anatomical reality, but a "best possible image" that differs from the reality to a greater or lesser degree.

ARTIFACTS

▶ Terminology

Prior to a discussion of different ultrasound artifacts, some important and common terms to describe ultrasound images, both static and moving, should be introduced. This terminology will enable the operator to describe the image, provide the information for medical records and to other health professionals, and better understand radiology and cardiology reports related to the ultrasound images (Table 3-6 and Figure 3-19).

▶ Artifacts and Image Alterations

The combination of complex processing, physical limitations, and partially valid assumptions is capable

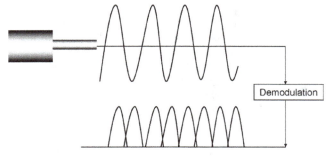

Figure 3-18 Demodulation converts all negative electrical impulses into positive ones with the same amplitude, making image formation possible, as negative electrical impulses cannot be processed further.

TABLE 3-4

List of Assumptions for Ultrasound Imaging

Assumptions	Validity
1. Ultrasound travels in a straight line from the transducer to the reflector and back.	Regrettably, this assumption is rarely valid. Although ultrasound pulses might approach the reflector in a relatively straight line, they probably will not strike the reflector at a 90° angle. Therefore, reflected echoes might never reach the transducer or return to it after being reflected from multiple other reflective boundaries.
2. The transmitted portion of the ultrasound continues to travel in a straight line, until it encounters another reflector, at which time the reflected echo will again return to the transducer in a straight line.	The transmitted portion of the pulse is the subject of refraction and is likely to continue its pass in a slightly different direction. It may also return to the transducer after encountering one or several secondary reflective boundaries.
3. Imaging ultrasound always strikes the reflector at a 90° angle.	This may be a valid assumption, but usually is not. It is also in stark contradiction to the next assertion regarding Doppler measurements if the single transducer is used for both.
4. Doppler ultrasound always strikes the moving reflector at a 0° angle.	This one is almost never correct and obviously contradicts the prior assumption if the same transducer is used for both imaging and Doppler.
5. All reflections arise only from the structures positioned along the axis of propagation of the ultrasound beam (pulse).	The axis of beam propagation itself is distorted by refraction, nonorthogonal reflections, and unexpected reflective boundaries.
6. The plane of 2D ultrasound sweep is very thin (has essentially no thickness).	This is incorrect. The ultrasound beam, just like a light beam, has a diameter and may simultaneously encounter and reflect off multiple structures.
7. The speed of sound in soft tissues is 1540 m/s.	This is incorrect. In fact, the human body does not contain any generic soft tissues. As the speed of sound is different in different tissues, and the distance to the reflector is calculated based on this assumption, this distance is never correct. Therefore, the position of the reflector is an estimated, and not a real, anatomical one.
8. The intensity of the reflection is related to the nature of the tissue.	The intensity of the reflection depends upon the interaction between multiple reflective boundaries and the ultrasound. Structures below the boundary with a higher difference in impedance may not be visualized (acoustic shadowing).
9. Two-dimensional ultrasound provides information in real time.	Depending on the temporal resolution of the ultrasound system and the depth of the reflector, the image formation is delayed and the motion of the reflective boundary is again an approximation of its real motion.

TABLE 3-5

Common Compromises Necessary to Obtain the "Best Possible Image"

Compromise	Reason	Operator Control
High vs. low frequency transducers	High frequency improves image quality, but limits the penetration.	Choose the appropriate transducer for the image depth and the view with the least depth.
High vs. low PRF	High PRF improves image quality, but limits the penetration.	Choose the view with the least depth that will adequately visualize the structure.
High vs. low transducer output	High transducer output improves signal-to-noise ratio, but may have more bioeffects.	Transducer output may be controlled by the operator in some systems.
Line frequency in the 2D image	More lines improve spatial resolution, but worsen temporal resolution.	Choose views with the narrowest sector that will adequately visualize the structure.
Multifocusing	Improves spatial resolution, but worsens temporal resolution.	Operator preference in system and transducer choice.
Image quality vs. Doppler	Best image at 90°, best Doppler at 0° incident angle.	Choose the view that will give an adequate information.
CW vs. pulsed or colored Doppler	CW measures high-flow velocity; pulsed is subject to aliasing, but provides sample location.	Choose both, when necessary to obtain complementary information.

CW, continuous wave; PRF, pulse-repetition frequency.

TABLE 3-6
Commonly Used Ultrasound Terminology

Term	Definition
Static Characteristics	
Anechoic	Also called "echo-free," and refers to the parts of the image that produce no returning signal. These occur below the boundary with high acoustic impedance (shadowing) or in liquid-filled structures, i.e., cysts.
Hypoechoic	A portion of the image may produce fewer returning echoes than the surrounding tissues, and appears less bright than the other parts of the image. An area of necrosis is a prime example.
Isoechoic	Refers to tissues with the same brightness and presumably produces similar echo return.
Hyperechoic	Portions of the image that appears either brighter than the surrounding tissues or brighter than expected. For example, the mitral valve as compared to the rest of the heart or carotid artery calcifications as compared to the normal artery.
Echohomogeneous	Any structure can be homo- or heterogeneous, depending on whether it has similar or different echo characteristics throughout.
Dynamic (Movement) Characteristics	
Akinetic	A structure or a part of an organ that should be moving, but does not (e.g., inferior wall of left ventricle in inferior myocardial infarction).
Hypokinetic	A structure that is moving less than expected (same example as for akinetic).
Diskinetic	A structure that is moving in the direction opposite to what is expected. Also known as paradoxical motion (e.g., the intraventricular septum in massive pulmonary embolism or the acute phase of left ventricular aneurysm).
Hyperkinetic	A structure that is moving too much compared with what is expected (i.e., left ventricle in patient with early hypovolemic shock).
Doppler Characteristics	
Laminar phasic	Characteristic of flow of reflectors and their position in the structure of travel. Normal venous flow.
Laminar pulsatile	Characteristic of flow of reflectors and their position in the structure of travel. Normal arterial flow.
Turbulent flow	Flow velocity depends on the cardiac structure or the caliber of the vessel, but normally will seldom exceed 2 m/s. Always abnormal, and sometimes described as mosaic in colored Doppler.

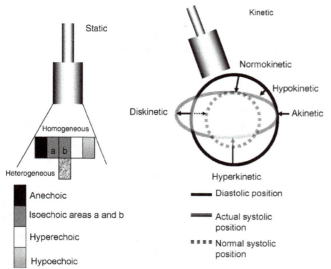

Figure 3-19 Image characteristics static (left) and kinetic (right).

of producing artifacts. Artifacts result from a discrepancy between the image interpretation and reality and include imaging errors, operator errors, and interpreter errors. Interpreter errors can be avoided by a solid knowledge of the ultrasound physics, image formation, ultrasound system, and human anatomy. With the exception of operator error, most common artifacts are caused by the discrepancy between the true physics of ultrasound and assumptions about image formation. Violations to the assumptions of image formation are known as acoustic artifacts. Most acoustic artifacts are seen on a single view and cannot be confirmed on subsequent views of the same anatomical structures. Others will disappear when corrective measures are taken by the operator. Persistent artifacts in multiple views might also signify system malfunctions and require a call to the manufacturer or service engineer. The most common ultrasound artifacts and their clinical significance are presented in Table 3-7.

TABLE 3-7
Common Artifacts and Their Clinical Significance

Artifact	Clinical Significance
Acoustic shadowing	When ultrasound reaches an object with very high acoustic impedance (attenuation), it will not be able to penetrate it any further. This will create acoustic shadowing, which is a linear anechoic or hypoechoic area covering deeper structures so that they cannot be visualized or displayed. Acoustic shadowing is used to diagnose high-attenuation objects such as gallstones or heavy calcified vessel walls. Another cause for acoustic shadowing is the refraction at the edge of a circular structure. An analogy is the circular appearance of the sun on a sunny day shining in your eyes. You can see very little the closer you get to it. This phenomenon is called shadowing by refraction (edge shadowing), and on the ultrasound image it will produce a hypoechoic line parallel to the sound beam. No anatomical structures will be visible in that "shadow." Anatomical edges of round organs such as the heart, kidneys, testicles, or a baby's head will be prone to produce such artifacts (Figure 3-20).
Reverberations and ring-down (comet-tail) artifacts	If the ultrasound reaches two reflectors, it might reflect multiple times like a candle standing between two mirrors. The resulting image will have a "Venetian blind" appearance, with equally spaced multiple lines perpendicular to the direction of the ultrasound beam's propagation. If the distance between the parallel lines diminishes, they may become confluent. Those merged reverberation artifacts are known as the "comet-tail" sign (Figure 3-21). These are solid hyperechoic lines that appear to visualize the ultrasound beam itself. Reverberations are common in echocardiography in the apical four-chamber view where the ultrasound beam is "bouncing" between layers of pericardium or between pericardium and epicardium, which are both high-impedance boundaries. In chest ultrasound, reverberation artifacts become clinically important. They are produced by the signal trapped between parietal and visceral pleura, which are both strong reflectors. The presence of reverberation artifacts implies that both pleural layers are in close proximity and virtually rules out pneumothorax. Normally, lung tissue is not visualized by contemporary ultrasound systems because the sound propagation speed in the lungs is way below the expected 1540 m/s (propagation speed error). But as the lung tissue becomes more dense from fluid accumulation (pulmonary edema) or inflammatory changes (pneumonia, ARDS) the speed of sound increases. This improves transmission of the ultrasound back to the transducer and converts distinct reverberation artifact lines into comet-tail artifacts. The number of comet-tail lines is thought by some to correlate with the degree of pulmonary edema or inflammatory changes and may become a useful diagnostic and prognostic tool in critically ill patients.
Enhancement	If the sound passes through an area of lower attenuation, structures located beneath appear hyperechoic. This hyperechoic band parallel to the ultrasound beam is known as an acoustic enhancement and will often be used to differentiate cysts (lower-attenuation structures) from cystic tumors and abscesses that have higher attenuation (Figure 3-22). The other type of enhancement, known as banding, occurs in the focal area of the single-focus transducers. It is a hyperechoic stripe perpendicular to the direction of the ultrasound beam. Banding became increasingly rare with modern transducers used in the portable ICU ultrasound machines.
Mirror image	The area of very high acoustic impedance may serve as an acoustic mirror deflecting the ultrasound beam to the side. The ultrasound system assumes that sound travels in a straight line, and thus is unable to recognize redirected beams as such. It will always place the image created by the deflected beam (mirror artifact) deeper than the correct anatomical position of the true reflector. This is because the redirected beam will take longer to reach the transducer (Figure 3-23). A high reflective boundary will be located between the anatomical reflector and the artifact.
Propagation speed errors	The ultrasound system assumes that the speed of sound in soft tissues is 1540 m/s. So if the actual propagation speed is higher, the reflector will be placed shallower, and if it is slower, deeper than the actual anatomical position. If the propagation speed differs significantly from the one assumed (i.e., silicone gel prosthesis or lung tissue), the position will vary significantly as well.
Refraction artifacts	If the sound strikes the boundary obliquely or if the propagation speed in two adjacent mediums differs, propagation with the bend or refraction will take place. The difference in propagation speed will compensate for the increased distance, and the reflection of the refracted beam will reach the transducer nearly simultaneously with the echo of the pulse that stuck the reflector with normal incidence. Therefore, the refraction artifact will be placed by the ultrasound system side by side with the true anatomical reflector (Figure 3-24). Because of this, one cannot say which one of the images is the reflector and which is an artifact.
Lobes	Lobes are caused by the parts of the ultrasound beam propagating in the direction other than the beam's main axis (violation of the Assumption 5 above) Because very few modern ICU ultrasound systems use mechanical or single PZT crystal transducers, side lobes specific to this kind of transducers will not be discussed further here. Commonly used array transducers produce the so-called grating lobes. Grating lobes are second copies of the reflector placed side by side with the reflector itself. They occur if the ultrasound beam is wider than the reflector itself. Use of tissue harmonic imaging greatly reduces the occurrence of this artifact.
Doppler artifacts	Two common Doppler artifacts are ghosting and cross talk. Ghosting is a Doppler shift produced by moving anatomical structures (i.e., pulsatile vessel wall), rather than the blood flow. Ghosting can be eliminated by rejecting low-level Doppler shifts with wall filters. Alternatively, ghosting can be helpful in identifying if the reflective boundary is moving, which in the case of pleural layers will rule out pneumothorax. Cross talk is a mirror image artifact as applied to the Doppler phenomenon. It can be caused by a high receiver gain or the Doppler incident angle of near 90°. It is seen as the identical flow pattern appearing above and below baseline and can be remedied by decreasing receiver gain or changing the incident angle. Strictly speaking, aliasing is another Doppler artifact but it was fully discussed previously and will not be discussed here.

ARDS, acute respiratory distress syndrome; ICU, intensive-care unit; PZT, lead zirconate titanate.

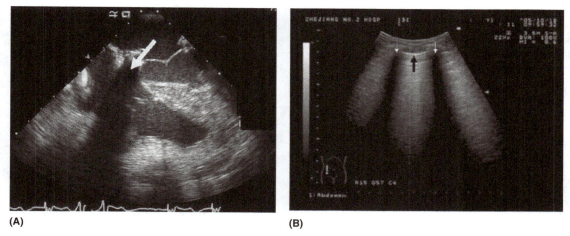

Figure 3-20 Two examples of acoustic shadowing. Part A is a transesophageal echocardiogram where shadowing of the severe calcification is preventing visualization of deeper structures (white arrow). In Part B rib calcifications are utilized to identify the pleural line (black arrow) formed by parietal and visceral pleura. Presence of motion (shimmering) in that location helps to rule out pneumothorax during ultrasound evaluation of the lung.

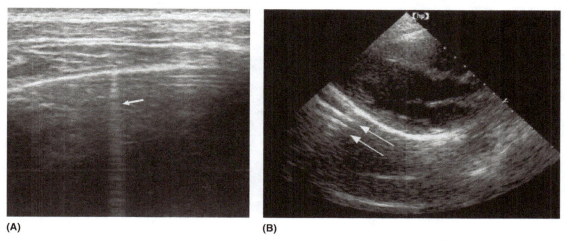

Figure 3-21 (**A**) Reverberation artifact on the lung ultrasound. "Comet-tail" sign helps to rule out pneumothorax (white arrow). Multiple similar artifacts may indicate an increase in lung stiffness due to congestion or inflammatory changes. (**B**) Classic reverberation artifacts (echocardiogram) are represented by the "Venetian blind" pattern produced by the pericardium and just causes the deterioration of image quality.

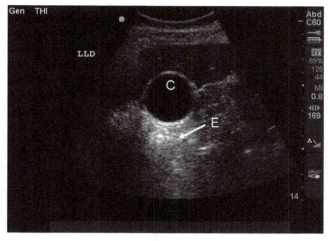

Figure 3-22 This image of a low-attenuation lesion (anechoic cyst C) shows a hyperechoic band parallel to the ultrasound beam, known as an acoustic enhancement (E), and will often be used to differentiate cysts (lower-attenuation structures) from tumors (high-attenuation structures) that will not produce this artifact.

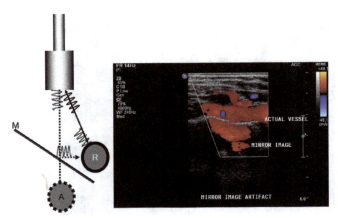 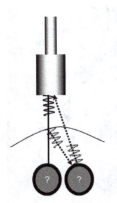 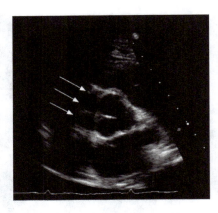

Figure 3-23 An ultrasound beam reaches anatomical reflector R by two routes, directly and after being reflected from a high-impedance boundary (mirror M). Because the reflected pulse takes longer to reach the transducer, the mirror artifact image A is placed deeper than the real reflector. Colored Doppler is also a subject to mirror image artifact as in this case of the carotid artery image.

Figure 3-24 Aortic duplication due to the refraction artifact (white arrows). Due to incomplete nature of duplication, the position of the artifact vs. anatomical position of the true reflector can be identified. This is not always the case. (Image courtesy of D. Adams, RDCS.)

SUGGESTED READING

Edelman SK. *Understanding Ultrasound Physics*. 3rd ed. Spring, TX: Esp Inc; 2004.

Hedrick WR, Hykes DL, Starchman DE. *Ultrasound Physics and Instrumentation*. 4th ed. St Louis, MO: Elsevier Mosby; 2005.

Kremkau FW. *Diagnostic Ultrasound: Principles and Instruments*. 7th ed. St Louis, MO: Saunders Elsevier; 2006.

Miele FR. *Ultrasound Physics and Instrumentation*. 4th ed. Forney, TX: Miele Enterpises; 2006.

Owen C, Zagzebski J. *Ultrasound Physics Review: A Q&A Review for the ARDMS Ultrasound Physics Exam*. Pasadena, CA: Davies Publishing Inc; 2008.

TRAINING IN CRITICAL CARE ULTRASONOGRAPHY

PAUL H. MAYO & ALEXANDER B. LEVITOV

In order to become competent in critical care ultrasonography (CCUS), the intensivist must access effective training, as competence is the goal of training. This chapter summarizes some aspects of training in CCUS that may be useful to two distinct groups: the frontline clinician who has decided to develop competence in CCUS and the faculty who are responsible for providing training to their colleagues.

Individual intensivists who seek training face different challenges depending on their function within the medical hierarchy. Physicians in training, such as residents or fellows, are in a good position, as they have the time and assignment to acquire a wide variety of skills intrinsic to critical care medicine, one of which includes CCUS. Only if there are no capable faculty available to provide them with training will they have difficulty in achieving this goal. Unfortunately, this is still the case in many fellowship training programs both in North America and Europe and will only be remedied in coming years by faculty development aided by the establishment of requirements for provision of training in CCUS at the fellowship level.

The attending level intensivist faces the challenge of obtaining training in CCUS while balancing the demands of the workplace, family life, and economic pressures. Some attending level intensivists come from an adverse training environment. They may work in a geographically isolated hospital surrounded by unfriendly colleagues from other specialties who are not interested in helping a co-worker develop a new skill. Others may be more fortunate and work in a hospital where knowledgeable radiology and cardiology colleagues are interested in providing local expertise for supervision of training.

There are several approaches that are effective when considering training. If a resident or fellow is in a program that provides formal training in CCUS, competence is achieved as a normal part of critical care training. If the program is not able to provide this, the fellow is in the same position as the attending who seeks training following their fellowship years. This group frequently develops competence using an "on the job" approach. In this case, the clinician works in a friendly training environment where they are supported by an informal network of colleagues.

Training in CCUS requires skills in image acquisition, image interpretation, and mastery of the cognitive elements of the field. Mastery of image acquisition is a key skill required for CCUS, as the frontline intensivist personally performs all parts of the ultrasound examination. Training in image acquisition requires partnering with a skilled ultrasonographer in combination with regular deliberate practice, initially on normal models followed by the scanning of patients. For "on the job" training, the learner may seek the help of highly skilled ultrasound technicians who, particularly in the United States, perform much of cardiology and radiology image acquisition. Widespread use of ultrasound technicians is common in the United States, while in Europe it is common for the physician to perform both image acquisition and interpretation. For training in image interpretation, the intensivist may partner with local experts from the disciplines of radiology or cardiology side. The cognitive elements required for competence in CCUS are now widely available in course materials, articles, and textbook formats. A self-designed program at the local level is both feasible and effective as a training option, but cannot be achieved if the intensivist works in an adverse training environment. The main obstacle to the "on the job" approach is that it is relatively inefficient compared to engaging in an organized training program that is specifically designed for mastery of CCUS.

HOW TO DEFINE COMPETENCE?

A clear definition of competence is a key element for training, as it defines the goals of training. If the goals of training are explicitly defined, this facilitates the development of a training program designed to provide competence. A definition of competence establishes specific learning objectives for both course design and bedside training, it leads to a definition of scope of practice and it is needed for the development of competency based testing.

In 2009, a working group from the American College of Chest Physicians (ACCP) and the Societe de Reanimation de Langue Francaise (SRLF) defined the elements of CCUS that were required for competence in CCUS.[1] The Statement on Competence in Critical Care Ultrasonography provides a roadmap for faculty who are tasked with developing training programs and for the individual intensivist who is interested in training in CCUS. While other working groups have developed important summaries of the field,[2,3,4] the ACCP/SRLF document is instead designed to address a basic question in developing training standards: what constitutes competence in CCUS. The Statement on Competence sets out the goals of training in a simple and user friendly manner, and is useful both for the individual who seeks training for competence in CCUS and for faculty who are responsible for the design of training systems. The document fills the need for an explicit definition of competence, so that it is designed to be used as a practical guide for goals of training.

The Statement on Competence describes a standard for competence that does not include many useful applications of ultrasonography that are discussed in this textbook. Instead, it defines a skill set that would meet the usual operational needs of a frontline intensivist. This should not discourage the learner from developing an advanced ultrasound skill that has utility to a specific practice situation.

HOW TO PROCEED WITH TRAINING?

In follow-up to the ACCP/SRLF Competence Statement, the European Society of Intensive Care (ESICM) organized an expert roundtable meeting to reach an international consensus on training in CCUS. Representatives from the Asia-Pacific, South America, the Middle East, and most countries of the European Union were in attendance. North America was represented by the ACCP, the American Thoracic Society, the Society for Critical Care Medicine (SCCM), and the Canadian Critical Care Society. The resulting document, entitled Training in Critical Care Ultrasonography, is designed to provide guidance to the critical care community in developing training in CCUS.[5] The working group recognized that there was a relative paucity of definitive literature on the subject of training except for some related to critical care echocardiography (CCE). As a result, the recommendations were formulated as suggestions to help guide training effort. However, there was agreement on several issues:

1. The ACCP/SRLF Statement on Competence was designated as the foundation document to guide training; i.e., the goals of training are explicitly defined in the Statement on Competence.
2. CCUS should be a required part of critical care training.
3. CCE should be divided into basic and advanced CCE. Basic CCE is a required part of general critical ultrasonography; advanced CCE requires an extensive course of study and is an optional component of training.
4. General CCUS (including basic CCE) requires no formal certification process to establish competence.
5. Advanced CCE requires a formal certification process to recognize competence.

The opinion of the working group was that CCUS should be considered as a routine part of the scope of practice of critical care, and so requires no special recognition through certification. The cost and complexity of developing the process of certification is prohibitive. Also, setting up a complex national level certification system would imply that other standard parts of critical care practice (e.g., vascular access, ventilator management, pleural access, and airway management) would logically be subjected to the same standard. This is not the case. As a result, it is unlikely that this type of certification will be developed in the United States or elsewhere.

Given the complexity of advanced CCE, this component of CCUS requires the development of a formal certification process. A certification process for advanced CCE would need to be developed and administered by a national level agency that is independent of any training group. In the United States, such Certification would be under the aegis of the National Board of Echocardiography. A process for certification in advanced CCE has already been developed in France and Australia. It is possible that this may occur in the United States. The Training Statement offers recommendations for the design of training in CCUS and advanced CCE that are summarized in Tables 4-1 and 4-2. These may helpful to both faculty and learners in the design of training.

In the absence of a process for certification in CCUS (with the exception of advanced CCE), determination of competence becomes an issue. One approach is to establish requirements for the number of studies and the duration of study needed to achieve competence. French investigators have been active in this field of research. Chalumeau-Lemoine et al. have studied the effectiveness of a training program for CCUS with positive results.[6] Vignon et al. have described a similar program related to basic CCE.[7] Charron et al. report that least 31 studies performed over a 6 month period is required to assure competence in transesophageal echocardiography (TEE).[8] These reports included a formal examination of competence to validate their results. The number or studies performed and the duration of study may have an uncertain relationship to competence, so that the summative testing of skill should be included into a training program. Competence based testing that focuses

TABLE 4-1
Summary of Recommendations for Training in Critical Care Ultrasonography*
1. **Theoretical program** Course design should include specific learning goals that are described in the ACCP/SRLF competence statement. The minimum number of hours for course design required to teach critical care ultrasonography (CCUS) and basic critical care echocardiography (CCE) is 10 h each, to be divided between lectures and didactic cases with image-based training.
2. **Format of the theoretical training** Both standard lecture format and Internet-based learning have advantages. Therefore, ideally both Internet-based learning and lecture format should be available to trainees, potentially in a blended fashion to allow them to take advantage of both. Lectures can include didactics and illustrative interactive cases.
3. **Required number of examinations to be performed by the trainee** There was no consensus on this issue. There is no data in the literature to identify a specific number of studies that need to be performed to reach the desired level of competence in CCUS with the exception that review of the literature suggests that 30 fully supervised transthoracic echocardiographic (TTE) studies is a reasonable training target to achieve competence in image acquisition. Tutored TTEs should be preferably performed in unstable patients to increase the probability of encountering abnormal findings. Trainees should learn CCUS with a locally qualified physician supervisor. This supervisor determines when the trainee has acquired competence in the practical bedside aspects of CCUS. The lack of consensus regarding numerical requirements can be compared to training in many other ICU techniques such as bronchoscopy or endotracheal intubation, for which no widely accepted quantitative targets have yet been established.
4. **How many cases of each clinical syndrome should be examined by the trainee?** There was no consensus on this issue. It is not reasonable to expect that each trainee will encounter all important clinical situations during the time course of his/her training in CCUS. Therefore, a comprehensive panel of important abnormal images with their clinical scenarios must be part of the didactic cases and interactive image interpretation sessions that are integral to training course design. This exposes the trainee to a wide variety of abnormal images in order that they are prepared for clinical situations. Abnormal images and their clinical scenarios may be presented in interactive lecture format, or through Internet-based methods.
5. **Is there a place for hands-on training on normal volunteers?** During initial practical training, hands-on training with normal volunteers is a convenient and effective method to teach key elements of image acquisition such as transducer manipulation, standard views, spatial orientation, and normal anatomy.
6. **What should be the format for documenting practical training in image acquisition and interpretation?** Each trainee should maintain a logbook of their scanning activity that includes reports of ultrasound studies performed and/or interpreted. Trainees should write reports of their image interpretation, and the reports should be cosigned by both trainee and supervisor to attest that the findings have been verified by a physician who is qualified in CCUS.
7. **Where should practical training take place, and who should supervise practical training in image acquisition and interpretation?** Initially, practical training may use normal models under the supervision of hands-on training faculty. In addition, training in CCUS requires a component of bedside scanning in the ICU under the direction of a supervisor who is competent in CCUS. The supervisor for practical training should be a locally qualified physician who regularly performs CCUS in the ICU environment. It is mandatory that a dedicated ultrasound machine be available in every ICU where training occurs.

*Adapted from the International Expert Statement on Training Standards for Critical Care Ultrasonography.

on the outcome rather than the process of training is one means of assuring that training has been effective. Competence based testing for CCUS requires the development of a clinically relevant examination of skill that includes bedside assessment of image acquisition.

INTERNATIONAL PATTERNS OF TRAINING IN CCUS

It is instructive to review what the approaches to training in CCUS that have been developed in different medical systems. Faculty tasked with training other intensivists may adapt these methods to local requirements.

There is difficulty in describing training patterns in Europe, as there is no single organization that determines standards for training in critical care. There is no equivalent to the American College of Graduate Medical Education (ACGME) that has the power to establish mandatory requirements for critical care training. Local standards are established within each country; so that what holds in Sweden, for example, has no relevance in Bulgaria. The author has witnessed strong interest in Europe in developing training in CCUS. The ESICM has been putting on courses at their international meeting that are well attended; the same holds for the International Symposium on Intensive and Emergency Medicine. As in the United States, the commitment to training varies by country, city,

TABLE 4-2
Summary of Recommendations for Training in Advanced Critical Care Echocardiography*

1. **Theoretical program**
   Course design should include specific learning goals as described in the ACCP/SRLF competence statement. The minimum number of hours for course design required to teach advanced critical care echocardiography (CCE) is 40 h, to be divided between lectures and didactic cases with image-based training.

2. **Format of the theoretical training**
   Both standard lecture format and Internet-based learning have advantages. Therefore, Internet-based learning and lecture format should be available to trainees, potentially in a blended fashion to allow them to take advantage of both. Lectures can include didactics and illustrative interactive cases.

3. **What is the required number of examinations to be performed by the trainee?**
   Trainees must acquire competencies in transthoracic echocardiography (TTE) and transesophageal echocardiography (TEE). There was a consensus that TEE is mandatory for advanced CCE. Review of the literature suggests that 150 fully supervised TTE studies and 50 fully supervised TEE studies are a reasonable training target to achieve competence in image acquisition and interpretation. Trainees should learn advanced CCE with a locally qualified physician supervisor. Using validated scoring system to evaluate acquisition of competencies at bedside has been proposed. A maximum period of 2 years is recommended to collect the appropriate number of echocardiographic studies.

4. **How many cases of each clinical syndrome should be examined by the trainee?**
   There was no consensus on this issue. It is not reasonable to expect that each trainee will encounter all important clinical situations during the time course of his/her training in advanced CCE. Therefore, a comprehensive panel of important abnormal images with their clinical scenarios must be part of the didactic cases and interactive image interpretation sessions that are integral to training program design. This exposes the trainee to a wide variety of abnormal images in order that they are prepared for clinical situations. Abnormal images and their clinical scenarios may be presented in interactive lecture format, or through Internet-based methods. Both TTE and TEE illustrative examples must be integrated in the training program.

5. **What should be the format for documenting practical training in image acquisition and interpretation?**
   Each trainee must maintain a logbook of their scanning activity that includes reports of studies performed and/or interpreted. Trainees should write reports of their image interpretation, and the reports be cosigned by trainee and supervisor to attest that the findings have been verified by a physician who is qualified in advanced CCE.

6. **Where should practical training take place, and who should supervise practical training in image acquisition and interpretation?**
   By definition, trainees have first to become competent in basic CCE. For that, practical training may initially use normal models under the supervision of hands-on training faculty. Subsequent training in advanced CCE requires bedside scanning by both transthoracic and transesophageal routes in the ICU under the direction of a supervisor who is competent in advanced CCE. The supervisor for practical training should be a locally qualified physician who regularly performs advanced CCE in the ICU environment. It is mandatory that a dedicated ultrasound machine with both transthoracic and transesophageal probes be available in every ICU where training occurs.

*Adapted from the International Expert Statement on Training Standards for Critical Care Ultrasonography.

and individual training program, so that it is difficult to summarize the situation in an organized manner.

The exception is in France, where the emphasis has been on developing a national level training program for both basic and advanced CCE. The French approach to providing training in both advanced and basic CCE is a model for others to follow. Initially, the SRLF, in cooperation with their cardiology colleagues, focused on developing a national level certification program targeted at critical care faculty who worked in the major teaching hospitals of France. Certification in advanced CCE required a 2-year program of study, one year of which was shared with cardiology trainees. In addition to the completion of formal course work, learners had to perform 220 transthoracic (TTE, transthoracic echocardiography) and 50 transesophageal (TEE) studies and pass a challenging high stakes board style examination. This initial training project yielded a group of expert level faculty, so that most teaching ICU faculty achieved the capability of training others in advanced CCE. As a next step, the requirements for training in advanced CCE were modified to reduce the number of TTE and TEE studies required (100 TTE and 25 TEE performed/25 TEE observed) with the total duration of study reduced to 1 year. This allowed both fellows and attendings to be trained by the initial group of core faculty to advanced level. As a final part of the national training program, the critical care faculty with advanced level training in CCE are now tasked with providing all critical care medicine fellows with training in basic CCE. The French approach holds that only some intensivist need be trained in advanced CCE, while all intensivists should be trained to basic level. It is likely that in coming years, all parts of CCUS will become a mandatory element of fellowship training in France. The success of the French approach to training in CCE reflects some unique features of how ICU services are organized in France, and may be difficult to duplicate in other countries that do not have the same level of centralized control over training of critical care fellows.

There are approximately 950 critical care fellows per year in the United States. The majority are enrolled in 3-year pulmonary/critical care programs, while a smaller proportion are in a surgical, anesthesiology, emergency medicine, or a straight critical care training track. Fellows are in an excellent position to obtain training in ultrasonography. A major problem is that many fellowship training programs lack faculty who have competence in the field, so that the fellows, though interested, have no one to train them. There are a number of fellowship programs that do have training faculty, but many do not. For example, in New York City, most fellowship programs have ultrasound capable faculty; in nearby cities, this is not the case. There is a well-developed ultrasound training faculty in critical care fellowship programs in Cleveland, Ohio and in Albuquerque, New Mexico. At the same time, many other programs are not able to provide faculty to train their fellows. This patchwork of training will likely improve in the next few years. The ACGME has mandated that training in certain aspects of CCUS must be included in fellowship training, and all components will be required in the foreseeable future. If this happens, fellowship programs will have to provide training or lose their accreditation, as the ACGME establishes national standards for training. More fellows are graduating with the skills to perform general CCUS. This junior group will be the faculty that trains the next generation of intensivists. The ACGME requirements will have the effect of increasing the number of ultrasound faculty so that in a few years, fellowship training in ultrasonography will be a routine component of the post graduate training programs.

The New York City experience is a case in point. In 2003, only a few critical care fellowship programs in the city were able to provide training in ultrasonography. In 2013, practically all fellowship training programs are doing so. The reason for this is that a few programs started to graduate fellows who were competent. Many of this original group took positions at nearby training programs and started to introduce ultrasonography training to the fellows in their new hospitals. This core group of faculty initiated a yearly 3-day training course for entry-level fellows that included training in image acquisition, image interpretation, and cognitive elements of the field. The fellows are removed from clinical responsibilities for the duration of the course. Faculty come with their fellows to the course, and are tasked with continuing their training in the hospital environment. Enrollment at the course has been consistent at 84 fellows per year, and interest in this cooperative training effort remains high from the fellowship programs in the City. Many of the current course faculty took the course when they were fellows. This is an example of a low-cost training system that could be adapted to local training needs.

There are approximately 6000 frontline attending level intensivists in the United States who require training in general CCUS. They face challenges in accessing adequate training. Heavy work schedules, economic pressures, and family responsibilities combine to make it difficult to commit the time required for training. Despite this, many attendings are committed to achieving competence as evidenced by the continued high attendance rates at large national courses in CCUS that are given by the ACCP and the SCCM. Over 2500 attending intensivists have taken the introductory course on CCUS given by ACCP, and there is no reduction in enrollment. The most common pathway that this author has observed is that the interested critical care clinician will take an introductory course, and then engage in self-directed learning in their own practice environment, often in cooperation with other motivated intensivists and with the support of their radiology and cardiology colleagues. This auto-didactic approach can be effective if the learner is motivated and organized in accessing cognitive material, has access to an adequate image library, and is helped by a friendly colleague to develop their scanning skills.

Unfortunately, some attendings work in an adverse training environment. This group has difficulty in achieving competence using a self-directed learning approach. The ACCP has developed a program that is designed to meet the needs of the attending that comes from an adverse training environment and for attending who seeks an effective and efficient means of obtaining competence. The certificate of completion includes a total of 7 days of course work that emphasizes hands on skills with image interpretation, a 20 hours internet based training sequence, a mandatory image portfolio collection that is reviewed by faculty, and an examination with a hands on image acquisition component.

Australia has a well-developed national level training program for certification in advanced CCE that includes a board type examination. In its present iteration, the number of studies required is considerably more than that required by the French system or by cardiology authorities in the United States. This reflects the Australian tradition of excellence in critical care training.

At present, this author is not aware of ongoing training programs designed to provide intensivists with competence in CCUS in China or Southeast Asia with the exception of Hong Kong, where the Health Authority is actively involved with introducing CCUS into their well-organized ICU system and critical care training programs. In India, the first national level course on CCUS took place at the All India Institute of Medical Science in New Delhi in 2012 and there is likely to be increasing training activity in India and in the Asia Pacific region in coming years.

CONCLUSION

Training in CCUS requires a mastery of image acquisition, image interpretation, and the cognitive elements of the field. The Competence Statement establishes specific learning objectives for training in CCUS, while the Training Statement offers recommendations that are helpful in the design of a program of study. Review of the various international approaches to training in CCUS is useful in developing local solutions to the challenge of training a new generation of intensivists in this important skill.

REFERENCES

1. Mayo PH, Beaulieu Y, Doelken P, et al. American College of Chest Physicians/La Société de Réanimation de Langue Française Statement on Competence in Critical Care Ultrasonography. *Chest.* 2009;135:1050–1060.
2. Volpicelli G, Elbarbary M, Blaivas M, et al. International liaison committee on lung ultrasound (ILC-LUS) for international consensus conference on lung ultrasound (ICC-LUS). *Crit Care Med: Focus Appl Ultrasound Crit Care Med.* 2007;35:S123–S307.
3. Volpicelli G, Elbarbary M, Blaivas M, et al. International evidence-based recommendations for point-of-care lung ultrasound. *Intensive Care Med.* 2012;38:577–591.
4. Labovitz AJ, Noble VE, Bierig M, et al. Focused cardiac ultrasound in the emergent setting: a consensus statement of the American Society of Echocardiography and American College of Emergency Physicians. *J Am Soc Echocardiogr.* 2010;23(12):1225–1230.
5. Cholley BP. International expert statement on training standards for critical care ultrasonography. *Intensive Care Med.* 2011;37:1077–1083.
6. Chalumeau-Lemoine L, Baudel JL, Das V, et al. Results of short-term training of naïve physicians in focused general ultrasonography in an intensive-care unit. *Intensive Care Med.* 2009;35:1767–1771.
7. Vignon P, Mücke F, Bellec F, et al. Basic critical care echocardiography: validation of a curriculum dedicated to noncardiologist residents. *Crit Care Med.* 2011;39:636–642.
8. Charron C, Vignon P, Prat G, et al. Number of supervised studies required to reach competence in advanced critical care transesophageal echocardiography. *Intensive Care Med.* 2013;39:1019–1024.

PEDIATRIC CRITICAL CARE: THE USE OF BEDSIDE ULTRASONOGRAPHY

WILLIAM TSAI, SHILPA AMARA, & ANTHONY D. SLONIM

Scan QR code or visit www.ccu2e.com for video in this chapter

INTRODUCTION

The pediatric intensive care unit (PICU), like other intensive care units (ICU), is a dynamic place that provides multidisciplinary care with the integration of numerous medical and surgical subspecialists who come together with a common goal—the care of a critically ill child. Predictably, the diseases span the spectrum of adult ICU care and range from acute illnesses such as septic shock and sepsis-related cardiomyopathy to hemorrhagic shock with traumatic visceral rupture. While the problems are similar to those encountered in adult ICUs, three additional layers of complexity are important to understand when caring for a critically ill child, namely age, size, and developmental status; all of these have relevance for critical care ultrasonography. First, many differential diagnoses encountered in the PICU are age dependent, which is important for the ultrasonographer to remember when performing ultrasound for diagnostic purposes on a child. Second, a child's size may range from <2 to >200 kg, which has important implications for the technical aspects of ultrasound procedures. Finally, children may not be able to cooperate with an examination or procedure like adults can, making the use of ultrasonography, a pain-free and noninvasive tool, an ideal method for extending one's physical examination. Bedside ultrasound is an important and evolving tool for pediatric intensivists and can be used to evaluate many disease processes, assist in procedural interventions, and assess for complications related to those procedures. While ultrasound technology has long been available, recent advancements have improved image quality and capabilities and have reduced equipment bulk, making point-of-care use in critical care areas considerably more feasible.[1] This chapter aims to provide a practical discussion on the use of bedside ultrasonography in the PICU.

DEVICES

Ultrasound use in the PICU ranges from being an aid for vascular access to being a versatile instrument that is able to perform an acute, comprehensive assessment of the critically ill child at the bedside and monitor response to critical treatment. Common indications for bedside ultrasound in the PICU are listed in Table 5-1.

Similarly, equipment also ranges from simple ultrasound with the use of a linear probe for vascular access to an instrument with multiple probes that can be manipulated and enhanced to provide the best visualization of cardiac, abdominal, vascular, and thoracic structures (see Chapter 3). Pediatric-sized probes are also available. Small hockey stick style linear probes have a small footprint and are able to provide excellent images in less accessible areas of the body such as the neck or axillae; small-phased array probes are also available for focused echocardiography but are infrequently necessary.

In some PICUs, a portable notebook-type ultrasound system is placed on a mobile cart with a curvilinear abdominal probe, a linear high frequency probe, and a low-frequency cardiac probe. These probes can be manipulated in terms of frequency, depth of ultrasound beam, and use of Doppler technology, but many systems have a very short power-on-to-scan-time and require very little manipulation to provide good images. They are lightweight, easily maneuvered, and have a very small footprint. These systems receive regular use in vascular access, thoracic and abdominal ultrasonography and focused echocardiography.

VASCULAR ACCESS

The use of procedural ultrasound in vascular access, namely central venous catheter placement, is more efficient and safer than techniques using palpation and landmarks.[2]

TABLE 5-1
Indications for the Use of Ultrasound in the Pediatric Intensive Care Unit
Procedural
Vascular access
Thoracentesis
Paracentesis
Pericardiocentesis
Focused echocardiography
Pericardial tamponade
Ventricular function
Volume status
Thoracic ultrasound
Pneumothorax
Pleural effusion
Abdominal ultrasound
Ascites/hemoperitoneum
Intraabdominal injury/trauma
Novel uses
Skeletal fractures
Intracranial pressure monitoring

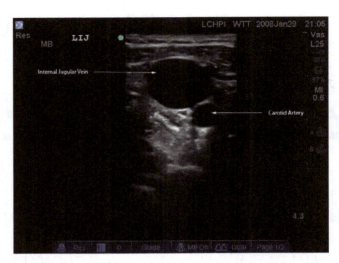

Figure 5-1 Left internal jugular vein with juxtaposed carotid artery.

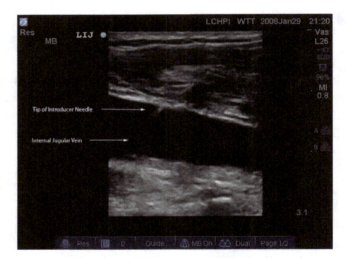

Figure 5-2 Internal jugular vein being accessed with an introducer needle.

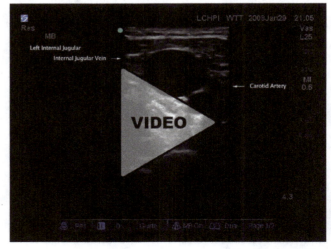

Video 5-1 Internal jugular–carotid artery relationships. View at www.ccu2e.com

Studies have demonstrated that the routine use of internal jugular central venous line (CVL) placement in children under ultrasound guidance improves speed and results in fewer attempts and fewer complications. Specifically, a study by Verghese et al.[3] investigating the use of ultrasound imaging to place internal jugular CVLs in infants prior to cardiac surgery found that imaging reduces the number of cannulation attempts, time to catherization, and number of carotid artery punctures, and improves the success rate for catheter placement. Similarly, a study by Alderson et al.,[4] which compared ultrasound-guided internal jugular cannulation with landmark techniques in infants, revealed that ultrasound assistance improves success rates and reduces time to cannulation. In addition, Maecken et al.[5] demonstrated that the inconsistent location and relationship between the internal jugular vein and carotid artery makes ultrasound guidance a useful tool.

Ultrasound guidance is beneficial in several ways. First, a survey of the vessels prior to deciding upon an access site is useful in children with vascular and anatomic abnormalities or those who have disease processes that predispose them to venous clotting or have undergone multiple cardiac catheterization procedures through access of the femoral vessels. Second, ultrasound helps confirm the position and relative position of the vein and its relationship to the artery and other anatomic structures (Figures 5-1, 5-2, and Video 5-1). Third, placement of the catheter using the landmark method or by palpating the artery can be imprecise, so ultrasound guidance may be used to improve specificity. Fourth, children, who tend to have smaller structures and more subcutaneous fat, frequently do not have reliable landmarks. Fifth, ultrasound can be used to confirm proper placement of the catheter (Figure 5-3). Finally, after difficult or repeated attempts to obtain vascular access, ultrasound can confirm whether a perivascular hematoma may

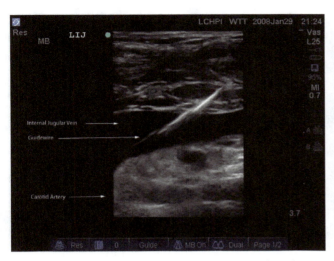

Figure 5-3 Internal jugular vein with an intraluminal guidewire.

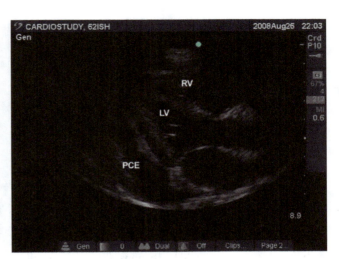

Figure 5-4 Pericardial effusion on echocardiogram. PCE = pericardial effusion; LV = left ventricle; RV = right ventricle. (From Longjohn M, Pershad J. Point-of-care echocardiography by pediatric emergency physicians. *Pediatr Emerg Care.* 2011;27:693.)

be impeding vessel cannulation (refer Chapter 27 for a step-by-step guide to the use of ultrasound in venous cannulation).

Video 5-2 shows a longitudinal image of an internal jugular vein with a guide wire in the lumen. Ultrasound-guided confirmation of vessel cannulation has been made prior to dilation of the vessel.

FOCUSED ECHOCARDIOGRAPHY

Focused or bedside echocardiography, combined with physical examination, has proven to improve clinical diagnosis and management of acutely ill patients. Point-of-care echocardiographic examination is typically geared towards answering a specific clinical question regarding the current state of hemodynamics and is generally shorter in duration than a traditional examination.[6] Data indicate that portable echocardiography performed by noncardiologists is largely accurate in diagnosing cardiac issues such as pericardial effusion (91%), left ventricular (LV) size (96%), and LV systolic function (96%).[7] Specifically, pericardial effusions appear as anechoic areas within the pericardial space (Figure 5-4), with right atrium and ventricle compression present in tamponade. Reduced LV function may be identified via observation of limited cardiac wall movement between diastole and systole.[8]

In the pediatric cardiac ICU, focused echocardiography aids in the diagnosis and management of pericardial effusion/tamponade, depressed cardiac function, hemodynamically significant pleural effusions, and aids in volume status assessment. It can also be performed quickly during the pulse check of advanced cardiac life support, to diagnose potential causes of cardiac arrest.[8] In addition, using more advanced techniques, right-sided heart failure can be rapidly evaluated with an assessment of right ventricular (RV) volume, tricuspid regurgitation, and paradoxical septal wall motion. These findings may be used to augment data from other hemodynamic measurements to confirm RV failure due to right ventriculotomy or pulmonary hypertension. Similar findings are seen in adult patients and older pediatric patients who have hemodynamically significant pulmonary embolism.

Transthoracic echocardiogram is the most widely used primary imaging technique for characterizing simple and complex structural cardiac defects,[9,10] and may be employed in a focused manner in the ICU. Importantly, it is noninvasive, universally available, and can provide detailed and quantifiable information on intracardiac morphology and function, valve gradients, pulmonary artery pressure, and chamber hypertrophy and enlargement at the bedside of the critically ill patient.[9,11] While transesophageal echocardiography may need to be used as an alternative in patients with poorer transthoracic windows, this is usually not an issue among pediatric patients.[9]

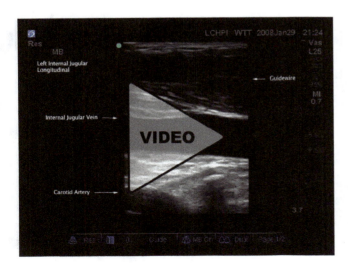

Video 5-2 Longitudinal internal-jugular with guidewire in vessel. View at www.ccu2e.com

TABLE 5-2
Focused Echocardiography

Cardiac function assessment
Left ventricular enlargement
Pericardial effusion
Inferior vena cava dynamics

The need to assess cardiac function may be underestimated in the general PICU.[12] The use of focused echocardiography may be useful in guiding patient management in undifferentiated, fluid-resistant hypotension. It allows the rapid assessment of global cardiac function, LV chamber dimensions, volume status, and identifies hemodynamically significant pericardial effusions (Table 5-2), all of which may influence management. Spurney et al.[7] demonstrated that with limited training and limited echocardiographic views (Figures 5-5 and 5-6), PICU physicians are capable of diagnosing significant pericardial effusions, decreased LV systolic function, and LV enlargement. Milner et al.[13] showed that children with altered mental status and tachycardia may be diagnosed with pericardial effusion and tamponade by cardiologist-performed bedside echocardiography, resulting in earlier diagnosis and improved outcomes. Focused bedside echocardiography also enables clinicians to perform serial bedside examinations and allows for important assessment and reassessment of the adequacy and efficacy of therapy (Videos 5-3 and 5-4).

The assessment of volume status in the PICU is extremely important, but assessments using physical examination may be inaccurate, particularly in the edematous child. Echocardiography has been validated for LV volume measurements, and assessment of LV end diastolic volume (LVEDV) on the parasternal short and long axes may guide volume management.[14] For example, an LV chamber with complete collapse or obliteration of the LV cavity guides

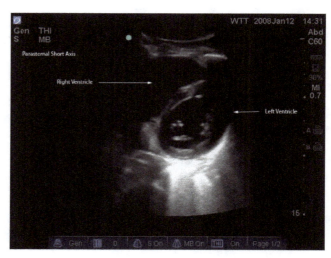

Figure 5-6 Parasternal short axis view of the heart during focused echocardiography.

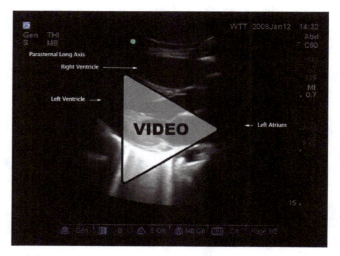

Video 5-3 Parasternal long-axis focused echocardiography. View at www.ccu2e.com

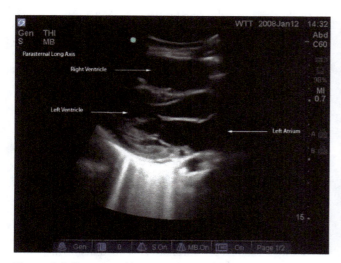

Figure 5-5 Parasternal long axis view of the heart during focused echocardiography.

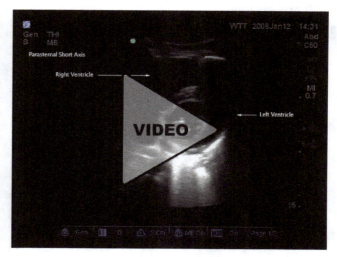

Video 5-4 Parasternal short-axis focused echocardiography. View at www.ccu2e.com

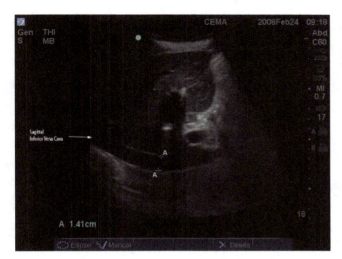

Figure 5-7 Assessment of IVC diameter.

management in a way that is markedly different than in a patient with a LV cavity that is clearly dilated and poorly functioning.

The assessment of inferior vena cava (IVC) diameter and its collapse during inspiration may also be used to assess volume status. This method has been validated in adults to differentiate right atrial (RA) pressures <10 mmHg or >10 mmHg.[15] IVC dilation without a normal reduction in caliber during inspiration usually indicates elevated RA pressures.[16] IVC measurements during mechanical ventilation are less reliable because of the IVC dilation that is normally seen while on the ventilator. However, a small diameter, or collapsed IVC will reliably exclude elevated RA pressures (Figure 5-7).[17,18] However, much of the research done on IVC dynamics has been performed on adult patients. More investigation into pediatric patients must be performed before widespread use of this technique can be validated with empirical evidence.

THORACIC ULTRASOUND

While it may seem that ultrasound of the chest would be of limited utility since air is a poor medium for conducting ultrasound waves, lung ultrasound is quite useful in the PICU for evaluating pneumothorax, pleural effusions, lung consolidation, and neonatal respiratory distress syndrome (RDS); specific sonographic signs for each of these conditions are outlined in Table 5-3.[19] Airway ultrasound may also be used to assist with endotracheal intubation.

▶ Pleural Effusion

Pleural effusion is frequently seen in critically ill patients, necessitating diagnosis and drainage for therapeutic purposes. Point-of-care diagnostic evaluation is useful in the ICU setting because it provides a rapid assessment of the size, quality, and location of the effusions, which appear as hypoechoic and homogenous structures present during

TABLE 5-3
Sonographic Signs on Lung Ultrasound
Pneumothorax
Presence of lung point(s)
Absence of lung sliding
Absence of B-lines
Absence of lung pulse
Pleural effusion
Space (usually anechoic) between parietal and visceral pleura
Respiratory movement of lung within the effusion (sinusoid sign)
Lung consolidation
Subpleural echo-poor region or one with tissue-like echotexture
Lung consolidation
Signs that vary by etiology and can help determine cause
Quality of deep margins of consolidation
Comet-tail reverberation artifacts
Presence of air bronchogram(s)
Presence of fluid bronchogram(s)
Vascular pattern within consolidation
Neonatal respiratory distress syndrome
Pleural line abnormalities
Absence of spared areas
Bilateral confluent B-lines

Source: From Volpicelli G, Elbarbary M, Blaivas M, et al. International evidence-based recommendations for point-of-care lung ultrasound. *Intensive Care Med.* 2012;38:577.

expiration and inspiration (Figures 5-8, 5-9, and Video 5-5). On dynamic video, the lung can be seen swinging into view with each ventilator breath (Video 5-6). Measurement of the intrapleural distance (i.e., distance between the lung and the posterior chest wall) can quantify the volume of the effusion, while ultrasound patterns can help assess the nature of the effusion; specifically, transudates are always anechoic, while exudates are often echoic and loculated.[20]

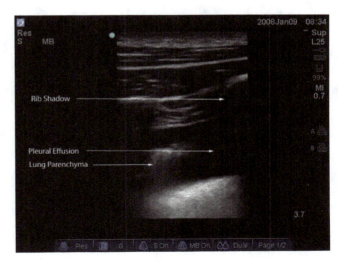

Figure 5-8 Simple pleural effusion.

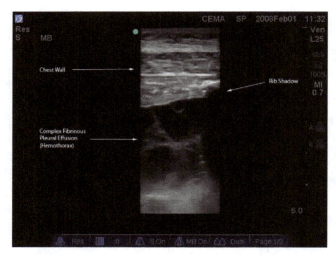

Figure 5-9 Complex pleural effusion.

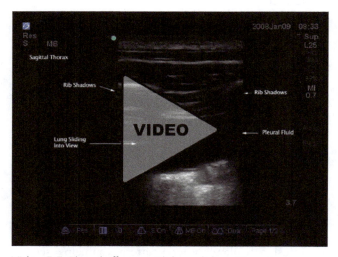

Video 5-5 Pleural effusion with lung sliding. View at www.ccu2e.com

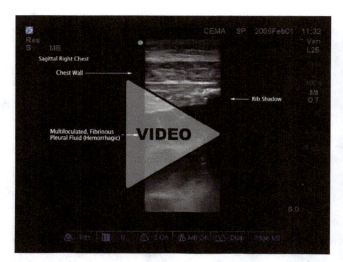

Video 5-6 Characteristics of a complex pleural effusion. View at www.ccu2e.com

Additionally, ultrasound-assisted drainage (i.e., thoracentesis) may be emergent and life saving in patients who are predisposed to hemodynamically significant pleural effusions (e.g., those with Fontan physiology). Studies in adults indicate that the routine use of ultrasound during thoracentesis significantly reduces complications such as pneumothorax and tube thoracostomy. While pediatric data are lacking, reason suggests that ultrasound-guided thoracentesis may be just as valuable, if not more so, due to smaller thorax sizes in children.[1]

▶ **Pneumothorax**

The assessment of pneumothorax can be extremely useful in those patients with a thoracic air leak. In healthy individuals, pleural sliding or shimmering (Figure 5-10) occurs on thoracic ultrasound when the visceral and parietal pleura are apposed to one another and slide past each other due to movements of the diaphragm or with mechanical ventilation. Dynamic images of pleural sliding are quite striking and its presence denotes the mobile apposition of the visceral pleura with the parietal pleura (Video 5-7). When lung sliding is eliminated, the beam cannot be transmitted through the injured parenchyma and only longitudinal reverberations of motionless pleural lines (i.e., A-lines) are seen on ultrasound (Figure 5-10).[20] Lack of sliding (Video 5-8) may suggest pneumothorax, although the clinician should still proceed through the differential diagnosis for lack of lung sliding (Table 5-4). Once pneumothorax has been confirmed, the transducer can be moved over the hemithorax to determine if loculation is present and to assess the extent of the pneumothorax (Figure 5-11). Thoracic ultrasound can help determine the best and safest place to insert a chest tube or pigtail drain.

Importantly, several studies have shown that bedside lung ultrasound is more efficient than chest radiography for diagnosing pneumothorax in emergency conditions. Indeed, one study conducted in trauma patients revealed

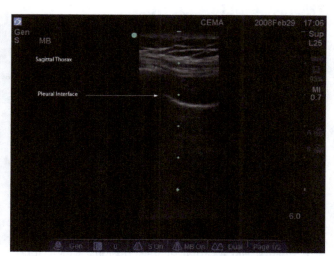

Figure 5-10 Pleural sliding.

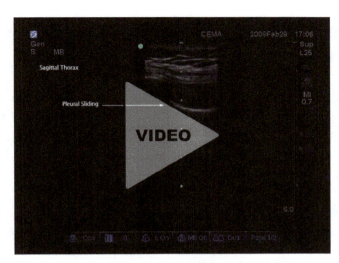

Video 5-7 Demonstration of pleural sliding. View at www.ccu2e.com

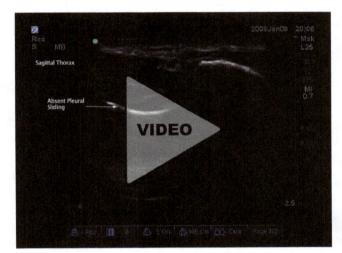

Video 5-8 Absent pleural sliding. View at www.ccu2e.com

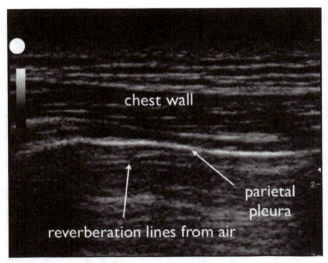

Figure 5-11 Pneumothorax. (From Pneumothorax by U/S. Sonographers Blog. http://wwwsonographersblog.blogspot.com/2010/01/pneumothorax-by-us.html. Accessed June 24, 2013.)

TABLE 5-4
Differential Diagnosis for Absence of Pleural Sliding
Pneumothorax
Pleural effusion
Pleural scarring
Poor respiratory effort
Mainstem intubation
Mainstem occlusion

a sensitivity and specificity of 86% and 97%, respectively, for lung ultrasound, versus 28% and 100%, respectively, for conventional chest radiography.[20]

▶ Lung Consolidation

Pulmonary edema, bacterial pneumonia, and pulmonary contusion (which is often identified in pediatric blunt chest trauma patients) all diminish lung aeration, thereby enabling ultrasounds to be transmitted towards the depth of the thorax. Lung consolidation presents as a poorly defined, wedge-shaped, hypoechoic structure, within which hyperechoic punctiform images representing air-filled bronchi may be observed (Figure 5-12). Among patients with bacterial pneumonia, preliminary data suggest that lung ultrasound may also be used to quantitatively assess pulmonary re-aeration following receipt of antimicrobial therapy.[20]

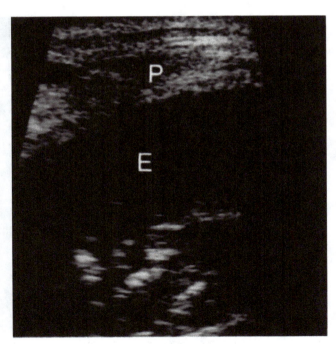

Figure 5-12 Lung consolidation with air-filled bronchi. P = posterior; E = effusion. (From Weinberg B, Diakoumakis EE, Kass EG, et al. The air bronchogram: sonographic demonstration. *AJR.* 147:593, 1986.)

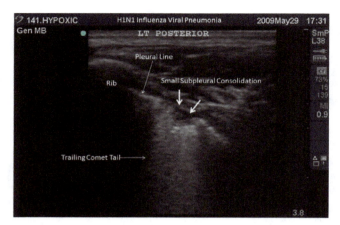

Figure 5-13 Viral pneumonia. (From Tsung JW, Kessler DO, Shah VP. Prospective application of clinician-performed lung ultrasonography during the 2009 H1N1 influenza A pandemic: distinguishing viral from bacterial pneumonia. *Crit Ultrasound J.* 2012;4:16.)

Unlike bacterial pneumonia, viral pneumonia and bronchiolitis typically present as small (less than 0.5 cm) subpleural consolidations on ultrasound, with echogenic vertical lines arising from the pleural line and spreading to the bottom of the ultrasound screen (Figure 5-13). Often referred to as B-lines or "comet-tail" artifacts, these lines have proven useful in distinguishing between bacterial and viral disease etiology.[21]

▶ Neonatal Respiratory Distress Syndrome

Lung ultrasound may also play a role in the diagnosis of neonatal RDS, a condition that occurs in premature infants with inadequate surfactant production and structural immaturity of the lungs. Neonatal RDS typically manifests as tachypnea, tachycardia, chest wall retractions, expiratory grunting, and cyanosis during breathing attempts. If left untreated, this condition may result in serious complications and death. Copetti et al.[22] found that neonatal RDS has a consistent appearance on ultrasound, which shows generalized alveolar-interstitial syndrome (vertical B-lines, or, in severe cases, echographic "white lung"), pleural line abnormalities (i.e., subpleural consolidations, thickening, irregularities, and coarse appearance), and an absence of areas with a normal pattern (i.e., spared areas). Investigators concluded that taken together, these ultrasonographic signs can distinguish neonatal RDS with a sensitivity and specificity of 100%.

▶ Airway Ultrasound

Finally, the use of ultrasound for verifying endotracheal tube position is still early in its evolution, but Galicinao et al.[23] reported a high success rate in confirming endotracheal intubation in children in the pediatric emergency department and PICU settings. In addition, investigators demonstrated specific instances where ultrasound was superior to CO_2 detection for determining tube placement. However, more research in this arena is necessary before it gains widespread use.

ABDOMINAL ULTRASOUND

Blunt abdominal trauma is another important indication for bedside ultrasound. Focused assessment with sonography in trauma (FAST) examination is a validated technique that aims to identify pathologic free fluid (usually blood) released from injured organs. Most research has been conducted in patients with abdominal injury and intraperitoneal fluid accumulation, but the FAST examination can also detect free fluid in the pleural and pericardial spaces. Specifically, free fluid of the hemoperitoneum or hemopericardium will appear anechoic against the more hyperechoic background of the solid organs (Figure 5-14). While abdominal computed tomography is the study of choice for stable patients with suspected traumatic abdominal organ injury, this method requires interpretation by specialists and subjects patients to ionizing radiation; it also requires patient transport to the radiology suite, which may not be possible in hemodynamically unstable patients. Conversely, the FAST scan can be performed at bedside by the treating clinician. Additionally, because radiation exposure is not a concern, the study may be repeated as necessary to evaluate progressing conditions, particularly after transfer from the Emergency Department to the PICU.[24]

It is important to note that FAST scanning in children is more challenging than in adults because children have a relatively higher incidence of solid organ injury without free fluid; as such, a negative FAST scan may not necessarily rule out organ injury. Indeed, although highly specific, reported FAST scan sensitivities in the pediatric population have ranged from 40% to 93%. Thus, this technique should always be used in conjunction with a thorough clinical history and physical examination.[24]

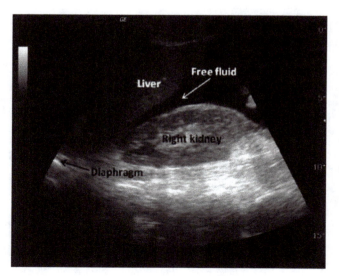

Figure 5-14 Abdominal FAST scan. (From Smith ZA, Postma N, Wood D. FAST scanning in the developing world emergency department. *SAMJ.* 2010;100:105.)

TABLE 5-5
Procedural Ultrasound
Vascular access
Central line placement
PICC line placement
Arterial line placement
Pericardiocentesis
Paracentesis
Thoracentesis
Airway intubation

PROCEDURAL ULTRASOUND

Interventional ultrasound may be used to guide simple invasive procedures, improving patient safety and reducing time to complete the procedure. Table 5-5 outlines specific critical care procedures where ultrasound guidance is useful. It is often used to assist with fluid drainage from spaces such as the pericardium (pericardiocentesis), pleural space (thoracentesis), joints (arthrocentesis), and peritoneum (paracentesis),[25] where it can identify optimal needle insertion point and depth (Figure 5-15). A study by Nazeer et al.[26] comparing traditional versus ultrasound-assisted paracentesis found that ultrasound guidance significantly improves procedure success rates. As mentioned earlier, bedside ultrasound can also be used to localize veins and guide central line placement in patients in whom cannulation may be difficult to perform.[25] Bedside ultrasound can also play an important role in airway imaging, such as that used for tracheal intubation. While a chest radiograph is the gold standard for confirming endotracheal tube position, it is often delayed and requires more handling than ultrasound. Studies have demonstrated good correlation between ultrasound and radiograph measurements when verifying tube positioning in newborns, and rapid confirmation via point-of-care ultrasound can prevent adverse outcomes such as hypoxemia, pneumothorax, lung collapse, and death.[27] Correct placement of the endotracheal tube in the trachea typically produces a dense hyperechoic shadowing, or 'comet-tail' appearance on ultrasound (Figure 5-16).

While critical care procedures have traditionally been performed without adjunctive measures, the use of ultrasound considerably enhances efficiency and safety. Not only does ultrasound identify the optimal access points, but it also demonstrates the anatomical relationships of internal structures and organs. While perhaps not as useful in patients with normal anatomy, it can be extremely useful in patients with abnormal anatomy or abnormal structural relationships. For example, in patients with hepatomegaly secondary to increased abdominal pressures, the insertion of a right-sided chest tube for an effusion or pneumothorax may come perilously close to the liver if the liver is encroaching into the chest. Abdominal ultrasound can help to identify the quantity and quality of ascitic fluid before attempting drainage. Figure 5-17 and Video 5-9 provide images of hemorrhagic ascites in a patient on extracorporeal membrane oxygenation (ECMO) who spontaneously bled into the peritoneum.

NOVEL USES

Finally, bedside ultrasound may be useful in patients with head trauma, as increased optic nerve sheath diameter, as measured by ultrasound, may be correlated with increased intracranial pressure (ICP). Indeed, ICP monitoring is a central component of critical care management for patients with severe brain injury. Point-of-care ultrasound provides a valuable and noninvasive assessment tool,

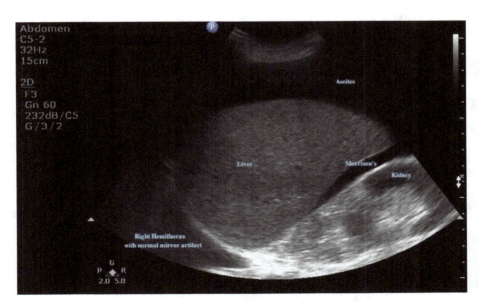

Figure 5-15 Ultrasound-guided paracentesis. (From Ultrasound guided paracenteses. Emory University School of Medicine. http://www.em.emory.edu/ultrasound/ImageWeek/paracentesis.html. Accessed June 24, 2013.)

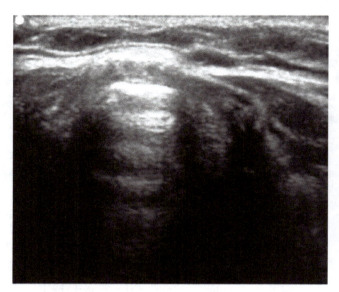

Figure 5-16 Correctly positioned endotracheal tube. (From Kajekar P, Mendonca C, Gaur V. Role of ultrasound in airway assessment and management. *Int J Ultrasound Appl Technol Perioper Care.* 2010;1:97.)

particularly among the pediatric population, where symptoms of elevated ICP may be nonspecific or indiscernible.[1]

CONCLUSION

Bedside ultrasound is an important and evolving tool for pediatric intensivists and can be used to evaluate many disease processes, assist in procedural interventions, and assess for complications related to those procedures. However, there are many artificial barriers to using bedside ultrasound in critically ill children. Such barriers include resistance from radiologic services, cardiologist opposition to limited focused emergency echocardiography, intensivist hesitancy to introduce ultrasound use when it was not required in the past, and difficulties associated with billing and liability; nonetheless, the use of ultrasound can enhance practice in the PICU and care for critically ill children in other settings as an extension of the physical examination.

Without proper training and expertise, however, the use of bedside ultrasonography may be misleading and may result in diagnostic and procedural errors. Thus, it is important that critical care practitioners gain experience in pediatric bedside ultrasonography.

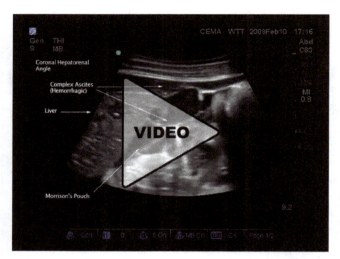

Video 5-9 Hemorrhagic ascites in an ECMO patient. View at www.ccu2e.com

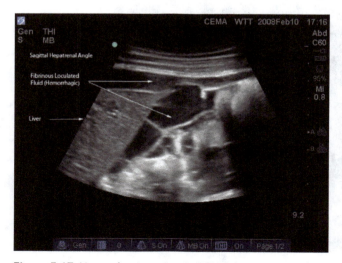

Figure 5-17 Hemorrhagic ascites in ECMO (extracorporeal membrane oxygenation) patient.

REFERENCES

1. Srinivasan S, Cornell TT. Bedside ultrasound in pediatric critical care: a review. *Pediatr Crit Care Med.* 2011;12:667.
2. Hind D, Calvert N, McWilliams A, et al. Ultrasonic devices for central venous cannulation; meta-analysis. *BMJ.* 2003;327:361.
3. Verghese ST, McGill WA, Patel RI, Sell JE, Midgley FM, Ruttimann UE. Ultrasound-guided internal jugular venous cannulation in infants: a prospective comparison with the traditional palpation method. *Anesthesiology.* 1999;91:71.
4. Alderson PJ, Burrows FA, Stemp LI, Holtby HM. Use of ultrasound to evaluate internal jugular vein anatomy and to facilitate central venous cannulation in paediatric patients. *Brit J Anaesth.* 1993;70:145.
5. Maecken T, Grau T. Ultrasound imaging in vascular access. *Crit Care Med.* 2007;35:S17.
6. Beaulieu Y. Specific skill set and goals of focused echocardiography for critical care clinicians. *Crit Care Med.* 2007;35:S144.
7. Spurney CF, Sable CA, Berger JT, et al. Use of hand-carried ultrasound device by critical care physicians for the diagnosis of pericardial effusions, decreased cardiac function, and left ventricular enlargement in pediatric patients. *J Am Soc Echocardiogr.* 2005;18:313.
8. Longjohn M, Pershad J. Point-of-care echocardiography by pediatric emergency physicians. *Pediatr Emerg Care.* 2011;27:693.
9. Stumper O. Imaging the heart in adult congenital heart disease. *BMJ Heart.* 1998;80:535.

10. Rice MJ, Sahn DJ. Transesophageal echocardiography for congenital heart disease: who, what, and when. *Mayo Clin Proc.* 1995;70:401.
11. Foster E. Congenital Heart Disease in Adults. *West J Med.* 1995;163:492.
12. Ceneviva G, Paschall JA, Maffei F, et al. Hemodynamic support in fluid-refractory pediatric septic shock. *Pediatrics.* 1998;102:e19.
13. Milner D, Losek JD, Schiff J, et al. Pediatric pericardial tamponade presenting as altered mental status. *Pediatr Emerg Care.* 2003;19:35.
14. Schiller NB, Shah PM, Crawford M, et al. Recommendations for quantitation of the left ventricle by two-dimensional echocardiography. American Society of Echocardiography Committee on Standards, Subcommittee on Quantitation of Two-Dimensional Echocardiograms. *J Am Soc Echocardiogr.* 1989;2:358.
15. Kircher BJ, Himelman RB, Schiller NB. Noninvasive estimation of right atrial pressure form the inspiratory collapse of the inferior vena cava. *Am J Cardiol.* 1990;66:493.
16. Feissel M, Michard F, Faller JP, et al. the respiratory variation in inferior vena cava diameter as a guide to fluid therapy. *Intensive Care Med.* 2004;30:1834.
17. Vieillar-Baron A, Chergui K, Rabiller A, et al. Superior vena caval collapsibility as a gauge of volume status in ventilated septic patients. *Intensive Care Med.* 2004;30:1734.
18. Barbier C, Loubieres Y, Schmit C, et al. Respiratory changes in inferior vena cava diameter are helpful in predicting fluid responsiveness in ventilated septic patients. *Intensive Care Med.* 2004;30:1740.
19. Volpicelli G, Elbarbary M, Blaivas M, et al. International evidence-based recommendations for point-of-care lung ultrasound. *Intensive Care Med.* 2012;38:577.
20. Bouhemad B, Zhang M, Lu Q, et al. Clinical review: bedside lung ultrasound in critical care practice. *Crit Care.* 2007;11:205.
21. Tsung JW, Kessler DO, Shah VP. Prospective application of clinician-performed lung ultrasonography during the 2009 H1N1 influenza A pandemic: distinguishing viral from bacterial pneumonia. *Crit Ultrasound J.* 2012;4:16.
22. Copetti R, Cattarossi L, Macagno F, et al. Lung ultrasound in respiratory distress syndrome: a useful tool for early diagnosis. *Neonatology.* 2008;94:52.
23. Galicinao J, Bush AJ, Godambe SA. Use of Bedside Ultrasonography for Endotracheal Tube Placement in Pediatric Patients: A Feasibility Study. *Pediatrics.* 2007;120:1297.
24. Levy JA, Noble VE. Bedside ultrasound in pediatric emergency medicine. *Pediatrics.* 2008;121:e1404.
25. Arienti V, Camaggi V. Clinical applications of bedside ultrasonography in internal and emergency medicine. *Inetrn Emerg Med.* 2011;6:195.
26. Nazeer SR, Dewbre H, Miller AH. Ultrasound-assisted paracentesis performed by emergency physicians vs the traditional technique: a prospective, randomized study. *Am J Emerg Med.* 2005;23:363.
27. Schmolzer GM, O'Reilly M, Davis PG, et al. Confirmation of correct tracheal tube placement in newborn infants. *Resuscitation.* 2013;84:731.

SECTION II

Cardiac Sonography in the ICU

GOAL-DIRECTED ECHOCARDIOGRAPHY IN THE ICU

SETH KOENIG, MANGALA NARASIMHAN, & PAUL H. MAYO

Scan QR code or visit www.ccu2e.com for video in this chapter

INTRODUCTION

This chapter reviews an important component of critical care ultrasonography (CCUS), which is basic critical care echocardiography (CCE). For purpose of the discussion, the term goal-directed echocardiography (GDE) and basic CCE are used interchangeably. They refer to a limited cardiac ultrasonography examination performed by the intensivist at bedside of the patient with hemodynamic failure in order to establish diagnosis and guide management of the shock state. The examination differs from cardiology-type echocardiography in the intensivist all aspects of the examination. Image acquisition, image interpretation, and application of the results are performed by the bedside clinician who is charge of the case. There is no delay in performance or interpretation of the study, nor is there any problem with clinical disassociation that occurs when the ultrasonographer is not directly involved with management of the case. GDE may be repeated as often as required by the clinical situation in order to track the evolution of disease and response to therapy.

THE GDE EXAMINATION

The ACCP/SRLF Statement of competence in CCUS defines GDE with transthoracic echocardiography (TTE) as constituting five views:[1] the parasternal long- and short-axis views, the apical four-chamber view, the subcostal long-axis four-chamber view, and the inferior vena cava (IVC) longitudinal view (Case 6-1). Color Doppler may be utilized in order to screen for significant valve dysfunction. The technique of obtaining these key views is reviewed in the chapter on TTE (Chapter 6). It may be difficult to obtain all five views in the critically ill patient, and so it is important to attempt all five in every patient. For example, patients on ventilatory support who are hyperinflated due to PEEP effect or obstructive airway disease may have inadequate parasternal and apical four-chamber views, and yet have a good quality subcostal view. If the IVC is not visible through an anterior sagittal approach, the examiner may need to scan from a lateral approach. A key aspect of GDE is its simplicity. The examination takes a only few minutes to perform, so that the intensivist may perform a rapid evaluation of shock state and immediately integrate the results into other key elements clinical evaluation: the history, the physical examination, and the laboratory analysis. There is no alternative method of assessing cardiac anatomy and function in the intensive care unit (ICU), given clinical reality of the ICU. For the frontline intensivist, mastery of GDE is an essential skill for the evaluation of the patient in shock.

The GDE examination may also be performed with transesophageal echocardiography (TEE). A typical set of images may be obtained from the midesophageal four-chamber view at 0°, the midesophageal three-chamber view at 120°, and the transgastric short-axis view at 0°. The superior vena cava view is preferred over the IVC view with TEE due to ease of use and its value at determination of preload sensitivity. The technique of obtaining these key views is reviewed in the chapter on TTE (Chapter 7). Though it is counter intuitive, skill at GDE using TEE may be easier to achieve compared to TTE; as the transducer movement is restricted to the esophagus, and the image planes are stereotypical. The image set that defines GDE with TEE not as fully established as that for TTE and several variations have been described, the latest of which can be performed with a miniaturized TEE probe that can be left in place for up to 72 h, allowing for repeated limited examinations. With this device, the GDE examination includes the SVC short-axis view, the midesophageal four-chamber view, and the transgastric view.

> **CASE 6-1**
> **Hypotension and Urosepsis**
>
> Goal-directed echocardiography (GDE) was performed on a patient who presented with hypotension and urosepsis. By definition, GDE must include the parasternal long-axis view, the parasternal short-axis view, the apical four-chamber view, subcostal long-axis view, and the inferior vena cava view. Videos 6-1A through E show a normal GDE. Based on these results, the critical care team categorized the shock state as distributive without evidence of obstructive, cardiogenic, or hypovolemic shock. Phenylephrine was the primary pressor agent given for vasoplegia of sepsis. As the IVC was greater than 2.5 cm in diameter without much respiratory variation, no further volume resuscitation was indicated. A follow-up GDE was performed which is shown in Case 6-7. The heart is not completely visualized on the subcostal view due to shadowing from bowel gas. There is a possible echogenic structure adjacent to the right atrial free wall on the apical four-chamber view that is not visible in other views. This would warrant referral for an advanced echocardiography examination.
>
> Video is available at www.ccu2e.com

TABLE 6-1
Competence in Basic CCE

Echocardiography: Required Cognitive Skills in Image Interpretation
Echocardiographic patterns
Global LV size and systolic function
Homogeneous/heterogeneous LV contraction pattern
Global RV size and systolic function
Assessment for pericardial fluid/tamponade
IVC size and respiratory variation
Basic color Doppler assessment for severe valvular regurgitation

LV, left ventricle; RV, right ventricle; IVC, inferior vena cava.

Source: Mayo PH, Beaulieu Y, Doelken P, et al. American College of Chest Physicians/La Société de Réanimation de Langue Française Statement on Competence in Critical Care Ultrasonography. Chest. 2009; 135(4):1050–1060.

The use of TEE for GDE is not a mandatory component of competence in of CCE for the reason that the technology is not yet widely available in many ICUs;[2] so that in North America and in many European countries, it is not common for intensivists to have access to TEE capability. Just as TTE is now much more widely available than a few years ago, it is likely that TEE will gradually become a standard ICU tool both for GDE and advanced CCE examinations.

TRAINING IN GDE

One question to ask is whether noncardiologists can be trained to perform GDE. The answer is unequivocally affirmative. Numerous studies have shown that noncardiologists at various levels of training can achieve mastery of GDE.[3-12] The American Society of Echocardiography has issued a position paper supporting GDE for use by emergency medicine physicians the principle of which applies equally well to intensivists.[13] Proficiency in GDE may be achieved by any interested intensivist providing the training program is well designed. Some recommendations regarding training in GDE are summarized in the chapter on training in CCUS of this textbook (Chapter 3). As with other aspects of CCUS, training in GDE requires the integration of training in image acquisition and image interpretation, with the cognitive elements of the field. Required cognitive elements that allow the clinician to make clinical decisions are summarized in Tables 6-1 and 6-2.

In terms of training program design for TTE, Manasia et al. reported that with 10 h of training, intensivists were able to perform GDE with results that were clinically relevant and that had strong correlation with cardiology performed studies.[14] Vignon et al. have described a program for training in GDE and concluded that 12-h training program that combined didactics, interactive clinical cases, and supervised hands-on training sessions for noncardiology residents was effective for reaching competence in basic CCE.[15,16] Regarding TEE, Benjamin et al. found that intensivists could perform GDE with results similar to cardiology performed TEE following an average of 10 supervised training studies.[17]

While is clear that intensivists can become skilled at GDE, it is important that the training program be well designed. The intensivist makes major clinical decisions that are predicated on the results of the GDE that may spell the difference between the life and death of the patient. The number of studies and duration of study may have uncertain relationship to the skill of the clinician in GDE. One means of assuring competence following training is to utilize rigorous competency based testing as a routine part of training program design.[18]

CLINICAL APPLICATIONS OF GDE

GDE should be a standard part of the assessment of the patient with hemodynamic failure. It is always combined with the history, the physical examination, and the laboratory assessment. It allows the intensivist for an immediate qualitative assessment of cardiac anatomy and function and so has effect on bedside management of the case in a variety of ways:

1. *Identification of an imminently life-threatening disease process:* The use of GDE allows the intensivist to identify an imminently life-threatening process where delay in diagnosis may result in the death of the patient and where urgent intervention may be lifesaving. Such situations include severe pericardial tamponade, major valve failure, massive pulmonary embolism, and the patient who is in severe shock while on inappropriate

TABLE 6-2
Competence in Basic CCE: Required

Cognitive Skills in Recognition of Clinical Syndromes

Clinical Syndromes	Echocardiographic Findings
Severe hypovolemia	Small, hyperdynamic ventricles
	Small IVC with wide respiratory variations
LV failure	Global LV systolic dysfunction
	Heterogeneous contractility pattern suggestive of myocardial ischemia
	LV cavity dilatation suggestive of chronic cardiac disease
RV failure	Acute cor pulmonale: RV dilatation and paradoxical septal motion[a]
	Isolated RV dilatation suggestive of RV infarct
	Associated findings: dilated, noncollapsible IVC
Tamponade	Pericardial effusion (regardless of size)[b]
	Right atrial/RV diastolic collapse
	Associated findings: dilated, noncollapsible IVC
Acute massive left sided valvular regurgitation	Normal LV cavity size (acute valvulopathy)
	Normal/hyperdynamic LV systolic function (LV volume overload)
	Massive color Doppler regurgitant flow[c]
Circulatory arrest	
During resuscitation	Tamponade or acute cor pulmonale (from massive pulmonary embolism)
	LV systolic function (cardiac standstill vs. severely depressed vs. hyperdynamic)
	Global LV systolic dysfunction
After successful resuscitation	Heterogeneous contractility pattern suggestive of myocardial ischemia

CCE, critical care echocardiography; LV, left ventricle; IVC, inferior vena cava; RV, right ventricle.

[a]Accurate identification of paradoxical septal motion may be challenging; acute cor pulmonale is mainly associated with ARDS or massive pulmonary embolism in critically ill patients.

[b]The rate of fluid accumulation within the pericardium rather than its volume determines the risk of tamponade; although echocardiographic findings are considered, the diagnosis of cardiac tamponade should be made on clinical grounds.

[c]The absence of apparent valvular regurgitation during color Doppler examination does not definitely rule out the diagnosis.

Source: Mayo PH, Beaulieu Y, Doelken P, et al. American College of Chest Physicians/La Société de Réanimation de Langue Française Statement on Competence in Critical Care Ultrasonography. Chest. 2009;135(4):1050–1060.

CASE 6-2
Severe Hypotension and Respiratory Failure

This goal-directed echocardiography (GDE) was performed on a patient who presented with severe hypotension and respiratory failure. Video 6-2A shows an attempt at the parasternal long-axis view. There are A lines with lung sliding. No cardiac structure is visible. Video 6-2B shows an attempt at the parasternal short-axis view. There are A lines with lung sliding. No cardiac structure is visible. Videos 6-2C1 and 6-2C2 show the apical four-chamber view. On 2D imaging, there is a possible defect in the interventricular septum (Video 6-2C1) that is confirmed with color flow Doppler (Video 6-2C2). Video 6-2D shows the subcostal long-axis view. There is a pericardial effusion with right atrial systolic compression and echogenic material in the effusion consistent with a hemopericardium. Video 6-2E shows the inferior vena cava (IVC) view. The IVC is enlarged. Case Figure 6-2 shows midsystolic right atrial collapse. Based on the GDE results, the patient was placed on an aortic balloon pump followed by emergency surgery that repaired an acute ventricular septal defect with an associated pseudoaneurysm and acute hemopericardium due to a left ventricular pseudoaneurysm. The patient made a full recovery. Early use of GDE identified an imminently life-threatening process that resulted in successful surgical intervention. It is common that some views of the GDE examination cannot be obtained, as in this patient due to hyperinflation. For this reason, it is important to attempt all five views. Frequently, the subcostal view is the best for patients with hyperinflation.

Video is available at www.ccu2e.com

inotropic support with end systolic effacement pattern. Though uncommon, each of these has a specific therapeutic response that may be lifesaving (Cases 6-2 through 6-5).

2. *Categorization of shock state and selection of initial management strategy:* The use of GDE allows the intensivist to rapidly categorize the hemodynamic failure. With the five standard views, the frontline intensivist to classifies the shock as cardiogenic, obstructive, hypovolemic, or distributive in pattern (Case 6-6). This categorization leads to logical selection of management strategy as well as search for etiology of abnormality. For example, the finding of normal cardiac function without evidence of preload sensitivity by analysis of IVC dynamics suggests that the patient has a distributive shock state. Further volume resuscitation and inotropic support are not indicated; vasopressors are the preferred agent to maintain blood pressure. The presence of severe left ventricular dysfunction with a large IVC suggests that inotropes are the indicated medication for the shock state. The presence of acute cor pulmonale pattern with shock results in immediate search for the cause of the right ventricular failure.

3. *Evolution of disease and response to therapy:* The use of repeated serial GDE allows the intensivist to

CASE 6-3
Acute Dyspnea and Hypotension

This goal-directed echocardiography (GDE) was performed on a patient who presented with acute dyspnea and hypotension. Videos 6-3A and 6-3B show the parasternal long-axis view. There is a mobile mass on the posterior mitral valve (MV) leaflet. Color flow Doppler shows severe mitral valve regurgitation. Video 6-3C shows the parasternal short-axis view. The left ventricular function is normal. Video 6-3D shows the apical four-chamber view. On this zoomed view, there is a mobile mass on the MV. Video 6-3E shows the subcostal long-axis view. This view is suboptimal for interpretation. Video 6-3F shows the inferior vena cava (IVC) view. The IVC diameter is large. Based on the GDE, major MV failure was identified. The patient was stabilized with an aortic balloon pump and underwent early and successful MV replacement. While the etiology of the MV failure cannot be determined by GDE, the examination identified an abnormality that required immediate escalation of support and cardiac surgery consultation. The parasternal short-axis view is off axis at times. This results from respiratory translational artifact. The subcostal view is not adequate for interpretation. It is common in the critically ill not to be able to obtain all views of the GDE examination.

Video is available at www.ccu2e.com

CASE 6-4
Severe Hypotension and Respiratory Distress

This goal-directed echocardiography (GDE) was performed on a patient who presented with severe hypotension and respiratory distress following a trans-Pacific flight. Video 6-4A shows the parasternal long-axis view. There is possible enlargement of the right ventricular (RV) outflow track. Video 6-4B shows the parasternal short-axis view. There is a "D" shaped left ventricle with possible enlargement of the RV. Video 6-4C shows the apical four-chamber view. There is a thrombus in transit in the right atrium, an enlarged RV, and McConnell's sign. Video 6-4D shows the subcostal long-axis view. There is a thrombus in transit in the right atrium and an enlarged RV. Video 6-4E shows the inferior vena cava view. There is a dilated IVC. Based on the GDE results, the patient underwent emergency surgical embolectomy with removal of the RA thrombus and multiple proximal pulmonary emboli. The patient made a full recovery. Early use of GDE identified an imminently life-threatening process that resulted in successful surgical intervention. Ideally, the interventricular septum should be orientated in the middle of the image for the apical four-chamber view. It is often difficult to obtain a good apical four-chamber view in the critically patient, due to problems with positioning the patient. When the RV is enlarged, it is also difficult to include both the RV and LV (left ventricle) in the same view.

Video is available at www.ccu2e.com

CASE 6-5
Progressive Hypotension

This goal-directed echocardiography (GDE) was performed for progressive hypotension. The patient presented with dyspnea and had a long history of hypertension. The admitting team treated the patient for congestive heart failure with diuretics. The patient developed hypotension and was started on dopamine. Escalating doses of dopamine resulted in further hypotension. The critical care team was called to evaluate the patient. Video 6-5A shows the parasternal long-axis view. The left ventricle (LV) is hyperdynamic with end-systolic effacement. Video 6-5B shows the parasternal short-axis view. The LV is hyperdynamic with end-systolic effacement. Video 6-5C shows the apical four-chamber view. The LV is hyperdynamic with end-systolic effacement. Video 6-5D shows the subcostal long-axis view. The LV is hyperdynamic with end-systolic effacement. Video 6-5E shows the inferior vena cava (IVC) view. The IVC diameter is small. This case is an example of inappropriate use of diuretics and an inotrope in a patient with an LV that was conditioned by long-term hypertension. Based on the GDE, the critical care team gave immediate volume resuscitation, changed the dopamine to phenylephrine, and administered a dose of intravenous beta-blocker. The hypotension was promptly corrected with these measures. Early use of GDE allowed identification of dangerous inappropriate therapy. The examiner had difficulty in obtaining a consistent on axis apical four-chamber view due to translational artifact from respiratory activity. This is a common problem in the critically ill patient with respiratory distress. For the intensivist with advanced critical care echocardiography skill, the diagnosis of end systolic effacement that has physiological consequence may be confirmed by placing a continuous wave Doppler interrogation line through the LV cavity using the apical four-chamber view. The Doppler envelope has a characteristic end-systolic peak velocity ("dagger shaped") profile, and the peak velocity is elevated (Case Figure 6-5). In this case, the end-systolic velocity gradient was 79 mmHg.

Video is available at www.ccu2e.com

---

follow the evolution of critical illness and response to therapy. The nature of critical illness is that it is a dynamic process, as is response to therapy (Case 6-7). The standard cardiology echocardiography approach does not typically include serial studies in close succession. This approach is routine with GDE. Early in the course of illness, GDE can easily be performed several times per day. As the patient becomes more stable, the frequency is reduced according to clinical requirements.

4. *Identification of coexisting diagnosis:* The use of GDE allows the intensivist to identify the presence of coexisting diagnosis that complicate the management of the primary process. This situation commonly occurs in the older patient or the patient with complex medical presentation. A typical example is the elderly patient with sepsis presentation who on GDE has evidence of severe aortic stenosis and severe left ventricular failure (Case 6-8). Though sepsis may be predominant cause of the shock state, early identification of the coexisting processes allows the intensivist to modify management strategy.

CASE 6-6
Hypotension with Left Ventricular Dysfunction

This goal-directed echocardiography (GDE) was performed on a patient with hypotension who had a known history of severe left ventricular (LV) dysfunction. Video 6-6A shows the parasternal long-axis view. There is severe global LV dysfunction. The valve anatomy is normal, but there is reduced mitral valve opening in diastole. A small pericardial effusion is present in association with a pleural effusion. Video 6-6B shows the parasternal short-axis view. This view confirms the findings of the parasternal long-axis view. Video 6-6C shows the apical four-chamber view. Endomyocardial definition is poor, so the image is suboptimal for interpretation. Video 6-6D shows the subcostal long-axis view. There is severe LV dysfunction. A small pericardial effusion is present. The echo free space in the near field represents ascites. Video 6-6E shows the inferior vena cava (IVC) view. The IVC is dilated. There is no video clip of the IVC, so respiratory variation cannot be determined. Based on the GDE results, the critical team categorized the shock state as cardiogenic in origin. Review of previous echocardiography reports showed no difference in LV dysfunction pattern. Obstructive and hypovolemic shock category were ruled with GDE. Review of the history, physical examination, and laboratory values identified no cause for coexisting distributive shock. The patient was treated for decompensated heart failure with diuretics and inotropic support and improved to baseline functional status. Following GDE, the critical care team called for advanced echocardiography study that included a dobutamine trial performed with multiple serial measurements of stroke volume and cardiac output with augmenting doses of dobutamine. This case emphasizes the importance of integrating all aspects of the clinical evaluation (history, physical examination, and laboratory results) with GDE. This allowed the team to exclude distributive shock. The GDE examination also identified that there was no need for volume resuscitation in this case and that there was a relative contraindication to its use as well. The apical four chamber is suboptimal, while the other views were sufficient to guide initial management. This supports the rule that every view of the standard GDE examination should be included when evaluating the patient in shock.

Video is available at www.ccu2e.com

CASE 6-7
Hypotension Related to Urosepsis

This goal-directed echocardiography (GDE) was performed 24 h following admission on a patient who presented with hypotension related to urosepsis. The initial GDE was normal (see Case 6-1). The patient was on norepinephrine at the time of the second GDE. Video 6-7A shows the parasternal long-axis view: There is severely reduced left ventricular function and segmental wall abnormality involving the inferolateral basal and midsegments. This is new from the initial GDE. Video 6-7B shows the parasternal short-axis view. This confirms the findings of the parasternal long-axis view. The apical four-chamber view is not shown due to inadequate image quality. Video 6-7C shows the subcostal long-axis view. There is severely reduced left ventricular (LV) function. Video 6-7D shows the inferior vena cava (IVC) view. The IVC is dilated. Video 6-7E shows the anterior chest lung examination. There are multiple profuse B lines present bilaterally. The GDE examination done 24 h after admission shows new severely reduced LV function with a segmental wall abnormality. This underlines the dynamic quality of GDE findings in the critically ill patient. In this case, the patient developed a sepsis cardiomyopathy. The team was concerned about the segmental wall abnormality. Cardiac enzymes and EKG were negative, and so that the segmental wall abnormality was a manifestation of the sepsis cardiomyopathy. The dilated IVC indicated that there would be no further benefit from volume resuscitation, while the profuse B line pattern informed that there was specific contraindication to further fluid infusion. The patient was continued on norepinephrine to provide both inotropic and pressor support and improved with antibiotics. A GDE performed two weeks later was normal. Sepsis cardiomyopathy is often fully reversible. The apical four-chamber view is often the most difficult to achieve in the critically ill patient, as demonstrated by this case.

Video is available at www.ccu2e.com

The question arises as to whether there is evidence showing clinical impact of GDE in the ICU.

LIMITATIONS OF GDE

It is important to recognize some of the limitations of GDE. Recognition may allow the ICU team to adjust their training and scanning strategy accordingly:

1. *Failure of image acquisition:* A major limitation of GDE by the TTE is failure of adequate image acquisition. Body habitus, tissue density, and difficulty in positioning the patient may result in suboptimal image quality. For this reason, it is important to attempt all of the views of GDE in every patient. Images that might be rejected out of hand by the cardiology echocardiographer may still be adequate for the intensivist. Improvement in machine design has reduced the number of inadequate images in medical critical care patients, but cardio thoracic and trauma patients present special challenges. The main indication for TEE in the ICU is in those patients who have inadequate TTE views.

2. *Limited image set:* The limited image set of GDE does not replace a full advanced level study. By design it does not rely on Doppler, and therefore cannot be used for assessment of hemodynamics. Identification of segmental wall abnormality, sophisticated measurement of valve function, or examination for congenital heart disease are not part of GDE. Training in GDE must therefore emphasize when it is appropriate to call for full echocardiography study.

3. *Failure of training:* Mastery of GDE requires training. To the neophyte scanner, GDE appears so straightforward

> **CASE 6-8**
> **Pneumonia with Septic Shock**
>
> This goal-directed echocardiography (GDE) was performed for an elderly patient with an established diagnosis of pneumonia with septic shock. Video 6-8A shows the parasternal long-axis view. There is severe reduction in left ventricular function (LV) with segmental wall abnormality involving the mid- and basal anterior septum. The aortic valve is hyperechoic and immobile consistent with aortic stenosis (AS). The mitral valve (MV) is hyperechoic and has reduced systolic opening. Video 6-8B shows the parasternal short-axis view. There is severe reduction in left ventricular function with segmental wall abnormality Video 6-8C shows the apical four-chamber view. There is severe reduction in left ventricular function. The anterolateral wall is not well seen. A right-sided pacer wire is in place. The apical subcostal view is not shown due to inadequate image quality. Video 6-8D shows the inferior vena cava (IVC) view. The IVC is dilated. This case demonstrates the importance of performing GDE in all patients with shock. The diagnosis of septic shock was made by history, physical examination, thoracic ultrasonography that identified pneumonia, and laboratory analysis. Standard treatment using the "sepsis bundle" approach would mandate substantial volume resuscitation in this situation. The GDE examination identified reduced LV function with segmental wall abnormality and significant AS. Vigorous volume resuscitation would not help this patient and could well be harmful. The presence of what might be severe AS with segmental wall abnormality, suggesting ischemic cardiac risk greatly complicates the medical management of this elderly patient. The GDE examination should be followed by an advanced critical care echocardiography examination in order to quantitate the severity of the AS as well as to further characterize the function of the MV.
>
> Video is available at www.ccu2e.com

that the enthusiastic learner may overestimate their abilities. With inadequate training in image acquisition, the intensivist may create an inaccurate result, as when a parasternal long view is off axis yielding a false impression of end-systolic effacement. Over rotation of the parasternal long-axis view may give a false D shaped ventricle. Inappropriate counterclockwise rotation of the probe in the apical four-chamber view will cause a dilated right ventricle to appear to be normal in size. Inadequate training in image acquisition will result in inaccurate classification of chamber size and function. Faculty who provide teaching in GDE have a special responsibility to providing rigorous training, as it is likely that a large number of intensivists will require competence in GDE.

4. *Difficulty with documentation:* The ease of use and strength of clinical may combine to present difficulty with documentation of GDE. In a busy multi-bed ICU where the intensivist staff performs GDE on a regular basis on 24/7, the number of studies may be so high as to make complete documentation of all studies a challenge. This may impact adversely on patient care when trying to compare the results of serial studies. In this situation, GDE becomes like physical examination; not every brief assessment can be captured. This is a departure from the standard paradigm of radiology and cardiology performed ultrasonography, where every study is fully documented. The solution to this problem may lie in the development of user-friendly image collection programs that interface by wireless connection to the ICU ultrasound machine, in order to facilitate reporting of results and image storage. As these become more widely available, the documentation issue will be less problematic. Integration of these data collection systems into ICU function requires training and buy-in by the intensivist staff.

5. *Over emphasis on GDE:* The use of GDE is so intuitively attractive that it may easily become the predominant ultrasound imaging modality in an ICU. In fact, GDE should be considered as a part of CCUS. It is best combined with the other elements of the discipline: thoracic, vascular diagnostic, screening abdominal, and procedure guidance. Faculty are responsible for designing training programs that include all aspects of CCUS.

CONCLUSIONS

GDE is a key skill for the intensivist, as it allows for rapid evaluation of hemodynamic failure. It requires skill at image acquisition, image interpretation, and knowledge of how to apply the results of the scan at the bedside of patient using five standard views: parasternal long axis, parasternal short-axis midventricular level, apical four chamber, subcostal long axis, and IVC long axis. The GDE examination is used to identify imminently life-threatening causes for shock, to categorize shock state, to develop rational management plan, to identify coexisting cardiac dysfunction that may complicate management of the primary process, and to follow the progression of the disease and therapy with serial scans. It is should be utilized with other components of critical ultrasonography and with other parts of the standard evaluation such as the history, physical examination, and laboratory evaluation.

REFERENCES

1. Mayo PH, Vieillard-Baron A, et al. American College of Chest Physicians/La Société de Réanimation de Langue Française Statement on Competence in Critical Care Ultrasonography. *Chest.* 2009;135:1050–1060.
2. Cholley B. International expert statement on training standards for critical care ultrasonography Expert Round Table on Ultrasound in ICU Mayo PH, subgroup leader. *Intensive Care Med.* 2011;37:1077–1083.
3. Mandavia DP, Hoffner RJ, Mahaney K, Henderson SO. Bedside echocardiography by emergency physicians. *Ann Emerg Med.* 2001;383:77–382.

4. Moore CL, Rose GA, Tayal VS, et al. Determination of left ventricular function by emergency physician echocardiography of hypotensive patients. *Acad Emerg Med.* 2002;9:186–193.
5. Vignon P, Chastagner C, François B, et al. Diagnostic ability of hand-held echocardiography in ventilated critically ill patients. *Critical Care.* 2003;7:R84–R91.
6. Randazzo MR, Snoey ER, Levitt MA, Binder K. Accuracy of emergency physician assessment of left ventricular ejection fraction and central venous pressure using echocardiography. *Acad Emerg Med.* 2003;10:973–977.
7. Lemola K, Yamada E, Jagasia D, Kerber RE. A hand-carried personal ultrasound device for rapid evaluation of left ventricular function: use after limited echo training. *Echocardiography.* 2003;20:309–312.
8. DeCara JM, Lang RM, Koch R, Bala R, Penzotti J, Spencer KT. The use of small personal ultrasound devices by internists without formal training in echocardiography. *Eur J Echocardiogr.* 2003;4:141–147.
9. Pershad J, Myers S, Plouman C, et al. Bedside limited echocardiography by the emergency physician is accurate during evaluation of the critically ill patient. *Pediatrics.* 2004;114:e667–e671.
10. Jones AE, Tayal VS, Sullivan DM, Kline JA. Randomized, controlled trial of immediate versus delayed goal-directed ultrasound to identify the cause of nontraumatic hypotension in emergency department patients. *Crit Care Med.* 2004;32:1703–1708.
11. Royse CF, Seah JL, Donelan L, Royse AG. Point of care ultrasound for basic haemodynamic assessment: novice compared with an expert operator. *Anaesthesia.* 2006;61:849–855.
12. Melamed R, Sprenkle MD, Ulstad VK, Herzog CA, Leatherman JW. Assessment of left ventricular function by intensivists using hand-held echocardiography. *Chest.* 2009;135:1416–1420.
13. Labovitz AJ, Noble VE, Bierig M, et al. Focused cardiac ultrasound in the emergent setting: a consensus statement of the American Society of Echocardiography and American College of Emergency Physicians. *J Am Soc Echocardiogr.* 2010;23:1225–1230.
14. Manasia AR, Nagaraj HM, Kodali RB, et al. Feasibility and potential clinical utility of goal-directed transthoracic echocardiography performed by noncardiologist intensivists using a small hand-carried device (SonoHeart) in critically ill patients. *J Cardiothorac Vasc Anesth.* 2005;19:155–159.
15. Vignon P, Dugard A, Abraham J, et al. Focused training for goal-oriented hand-held echocardiography performed by noncardiologist residents in the intensive care unit. *Intensive Care Med.* 2007;33:1795–1799.
16. Vignon P, Mücke F, Bellec F, et al. Basic critical care echocardiography: validation of a curriculum dedicated to noncardiologist residents. *Crit Care Med.* 2011.
17. Benjamin E, Griffin K, Leibowitz AB, et al. Goal-directed transesophageal echocardiography performed by intensivists to assess left ventricular function: comparison with pulmonary artery catheterization. *J Cardiothorac Vasc Anesth.* 1998;12:10–15.
18. Charron C, Prat G, Caille V, et al. Validation of a skills assessment scoring system for transesophageal echocardiographic monitoring of hemodynamics. *Intensive Care Med.* 2007;33:1712–1718.

TRANSTHORACIC ECHOCARDIOGRAPHY: IMAGE ACQUISITION

JOSE CARDENAS-GARCIA & PAUL H. MAYO

Scan QR code or visit www.ccu2e.com for video in this chapter

INTRODUCTION

Transthoracic echocardiography (TTE) has major application in the intensive care unit (ICU). Proficiency in TTE allows the intensivist to determine the diagnosis of cardiopulmonary failure, develop management strategies, and follow the results of therapeutic interventions with serial examinations. By definition, critical care echocardiography (CCE) is performed by the intensivist in the ICU. The clinician personally acquires and interprets the image at the bedside and uses the information to immediately guide management. It follows that the intensivist must have a high level of skill in image acquisition that requires knowledge of ultrasound physics, machine controls, and transducer manipulation. This chapter reviews important elements of image acquisition with emphasis on transducer manipulation. The reader is referred to Chapters 2 and 3 for a comprehensive discussion of physics and machine controls.

BASIC AND ADVANCED CCE

Proficiency in CCE can be separated into basic and advanced levels. Basic CCE is performed as a goal-directed examination using a limited number of views (see Chapter 6). It is designed to answer specific clinical questions at the bedside. Proficiency in advanced CCE requires a high level of skill in all aspects of image interpretation and acquisition. Advanced CCE allows a comprehensive evaluation of cardiac anatomy and function using two-dimensional (2D) imaging and Doppler echocardiography. Both basic and advanced CCE require skill in image acquisition.

▶ Technical Issues

The performance of TTE has challenges that relate to the fact that the heart is surrounded by lung and ribs, both of which block ultrasound transmission. Since ribs block ultrasound, cardiac transducers are designed with a small footprint to scan through the rib interspace. During scanning, left arm abduction may increase the size of the interspace. Aerated lung also blocks ultrasound, so that placing the patient in the left lateral decubitus position may be helpful. In this position, the heart is moved from behind the sternum and the left lung moves laterally, thus exposing more of the heart for examination. While the left lateral decubitus view improves visualization from the parasternal and apical views, the supine position is best for the subcostal examination.

The critically ill patient may be difficult to place in a favorable scanning position. Patients on ventilatory support, particularly when hyperinflated, may have poor parasternal and apical windows. Very often, the subcostal view yields the only acceptable image. TTE image quality may be poor in the edematous or muscular patient. Obesity presents a special challenge, as it attenuates the penetration of ultrasound. In addition, abdominal obesity elevates the diaphragm, particularly when the patient is supine and when passive on ventilatory support. The heart is then rotated into a more vertical position. This makes it difficult to obtain properly orientated parasternal views. The presence of chest dressings, wounds, or subcutaneous air also degrade TTE image quality. Transesophageal echocardiography (TEE) is an alternative in the patient who fails TTE. Artifacts in echocardiography relate, in part, to the fact that the heart is a highly mobile organ in constant motion within the thorax. Translational, torsional and rotational movement of the heart may be misinterpreted as reflecting actual cardiac contractile function.

In addition to these challenges, CCE is performed in a difficult operating environment. The patient is often surrounded by multiple ICU devices, so that positioning of the machine and operator may be difficult. The light level in the patient room is often too bright for optimal screen display. The echocardiographer is under pressure to complete the examination rapidly, because the patient is critically ill and other patients demand attention. The results of the study frequently require immediate response so that image acquisition and interpretation must be accurate. The intensivist should always attempt to obtain the best image quality. However, image quality may be limited in the critically ill and may be below the standards mandated by standard cardiology echocardiography practice.

Advanced CCE requires that the intensivist has proficiency in Doppler measurement. The physics of Doppler measurement are covered in detail in Chapter 2 and its clinical applications in other chapters of the book. The technical issues related to Doppler include the following:

1. Doppler measurements are angle dependent; therefore, the best angle of Doppler interrogation may not be necessarily obtained from standard imaging orientation. The examiner should feel free to use nonstandard 2D image views if required for optimal Doppler measurement.
2. A poor quality 2D image (e.g., related to obesity or edema) does not preclude good quality Doppler measurements. The examiner should always attempt standard Doppler analysis even if the 2D image is suboptimal.
3. Continuous wave (CW) Doppler has range ambiguity but is able to measure high velocity of blood flow. Pulsed wave (PW) Doppler is able to measure blood flow velocity in a small sample area, but due to aliasing phenomena, it cannot measure high blood flow velocity.
4. Color flow Doppler has specific pitfalls. It is gain sensitive such that over and under gaining will over or under estimate the severity of vascular regurgitation, respectively. It is subject to the aliasing phenomena. Color Doppler jets that are directed along the wall of the atrium systematically underestimate the severity of regurgitation.

▶ Nomenclature

TTE examines the heart in tomographic planes obtained by positioning the transducer and "slicing" the heart through different planes. By obtaining multiple views of the heart, the examiner integrates the information to yield a comprehensive evaluation of cardiac anatomy and function. The addition of Doppler analysis gives important information related to cardiac pressures and flows. The American Society of Echocardiography (ASE) has defined the standard tomographic views of the heart.[1] The three standard image planes are as follows:

1. The long-axis plane is parallel to the long axis of the left ventricle (LV). This is defined by a line that goes through the LV apex and the center of the base of the LV intersecting with the center of the aortic valve (AV).
2. The short-axis plane is perpendicular to the long-axis plane.
3. The four-chamber plane is perpendicular to both the short- and long-axis views. This is defined by a plane that goes through the LV apex and intersects the LV and right ventricle (RV) and atria.

The various tomographic planes of TTE are characterized by the position of the transducer required to obtain the image (the window) and the resulting image plane (the view). Transducer manipulation occurs as follows:

1. *Move:* The transducer is shifted to a different position on the thorax.
2. *Tilt:* The transducer is tilted or rocked along the same tomographic plane without moving it.
3. *Angle:* Without moving the transducer, angulation is changed to obtain adjacent tomographic planes.
4. *Rotate:* The transducer is rotated without moving, tilting, or angling it in order to obtain orthogonal tomographic planes.

Image orientation is standardized for adult TTE. The transducer position is projected at the top of the screen. The image orientation marker is set to the upper right of the screen. In the long-axis view, superior or cephalad cardiac structures project to the right of the screen. In the short-axis view, left-sided cardiac structures project to the right side of the screen. This is reverse to the orientation used for abdominal, thoracic, and vascular ultrasonography.

The basic or goal-directed CCE examination includes five views without Doppler analysis, while the advanced CCE examination includes a minimum of 14 views of the heart with comprehensive Doppler measurements. At each view, the examiner may choose to obtain one or more tomographic planes by tilting and angling the transducer. There is no officially sanctioned sequence for image acquisition. However, regardless of the sequence used; the intensivist should use a methodical approach to image acquisition for initial examination. The examination should be performed in standard sequence, as this reduces the likelihood that views will be omitted. Typically, CCE uses sequential follow-up examinations of the heart to check for response to therapy, progression or regression of disease, and new problems. Follow-up examinations may be very limited in scope. Certain situations do not permit any but the briefest examination. For example, echocardiography performed during cardiopulmonary arrest may include only several seconds of a subcostal view during a pulse check.

THE TTE EXAMINATION

In the previous chapter, the authors reviewed the concept of basic critical care echocardiography (CCE). It is likely that most readers of this chapter will be interested in this important application of CCE, and they will not choose to develop competence in advanced CCE. The basic CCE examination is a mandatory part of training in general critical care ultrasonography, whereas advanced CCE is not.[2] The intensivist needs to decide what skill level in echocardiography is required for their practice. Therefore, this chapter is divided into two parts. The first part focuses on image acquisition needed for basic CCE, the second reviews the complex image set relevant to advanced CCE.

THE BASIC CCE EXAMINATION

The basic CCE examination consists of the following views:[3]

a. Parasternal long axis
b. Parasternal short axis at the midventricular level
c. Apical four-chamber view
d. Subcostal four-chamber view
e. Inferior vena cava (IVC) view

What follows is a description of transducer use required to obtain the standard views of the basic CCE examinations. The discussion does not include a detailed review of Doppler measurements, beyond the use of color Doppler for screening purposes, as these are not part of the basic CCE.

▶ Parasternal Long-Axis View

The transducer is placed in the left 3rd, 4th, or 5th intercostal space adjacent to the sternum and held perpendicular to the skin surface, with the transducer index mark pointing to the patient's right shoulder (Figure 7-1 and Case 7-1). Movement of the transducer in either caudal or cephalad direction brings the parasternal long axis into view. The transducer should be moved in small increments to obtain the best tomographic view. With minor movement and angulation, the examiner seeks a view that bisects the mitral valve (MV), the AV and that includes the LV cavity in its longest axis. The LV apex is not visible in the parasternal long-axis view. The image should be orientated so that the ascending aorta is displayed on the right, with the LV cavity on the left of the screen. The right ventricular outflow tract (RVOT) and chest wall appear at the top of the screen. Posterior structures, such as the left atrium (LA), the pericardium, and descending aorta, appear at the bottom of the screen. While the perfect long-axis view displays the heart horizontally on the screen, technical limitations such as patient positioning, body habitus, mechanical ventilation, and examiner inexperience may yield a more vertical view of the heart.

Echocardiographic findings

Qualitative assessment of ejection fraction (EF); RVOT/LV wall thickness, size and function; LV segmental wall function; septal kinetics; LA chamber size; and evaluation of AV/MV anatomy with screening color Doppler analysis, descending aorta, and pericardial space.

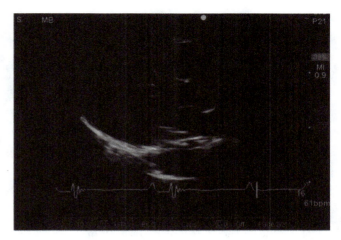

Figure 7-1 The parasternal long-axis view.

Pitfalls of the parasternal long-axis view

For the basic CCE echocardiographer, the pitfalls of this view include the following:

1. *Inaccurate assessment of RV size:* This is because the parasternal long-axis view affords a view of the RVOT and so cannot be used to determine RV size. The apical four-chamber and subcostal views are used for assessment of RV size.

2. *Inaccurate assessment of LV size and function:* Off-axis views of the LV due to rotation or angulation may

---

CASE 7-1

Parasternal Long-axis View

Video 7-1A shows the parasternal long-axis view and demonstrates the importance of performing the initial view with a depth setting that allows visualization of structures posterior to the heart. In this case, there is a pleural effusion with atelectatic lung floating within it. This would be missed if the depth setting were set initially to place the heart in central screen position. Video 7-1B has the depth setting adjusted to place the heart in central screen position. There is severe reduction of left ventricular (LV) function with a segmental wall abnormality involving the anterior septum. The septum is thin and the LV cavity is dilated suggesting chronic LV dysfunction related to ischemic injury. Diastolic excursion of the anterior mitral valve (MV) is reduced consistent with reduced LV function. Chamber size and wall thickness would require formal measurement with M-mode or direct caliper measurement. Videos 7-1C1 and 7-1C2 demonstrate color Doppler interrogation of the MV and aortic valve, respectively, with what is likely moderate mitral regurgitation (MR). The examiner is required to enlarge the color grid to cover the entire left atrium in order to give an more accurate qualitative estimate of the severity of the MR. The cause of the MR is not evident by morphological pattern, while the segmental wall abnormality suggests the possibility of ischemic origin.

Video is available at www.ccu2e.com

lead to erroneous assessment of LV size and function. In particular, the LV may appear to be hyperdynamic with end-systolic effacement; if the transducer is not orientated to identify the largest LV cavity and aligned through the midpoint of the AV and MV.

3. *Inaccurate assessment of MV and AV function:* The MV and AV may appear to be anatomically normal on 2D view, but can have substantial degrees of regurgitation discernible only with color or spectral Doppler analysis. Proficiency in basic CCE does not allow the examiner to reliably exclude severe valvular regurgitation. Color Doppler has limitations not intuitively obvious to the inexperienced examiner. These include gain settings ("dial a jet"), wall jet effect (Coanda effect), angle effect (both of transducer and by Doppler interrogation angle relative to the jet), and shadowing by surrounding structures such as a prosthetic valve apparatus or a calcified annulus.

4. *Inaccurate assessment of pericardial and pleural effusion:* Identification of a pleural effusion requires that the depth setting on the ultrasound machine be increased such that the structures posterior to the heart are visualized. A pleural effusion will be seen as a relatively hypoechoic space posterior to the LV and posterior to the descending aorta. A pericardial effusion will track anterior to the descending aorta.

▶ Parasternal Short-Axis Midventricular View

From the parasternal long-axis view, the transducer is rotated 90° clockwise without angulation or tilting. This results in cross-sectional views of the heart. A good short-axis view follows from a good long-axis view. Rotation of the transducer may be achieved using a two-handed approach, keeping the transducer hand steady while rotating with the other hand will give the best results. The transducer is rotated until the short axis of the heart is obtained with the transducer index mark pointing towards the left shoulder. By angling the transducer along a right-shoulder-to-left-hip axis, multiple tomographic views of the heart may be obtained. For the basic CCE examination, the only view that is required is the midventricular tomographic plane (papillary muscle level) (Figure 7-2 and Case 7-2).

Echocardiographic findings

Qualitative assessment of EF, RV/LV wall thickness, LV segmental wall function, RV/LV chamber size and function, septal kinetics, and pericardial space.

Pitfalls of the parasternal short-axis midventricular view

For the basic CCE echocardiographer, the pitfalls of this view include the following:

1. *Inaccurate assessment of LV configuration:* The normal LV should be circular in short axis. An elliptical

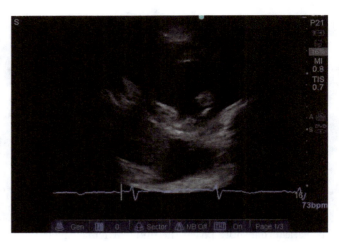

Figure 7-2 The parasternal short-axis view midventricular view.

appearance results from an off-axis view related to a nonperpendicular tomographic plane or under/over rotation of the transducer. An off-axis view may result in inaccurate diagnosis of segmental wall contraction abnormality or septal flattening ("D" shaped heart). The supine position, ventilatory support with lack of diaphragmatic movement, obesity, and elevation of intra-abdominal pressures may all cause the heart to

---

CASE 7-2

Parasternal Short-axis View at the Midventricular Level

Video 7-2A shows a parasternal short-axis view at the midventricular level. Left ventricular (LV) function is normal. The right ventricle is normal in size and there is no septal dyskinesia. Video 7-2B shows normal LV function but with increased LV wall thickness. There is also a circumferential pericardial effusion. Strictly speaking, ventricular hypertrophy requires a formal measurement of ventricular muscle mass that requires a series of specific measurements that are not within the purview of basic critical care echocardiography. The intensivist should report increased wall thickness consistent with ventricular hypertrophy, and consider alternative causes for increased wall thickness. In this case, the patient had advanced amyloidosis. Video 7-2C shows severe LV dysfunction with segmental wall abnormality. The anterior mid septum is akinetic while the inferior and lateral walls are contracting although to reduced extent. The anterior and anterolateral walls are not well visualized due to a rib shadow. Adequate image quality in all views is frequently not possible in the critically ill. The subcostal short-axis view would be an alternative. Video 7-2D shows severe LV dysfunction with a segmental wall pattern. The septal function is very reduced as is the anterior wall, suggesting a left anterior wall infarction, while the inferior, infero lateral, and anterolateral segments are reduced in function but to lesser extent. There is a pleural effusion with atelectatic lung within it. At the end of the clip, the tomographic plane changes to the mitral level. This resulted from respiratory translation movement of the heart, which is a common artifact of echocardiography performed in the patient with respiratory distress.

Video is available at www.ccu2e.com

be rotated such that the long-axis view tends to result in a more vertical position of the heart in the critically ill. This results in an off-axis view of the LV in the transverse scanning plane. This cannot be corrected by transducer manipulation. An alternative method of obtaining a short-axis view of the LV is to use the subcostal approach.

2. *Inability to visualize the RV free wall:* Estimates of RV size require visualization of the RV wall, which may be difficult in the parasternal short-axis view of the LV. The apical four-chamber and subcostal views are superior for assessment of RV size and function.

▶ Apical Four-Chamber View

The transducer is placed at the anatomic apex of the LV with the tomographic plane bisecting the ventricles and atria (Figure 7-3 and Case 7-3). Ideally, the patient should be placed in the left lateral decubitus position. This is often difficult in the critically ill patient. The window for the apical four-chamber view is frequently small and difficult to locate. A good starting position is infero-laterally to the nipple with the transducer index mark pointing 3 to 4 o'clock position. The septum should be orientated vertically in the center of the screen, and the tomographic plane adjusted such that it bisects the apex, the ventricles, and the atria.

Echocardiographic findings

Qualitative assessment of EF; RV/LV wall thickness, size and function; LV segmental wall function; septal kinetics; right atrium (RA) and LA chamber size; evaluation of tricuspid valve (TV) and MV anatomy with screening color Doppler analysis; and pericardial space.

Pitfalls of the apical four-chamber view

For the basic CCE echocardiographer, the pitfalls of this view include the following:

1. *Off-axis image:* The apical four-chamber view is the most difficult for the basic-level echocardiographer to obtain.

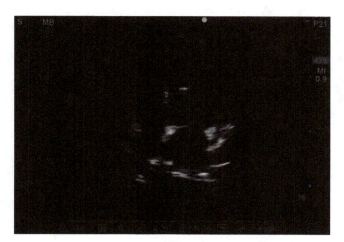

Figure 7-3 The apical four-chamber view.

> **CASE 7-3**
> **Apical Four-chamber View**
>
> Video 7-3A shows an apical four-chamber view (AP4). While the septum is centrally orientated, the left ventricle is foreshortened. This was the best view that could obtained in this obese patient on ventilatory support, continuous hemofiltration, and high-dose pressors. The intensivist faces major obstacles in obtaining the apical views related to patient habitus, supine position, respiratory translational artifact, and ICU equipment that blocks good scanning position. In this case, there is moderate right ventricular (RV) enlargement with normal RV free wall function. At times, the intra-atrial septum bows into the left atrium, suggesting elevation of right atrial pressures. The subcostal long-axis view would be obligatory alternative view to examine RV wall thickness and septal kinetics. Video 7-3B shows mild mitral regurgitation (MR) by color Doppler, but with a wall jet pattern. A MR wall jet is known to result in an underestimate of the severity of MR. This mandates examination of multiple views and, if indicated, advanced methods for determining the severity of the MR. In this case, the wall jet pattern was seen in multiple views, but the MR was determined to be moderate in severity by vena contracta measurement. Video 7-3C shows mild to moderate tricuspid regurgitation. The jet is well oriented for measurement of the TR velocity. Other views showed a similar degree of TR.
>
> Video is available at www.ccu2e.com

There are three key goals to adequate image quality. First, the position of the septum should be in the center of the screen. Second, the tomographic plain should bisect the anatomical apex as well as bisecting the midpoint of the MV and TV orifices. Finally, the transducer rotation should be adjusted such that the RV size is maximal. As LV to RV size ratio is important measurement of basic CCE, proper orientation is critical. An off-axis view may result in an inability to visualize the RV free wall, and counterclockwise transducer rotation may result in underestimation of RV size. The subcostal view is the best alternative approach in the case of sub-optimal image quality in the apical four-chamber view position.

▶ Subcostal Four-Chamber View

This view is best obtained with the patient lying supine. The transducer is placed just below the xiphoid process, pointing toward the left shoulder. The transducer index mark is orientated to the 3 to 4 o'clock position. This view requires the transducer to be held on its top surface, as some or most of its bottom surface will be contacting the patient. This yields a four-chamber view, with the tomographic plane sectioning the heart from the right side through to the left (Figure 7-4 and Case 7-4).

Echocardiographic findings

Qualitative assessment of EF; RV/LV wall thickness, size and function; LV segmental wall function; septal kinetics;

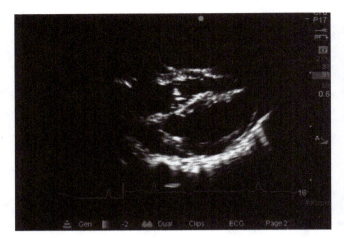

Figure 7-4 The subcostal long-axis view.

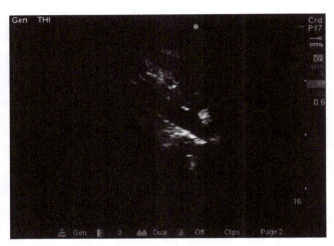

Figure 7-5 The inferior vena cava long-axis view.

evaluation of TV/MV anatomy with screening color Doppler analysis; and pericardial space.

Often the subcostal view is the best quality image of the basic CCE. In the hyperinflated patient on ventilatory support may be the only obtainable image. During cardiopulmonary resuscitation sequence, it is the preferred image plane for rapid assessment of cardiac function during brief pulse checks.

Pitfalls of the subcostal four-chamber view

For the basic CCE echocardiographer, the pitfalls of this view include the following:

1. *Off-axis view:* The tomographic plane should be orientated such that the RV and LV size are maximal and both atria are visible. The subcostal view is particularly susceptible to translational artifact that occurs with the respiratory cycle. The heart can be pushed out of plane in patients who are in respiratory distress or on mechanical ventilatory support.

▶ IVC Longitudinal View

There are several methods of obtaining the IVC longitudinal view. One method is, from the subcostal four-chamber view, to rotate the transducer counter clockwise until the transducer index marker is in the 12 o'clock position followed by angulation of the tomographic plane towards the right (Figure 7-5 and Case 7-5). Alternatively, the transducer can be moved directly to a right paramedian longitudinal plane, either on subscostal or transcostal position to locate the target structure. If bowel gas or surgical dressing block this window, the transducer may be moved to the right midaxillary line with the tomographic cut orientated in sagittal plane.

CASE 7-4

Subcostal Long-axis View

Video 7-4A shows a subcostal long-axis view. The right ventricle (RV) and right atrium (RA) are enlarged. The RV free wall is thickened, suggesting that the RV has been under chronic load. This would require M-mode or caliper based measurement, if there was need for quantitative purposes. The intra-atrial septum is bowed into the left atrium, suggesting elevation of RA pressure. This is supported by the presence of a dilated coronary sinus. The left ventricular (LV) function is normal; although at a qualitative level, it appears to be compressed by the RV. Video 7-4B shows a color Doppler grid positioned over the intra-atrial septum, with the purpose of checking for a patent foramen ovale in this patient with severe hypoxemic respiratory failure. There was no color Doppler evidence of right to left shunt. This was confirmed with agitated saline contrast injection. At times, the LV seems to have end-systolic effacement. This is an artifact of respiratory translational artifact that is a common feature of critical care echocardiography performed on the acutely dyspneic patient.

Video is available at www.ccu2e.com

CASE 7-5

Inferior Vena Cava Long-axis View

Video 7-5A shows a small diameter inferior vena cava (IVC) in longitudinal axis. Video 7-5B shows a large IVC without respiratory variation. Video 7-5C shows a problem with the measurement that occurs in patients with translational artifact due to movement of the IVC in and out of the tomographic plane. If the examiner is trying to reliably measure a 12% variation of IVC size as a determinant of preload sensitivity, true respiratory variation may be difficult to distinguish from translational artifact. Examination of variation in superior vena cava size with transesophageal echocardiography is an effective alternative. Respirophasic diameter variation of the IVC has utility in determination of preload sensitivity, if the patient is on mechanical ventilatory support without spontaneous respiratory effort. The diameter alone may have some value in this determination, but only at the extremes of size.

Video is available at www.ccu2e.com

Echocardiographic findings

Determination of preload sensitivity (see Chapter 10).

Pitfalls of the IVC longitudinal view

For the basic CCE echocardiographer, the pitfalls of this view include the following:

1. *Misidentification of the aorta for the IVC:* The aorta is to the left of the midline and directed posteriorly. The IVC is to the right of the midline, it is closely associated with the liver, and it passes through the diaphragm into the heart.
2. *Off-axis view:* Determination of preload sensitivity requires an accurate measurement of IVC diameter. The scanning plane must be orientated along the midline of the IVC and along its longitudinal axis in order to assure accurate diameter measurement.
3. *Translational artifact:* Preload sensitivity is determined by IVC diameter change when the patient is on ventilatory support without spontaneous respiratory effort. When the ventilator cycles, the liver is displaced by diaphragmatic movement. This may move the IVC out of the initial scanning plane, giving the impression of diameter change that actually is a translational artifact. This is an important consideration, because preload sensitivity may be determined by IVC diameter change. Translational artifact may result in a spurious measurement.

THE ADVANCED CCE EXAMINATION

The majority of intensivists will develop skill in basic CCE but do not need higher level capability. A minority based upon practice needs will develop competence in advanced CCE. This section reviews the views that are required for the advanced CCE examination.

▶ Parasternal Long-Axis View

Echocardiographic findings

In addition to the features already described in the basic CCE section, standard M-mode measurements, measurement of left ventricular outflow tract (LVOT) diameter for SV calculation, measurement of LA volume, and detailed assessment of valve morphology and function.

▶ Right Ventricular Inflow and Outflow Long-Axis Views

From the parasternal long-axis view, the transducer is angled medially (Figure 7-6 and Case 7-6). This shifts the tomographic plane to display the RV, TV, and RA. An adequate RV inflow image shows only the RV and not the LV. The anterior and septal leaflets of the TV are visible. Care must be taken to start with an on axis parasternal long-axis view in order to visualize the right ventricular inflow and outflow views. To obtain the outflow view, the intensivist moves the transducer slightly medially toward the sternum, while tilting towards the base of the heart and rotating the transducer clockwise. This results in a long-axis view of the RVOT, the pulmonic valve (PV), and the pulmonary artery (PA).

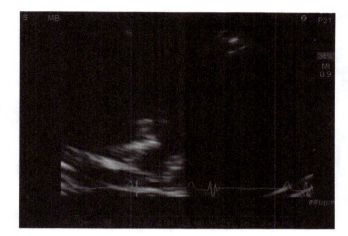

Figure 7-6 The right ventricular inflow view.

CASE 7-6

Right Ventricular Inflow View

Video 7-6A shows the right ventricular inflow view. The anterior tricuspid leaflet is morphologically normal, but the septal leaflet is obscured by an echogenic focus. It does not have the appearance of a vegetation or catheter, but instead is an artifact. Artifacts are common and represent a challenge to the examiner both at basic and advanced training level. The key observation here is that the part of the artifact is not moving in synchrony with surrounding structures and has no other reasonable explanation. In addition, it was not visible on any other view. Video 7-6B shows color Doppler interrogation of the tricuspid valve with what is mild to moderate tricuspid regurgitation (TR), although other views will need to be examined. The directionality of the color jet is ideal for measurement of the trans-valvular velocity gradient, which would allow an estimate of pulmonary artery systolic pressure. The TR jet velocity would need to be measured from other views as well.

Video is available at www.ccu2e.com

Echocardiographic findings

Evaluation of TV/PV anatomy and function and RA/RVOT anatomy; color and spectral Doppler analysis for measurement of TV/PV regurgitation, cardiac pressures (i.e., for estimate of pulmonary systolic pressures).

▶ Parasternal Short-Axis View

By angling toward the base of the heart, the aortic level (Figure 7-7 and Case 7-7) comes into view. This short-axis view results in a cross section of the AV. Medial tilting shows the TV, while lateral tilting and superior

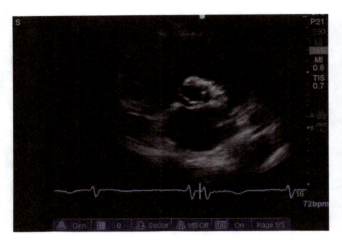 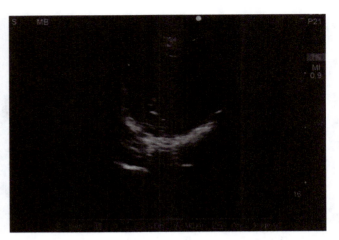

Figure 7-7 The parasternal short-axis view aortic valve level. Figure 7-8 The parasternal short-axis view mitral valve level.

CASE 7-7
Parasternal Short-axis View at Aortic Valve Level

Video 7-7A shows the aortic valve (AV), the tricuspid valve (TV), and the pulmonic valve (PV) in the parasternal short-axis AV view. The AV has three leaflets, which are morphologically normal. Video 7-7B shows no evidence of AV regurgitation with color Doppler. Video 7-7C shows mild tricuspid regurgitation (TR) with color Doppler, but the jet appears truncated. The TR velocity gradient would be measured at this site as matter of routine, but several other views would be required before any conclusion could be made concerning the severity of the TR or the velocity gradient. Video 7-7D shows mild pulmonic regurgitation with a regurgitant jet that is well positioned for Doppler interrogation, in order to estimate pulmonary artery diastolic pressure. Video 7-7E shows the main pulmonary artery (MPA). It is difficult to obtain this view in adult patients, but if obtained, it can be used for Doppler interrogation of MPA outflow, to measure PA diameter (enlarged in this case), and occasionally to identify pulmonary emboli.

Video is available at www.ccu2e.com

CASE 7-8
Parasternal Short-axis View at Mitral Valve Level

Video 7-8A shows a parasternal short-axis view at the mitral valve (MV) level. The main utility of this study is to assess segmental wall function of the basal segments, which are normal in this case. MV function may be observed as well, although other views may be more helpful. Video 7-8B shows severely reduced left ventricular (LV) function without segmental wall abnormality (acknowledging the poor basal anterior and basal anterolateral wall visualization). In conjunction with the reduced LV function, there is reduced opening of the MV. Video 7-8C demonstrates a less common cause of reduced MV opening related to mitral stenosis. Planimetry of the MV opening is one method of measuring the severity of MS, although it requires attention to gain, angle, and cross section; Doppler based methods should also be utilized.

Video is available at www.ccu2e.com

---

angling of the transducer permits visualization of the PV and proximal PA. Angling the transducer inferiorly results in a cross-sectional view of the anterior and posterior leaflets of the MV (Figure 7-8 and Case 7-8). More inferior angulation of the transducer results in a cross section of the LV at the level of the anterolateral and posteromedial papillary muscles (Figure 7-2 and Case 7-2). A cross-sectional view of the apex finishes the parasternal short-axis examination (Figure 7-9 and Case 7-9).

Echocardiographic findings

In addition to the features already described in the basic CCE section, detailed evaluation of anatomy and function of MV/TV/PV/AV with 2D imaging, and CW/PW/color Doppler; LV/RV function, detailed segmental wall function using ASE segments measurement of intracardiac pressures; and evaluation of pericardial space.

▶ Apical Four-Chamber View
Echocardiographic findings

In addition to the features already described in the basic CCE section, detailed evaluation of anatomy and function of MV/TV with CW/PW/color Doppler; LV/RV function including Simpson's SV/EF, tricuspid annular planar systolic excursion, detailed segmental wall function using ASE segments, measurement of intracardiac pressures, tissue Doppler of valve annulus, Doppler measurements of pulmonary venous flow; and pericardial space (Figure 7-3 and Case 7-3).

▶ Apical Five-Chamber View

From the apical four-chamber view, the transducer is angled anteriorly to obtain an image of the LVOT and AV (Figure 7-10 and Case 7-10).

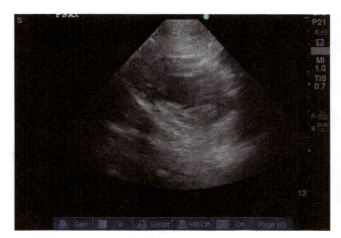

Figure 7-9 The parasternal short-axis view apical level.

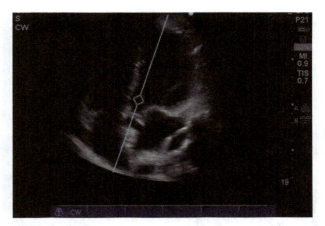

Figure 7-10 The apical five-chamber view.

CASE 7-9
Parasternal Short-axis View at the Apical Level

Video 7-9 shows a parasternal short-axis view at the apical level. The left ventricular function is normal. There is significant respiratory translational artifact, such that the heart moves between the apical and midventricular tomographic planes in respirophasic pattern. At the apical level, there are four wall segments instead of the six that are assigned at the mid and basal levels. The main utility of this view is to examine segmental wall function.

Video is available at www.ccu2e.com

CASE 7-10
Apical Five-Chamber View

Video 7-10A shows an apical five-chamber (AP5) view with the Doppler sample volume positioned to measure stroke volume. The actual measurement will be made with pulsed wave Doppler, rather than continuous wave Doppler. An alternative method is to use the apical three-chamber view. Video 7-10B shows the AP5 view with mild aortic regurgitation (AR). This view may be used to make Doppler measurements to estimate the severity of AR and with AR, to estimate left ventricular end diastolic pressure.

Video is available at www.ccu2e.com

Echocardiographic findings

Measurement of SV using PW Doppler, determination of preload sensitivity by dynamic indices (see Chapter 10), and detailed evaluation of anatomy and function of AV with CW/PW/color Doppler.

▶ Apical Two-Chamber View

From the apical four-chamber view position, the transducer is rotated counterclockwise approximately 60° without movement, angulation, or tilting to obtain a view of the LV and LA (Figure 7-11 and Case 7-11).

Echocardiographic findings

Detailed evaluation of anatomy and function of MV with CW/PW/color Doppler; LV function including Simpson's SV/EF, detailed segmental wall function using ASE segments, measurement of intracardiac pressures, and pericardial space.

▶ Apical Three-Chamber View

From the apical two-chamber view, the transducer is rotated counterclockwise approximately 60° without movement, angulation, or tilting to obtain a view of the LV,

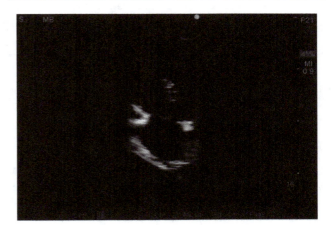

Figure 7-11 The apical two-chamber view.

CASE 7-11
Apical Two-Chamber View

Video 7-11A shows an apical two-chamber view. Video 7-11B shows the same image with color Doppler. The main utility of this view is to assess segmental wall function, but it can also be used to make Doppler measurements of mitral function and to examine the morphology of the mitral valve. As with other apical views, it is often difficult to obtain an on axis image of this view in the critically ill patient.

Video is available at www.ccu2e.com

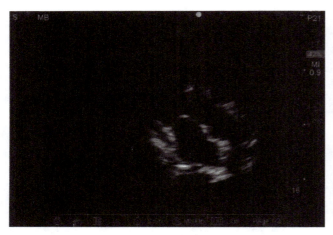

Figure 7-12 The apical three-chamber view.

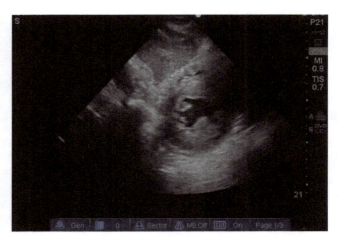

Figure 7-13 The subcostal short-axis view.

CASE 7-12
Apical Three-Chamber View

Video 7-12A shows an apical three-chamber view. Video 7-12B shows the same image with color Doppler. The main utility of this view is to assess segmental wall function, but it can also be used to make Doppler measurements of mitral and aortic valve function and to examine the morphology of the both valves. It is an alternative to the apical five-chamber view for measurement of stroke volume. Overall left ventricular function is normal. There is possibility of apical hypokinesis, but near field resolution is suboptimal. Other views showed normal apical function. As with other apical views, it is often difficult to obtain an on axis image of this view in the critically ill patient.

Video is available at www.ccu2e.com

CASE 7-13
Subcostal Short-axis View at Midventricular Level

Video 7-13 shows the subcostal (SC) short-axis view at the midventricular level. Left ventricular (LV) function is normal. The LV wall thickness is abnormal consistent with hypertrophy. The right ventricular free wall is also of abnormal thickness. Standard measurements by M-mode of caliper technique are required for a quantitative statement. The SC short-axis view gives similar information as the parasternal short-axis midventricular view, and is often the only such view that is available in the critically ill patient on ventilatory support.

Video is available at www.ccu2e.com

LA, RV, LVOT, AV, and ascending aorta (Figure 7-12 and Case 7-12). The view is similar to the parasternal long-axis view except that the apex is in the near view.

Echocardiographic findings

Detailed evaluation of anatomy and function of MV/AV with CW/PW/color Doppler; LV function including measurement of SV using PW Doppler, detailed segmental wall function using ASE segments, measurement of intracardiac pressures; and pericardial space.

▶ Subcostal Four-Chamber View
Echocardiographic findings

In addition to the features already described in the basic CCE section, detailed evaluation of anatomy and function of MV/TV with CW/PW/color Doppler; LV/ RV function, detailed segmental wall function using ASE segments, measurement of intracardiac pressures, LA/RA size, intraatrial septal anatomy and function, observation of right sided agitated saline contrast injection; and pericardial space (Figure 7-4 and Case 7-4).

▶ Subcostal Short-Axis View

From the subcostal four-chamber view, the transducer is rotated counterclockwise 90° without movement, angulation, or tilting to obtain a cross section of the LV similar to that obtained with the parasternal short-axis midventricular view (Figure 7-13 and Case 7-13). Slight counterclockwise rotation yields a long-axis view of the RVOT, PV, and main pulmonary artery to its bifurcation (Figure 7-14 and Case 7-14).

Echocardiographic findings

Evaluation of LV/RV function, detailed segmental wall function using ASE segments, evaluation of anatomy and function of PV with CW/PW/color Doppler.

▶ IVC Longitudinal View
Echocardiographic findings

In addition to the features already described in the basic CCE section, estimate of right atrial pressure, and Doppler analysis of the hepatic venous flow (Figure 7-5 and Case 7-5).

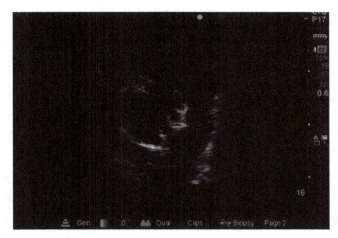

Figure 7-14 The subcostal main pulmonary artery view.

CASE 7-14

Subcostal Main Pulmonary Artery View

Video 7-14 shows a subcostal main pulmonary artery (MPA) view. The color Doppler grid is placed over the tricuspid valve where there is a truncated color Doppler tricuspid regurgitation (TR) jet. Other views are indicated in order to grade the severity of the TR and to measure the TR jet velocity. Visualization of the MPA allows Doppler interrogation of the MPA, measurement of MPA diameter, and occasional identification of pulmonary emboli.

Video is available at www.ccu2e.com

▶ Suprasternal and Supraclavicular Views

These are uncommon views for the advanced CCE and may be reviewed in standard textbooks. The transducer is placed in the suprasternal or supraclavicular area with the scanning plane directed toward the heart and great vessels. The transducer may be manipulated in order to obtain the axis appropriate to the study question. These views are not part of the basic CCE examination.

Echocardiographic findings

Evaluation of aorta anatomy, and CW/PW/color Doppler analysis of AV flow, aortic, and superior vena cava flow.

CONCLUSION

Competence in basic and advanced CCE requires skill in image acquisition, as the frontline intensivist personally performs and interprets the echocardiogram at the bedside of the critically ill patient. Proficiency at transducer manipulation is therefore a mandatory part of proficiency in CCE. This chapter reviews transducer manipulation and serves as a guide for the intensivist interested in developing skill at CCE.

REFERENCES

1. Henry WL, DeMaria A, Gramiak R, et al. Report of the American Society of Echocardiography committee on nomenclature and standards in two-dimensional echocardiography. *Circulation.* 1980;62:212–217.
2. Cholley BP. International expert statement on training standards for critical care ultrasonography. *Intensive Care Med.* 2011;37:1077–1083.
3. Mayo PH, Beaulieu Y, Doelken P, et al. American College of Chest Physicians/La Société de Réanimation de Langue Française Statement on Competence in Critical Care Ultrasonography. *Chest.* 2009;135:1050–1060.

TRANSESOPHAGEAL ECHOCARDIOGRAPHY: IMAGE ACQUISITION AND TRANSDUCER MANIPULATION

Scan QR code or visit www.ccu2e.com for video in this chapter

VIERA LAKTICOVA & PAUL H. MAYO

INTRODUCTION

The value of performing transesophageal echocardiography (TEE) in the intensive care unit (ICU) is well established. Although transthoracic echocardiography (TTE) is a useful diagnostic tool in the ICU, TEE has superior diagnostic accuracy and therapeutic impact in several clinical situations, particularly for patients in shock states.[1-3] Several authors have demonstrated that TEE findings lead to major therapeutic decisions between 43% and 68% of the time.[1,4-6] TEE produces good image quality due to the position of the probe proximate to the heart, allowing for the use of higher frequency ultrasound with superior resolution of cardiac structures than with TTE. Although improvements in imaging, software, and portable systems have reduced the rates of inadequate image quality seen with TTE, there remain a significant percentage of patients in the ICU whose image quality with TTE is inadequate. Many factors account for this including inadequate patient positioning, lung hyperinflation, obesity, edema, and the presence of chest devices, wounds, and dressings. TTE results in adequate image quality in approximately 55% of mechanically ventilated ICU patients, with the remaining 23% and 22% of studies being of suboptimal and poor quality, respectively.[3] In addition to overcoming poor image quality of TTE, TEE is often necessary for the evaluation of specific diagnoses in the ICU such as endocarditis, identifying an embolic source, intracardiac shunt, aortic dissection, and loculated pericardial effusion. For hemodynamic assessment, TEE is the only method to assess superior vena cava (SVC) variation, a predictor of volume responsiveness.[7] When compared with helical computed tomography (CT), TEE has good sensitivity and specificity for central pulmonary embolism (PE) associated with right ventricular dilatation.[8,9]

Critical care TEE differs from standard cardiology TEE in several ways. Typically, TEE performed by a cardiologist is an elective procedure, which has specific indications such as the evaluation for left atrial appendage thrombus, diagnosis of congenital heart disease, identification of valvular abnormalities such as endocarditis, and assessment of prosthetic valve function. Most often, the patient is not on ventilatory support and the procedure is performed outside of the ICU. In comparison, critical care TEE emphasizes hemodynamic evaluation of cardiopulmonary failure. It is a useful diagnostic tool allowing differentiation between shock subtypes in the critically ill while replacing invasive procedures such as the insertion of a pulmonary artery catheter. Because this chapter is written for the intensivist, our emphasis will be on utilization of TEE in the critical care setting rather than focusing on a cardiology type TEE examination.

Critical care TEE is routinely performed in large ICUs in Europe; for example, in Hospital Ambroise-Pare in Boulogne and the Erasme University Hospital in Brussels, where it is considered a routine procedure for the assessment of the shock state. In France, there is a well-defined training sequence for attendings and fellows developed by Societe de Reanimation de Langue Francaise that includes training in critical care TEE. In Australia, TEE is also is a common tool for the assessment of hemodynamic failure in the ICU. By comparison, critical care TEE is not widely used by intensivists in North America with the exception of cardiac anesthesiologists who have responsibility within an ICU. One reason for this dichotomy is that in the Europe, critical care specialists come from a variety of training backgrounds including cardiology. As a result, some intensivists have formal cardiology training in echocardiography before entering critical care subspecialty training. In the United States, formal training for critical care fellows in TEE is still very uncommon.

INDICATIONS FOR TEE

The most common indications for critical care TEE are as follows:

1. Assessment of hemodynamic failure, if TTE views are inadequate.

   Echocardiography is a primary tool for the evaluation of shock in the ICU. There is logic to the consideration that early echocardiography should be a mandatory component of initial and continuing assessment of all patients with hemodynamic failure.[10] This being the case, TEE is indicated when TTE views are inadequate due to factors such as obesity, edema, heavy musculature, dressings, wounds, or hyperinflation. Critical care TEE is particularly useful in certain circumstances for the evaluation of hemodynamic failure where even good quality TTE images may not answer clinical questions such as:

   a. Identification of preload sensitivity. There are a variety of validated methods for the assessment of preload sensitivity using TTE (see Chapter 9). On occasion these may yield equivocal results. Using TEE, the evaluation of size variation in the SVC during mechanical ventilation cycling is easy to perform and may allow the clinician to clarify an ambiguous TTE result in order to identify preload sensitivity.

   b. Identification of PE. Central PE can be visualized with TEE, whereas TTE is not as effective for this application.

   c. Unexplained hypoxemia. Intracardiac shunt (e.g., patent foramen ovale with high right-sided pressures) may be assessed using agitated saline injection. TTE imaging is frequently inadequate, while TEE has excellent image quality for this application.

   d. Identification of aortic dissection. TTE offers only a limited view of the ascending aorta, while TEE allows imaging of the ascending and descending aorta.

   e. Cardiac arrest. TEE can be used to assess the etiology and adequacy of resuscitation efforts during cardiac arrest on a continuous basis, whereas TTE is limited to a brief subcostal view during pulse checks.

2. Other questions that cannot be definitively answered with TTE regardless of image quality. These include an examination for intracardiac thrombus, subtle valvular abnormalities (e.g. vegetation), and detailed Doppler analysis of pulmonary venous inflow. Examination for this type of abnormality represents an overlap with the skill set that is typical for cardiology TEE, but that can be mastered by the intensivist.

TRAINING FOR CRITICAL CARE TEE

Similar to other aspects of critical care ultrasonography, training in critical care TEE includes the mastery of image acquisition, image interpretation, and the cognitive elements of the field (see Chapter 4). Competence in TTE is helpful in training for TEE, as the learner is already familiar with the echocardiographic anatomy. As with all forms of critical care, skill in image acquisition is gained only through practice. Charron et al. report that trainees developed competence in critical care TEE following the performance of approximately 31 supervised studies. In this study, the authors describe a competency-based examination that is a model for fellowship programs to follow in order to assure that training has been successful.[11,12] Sophisticated TEE simulators are available to aid in the acquisition of transducer manipulation skills prior to scanning an actual patient.

PATIENT SELECTION AND PREPARATION

One of the distinguishing points between cardiology and critical care TEE is that intensivists do not generally perform TEE unless the patient is on mechanical ventilatory support. Therefore, the discussion on patient preparation will be limited to the patient who is intubated and on ventilatory support.

TEE is a minimally invasive and safe procedure with a few definite risks.[13] Because, by definition, the patient has an endotracheal tube in place, the risk of airway complication in the mechanically ventilated patient in the ICU is low when compared with the performance of cardiology TEE. Other complications are rare, and include esophageal abrasion, perforation, and bleeding. These can be avoided by appropriate patient selection and by minimizing the rotational movement of the endoscope tip while under flexion (see section Transducer Manipulation).

TEE is contraindicated in the setting of esophageal disease such as esophageal varices, strictures, bleeding, recent surgery, tumor, or diverticula. It is important that an accurate history is obtained that addresses the risk of esophageal injury during TEE. If such conditions are present, a barium swallow or endoscopic evaluation of the esophagus is recommended prior to the procedure.[13] Coagulopathy or thrombocytopenia is a relative contraindication to TEE. If the clinical situation permits, significant abnormalities should be corrected.

ENDOTRACHEALLY INTUBATED PATIENTS

Since mechanically ventilated patients have a secure airway that facilitates intubation, they require minimal airway preparation. Our approach is to augment intravenous sedation so that the patient is deeply sedated during the TEE examination. The patient is monitored with an electrocardiogram (ECG), arterial blood pressure, and oxygen saturation. An ECG signal should be displayed on the TEE ultrasound screen at all times. We recommend that the patient not be spontaneously breathing during the procedure, which may require transient use of a neuromuscular blocking agent. This is important when assessing preload sensitivity with TEE.

PROBE INSERTION

In most patients, the probe can be inserted blindly. The well-lubricated probe is introduced through a mouthpiece in the midline with the transducer surface facing the tongue. It is advanced with gentle forward force and with gradual anteflexion of the device. Flexion of the neck may facilitate insertion into the esophagus.

On occasion, blind insertion is unsuccessful, with the operator encountering significant resistance to forward movement of the probe. In this case, we recommend use of an intubating laryngoscope to expose the esophageal opening. A video laryngoscope is particularly useful in this situation. The TEE probe is then introduced under direct visualization. If the patient has a gastric tube in place, this may need to be removed in order to improve image quality.

EQUIPMENT

The modern TEE probe utilizes a multicrystal, phased-array transducer placed at the tip of a flexible endoscope. The probe can be advanced within the esophagus and positioned directly posterior to the heart, with excellent resolution of cardiac structures.

Historically, TEE probes were equipped with a monoplane transducer that could provide only a single-plane view of the heart that was transverse in orientation. The development of multiplane probes allowed the transducer to be rotated to any position between 0° and 180°. This provides multiple views of the heart when combined with movements of the endoscope such as advancement, turning, or flexion.

An advantage of the proximity of the TEE probe to the heart is that it enables the use of ultrasound frequencies between 5 and 7.5 MHz. This results in superior resolution of posterior cardiac structures when compared with TTE. However, anterior cardiac structures may require reduction in the ultrasound frequency for better penetration, at the expense of reduced resolution. The frequency of the transducer is adjusted according to the distance to the imaging target.

TRANSDUCER MANIPULATION

It is important to standardize the description of operator manipulation of the probe, particularly for communication when two operators are involved with scanning. Each TEE view requires a specific position and orientation of the transducer with respect to the heart. The American Society of Echocardiography (ASE) recommends that the following terms be used to describe transducer movement.

1. Advancement/withdrawal of probe: This is accomplished by moving the probe in and out of the esophagus (the depth of insertion is noted on the shaft of the endoscope).
2. Flexion of probe from the neutral position in four directions: This is accomplished by rotation of the control knobs on the shaft of the endoscope. Rotation of the large knob results in anteflexion of the probe face (moving the face of the probe in an anterior/superior-directed view) or retroflexion of the probe face. Rotation of the small knob results in right or left flexion of the probe face.
3. Turning of the probe to the right or left side: This is accomplished by twisting the shaft in a counterclockwise (to look towards the left side of patient) or clockwise motion (to look towards the right side of patient).
4. Rotation: This is accomplished by changing the plane of orientation of the crystal within the probe. If the operator is standing to the left of the patient and looking down at the patient, the face of the transducer will be facing anteriorly, that is, toward the operator. Rotation of the transducer beam plane occurs in a counterclockwise fashion via an electronic switch that allows for 1° incremental changes. The exact orientation of the transducer is represented by the angle indicator on the screen with values between 0° and 180°.

ORIENTATION OF TEE VIEWS

Knowledge of the standard TEE view orientation relies on two main principles:

1. The ultrasound beam originates from behind the heart. The top or "apex" of the screen displays structures closest to the esophagus, that is, the atria and great vessels when the endoscope is in a neutral position within the esophagus; and the inferior wall of the heart, when it is anteflexed from within the stomach. Structures in the far field of the screen represent anterior cardiac structures. The one exception to this convention is the deep gastric apical four-chamber view, which results in the apex of the heart being projected at the top of the screen.
2. The orientation is described by the degree rotation of the ultrasound beam plane. For example, 0° pertains to the transverse plane, with the leftmost part of the screen pertaining to the rightmost part of the patient (similar to the orientation of a chest x-ray). Increasing the degree rotation corresponds to a counterclockwise rotation of the scan plane; thus, a 90° view results in a longitudinal view, with superior structures to the right of the screen and inferior structures to the left of the screen.

The operators should be familiar with the degree of orientation of the four primary TEE views: (1) 0°: transverse plane, (2) 45°: short-axis view of aortic valve (AV), (3) 90°: oblique, long-axis view, and (4) 135°: "true" long-axis view. These four primary views, when combined with turning and flexion, can produce all of the standard ASE views.

TEE EXAMINATION

The number and sequence of views required for a critical care TEE examination have not been standardized. In its simplest iteration, the examination can be as limited as that of the goal-directed TTE examination. Benjamin et al.

reported on the use of a monoplane pediatric probe by intensivists.[4] Their protocol required four views with three quantitative assessments. Examinations were completed in 12 minutes, and resulted in therapeutic changes in 52% of cases. Intensivists easily developed skill at this type TEE examination. Along these lines, there is now available a miniaturized disposable TEE probe developed for limited assessment of hemodynamic function. Due to its small diameter and flexibility, it may be left indwelling for up to 72 hours, which allows for regular reassessment of hemodynamic status. Vieillard-Baron et al. have demonstrated its safety and feasibility in the ICU,[14] and it has a short learning curve relative to standard TEE. The device is designed to rapidly and repeatedly obtain three basic views for hemodynamic assessment: the transverse SVC view, the four-chamber view, and the gastric short-axis view. Vieillard-Baron et al. described three views with four qualitative assessments.[15] These qualitative assessments were similar to results obtained quantitatively in the same patient. These studies support the concept of goal-directed echocardiography.

In some clinical situations, a comprehensive TEE examination is indicated. In critical care practice, it is neither necessary nor practical to perform a comprehensive TEE examination in all patients. This is an important consideration when evaluating the acutely ill patient with severe hemodynamic failure in a busy ICU environment or when using TEE as a monitoring tool. Vieillard-Baron et al. have described the use of serial daily TEE examinations in sepsis with circulatory failure using a limited number of views for the purpose of guiding volume resuscitation and inotrope/pressor use.[16]

The limited or goal-directed approach may have particular application for rapid assessment of the very unstable patient and for brief repeated examinations to determine response to therapy or evolution of disease. Full competence in critical care TEE is part of advanced critical care echocardiography, and requires that the intensivist be proficient in performing a comprehensive TEE examination as well as limited goal-directed approach.

The complete TEE examination as defined by the ASE consists of 28 standard views.[17] Obtaining all views in every examination requires a significant amount of time, which may not always be practical in the ICU. By convention, cardiologists generally perform a complete TEE examination with full assessment of all cardiac structures. In comparison, the intensivist may perform the TEE for a specific indication, such as the determination of preload sensitivity or identification of acute cor pulmonale pattern. If indicated, the comprehensive cardiology type TEE examination may still be performed.

Because the chapter is intended for intensivists, we will not review all components of the complete TEE examination as performed by cardiologists. Instead, we describe an examination designed to rapidly assess hemodynamic

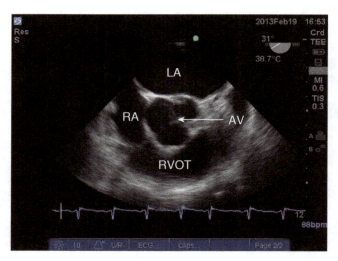

Figure 8-1 Aortic valve short-axis view. AV, aortic valve; LA, left atrium; RA, right atrium; RVOT, right ventricular out flow tract.

function that is used by the critical care group at Hospital Ambroise-Pare in Boulogne, France, headed by Dr. Vieillard-Baron.[11,12] There are many variations that can be proposed for this type of TEE examination in terms of the sequence and the views that can be obtained. It is important for the development of the field to adapt a standard examination sequence, so that training standards and competency-based testing are comparable across international borders. The French hemodynamic TEE examination fulfills these requirements, and it is what we propose as a minimum standard for the intensivist. Other elements of the TEE examination may be included when indicated. An added advantage to using the French approach is that it permits standardization of competency-based testing, an issue of importance for faculty engaged in training fellows in critical care TEE.

TEE VIEWS

1. *Midesophageal AV short-axis view with and without color Doppler* (Figure 8-1)

Rotation: 30°–45°

Transducer positioning: In neutral position, the probe tip is advanced into the esophagus until the AV appears in short axis. If the AV is not in the center of the screen, the operator may turn probe in the appropriate direction to place the target in central screen position. At the 0° position, the beam plane does not achieve a true short axis due to the tangential course of the aorta as it leaves the heart. To achieve a true short axis of the AV, the beam plane is rotated to approximately 30–45°, so that all three AV leaflets and commissures with a coaptation point are seen.

Clinical utility: Aortic and periaortic valve anatomy and function, ascending aorta anatomy, and left atrial anatomy. See Case 8-1.

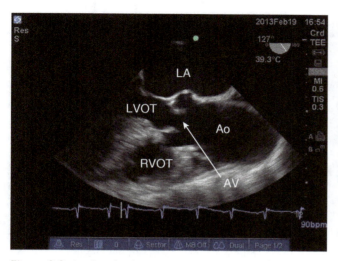

Figure 8-2 Aortic valve long-axis view. AV, aortic valve; Ao, ascending aorta; LA, left atrium; LVOT, left ventricular out flow tract; RVOT, right ventricular out flow tract.

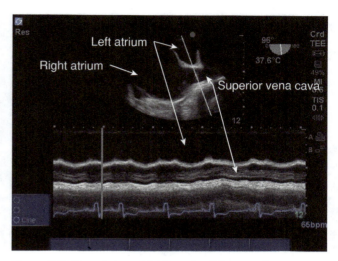

Figure 8-3 Bicaval view with M-mode of the superior vena cava. Structures are as indicated.

2. *Midesophageal AV long-axis view with and without color Doppler* (Figure 8-2)

   Rotation: 120°–135°

   Transducer positioning: From the short axis, the beam plane is rotated an additional 90° until the entire course of the left ventricular outflow tract (LVOT), AV, and the proximal ascending aorta are seen. This may require slight turning of the probe to obtain an on axis image.

   Clinical utility: Aortic and periaortic valve anatomy and function, ascending aorta anatomy, and left atrial anatomy. See Case 8-1.

3. *Midesophageal bicaval view* (Figure 8-3)

   Rotation: 0° and 90°

   From the AV long-axis view, the beam plane is rotated back to 0°, and the probe is turned in a clockwise rotation until the superior vena cava (SVC) or high right atrium (RA) is placed at the center of the screen. The transducer beam plane is then rotated to 90°, in order to visualize the SVC and RA in longitudinal axis. It may be necessary to turn, withdraw, or advance the probe to achieve an optimal view.

   Clinical utility: SVC thrombus, SVC catheter position, assessment of volume responsiveness, RA anatomy, identification of interatrial connection using agitated saline injection. See Case 8-2.

CASE 8-1
Hypotension and Urosepsis

This transesophageal echocardiogram (TEE) was performed on a patient who presented with hypotension and urosepsis with poor-quality transthoracic echocardiography (TTE) views. In the short-axis view, the aortic valve (AV) has no anatomic abnormality and color Doppler interrogation reveals no regurgitation (Video 8-1A and 8-1B). This is confirmed in the long-axis view of the AV (Video 8-1C). There is a left atrial mass, which was an unanticipated finding. A common indication for TEE is in the patient with hemodynamic failure where TTE views are of poor quality. The examination includes the assessment of valve function to look for a lesion that will complicate management or for the occasional unanticipated finding of catastrophic valve failure causing the shock state. In this case, the AV was normal. The unanticipated finding of a left atrial mass reminds the intensivist to remain alert for incidental findings that are separate from the primary structure of interest. The mass was a sarcoma.

Video is available at www.ccu2e.com

CASE 8-2
Hypotension

This transesophageal echocardiogram (TEE) was performed on a patient who presented with hypotension and poor-quality transthoracic echocardiography views. The patient was on ventilatory support and without any spontaneous breathing effort. The bicaval view shows a pacer wire in the superior vena cava (SVC) with adherent masses consistent with pacer wire thrombi (Video 8-2). At the end of the video clip there is possible reduction in SVC size. This could reflect preload sensitivity or respiratory translational artifact. An M-mode tracing of the SVC shows no respiratory variation indicating absence of preload sensitivity (Figure 8-3). The bicaval view of the SVC has major utility for determination of preload sensitivity. To make the measurement of respiratory variation, the patient must be passive in their interaction with the ventilator; but this is usually the case during performance of the TEE. The incidental finding of pacer wire thrombi complicates management of the case, as an argument can made in favor of anticoagulation. The unanticipated finding of the thrombi reminds the intensivist to remain alert for incidental findings that are separate from the primary structure of interest.

Video is available at www.ccu2e.com

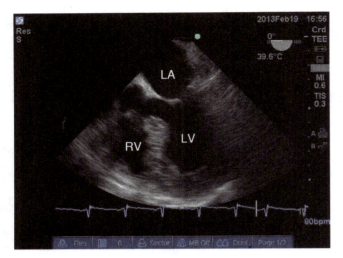

Figure 8-4 Four-chamber view. LA, left atrium; LV, left ventricle; RV, right ventricle.

4. *SVC M mode view* (Figure 8-3)

   Rotation: 90°
   The M-mode cursor is placed across the SVC in order to record respiratory variation in the SVC.
   Clinical utility: Assessment of preload sensitivity. See Cases 8-2

5. *Midesophageal four-chamber view with and without color Doppler* (Figure 8-4)

   Rotation: 0°
   From the bicaval view, the beam plane is rotated back to 0°, and the probe is turned counterclockwise until the mitral valve (MV) is in central screen position. The probe is then advanced slightly until a four-chamber view is achieved. Retroflexion of the probe may be required to optimize the view of all four chambers.
   Clinical utility: RV and LV chamber size and function, anatomy and function of the tricuspid valve and MV, inferoseptal and anterolateral left ventricular (LV) wall contractility. See Cases 8-3 to 8-6.

6. *Midesophageal long-axis view with and without color Doppler* (Figure 8-5)

   Rotation: 90–120°
   From the four-chamber view with the LV in the central screen position, the beam plane is rotated to 90–120° in order to obtain a three-chamber view.

CASE 8-3

Unexplained Hypotension

This transesophageal echocardiogram (TEE) was performed on a patient who presented with unexplained hypotension and poor-quality transthoracic echocardiography (TTE) views. The left ventricular function is normal, as is the size and function of the right ventricle (Video 8-3A). There is no pericardial effusion and the mitral valve anatomy is normal without major mitral regurgitation (Video 8-3B). A common indication for TEE is when TTE is not of adequate quality to answer the clinical question at hand. In this case, TEE results did not establish a cause for the shock state. Was the study of clinical utility; or was it, being normal, unnecessary? A normal result is a useful result, as it allows the intensivist to rapidly exclude a variety dangerous diagnoses. The TEE results suggest that the patient has distributive shock and that treatment with pressor agents is indicated without use of inotropic support. Determination of preload sensitivity will require other TEE views. The patient had septic shock as a final diagnosis.

Video is available at www.ccu2e.com

CASE 8-4

Fever, Elevated White Count, and Hypotension

This transesophageal echocardiogram (TEE) was performed on a patient who presented with fever, elevated white count, and hypotension with poor-quality transthoracic echocardiography views. The left ventricular function is normal, but the right ventricle (RV) is dilated (Video 8-4A). There is trace mitral regurgitation (Video 8-4B), and an indeterminate amount of tricuspid regurgitation, as a wall jet is present (Video 8-4C). This patient presented with septic shock. The TEE examination showed a dilated RV. This prompted the critical care team to search for additional diagnosis, and led to discovery of pulmonary emboli related to deep venous thrombosis diagnosed by the intensivist with a bedside study. The presence of RV dilation represents a specific contraindication to volume resuscitation unless there is other definitive indication of preload sensitivity. Early performance of TEE established a dual diagnosis for the shock state, and allowed the team to avoid inappropriate volume resuscitation.

Video is available at www.ccu2e.com

CASE 8-5

Hypotension and Severe LV Failure

This transesophageal echocardiogram (TEE) was performed on a patient who presented with hypotension, a history of severe left ventricular (LV) failure, and poor-quality transthoracic echocardiography (TTE) views. There is severe LV dysfunction with evidence of segmental wall abnormality (Video 8-5). The anterolateral wall is contracting to some extent, while the inferoseptum is akinetic. This was noted on other views. The segmental wall abnormality suggests an ischemic pattern, although it is not diagnostic. The image is somewhat off axis, and would be supplemented by several other images. A more complete hemodynamic assessment would require measurement of the LV stroke volume (SV) (see Cases 8-11 and 8-12), as LV dysfunction with severe reduction of ejection fraction may not necessarily be associated with a reduction of SV.

Video is available at www.ccu2e.com

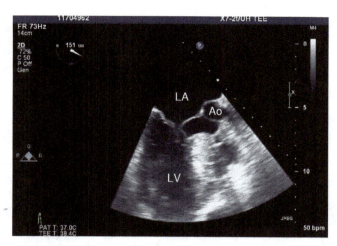

Figure 8-5 Three-chamber view. Ao, aorta; LA, left atrium; LV, left ventricle.

Clinical utility: RV and LV chamber size and function, anatomy and function of the MV and AV. LVOT anatomy, anteroseptal and inferolateral LV wall contractility. See Case 8-7.

7. *MV inflow*

Rotation: 0°

In the four-chamber view, the pulsed wave Doppler sample volume is placed at the opening of the MV valve tips and MV inflow is measured.

Clinical utility: Assessment of LV diastolic function (estimate of left atrial pressure and grading of diastolic dysfunction). See Case 8-8.

CASE 8-6
Fever, Severe Dyspnea, Hypotension, and Bilateral Diffuse B Lines with Smooth Pleural Surface

This transesophageal echocardiogram (TEE) was performed on a patient who presented several days of fever, sudden onset of severe dyspnea, hypotension, bilateral diffuse B lines with smooth pleural surface, and inadequate transthoracic echocardiography (TTE) views. There is a mitral valve (MV) vegetation with a flail leaflet (Video 8-6A). The mitral regurgitation (MR) by color Doppler does not appear severe on this view, but the color Doppler jet suggests a wall jet pattern (Video 8-6B). Wall jets systematically underestimate the severity of MR. Other measurements such as vena contracta or regurgitant fraction and volume would need to be performed for quantitative measurement of the MR. The combination of acute respiratory failure, evidence of acute cardiogenic pulmonary edema on lung ultrasonography examination with hypotension prompted the critical care team to consider catastrophic valve failure. Prompt identification of the MV failure led to insertion of an aortic balloon pump and lifesaving surgical intervention. An early TEE examination was indicated in view of the nondiagnostic TTE examination.

Video is available at www.ccu2e.com

CASE 8-7
Hypotension and Ventilatory Support

This transesophageal echocardiogram (TEE) was performed on a patient who presented with hypotension, while on augmenting doses of dobutamine and diuretics and ventilatory support that included PEEP. Transthoracic echocardiography views were inadequate. There is systolic anterior motion of the anterior mitral leaflet (SAM) (Video 8-7A) and turbulent flow pattern in the left ventricular outflow track (LVOT) on color Doppler (Video 8-7B). Although not a common finding, SAM may have hemodynamic consequence if combined with inotropic support, diuresis, and mechanical ventilatory support that tends to reduce venous return and preload. As the LVOT obstruction worsens due to the SAM, the MR may also worsen due to displacement of the anterior leaflet. TEE allowed identification of this pattern. The critical care team responded by giving volume and switching to phenylephrine with improvement of hemodynamics.

Video is available at www.ccu2e.com

---

8. *Tissue Doppler Imaging (TDI) of lateral MV annulus*

Rotation: 0°

In is the four-chamber view, the TDI sample volume is placed on the lateral MV annulus and the TDI velocities are measured.

Clinical utility: Assessment of LV diastolic function (estimate of left atrial pressure and grading of diastolic dysfunction). See Case 8-8.

9. *Transgastric midpapillary short-axis view* (Figure 8-6)

Rotation: 0°

The probe is advanced into the stomach and anteflexed. This results in a short-axis view of the LV similar

---

CASE 8-8
Respiratory Failure, Bilateral B Lines, and Reduced LV Function

This transesophageal echocardiogram was performed on a patient with respiratory failure and bilateral B lines on lung ultrasonography with reduced left ventricular (LV) function. Case Figure 8-8A is of the mitral valve diastolic inflow and is a required measurement when using the standard algorithm for estimating left atrial pressures in the patient with reduced LV function (see Chapter 9). The E/A ratio is 1.5, so that the mitral valve annular velocity is required to give an estimate of LAP. Case Figure 8-8B is of the lateral mitral annular velocity measured with tissue Doppler imaging of the same patient. This is a required measurement when using the standard algorithm for estimating left atrial pressures in the patient with reduced LV function (see Chapter 9). The e' velocity is 11.6 cm/s. So the E/e' ratio is 5.8. The LAP is normal. The bilateral B lines are not caused by elevation of LAP, but rather by a primary lung process.

See entire case at www.ccu2e.com

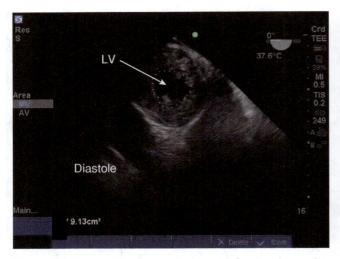 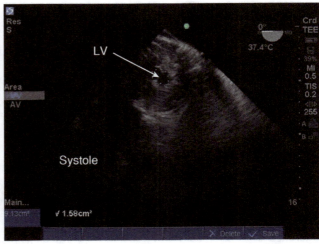

Figure 8-6 Transgastric short-axis view with fractional area change measurements. LV, left ventricle.

to the TTE parasternal short-axis midventricular view at the papillary muscle level.

Clinical utility: LV chamber size, function, and segmental wall motion analysis, RV size and function, septal kinetics. See Case 8-9.

10. *Fractional area change* **(FAC%)** (Figure 8-6)

   Rotation: 0°

   The FAC% is performed from the transgastric mid-papillary short-axis view. A frozen image of the LV cavity is performed in systole and in diastole. Using the cursor function, the area of the LV cavity at the papillary muscle level is measured.

   The FAC% is calculated as (EDA-ESA)/EDA, where EDA is end-diastolic area and ESA is end-systolic area.

   Clinical utility: Assessment of LV systolic function. See Case 8-10.

11. *Transgastric long-axis view* (Figure 8-7)

   Rotation: 120°

   From the transgastric short-axis view, the transducer beam plane is rotated to 120° in order to expose the LVOT. The pulsed wave Doppler sample volume is placed within LVOT to measure the LVOT velocity time integral (VTI).

   Clinical utility: Calculation of LV stroke volume variation in the stroke volume during ventilator cycling. See Case 8-11.

CASE 8-9

Two Patients with Unexplained Hypotension

Video 8-9A was performed on a patient with unexplained hypotension and poor-quality transthoracic echocardiography (TTE) views. Overall left ventricular function (LV) and septal kinetics are normal. There is end systolic effacement of the left ventricle (LV). Video 8-9B was performed on a patient with unexplained hypotension and pulmonary artery hypertension with poor-quality transthoracic echocardiography (TTE) views while on ventilatory support that included PEEP of 15 cm H$_2$O. There is septal flattening at the end of systole and during diastole. The transgastric short-axis view is often easy to obtain and gives a useful assessment of overall LV function, as well as septal kinetics. The patient in Video 8-9A had distributive shock due to sepsis with end systolic effacement of the LV cavity. The critical care team assessed preload sensitivity and gave volume resuscitation to the patient while treating the hypotension with phenylephrine. Regarding the patient in Video 8-9B, the late systolic flattening of the septum reflected the prolonged right ventricular (RV) ejection caused by the pulmonary hypertension (pressure overload of the RV), while the diastolic septal flattening was caused by severe tricuspid regurgitation (volume overload of the RV). The critical care team gave diuretics to the patient and took measures to reduce RV afterload by reducing PEEP with ventilator adjustment.

Video is available at www.ccu2e.com

CASE 8-10

Calculation of FAC in Patient with Unexplained Hypotension

This transesophageal echocardiogram was performed on a patient with unexplained hypotension. The images show the left ventricle using the transgastric short-axis view in systole and diastole. The endomyocardial borders are traced (not including the papillary muscles) to derive the fractional area change (FAC). The FAC% is calculated as (EDA—ESA)/EDA, where EDA is end-diastolic area (Case Figure 8-10A) and ESA is end-systolic area (Case Figure 8-10B). In this case, this FAC is 83%. An FAC above 48% is normal. The FAC is an index of overall LV function that is straightforward to perform when compared to the complexity of the formal Simpson's measurement. The transgastric short-axis view is generally easy to obtain, and the planimetry can be done quickly. A problem with the measurement occurs if there is segmental wall abnormality as the FAC measurement reflects function only at the mid segmental level.

See entire case at www.ccu2e.com

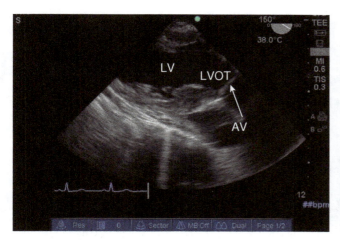

Figure 8-7 Transgastric long-axis view. AV, aortic valve; LV, left ventricle; LVOT, left ventricular out flow tract.

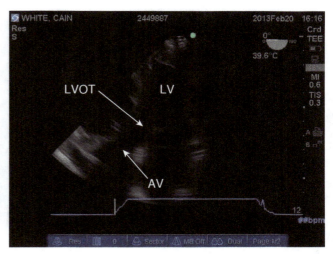

Figure 8-8 Deep gastric long-axis view. AV, aortic valve; LV, left ventricle; LVOT, left ventricular out flow tract.

An alternative method to measure the LVOT VTI is from the deep gastric view. The probe is inserted at 0° to the apex of the heart and fully anteflexed until the LVOT is identified. This is similar to the TTE five-chamber view. The pulsed wave sample volume is placed in the LVOT to measure the VTI (Figure 8-8) (Case 8-12).

12. *Midesophageal ascending aorta short-axis view (including main pulmonary artery (MPA) VTI (Figure 8-9)*

    Rotation: 0°
    Probe is withdrawn until the right pulmonary artery (RPA) is identified, which is immediately above the left atrium. Once the RPA is visualized, the probe is rotated counterclockwise with some increased beam plane angle until the MPA is seen. This may require adjustment of probe flexion. The pulsed wave sample volume is placed in MPA in order to measure the MPA VTI.

The left pulmonary artery is difficult to visualize due to interposition of the air filled trachea. This view is also useful for imaging the ascending aorta.

Clinical utility: Anatomy of the MPA and RPA, examination for proximal PE, measurements derived from MPA VTI, anatomy of the ascending aorta. See Case 8-13.

Additional views: The preceding views should be considered a minimum standard for hemodynamic assessment by TEE. There are a variety of other views that have utility for intensivist and may be used depending on the clinical situation. For example, measurement of pulmonary venous inflow, and observation of the left atrial appendage may have indicated. Examination of

---

CASE 8-11

Septic Shock

This transesophageal echocardiogram (TEE) was performed on a patient with septic shock and poor-quality transthoracic echocardiography (TTE) views. Video 8-11 shows a good-quality transgastric long-axis view at 150° that allowed measurement of the left ventricular outflow track (LVOT) velocity time index (VTI). It was 20.4 cm, which is normal range (Video 8-11). Measurement of the LVOT VTI is a key measurement of both the TEE and TTE examination, as it permits calculation of the LV stroke volume (SV). As a qualitative statement, a LVOT VTI of 18 to 22 cm indicates a normal SV. For quantitative SV, the area of the LVOT must be measured (see Chapter 9). Variation of LVOT VTI may also be used for determination of preload sensitivity providing that the patient is passive on the ventilator with a regular cardiac rhythm and is without right ventricular dysfunction. The long-axis view of the LVOT is generally found between 120° and 150° of rotation.

Video is available at www.ccu2e.com

CASE 8-12

Septic Shock with History of LV Failure

This transesophageal echocardiogram (TEE) was performed on a patient with septic shock with a history of left ventricular failure and poor quality transthoracic echocardiography (TTE) views. Video 8-12 shows a deep gastric long-axis view at 0° that allowed measurement of the left ventricular outflow track (LVOT) velocity time index (VTI) (Video 8-12). It was 11.5 cm, which is well below normal range. Measurement of the LVOT VTI is a key measurement of both the TEE and TTE examination, as it permits calculation of the LV stroke volume (SV). As a qualitative statement, a LVOT VTI of 18–22 cm indicates a normal SV. For quantitative SV, the area of the LVOT must be measured (see Chapter 9). Variation of LVOT VTI may also be used for determination of preload sensitivity providing that the patient is passive on the ventilator with a regular cardiac rhythm and is without right ventricular dysfunction. The deep gastric view of the LVOT is often difficult to obtain. The critical care team measured the LVOT area, calculated the SV, and determined the cardiac index was critically compromised in this patient. Dobutamine was effective in improving hemodynamics.

Video is available at www.ccu2e.com

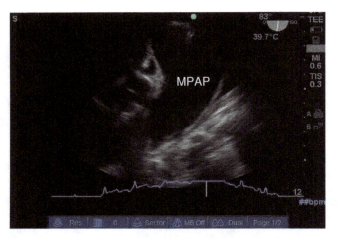

Figure 8-9 Main pulmonary artery view. MPAP, main pulmonary artery.

the aorta may be performed if aortic pathology is of concern.

Descending aorta:

Rotation: 0°

From the short-axis transgastric view, the probe is turned clockwise approximately 180° in order to identify the descending aorta. The transducer is withdrawn to examine the entire descending thoracic aorta. At regular intervals, the transducer can be rotated to 90° to achieve a longitudinal view of aorta. During probe withdrawal, the posteromedial left pleural space may be examined for pleural effusion and lung pathology such as consolidation.

Aortic arch:

Rotation: 0°

In order to image aortic arch, starting at the proximal descending thoracic aorta, the probe is further withdrawn with gradual clockwise turning of the probe in order to image aortic arch. Frequently, air-filled trachea will block full visualization of aortic arch.

PROBE CLEANING

The endoscope should be cleaned according to institutional policy.

CASE 8-13

Unexplained Hypotension

This transesophageal echocardiogram (TEE) was performed on a patient with hypotension and poor quality transthoracic echocardiography (TTE) views. Video 8-13 shows a dilated main pulmonary artery (MPAP). This view is used to measure the MPAP systolic velocity envelope. A short acceleration time (AT) and a biphasic contour would be suggestive of pulmonary artery hypertension (see chapter 11).

Video is available at www.ccu2e.com

CONCLUSION

TEE is useful in the ICU, particularly when TTE image quality is suboptimal. The intensivist may use TEE in a goal-directed fashion for rapid assessment of hemodynamic failure and to guide ongoing therapy of the critically ill patient. Depending on the clinical circumstance, the intensivist may choose to perform a more comprehensive examination that focuses on hemodynamic assessment of the patient with shock. This requires mastery of transducer manipulation, cardiac anatomy, and knowledge of standard views.

REFERENCES

1. Vignon P, Mentec H, Terre S, Gastinne H, Gueret P, Lemaire F. Diagnostic accuracy and therapeutic impact of transthoracic and transesophageal echocardiography in mechanically ventilated patients in the ICU. *Chest.* 1994;106:1829–1834.
2. Huttemann E, Schelenz C, Kara F, Chatzinikolaou K, Rein-hart K. The use and safety of transoesophageal echocardiography in the general ICU—a minireview. *Acta Anaesthesiol Scand.* 2004;48:827–836.
3. Huttemann E. Transesophageal echocardiography in critical care. *Minerva Anestesiol.* 2006;72:891–913.
4. Benjamin E, Griffin K, Leibowitz AB, et al. Goal-directed transesophageal echocardiography performed by intensivists to assess left ventricular function: comparison with pulmonary artery catheterization. *J Cardiothorac Vasc Anesth.* 1998;12:10–15.
5. Colreavy FB, Donovan K, Lee KY, Weekes J. Transesophageal echocardiography in critically ill patients. *Crit Care Med.* 2002;30:989–996.
6. Poelaert JI, Trouerbach J, De Buyzere M, Everaert J, Colardyn FA. Evaluation of transesophageal echocardiography as a diagnostic and therapeutic aid in a critical care setting. *Chest.* 1995;107:774–779.
7. Vieillard-Baron A, Chergui K, Rabiller A, et al. Superior vena caval collapsibility as a gauge of volume status in ventilated septic patients. *Intensive Care Med.* 2004;30:1734–1739.
8. Vieillard-Baron A, Qanadli SD, Antakly Y, et al. Transesophageal echocardiography for the diagnosis of pulmonary embolism with acute cor pulmonale: a comparison with radiological procedures. *Intensive Care Med.* 1998;24:429–433.
9. Krivec B, Voga G, Zuran I, et al. Diagnosis and treatment of shock due to massive pulmonary embolism: approach with transesophageal echocardiography and intrapulmonary thrombolysis. *Chest.* 1997;112:1310–1316.
10. Schmidt GA, Koenig S, Mayo PH. Shock: ultrasound to guide diagnosis and therapy. *Chest.* 2012;142: 1042–1048.
11. Charron C, Prat G, Caille V, et al. Validation of a skills assessment scoring system for transesophageal echocardiographic monitoring of hemodynamics. *Intensive Care Med.* 2007;33:1712–1718.
12. Charron C, Vignon P, Prat G, et al. Number of supervised studies required to reach competence in advanced critical care transesophageal echocardiography. *Intensive Care Med.* 2013;39:1019–1024.

13. Milani RV, Lavie CJ, Gilliland YE, Cassidy MM, Bernal JA. Overview of transesophageal echocardiography for the chest physician. *Chest*. 2003;124:1081–1089.
14. Vieillard-Baron A, Slama M, Mayo P, et al. A pilot study on safety and clinical utility of a single-use 72-hour indwelling transesophageal echocardiography probe. *Intensive Care Med*. 2013;39:629–635.
15. Vieillard-Baron A, Charron C, Chergui K, Peyrouset O, Jardin F. Bedside echocardiographic evaluation of hemodynamics in sepsis: is a qualitative evaluation sufficient? *Intensive Care Med*. 2006;32:1547–1552.
16. Vieillard-Baron A, Caille V, Charron C, Belliard G, Page B, Jardin F. Actual incidence of global left ventricular hypokinesia in adult septic shock. *Crit Care Med*. 2008;36:1701–1706.
17. Hahn RT, Abraham T, Adams MS, et al. Guidelines for performing a comprehensive transesophageal echocardiographic examination: recommendations from the American Society of Echocardiography and the Society of Cardiovascular Anesthesiologists. *J Am Soc Echocardiogr*. 2013;26:921–964.

ECHOCARDIOGRAPHIC ASSESSMENT OF LEFT VENTRICULAR SYSTOLIC AND DIASTOLIC FUNCTION

Scan QR code or visit www.ccu2e.com for video in this chapter

ALEXANDER B. LEVITOV, PAUL H. MAYO, & LOUIS VASTARDIS

Left ventricular (LV) dysfunctions (systolic and diastolic) are common in the critically ill patient. They may be due to preexistent disease (e.g., coronary artery disease [CAD]) or acquired as a part of a clinical syndrome responsible for the intensive care unit (ICU) admission (e.g., septic cardiomyopathy). Clinical examination alone or in combination with chest radiography may be insufficient for assessing LV function in the ICU. Echocardiography will provide crucial information; thus, echocardiographic assessment of LV function is necessary in nearly all ICU patients. Other technologies, such as bioreatance (NICOM) and thermo or marker dilution (LiCO, PICO), may provide additional information that can also be useful. Indwelling Doppler devices assessing aortic blood flow have been utilized with variable degree of success. Finally, carotid artery blood flow measured ultrasonographically has been recently suggested as an alternative to more technically challenging analysis of the transaortic stroke volume (SV) (cardiac output [CO]). All of these methods assist in assessing the LV.

TRANSTHORACIC ECHOCARDIOGRAPHY VERSUS TRANSESOPHAGEAL ECHOCARDIOGRAPHY—HAND-HELD DEVICES

Transthoracic echocardiography (TTE) is the modality most frequently utilized in the ICU. In spite of being operator dependent TTE will usually provide clinically useful information that alters the plan of care in nearly 50% of critically ill patients. It is noninvasive, has virtually no contraindications, can be repeated as often as necessary to reevaluate cardiac function after therapeutic interventions (volume resuscitation, inotropic support, vasoconstrictors), and usually requires no more then 5 min to acquire clinically relevant information about cardiac function by the experienced operator.[1] Moreover, it is easy to train intensivists in TTE. Newer generations of the handheld, pocket sized, battery-powered devices are now available and are simple and convenient to operate. They can provide a focused qualitative assessment of the LV systolic function. Handheld devices can be also valuable in ultrasound-guided thoracentesis, paracentesis, and abdominal examination. The role and utility of these devices in the assessment of the hemodynamically unstable ICU patient is still evolving.

Transesophageal echocardiography (TEE) is often considered superior to TTE in the ICU. TTE frequently provides poorer image quality in postoperative patients due to mechanical ventilation (positive end-expiratory pressure [PEEP] >15 cm of H_2O), inability to position the patient, lack of patient cooperation, chest wall edema and obstructed views due to wound dressings, chest tubes, drains, and an open chest or abdomen. In the critical care setting, TTE leads to a successful examination in 50% of attempts,[2,3] in contrast to 90% with TEE.[4,5] There are, however, challenges to the routine performance of TEE in the ICU. The TEE examination requires additional time and expertise when compared with the TTE examination. There is a small, but definite list of absolute and relative contraindications (Chapter 8). Insertion of the probe into the esophagus carries with it a risk of loss of the airway. Additionally, TTE carries with it a small but real risk, in the order of 0.01%, of significant complications such as esophageal perforation.

Regardless of what modality is used to perform the examination, it is important that the examination be as complete as the training of the practitioner allows. If the initial point of care examination is technically limited or there is doubt as to the findings, the examination should be followed as soon as possible with a comprehensive examination by a more experienced operator. A comprehensive examination is less likely to miss an unexpected diagnosis. With practice, a complete examination may be performed in minutes.

A reasonable strategy is to first focus on the areas or structures of interest as directed by the clinical presentation. Once the immediate question is answered, this should be followed by a complete examination. Items of lesser interest may then be reexamined in a more leisurely manner. Guidelines exist that standardize the images captured on both the TTE and TEE examinations.[6] These are important in assuring that all structures are viewed from multiple angles, allowing each individual structure to be completely and accurately assessed and documented as needed. The standardized views also assure that no structure is missed in the examination and provide the common language that allows practitioners to communicate their findings with each other and all members of the treatment team.

LV SYSTOLIC FUNCTION

Not less than 36% of all critically ill patients have reduced LV systolic function during their ICU stay. In the past, systolic function and particularly assessment of LV ejection fraction (LVEF) was overstated at the expense of diastolic function and volume responsiveness. This was partially due to historical connection of the bedside ultrasonography of the heart to classical cardiac echocardiography and the statistical importance of CAD to the latter. Recently, diastolic function, venous return and right ventricular function are increasingly recognized as major contributors to hemodynamic stability (see below). Nonetheless, LVEF assessment is still an important pert of the point of care cardiac evaluation. Thus, assessment of LV systolic function and its changes over time are quite helpful in therapeutic decision-making for the critically ill patient. Global LV systolic function is important because many diseases of the critically ill, and in particular sepsis, may lead to global rather than focal ventricular dysfunction. The presence of focal or regional wall motion abnormalities during the initial evaluation may indicate preexistent CAD, while the appearance of new or worsening wall-motion abnormalities may be indicative of the ischemic changes due to hypoxia or superimposition of myocardial infarction. Regardless, information on global and regional LV function is of critical importance in the clinical decision making throughout the ICU stay and may be useful in both early and later stages where challenging liberation from mechanical ventilation or inotropic medication may be explained and a causative lesion appropriately treated.

Echocardiography is largely a two-dimensional (2D) method of viewing a three-dimensional (3D) structure. A minimum of two orthogonal views should be performed for each structure of interest before making a diagnostic or a therapeutic decision. This is specifically mandated for a quantitative LVEF calculation by a biplane Simpson's method where evaluation in the apical four-chamber and two-chamber (perpendicular) views is mandatory.

Ventricular systolic function depends on both preload and afterload. Estimates of systolic function should be performed under different loading conditions to ascertain the true function. Once again, this demonstrates the importance of obtaining serial assessments rather than single snapshot views. Responses to passive leg raising or volume challenge are two methods of determining LV contractility relation to loading conditions (see Chapter 10).

Segmental wall-motion abnormality assessment and regional LV function should be performed using visual identification with a standardized 17-segment model simultaneously with global LV function evaluation. Qualitative, semi-quantitative and quantitative measures are used for assessing global LV systolic function. LVEF by visual assessment or biplane Simpson's methods, and linear M-mode measurements (i.e., fractional shortening) can be evaluated by TTE in initial stages or adopting ultrasonography into clinical ICU practice. Once Doppler techniques become familiar to the operator velocity–time integral (VTI) can be included and provide additional information on SV and CO independent of LVEF measurements. All of the methods, once integrated into clinical practice will provide a reliable set of tools with low-variability and high-quality bedside information. The most commonly used methods will now be discussed. It is incumbent upon the intensivist echocardiographer to be familiar with the advantages and limitations of all methods used in the assessment of LV systolic function.

QUALITATIVE ASSESSMENT OF LV SYSTOLIC FUNCTION

The most important and commonly used method of assessing LV global and focal wall motion is by a qualitative assessment in multiple views. This method is extremely effective, rapid, and consistent with nuclear scanning studies when done by an experienced echocardiographer. The result is both an assessment of regional wall motion and an overall assessment of LV function usually expressed in terms of an estimated ejection fraction (EF). To help interpret LV systolic function, several questions should be asked:

- Is the ventricle adequately filled? (See chapter 10)
- Is the ventricle's contractile function adequate?
- Is the ventricular contractility uniform throughout the coronary artery distributions and if present can regional wall motion abnormalities be attributed to the specific coronary artery.

Qualitative LV systolic function can be adequately performed with portable and pocket size ultrasound systems.

▶ Visual Assessment with a Standard 17-Segment Model

In an effort to have a uniform nomenclature for the LV function derived from multiple assessment modalities such as cardiac magnetic resonance imaging (MRI), echocardiography, nuclear scanning, and angiography, the American Heart Association produced a consensus statement suggesting that the LV be divided into 17 different segments.[7]

CHAPTER 9 ECHOCARDIOGRAPHIC ASSESSMENT OF LEFT VENTRICULAR SYSTOLIC AND DIASTOLIC FUNCTION 91

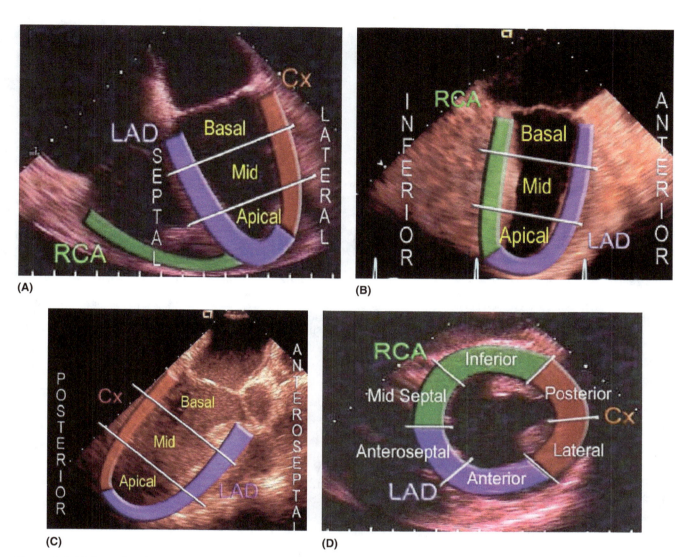

Figure 9-1 (**A**) Four-chamber view showing the coronary artery distribution and the corresponding LV segments. The septal wall (anterior 1/3) is supplied by the left anterior descending (LAD) artery; lateral wall is supplied by the circumflex artery (Cx). (**B**) Two-chamber view showing the coronary artery distribution and the corresponding left ventricular segments. The base, mid, and apical segments of anterior wall are supplied by the LAD artery and the inferior wall is supplied by the right coronary artery. (**C**) Oblique view of the LV showing the anteroseptal and posterior segments. The base, mid, and apex of the anteroseptal wall and posterior wall are supplied by the LAD and left circumflex (Cx) arteries, respectively. (**D**) Midpapillary short-axis view of the left ventricle (LV) showing the three arterial distribution and corresponding segments. This is the midpapillary transgastric short-axis view of the LV showing the LAD supplying the midanterior and anteroseptal segments, Cx supplying midlateral and posterior segments of the lateral wall, and RCA supplying midseptal and inferior segments of the LV. Cx, left circumflex coronary artery; LAD, left anterior descending artery; RCA, right coronary artery. (Reproduced with permission from Dr. Martin London's Web site www.ucsf.edu/teeecho.)

The LV is divided into basal, midcavity, and apical segments along the long axis of the heart. Each segment is then further divided into six in the basal, six in the midcavity, and four in the apical segments, and an apical cap is included as the 17th segment. The corresponding coronary arterial distribution is shown in Figure 9-1.

The left anterior descending (LAD) coronary artery supplies the anterior wall of the heart and anterior two thirds of the interventricular septum. The left circumflex artery (LCx) supplies the lateral wall of the LV. The right coronary artery (RCA) supplies the posterior third of the interventricular septum and inferior wall of the LV. A semiquantitative assessment can be performed using a wall-motion score or index. The LV contractility is dependent on movement of the base toward the apex, thickening of the wall segments, and a spiral squeeze or rotational movement of the LV. Thickening of the wall segments and the endocardial excursion of the LV segment are important to assess the wall motion. The wall-motion score is described here:

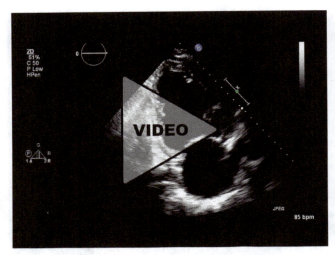 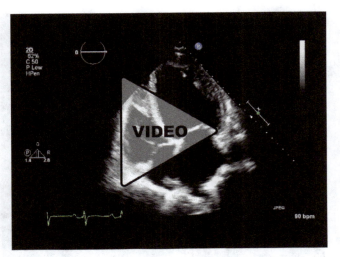

Video 9-1 Cardiac recording in apical two-chamber view for biplane Simpson's calculations of LV systolic function (SV, LVEF%). LVEF, left ventricular ejection fraction; LV, left ventricle; SV, stroke volume. View at www.ccu2e.com

Video 9-2 Cardiac recording in apical four-chamber view for biplane Simpson's calculations of LV systolic function (SV, LVEF%). Notice apical two- and four-chamber views are in the planes perpendicular to each other, thus providing reasonable volume estimates. LVEF, left ventricular ejection fraction; LV, left ventricle; SV, stroke volume. View at www.ccu2e.com

1. Normal (>30% endocardial excursion and >50% wall thickening)
2. Mild hypokinesis (10–30% endocardial excursion and 30–50% wall thickening)
3. Severe hypokinesis (<20% endocardial excursion and <30% wall thickening)
4. Akinesis (no endocardial excursion and <10% wall thickening)
5. Dyskinesis (moves paradoxically-outwards during systole)

The wall-motion score index is defined as the wall-motion score/number of segments. This is a subjective assessment and does not have a true linear relationship. A stunned myocardium without a perfusion defect can exhibit wall-motion abnormality. Multiple views must be obtained to truly define the degree of LV impairment and the arterial distribution involved. Endocardial excursion alone may be due to tethered myocardium, and a change in wall thickness is a precise indicator of ischemia.[8] The reproducibility of wall thickening measurements was evaluated, which led to the following conclusions:

1. It is difficult to obtain consistent data on wall thickening in the longitudinal plane.
2. Multiple measurements are necessary to reduce variability.
3. It is necessary to ensure that borders, locations, and angles are carefully defined.[9]

QUANTITATIVE ASSESSMENT OF LV SYSTOLIC FUNCTION WITH ECHOCARDIOGRAPHY

Quantitative techniques of ventricular assessment allow for a more measurable and arguably less biased assessment of the ventricle. These techniques have their advantages and their limitations.

▶ Volumetric Ejection Fraction, SV, and CO by Biplane Simpson's Method

SV is obtained by calculating the difference between the end-diastolic volume (EDV) and end-systolic volume (ESV). SV = ESV/EDV. EF is defined as SV divided by the EDV. EF = SV/EDV %. CO can be quantified by multiplying SV by the heart rate (HR). CO = SV × HR. The American Society of Echocardiography (ASE) recommends the modified Simpson's method.[10] This method calculates ESV, EDV, SV, and EF in two planes and averages them. With TTE apical four- and two-chamber views are utilized as located in the planes perpendicular to each other (Videos 9-1 and 9-2). Endocardial borders need to be well visualized to trace them out. Representative frames are chosen at the end of systole (Figures 9-2 and 9-3) and diastole (Figures 9-4 and 9-5) and endocardial borders traced. End systole and end diastole are identified by the position and motion of mitral valve leaflets in two subsequent frames or less reliably by the EKG or the LV visible cavity size (smallest vs. largest) (Table 9-1). When using TEE, the midesophagus four-chamber, and two-chamber planes can be used for the same purpose (Figure 9-6). Most ultrasound systems will automatically calculate EDV, ESV, and EF. The CO can be calculated manually if not so provided.

However, this method has limitations:

- Mitral annular calcifications commonly interfere with border detection.
- The LV apex is frequently foreshortened and ASE specifically warns of four-chamber foreshortening.

- Lateral wall dropouts can occur in the four-chamber view, as the ultrasound beam is parallel to the lateral wall.
- The trabeculations in the LV can also interfere with border detection and should be partially included in EDV tracings.
- Endocardial border definition is extremely important to assess LV function. In some patients with conditions such as obesity or emphysema, it is often difficult to define the endocardial borders. Contrast echocardiography[11] plays an important role in such patients. Acoustic quantification[12] differentiates the tissue from blood and automatically outlines the endocardial border in some newer ultrasound systems.
- Finally visual estimation "eyeballing" of the EF is often dismissed as operator dependent and unreliable. However when EF is visually estimated by the experienced echocardiographer without formal calculations, there seems to excellent correlation with formal measurements.[13]

TABLE 9-1

Identification of the End Systolic and End Diastolic Frames for Tracing to Assess LV Function by the Biplane Simpson's Method

Cardiac Phase	Frame	Next Frame	EKG
End systole	MV closed	MV starts to open	T wave appears
End diastole	MV opened	MV starts to close (Systolic coaptation)	QRS complex appears

LV, left ventricle; MV, mitral valve.

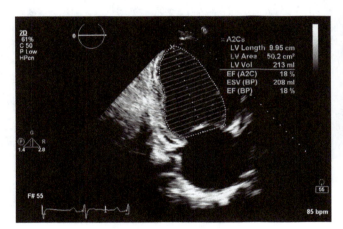

Figure 9-2 Endocardial borders are traced in systole in apical two-chamber view.

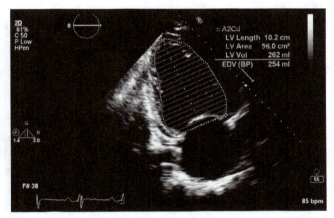

Figure 9-4 Endocardial borders are traced in diastole in apical two-chamber view.

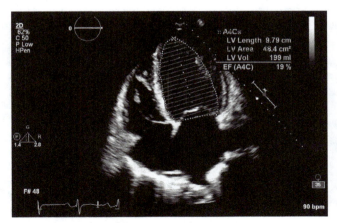

Figure 9-3 Endocardial borders are traced in systole in apical four-chamber view. Note that ejection fraction is automatically calculated by the ultrasound system.

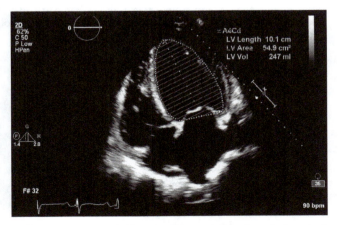

Figure 9-5 Endocardial borders are traced in diastole in apical four-chamber view. Note that Left ventricular diastolic volume is automatically calculated by the ultrasound system.

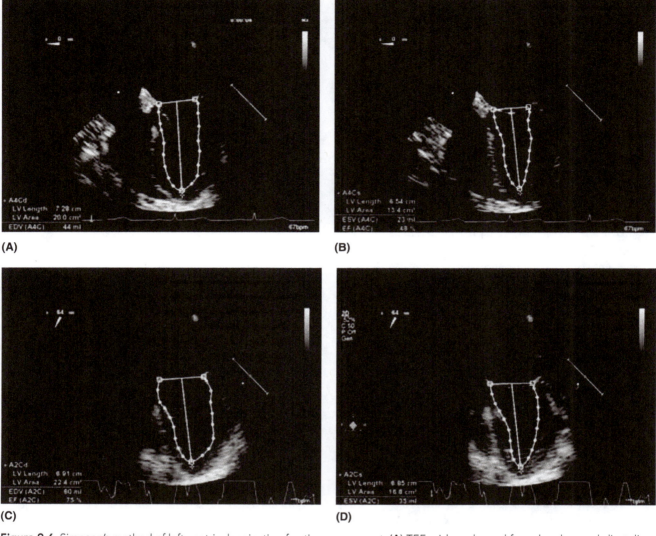

Figure 9-6 Simpson's method of left ventricular ejection fraction assessment. (**A**) TEE midesophageal four-chamber end-diastolic frame: LV at end-diastole frame is frozen. The endocardial border is traced out to get the end-diastolic dimension. (**B**) Midesophageal four-chamber end-systolic frame: the LV frame at end-systole is frozen. The endocardial border is tracked in the machine. (**C**) Midesophageal oblique two-chamber end-diastolic frame: the LV frame at end-diastole is frozen in this oblique view, adding another dimension to the previous measurements. The endocardial border is tracked in the machine. (**D**) Midesophageal oblique two-chamber end-systolic frame: the LV frame at end-systole is frozen. The endocardial border is tracked in the machine in this two-chamber view, giving an added dimension to the previous calculation. LV, left ventricle.

▶ Calculation of SV and CO by Pulsed-Wave Doppler

Figures 9-7 and 9-8. See also Video 9-3. Calculation of stroke volume and cardiac output with pulsed-wave Doppler (PWD) by TTE. A pulmonary artery catheter has been used to measure CO in the ICU. However, with the current evidence not favoring this modality, echocardiography has a critical role in assessing CO in the ICU. Both the right and left ventricular COs can be measured using echocardiography. LV CO measurement is reproducible and accurate.

Heart rate can be measured using the electrocardiogram or from one VTI to another VTI. This is automatically stored in the echo machine. When blood is ejected from the LV into the cylindrical aorta, the SV is calculated from the height over time of this blood column, which is the VTI. Thus, VTI forms the sides of a bullet like cylinder representing the SV. The base of this cylindrical output is formed by the left ventricular outflow tract (LVOT). LVOT cross-sectional area (SCA) can be easily calculated. SCA = $\pi \times R^2$ (where R is the LVOT radius). SV= VTI × CSA = VTI × π (3.14) × $(R)^2$. In TTE, VTI is traced with a PWD in the apical 5 chamber view at LVOT level (Figure 9-7). LVOT diameter ($R \times 2$) is measured in parasternal long axis view (Figure 9-8 and Video 9-3). With notable exception of "super portables" most bedside ultrasound systems will automatically calculate SV and thus CO utilizing the above formulas after the input of the VTI and the LVOT diameter.

With TEE, VTI is traced with PWD assessing the flow at the LVOT through a deep transgastric aortic valve view or

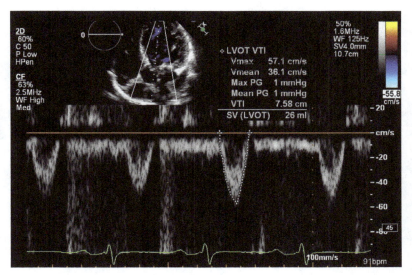

Figures 9-7 Velocity–time integral (VTI) is obtained in apical five-chamber view using pulse wave (PW) Doppler. Note that left ventricular outflow tract (LVOT) diameter (next figure) has been already recorded and the system is exhibiting stroke volume (SV) (diminished to 26 mL). With the heart rate of 50 beats a minute cardiac output is diminished to 1.300 mL.

transgastric aortic valve long-axis view (Figure 9-9). Tracing this PWD wave from the LVOT will provide the LVOT VTI. The assumption made here is that the area measured for the calculation of SV is constant during systole. A small error in radius measurements at LVOT will amplify the error because it is squared. To minimize this error, the depth of the image should be reduced and LVOT amplified. The next assumption is that flow across the LVOT is laminar. The validity of this assumption is demonstrated by the narrow velocity band and smooth spectral signal on pulsed Doppler recordings. The flat velocity profile is confirmed by moving the sample volume across the flow stream in two orthogonal views to demonstrate uniform velocities at the center and at the edges of the flow stream. Importantly, the Doppler beam angle should be parallel to the flow or within 20°. The Doppler signal is recorded at a parallel intercept angle to flow, resulting in an accurate measurement of velocity (Cos 0 = 1). It is important to remember that for Doppler measurements the angle of interrogation should be parallel to flow, while for the 2D or M-mode measurements the interrogating beam should be perpendicular to the structure of interest. The LVOT diameter and the PWD should be evaluated from the same anatomic site to assure that spatial and temporal relationships of interrogating pulsed-wave Doppler are maintained. This error can be minimized by choosing the area proximal to the aortic valve as the point of interest and used as a routine method of measurement. Since there can be

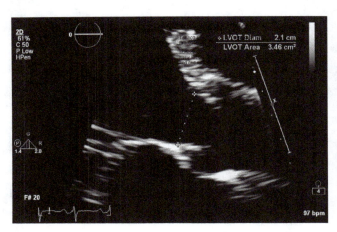

Figures 9-8 Measuring left ventricular outflow tract (LVOT) diameter (D) in parasternal long-axis view. LVOT is measured at the attachment of the aortic valve cusps (right coronary cusp on the top and noncoronary cusp on the bottom). $R = 1/2\ D$ (LVOT surface area $= \pi \times R^2$). LVOT is assumed to be circular. $SV = VTI \times LVOTR^2$. LVOTR, left ventilatory outflow tract radius; VTI, velocity–time integral; SV, stroke volume.

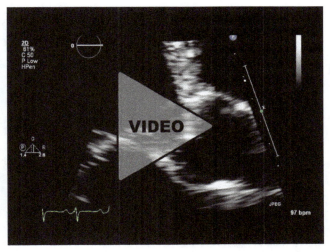

Video 9-3 Recording of the LVOT in parasternal long-axis view. LVOT diameter/radius measurements for the calculation of stroke volume and cardiac output with pulsed-wave Doppler (PWD) are done at the attachment of the aortic cusps (see Figure 9-8). Note poor aortic cusps separation due to decreased LV systolic function (LVEF%). LVEF, left ventricular ejection fraction; LV, left ventricle; LVOT, left ventricular outflow tract. View at www.ccu2e.com

SECTION II CARDIAC SONOGRAPHY IN THE ICU

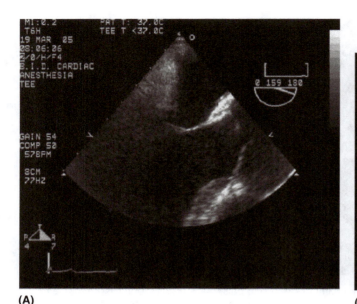

(A)

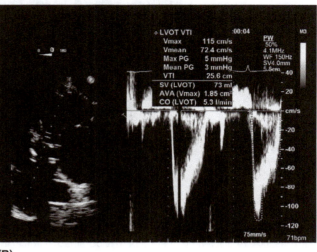

(B)

Figure 9-9 (A) Stroke volume measurement by **TEE**: calculation of left ventricular outflow tract (LVOT) diameter; decreasing the depth gives an enlarged view of the LVOT. This minimizes error in calculating the LVOT measurements. (B) Calculation of stroke volume: VTI measurement across LVOT. The LVOT is aligned parallel to the Doppler (in this TEE view, it is deep transgastric view); a pulsed-wave Doppler is placed at the same spot as the LVOT measurement to obtain a clean envelope. This is traced to calculate the VTI measurement. LVOT, left ventricular outflow tract; TEE, transesophageal echocardiography; VTI, velocity–time integral.

dynamic changes in heart rate, the measurements should be performed at the same time and all measures should be repeated when evaluating CO at a different point of time.

▶ RV SV Measurements

With TEE, it is common to utilize LVOT as the primary site, followed by the main pulmonary artery and the right ventricular outflow tract (RVOT) (Figure 9-10). With TTE, SV can be measured at the aortic valve leaflet tips or in the ascending aorta. Ascending aortic diameter is measured from a parasternal long-axis view and flow from the suprasternal notch or the apical TTE view. Transmitral SV can be measured as well with the pulsed Doppler at the mitral leaflet tips. Because of the complex mitral valve geometry and increasing assumptions, it is uncommon to use this site as a routine for CO evaluation. In the right side of the heart, the tricuspid valve or pulmonary artery can be used to measure SV. Right ventricular CO is possible to measure and the pulmonary valve output can be measured just as described for the LV (Figure 9-10). However, the main pulmonary artery diameter measurements are not always fixed and vary depending upon the view. Also, it is not always possible to achieve the right ventricular output flow parallel to the Doppler (PWD).

SEMIQUANTITATIVE METHODS

▶ Fractional Shortening and M-Mode Derived Modality

This is a one-dimensional (1D) measurement of LV global systolic function (Figure 9-11).[10,14] M-mode across the LV midpapillary axis is obtained (Video 9-4). A freeze-frame analysis of this M-mode is used to calculate fractional shortening (Figure 9-11). Ventricular internal dimensions are measured from the leading edge to the leading edge of interest. The advantage of this method is that it is quick and fairly reproducible. The M-mode provides a very high time resolution and delineates the endocardial borders well. This is a basic, crude estimate of

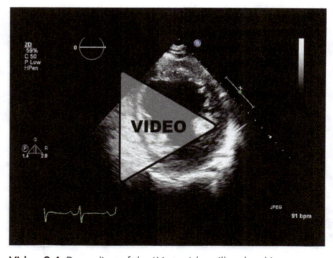

Video 9-4 Recording of the LV at midpapillary level in parasternal short axis view for linear (M-mode) assessment of left ventricular function by TTE. LVEF is decreased by visual estimation and calculations (see Figures 9-11 and 9-12). TTE, transthoracic echocardiography; LVEF, left ventricular ejection fraction; LV, left ventricle. View at www.ccu2e.com

CHAPTER 9 ECHOCARDIOGRAPHIC ASSESSMENT OF LEFT VENTRICULAR SYSTOLIC AND DIASTOLIC FUNCTION

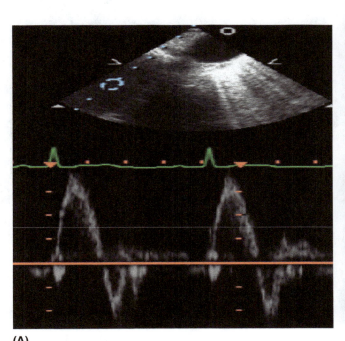
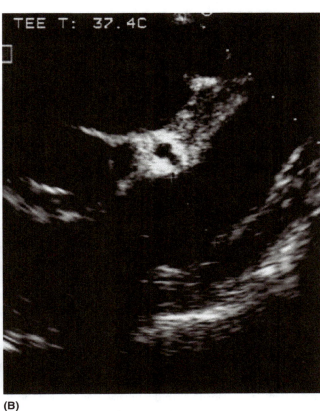

Figure 9-10 (**A**) Stroke volume measurement sites: pulmonary artery from the aortic arch view; in this **TEE** view, the probe is placed in the aortic arch and rotated 20°–40°. The main pulmonary artery appears on the left and aligns parallel to the pulsed-wave Doppler interrogation. (**B**) Stroke volume measurement sites: pulmonary artery from the midesophageal inflow–outflow view; in this right ventricular view, one can appreciate that the pulmonary artery is not aligned parallel to the pulsed-wave Doppler interrogation. This can lead to error in measurements, as explained in the text. TEE, transesophageal echocardiography.

LV global systolic function, with the normal range being 25–45%. However, this method could easily be prone to error if focal wall-motion abnormalities exist. An oblique cut of the 1D plane can lead to errors in length measurements. It is important to keep in mind these caveats and the potential overestimation or underestimation of this measurement. Adding another dimension to this semi-quantitative method may improve the evaluation of global function.

Though widely used previously and reliable for relatively uniformed changes in the LV systolic function, M-mode linear measures of LV function are problematic when there is a marked regional difference in the LV function. This is often the case with critically ill patients with sepsis, hypertension or obesity, as well as with unrecognized or recognized CAD. Thus, previously used Teichholz (Figure 9-12) or Quinones methods of calculating LV EF from the M-mode are no longer recommended by ASE. Such calculations are still available in most ultrasound systems and can be used by the intensivist at the bedside based upon clinical discretion. Similar information can be obtained by TEE (Figure 9-13).

Figure 9-11 Linear end diastolic volume calculations by TTE. M-mode is obtained in parasternal short-axis view at midpapillary level. Note linear (broken line) curser position in end-diastole in two-dimensional and M-mode recording. Ultrasound system has calculated end diastolic volume (360 mL). TTE, transthoracic echocardiography.

▶ Fractional Area Change

This is a 2D measure of LV systolic function. One of the prerequisites for obtaining these values is to have adequate endocardial border definition. Detection of the endocardium

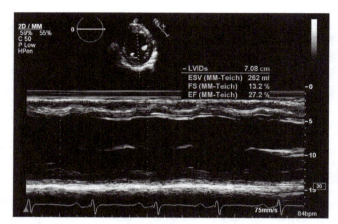

Figure 9-12 Linear shortening (FS) and ejection fraction (EF) calculations by TTE. M-mode is obtained in parasternal short-axis view at midpapillary level. Note linear (broken line) curser position in end-systole in two-dimensional and M-mode recording. Ultrasound system has calculated SF = 13.2% and EF = 27.2% (both diminished) using diastolic data from the previous frame (Figure 9-11). TTE, transthoracic echocardiography.

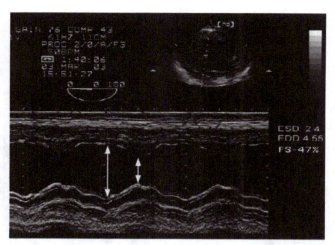

Figure 9-13 Fractional shortening by TEE: M-mode is recorded at midpapillary transgastric short-axis view of the LV, a high-resolution time frame is obtained. When this frame is frozen, end-diastolic and end-systolic lengths can be measured and lead to fractional shortening measurements. EDD, end-diastolic diameter; ESD, end-systolic diameter; FS, fractional shortening; LV, left ventricle; PLAX, parasternal long-axis view; TTE, transthoracic echocardiography.

throughout the entire view can be time consuming, especially if the borders are not well visualized. Fractional area change can be used to quantify EF[15] (Figure 9-14). This measure is heavily dependent on afterload and slightly dependent on preload. A midpapillary, transgastric short-axis view to calculate FAC has demonstrated close correlation to radionuclide angiography and scintigraphy.[16]

▶ Three-Dimensional Assessment of LV Function and Volume

Reconstruction of real-time images can provide 3D image of the LV. When reconstruction is performed, a series of 2D images are obtained at a standard of 3° or 5° with a stationary transducer. The number of planes and the quality of 2D images will determine the quality of 3D image. Development of the matrix-array transducer has led to acquisition of images from many lines of sight simultaneously to reconstruct a volume of ultrasound data in real time. They are still insufficient to display the entire adult LV. To obtain the entire LV, a series of component volumes of the heart are obtained over consecutive cardiac cycles and then integrated to obtain a larger volume.

LV volume and function can be calculated from the 3D approach and is a more accurate representation (compare

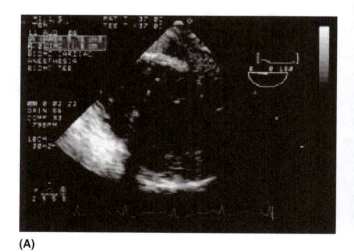
(A)

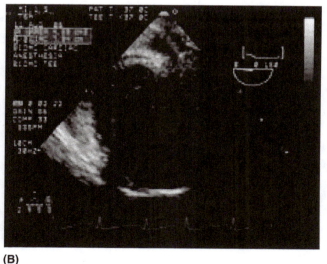
(B)

Figure 9-14 (A) Fractional area calculation: end-diastole frame. Midpapillary short-axis view of the LV is frozen at the end of diastole. The endocardial border is traced, which gives the end-diastolic area an extra dimension, unlike fractional shortening. (B) Fractional area calculation: end-systole frame. Midpapillary short-axis view of the LV is frozen at the end of systole. The endocardial border is traced. LV, left ventricle.

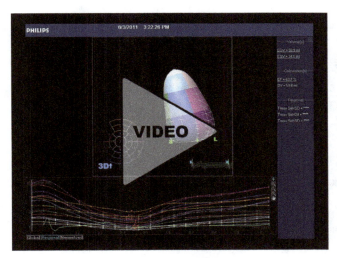

Video 9-5 Three-dimensional echocardiogram recording of the normal left ventricular systolic function. View at www.ccu2e.com

Videos 9-5 and 9-6). The 3D approach compares favorably with MRI and is accurate with less interobserver variability.[17,18] This is understandable, as unlike M-mode or 2D, there are fewer assumptions made. Because the volume estimation is more accurate, changes in volume estimates with systole will also be accurate and result in a reliable estimation of LVEF. There are some limitations with this approach. Line-density in a 3D volume is much lower than in a 2D image, and more interpolation is often necessary. When the acquisition is from a fixed transducer position alignment with various structures, it is often not ideal and results in a poor image.[19] Movement of the heart with breathing and arrhythmias can often result in image artifacts. With a progressive reduction in analysis time and the availability of improved technology, 3D is likely to become the preferred method for assessing LV volume and function in critically ill patients in the future.

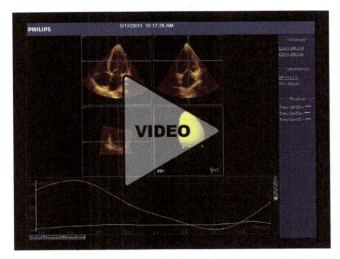

Video 9-6 Three-dimensional echocardiogram recording of the severely reduced left ventricular systolic function (compare to Video 9-5). View at www.ccu2e.com

ASSESSMENT OF LV DIASTOLIC FUNCTION

The intensivist with skill at advanced critical care echocardiography (CCE) is able to identify and grade diastolic function using techniques that are standard to cardiology echocardiography. As the measurements require skill at Doppler, they are not part of the basic CCE examination. In critical care practice, the assessment of left side filling pressures has clinical utility, as an elevated left atrial pressure (LAP) is associated with cardiogenic or hydrostatic pulmonary edema. With the patient on ventilatory support with bilateral granular radio-density pattern, a key differential is whether the disease process is caused by cardiac disease (cardiogenic pulmonary edema) or caused by primary lung injury. Identification and grading of diastolic function has less clinical utility for the intensivist, so the discussion will start with measurement of left-sided filling pressures.

▶ Measurement of LV Filling Pressures

Echocardiography allows for a clinically relevant estimate of LAP without the use of a pulmonary artery catheter. The latter was a dominant tool in ICU practice, but it has now been superseded by ultrasonography. While the measurement of left-sided filling pressures is not relevant to a determination of preload sensitivity,[20,21] it is important in determining whether the patient has respiratory failure related to hydrostatic pulmonary edema. The distinction between heart failure and primary lung injury as the cause for respiratory dysfunction has major implications for management strategy.

▶ Measurement Technique

The American Society of Echocardiography (ASE) has published a useful statement entitled Recommendations for the Evaluation of LV Diastolic Function by Echocardiography.[22] The document presents two well-designed algorithms that allow the frontline intensivist to determine a qualitative estimate of LAP (Figures 9-15 and 9-16).

As a first step, the intensivist determines by 2D echocardiography the LV EF. For those patients with an EF less than 40%, mitral inflow is measured by placing the PWD sample volume between the tips of the mitral valve (MV) leaflets from the apical four-chamber view. This allows measurement of the E wave velocity, the E wave deceleration time, the A wave velocity and the E/A ratio (Figure 9-17). If the E wave velocity is less than 50 cm/s and the E/A ratio is less than 1, the LAP is normal. If the E/A ratio is greater than 2 and the deceleration time is less than 150 ms, the LAP is elevated. If neither pattern holds, the E/e' ratio is measured, where e' is the velocity of the lateral mitral annulus during diastole measured with tissue Doppler imaging (Figure 9-18). If E/e' is less than 8, the LAP is normal; if the E/e' is greater than 15, the LAP is elevated. If E/e' is between these values, there are a series of further measurements that must be made. Except for measurement of the pulmonary artery

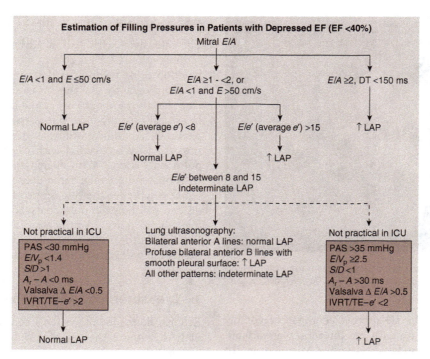

Figure 9-15 This figure is a modification of the American Society of Echocardiography algorithm for estimation of left atrial pressure (LAP) in patients with reduced left ventricular function. Measurement of mitral valve inflow and mitral annular velocity allows the intensivist to identify an elevated or normal LAP in some cases, but may yield an indeterminate result. The ultrasonographer is then required to make a series of complex measurements that are listed in the figure. Given the time constraints and difficult imaging conditions in the intensive care unit, these are not practical for the frontline intensivist to perform. Instead, lung ultrasonography may be incorporated into the study to estimate LAP. (Adapted from Nagueh SF, Appleton CP, Gillebert TC, et al. Recommendations for the evaluation of left ventricular diastolic function by echocardiography. *J Am Soc Echocardiogr.* 2009;22:107–133.)

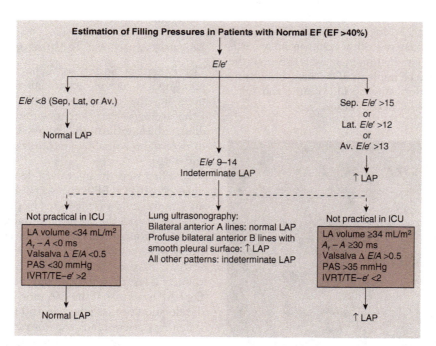

Figure 9-16 This figure is a modification of the American Society of Echocardiography algorithm for estimation of left atrial pressure (LAP) in patients with normal left ventricular function. Measurement of mitral valve inflow and mitral annular velocity allows the intensivist to identify an elevated or normal LAP in some cases, but may yield an indeterminate result. The ultrasonographer is then required to make a series of complex measurements that are listed in the figure. Given the time constraints and difficult imaging conditions in the intensive care unit, these are not practical for the frontline intensivist to perform. Instead, lung ultrasonography may be incorporated into the study to estimate LAP. (Adapted from Nagueh SF, Appleton CP, Gillebert TC, et al. Recommendations for the evaluation of left ventricular diastolic function by echocardiography. *J Am Soc Echocardiogr.* 2009;22:107–133.)

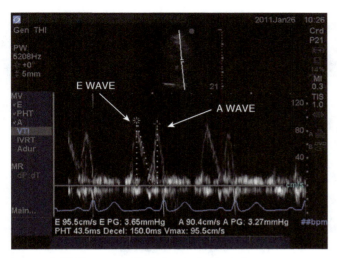

Figure 9-17 This image shows a mitral valve inflow tracing. Measurement of the Doppler velocity profile. This measurement is required when estimating left atrial pressures and for assessing diastolic function of the left ventricle.

systolic pressure (PASP), they may be impractical for routine bedside use in the ICU.

For those patients with normal LVEF greater than 40%, the algorithm does not call for measurement of mitral valve inflow. Rather, the E/e' ratio is the initial measurement. If the ratio is less than 9, the LAP is normal; if it is greater than 14, the LAP is elevated. If it is between these values, there are a series of further measurement that must be made. Except for measurement of the PASP, they may be impractical for routine bedside use.

▶ **Problems with Measurement of LV Filling Pressures**

The measurement scheme proposed by the ASE algorithm is useful to the intensivist if the determination of LAP can

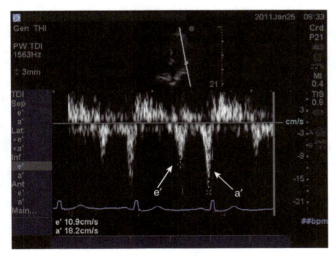

Figure 9-18 This image shows the tissue Doppler imaging of the lateral mitral annulus. This measurement is required when estimating left atrial pressures and for assessing diastolic function of the left ventricle.

derived from MV inflow, e', and PASP. Otherwise, the additional measurements required may be too time consuming for the frontline intensivist to accomplish; and they require good image quality that may not be readily achievable at the bedside (unless TEE is performed). The type of study required is more relevant to a cardiology echocardiography laboratory.

Using the ASE approach, the LAP measurement does not give a quantitative result. Rather, it is designated as normal or elevated. The implication of an elevated value is that the patient is at risk for hydrostatic pulmonary edema. The lack of a specific value for LAP is not of particular importance, as the exact value of LAP has limited value in determining preload sensitivity. An elevated value of LAP has particular importance in identifying whether the patient may have cardiogenic pulmonary edema.

▶ **Alternative Methods**

Lung ultrasonography allows the intensivist to distinguish between cardiogenic pulmonary edema and primary lung injury. The finding of anterior A lines with sliding lung indicates that the pulmonary artery occlusion pressure is less than 18 mmHg and probably less than 12 mmHg.[22] The finding of profuse bilateral anterior B lines with smooth pleural line morphology is highly suggestive of cardiogenic pulmonary edema, whereas focal anterior B lines, whether unilateral or bilateral with irregular pleural line morphology, strongly suggests a primary pulmonary process (See chapter on lung ultrasonography).[23] Lung ultrasonography should be routinely paired with echocardiography when assessing for the possibility of cardiogenic pulmonary edema. The combination of the two modalities allows the intensivist to reliably determine whether the patient has primary lung disease or cardiogenic pulmonary edema.

▶ **Assessment of Diastolic Function**

The ASE Statement presents an algorithm that allows the intensivist to identify normal and to grade patterns of abnormal diastolic function (Figure 9-19).[24] The measurement scheme requires the measurement of the MV inflow E wave velocity, the mitral annular e' velocity, and the LA volume. The LA volume requires use of the modified Simpson's formula to calculate the area of the LA in two orthogonal views. If initial measurements do not indicate normal diastolic function, additional measurements are used to assign a grade to the diastolic dysfunction. They may be impractical for routine bedside use in the ICU.

▶ **Problems with Measurement of Diastolic Function**

While E wave and e' velocity may be easily determined, the measurement of LA volume adds time to the examination. If the resulting pattern is not consistent with normal diastolic function, some of the additional measurements required by the algorithm are impractical for use

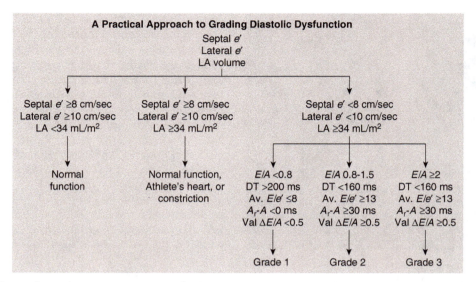

Figure 9-19 This figure shows the American Society of Echocardiography algorithm for grading diastolic function. (Adapted from Nagueh SF, Appleton CP, Gillebert TC, et al. Recommendations for the evaluation of left ventricular diastolic function by echocardiography. *J Am Soc Echocardiogr.* 2009;22:107–133.)

in the ICU, excepting the A wave velocity and the E wave deceleration time. This is compounded by the fact that, compared to the measurement of LAP, identification of the grade of diastolic function may not have immediate application for the frontline intensivist who is managing the patient with cardiopulmonary failure beyond indicating that the patient is at risk for pulmonary edema under certain cardiac loading conditions. Detailed assessment of diastolic function is generally of interest to the cardiologist rather than the intensivist. That being said, the intensivist with skill at advanced critical care echocardiography must have comprehensive knowledge of both the measurements required and their clinical utility. The reader is referred to standard Cardiology textbooks for comprehensive discussion of diastolic function.

REFERENCES

1. Jensen MB, Sloth E, Larsen KM, Schmidt MB. Transthoracic echocardiography for cardiopulmonary monitoring in intensive care. *Eur J Anaesthesiol.* 2004;21:700–707.
2. Pearson AC. Noninvasive evaluation of the hemodynamically unstable patient: the advantages of seeing clearly. *Mayo Clin Proc.* 1995;70:1012–1014.
3. Cook CH, Praba AC, Beery PR, Martin LC. Transthoracic echocardiography is not cost-effective in critically ill surgical patients. *J Trauma.* 2002;52:280–284.
4. Pearson AC, Castello R, Labovitz AJ. Safety and utility of transesophageal echocardiography in the critically ill patient. *Am Heart J.* 1990;119:1083–1089.
5. Oh JK, Seward JB, Khandheria BK, et al. Transesophageal echocardiography in critically ill patients. *Am J Cardiol.* 1990;66:1492–1495.
6. Shanewise JS, Cheung AT, Aronson S, et al. ASE/SCA guidelines for performing a comprehensive intraoperative multiplane transesophageal echocardiography examination: recommendations of the American Society of Echocardiography Council for Intraoperative Echocardiography and the Society of Cardiovascular Anesthesiologists Task Force for Certification in Perioperative Transesophageal Echocardiography. *Anesth Analg.* 1999;89:870–884.
7. Cerqueira MD, Weissman NJ, Dilsizian V, et al. Standardized myocardial segmentation and nomenclature for tomographic imaging of the heart: a statement for health-care professionals from the Cardiac Imaging Committee of the Council on Clinical Cardiology of the American Heart Association. *Circulation.* 2002;105:539–542.
8. Buda AJ, Zotz RJ, Pace DP, Krause LC. Comparison of two-dimensional echocardiographic wall motion and wall thickening abnormalities in relation to the myocardium at risk. *Am Heart J.* 1986;111:587–592.
9. Konstadt SN, Abrahams HP, Nejat M, Reich DL. Are wall thickening measurements reproducible? *Anesth Analg.* 1994;78:619–623.
10. Roberto M. Lang, Michelle Bierig, Richard B. Devereux, MD et al. Recommendations for Chamber Quantification: A Report from the American Society of Echocardiography's Guidelines and Standards Committee and the Chamber Quantification Writing Group, Developed in Conjunction with the European Association of Echocardiography, a Branch of the European Society of Cardiology. *J Am Soc Echocardiogr.* 2005;18:1440–1463.
11. Mulvagh SL, DeMaria AN, Feinstein SB, et al. Contrast echocardiography: current and future applications. *J Am Soc Echocardiogr.* 2000;13:331–342.
12. Mor-Avi V, Vignon P, Koch R, et al. Segmental analysis of color kinesis images: new method for quantification of the magnitude and timing of endocardial motion during left ventricular systole and diastole. *Circulation.* 1997;95:2082–2097.
13. Folland ED, Parisi AF, Moynihan PF, Jones DR, Feldman CL, Tow DE. Assessment of left ventricular ejection

fraction and volumes by real-time, two-dimensional echocardiography. A comparison of cineangiographic and radionuclide techniques. *Circulation*. 1979;60:760–766.
14. Vuille C, Malvern WA. Left ventricle I: general considerations, assessment of chamber size and function. In: Malvern WA, ed. *Principles and Practice of Echocardiography*. 2nd ed. Philadelphia, PA: Lea & Febiger; 1994.
15. Abel MD, Nishimura RA, Callahan MJ, et al. Evaluation of intraoperative transesophageal two-dimensional echocardiography. *Anesthesiology*. 1987;66:64–68.
16. Clements FM, Harpole DH, Quill T, Jones RH, McCann RL. Estimation of left ventricular volume and ejection fraction by two-dimensional transoesophageal echocardiography: comparison of short axis imaging and simultaneous radionuclide angiography. *Br J Anaesth*. 1990;64:331–336.
17. Chan J, Jenkins C, Khafagi F, Du L, Marwick TH. What is the optimal clinical technique for measurement of left ventricular volume after myocardial infarction? A comparative study of 3-dimensional echocardiography, single photon emission computed tomography, and cardiac magnetic resonance imaging. *J Am Soc Echocardiogr*. 2006;19:192–201.
18. Sugeng L, Mor-Avi V, Weinert L, et al. Quantitative assessment of left ventricular size and function: side-by-side comparison of real-time three-dimensional echocardiography and computed tomography with magnetic resonance reference. *Circulation*. 2006;114:654–661.
19. Picard MH, Popp RL, Weyman AE. Assessment of left ventricular function by echocardiography: a technique in evolution. *J Am Soc Echocardiogr*. 2008;21:14–21.
20. Kumar A, Anel R, Bunnell E. Pulmonary artery occlusion pressure and central venous pressure fail to predict ventricular filling volume, cardiac performance, or the response to volume infusion in normal subjects. *Crit Care Med*. 2004;32:691–699.
21. Michard F, Teboul JL: Predicting fluid responsiveness in ICU patients: a critical analysis of the evidence. *Chest*. 2002;121:2000-2008.
22. Nagueh SF, Appleton CP, Gillebert TC, et al. Recommendations for the evaluation of left ventricular diastolic function by echocardiography. *J Am Soc Echocardiogr*. 2009;22:107–133.
23. Lichtenstein DA, Mezière GA, Lagoueyte JF, Biderman P, Goldstein I, Gepner A. A-lines and B-lines: lung ultrasound as a bedside tool for predicting pulmonary artery occlusion pressure in the critically ill. *Chest*. 2009;136:1014–1020.
24. Copetti R, Soldati G, Copetti P. Chest sonography: a useful tool to differentiate acute cardiogenic pulmonary edema from acute respiratory distress syndrome. *Cardiovasc Ultrasound*. 2008;6:16.

ECHOCARDIOGRAPHIC EVALUATION OF PRELOAD RESPONSIVENESS

ALEXANDER B. LEVITOV & PAUL E. MARIK

Scan QR code or visit www.ccu2e.com for video in this chapter

INTRODUCTION

Shock (hemodynamic failure) is ubiquitous in the modern intensive care unit (ICU). Venodilation, transudation of fluid from the vascular space into the interstitium and increased insensible losses will all result in hypovolemia in the course of patients with sepsis. Absolute hypovolemia is defined as a reduction of total circulating blood volume, while relative hypovolemia is an inadequate distribution of blood volume between the central and peripheral compartments.

Early goal-directed therapy emphasizes aggressive fluid resuscitation of septic patients during the initial 6 h of presentation. Persistent hypotension after initial fluid resuscitation is common and poses the dilemma of whether the patient should receive additional fluid boluses, positive inotropic agent or a vasopressor. Persistent signs of organ hypoperfusion such as oliguria make timely decision making crucial. While a number of technologies including pulse counter analysis, transpulmonary thermodilution, and bioreatance have all shown promise in the evaluation of volume status of septic patients, bedside ultrasonography has already established itself as a useful tool for evaluating cardiac function. Applying the same echocardiographic techniques to dynamically assess the physiological response to spontaneous or mechanical ventilation, bedside maneuvers and the response to therapeutic interventions will likely become a cornerstone of hemodynamic monitoring in the modern ICU. This chapter reviews the utility of echocardiography for identification of the volume-responsive patient with hemodynamic failure.

BENEFITS AND PITFALLS OF FLUID RESUSCITATION

When hypovolemia (either absolute or relative) is present, fluid resuscitation will provide benefit to the patient by increasing venous return, left ventricular diastolic volume, cardiac output, arterial blood pressure, and ultimately tissue perfusion. The rapidity with which euvolemia is reestablished may be a decisive factor in the eventual outcome. That being said, there is an increasing body of evidence suggesting that fluid resuscitation is not without serious and possibly lethal complications. Those complications may be related to preexisting conditions such as systolic or diastolic heart failure, acute cor pulmonale (ACP), or the development of sepsis-related cardiac dysfunction. In patients with ACP, volume resuscitation may be particularly harmful as it may cause further right ventricular (RV) enlargement and left ventricle (LV) compression, thus worsening the shock state (see Chapter 11 and Videos 10-1 and 10-2). ACP can be readily recognized by the clinician with basic-level echocardiography skills. Extravasation of prescribed fluids may result in worsening of acute respiratory distress syndrome (ARDS) and prolonged mechanical ventilation. Anemia and clotting disorders occur with hemodilution. Excessive fluid resuscitation can be positively correlated with increased mortality in the ICU. Given the risk to benefit ratio of volume expansion, the key question is whether the patient would benefit from additional fluid boluses. It is essential to make this determination as clinical studies have repeatedly demonstrated that only about 50% of hemodynamically unstable ICU patients are volume responsive (see definitions below).

FLUID CHALLENGE VERSUS VOLUME RESPONSIVENESS

Previously this key question was answered by administering a "fluid challenge" of 30 mL/kg of crystalloid solution and the patients' clinical (blood pressure, heart rate, urine output) and hemodynamic response (central venous pressure [CVP], pulmonary artery occlusion pressure [PAOP]) to the challenge was evaluated. Importantly, because a fluid

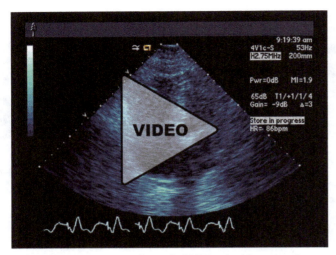

Video 10-1 Acute cor pulmonale (ACP) apical four-chamber view. Note dilated right ventricle (RV) is now an apex forming chamber. View at www.ccu2e.com

challenge has to be given to assess volume responsiveness and hypervolemia is associated with significant complications, it is possible, that the increases in mortality associated with invasive hemodynamic monitoring may be attributed to this approach. Given the increased mortality associated with excessive fluid resuscitation it seems prudent to predict the response to a fluid bolus prior to administering the bolus; a concept known as volume responsiveness.

The standard definition of volume responsiveness is a >15% increase in cardiac output in response to volume expansion. Although the volume of the fluid bolus has not been well standardized, a volume of between 500 mL and 1000 mL of crystalloid solution has been most studied. One or more baseline hemodynamic parameters are measured and evaluated for the ability to discriminate between responders and nonresponders.

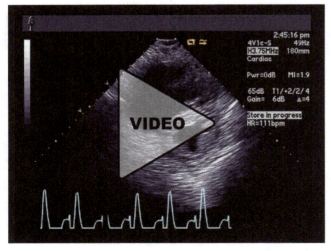

Video 10-2 Acute cor pulmonale (ACP) parasternal short-axis view, note left ventricular (LV) compression by the dilated right ventricle (RV). View at www.ccu2e.com

STATIC PARAMETERS

A static parameter is measured under a **single-ventricular loading** condition and is presumed to reliably estimate the preload of the right ventricle (RV), LV, or both ventricles (Figure 10-1). This estimation is used to evaluate the probability of responsiveness to ventricular filling, by assuming that a lower preload increases the probability of a response to volume expansion. Several static parameters of ventricular preload have been used in the ICU; some are based on direct pressure measurements, while others use echocardiographic indices.

▶ Static Pressure Parameters

The traditional approach to fluid resuscitation consists of measuring a pressure parameter such as the CVP or pulmonary artery occlusion pressure (PAOP) together with a cardiac output determination. The clinician would then prescribe a "fluid challenge" and reassess the above-mentioned parameters. This approach has been largely discredited by the data suggesting a poor or no correlation between the CVP or PAOP and volume responsiveness as well as intravascular volume. Nevertheless, the vast majority of intensivists still utilize the CVP to assess volume status and the major critical care societies advocate for CVP as a measure of successful fluid resuscitation. Multiple studies have demonstrated that the response to a fluid challenge even in healthy volunteers cannot be predicted by either the CVP or PAOP. In a study by Kumar et al. in healthy subjects, static indices of ventricular preload (CVP, PAOP, left ventricular end diastolic volume [LVEDV] index, right ventricular end diastolic volume [RVEDV] index) and cardiac performance indices (cardiac index, stroke volume [SV] index) were measured before and

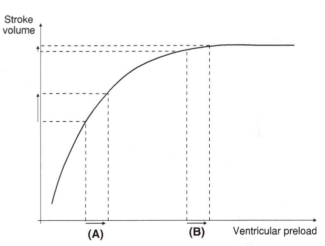

Figure 10-1 (**A**) The Frank–Starling curve indicating a patient with preload responsiveness; the increase of preload is followed by a significant increase of stroke volume, indicating that the patient is in the ascending part of the Frank–Starling curve. (**B**) A patient without preload responsiveness; the increase of preload is not followed by a significant increase of stroke volume, indicating that the patient is in the horizontal part of the Frank–Starling curve.

after 3 L of normal saline loading. In this study, there was no correlation between baseline static pressure parameters and changes in the cardiac performance indices (cardiac index, SV index) after fluid loading. Similarly, there was no correlation between changes in the CVP and PAOP and changes in cardiac performance. A meta-analysis by Coudray et al. reviewed five studies on a mixed population of spontaneously breathing critically ill patients and demonstrated the absence of a correlation between the initial PAOP and the response to a crystalloid infusion (an average of 1 L).

▶ Static Echocardiographic Parameters

Noninvasive echocardiography has advantages over pressure-derived parameters particular those obtained from CVP catheters or pulmonary artery catheterization. Transthoracic echocardiography (TTE) is preferred; however, in certain circumstances transesophageal echocardiography (TEE) may be required. The CVP and PAOP (left atrial pressure) can be approximated by echocardiography. In spontaneously breathing patients, there is a fairly good correlation between the size of the inferior vena cava (IVC) and the CVP. However, Feissel et al. demonstrated that the absolute IVC size failed to predict fluid responsiveness in patients with septic shock.

Left atrial pressure (left ventricular end diastolic pressure [LVEDP], PAOP) estimates involving the use of Doppler mitral flow, E/A ratio, pulmonary venous flow, tissue Doppler (E/e′ ratio) or colored coded Doppler (E/V_p ratio) may be helpful. While beyond the expertise level of most American intensivists, the estimated left atrial pressure (LVEDP, PAOP) can be estimated, utilizing formulas: LAP = 1.9 + 1.24 × E/e′ (mmHg) or LAP = E/e′ + 4 (mmHg) as a part of a comprehensive echocardiographic examination performed by an experienced operator. However, it is also worth noting that the PAOP fails to predict volume responsiveness whether measured directly or by echocardiography. The RV and LV diastolic diameter or area has been used as a measure of preload. However, Tavernier et al. and Feissel et al. have demonstrated that LV size (left ventricular end-diastolic area [LVEDA]) are not useful predictors of fluid responsiveness in patients on mechanical ventilation, unless the LV is very small and hyperkinetic (Figure 10-2 and Videos 10-3 and 10-4). A meta-analysis by Marik et al. demonstrated the failure of the LVEDA to predict volume responsiveness in mechanically ventilated patients.

Generally speaking, static parameters appear to be poor predictors of volume responsiveness except in patients with relatively obvious hypovolemia, which is an uncommon event in the modern ICU. It can be concluded that standard static indices of preload are not useful in predicting volume responsiveness in ICU patients. This observation may be due to dynamic changes in left (LV) and to a lesser degree RV

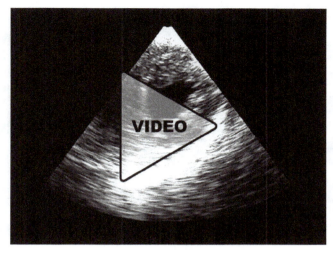

Video 10-3 Minimally invasive TEE short transgastric view of the LV. Note decrease LV diastolic area (LVDA). This patient appears hypovolemic and is likely to benefit from volume resuscitation. TEE, transesophageal echocardiography; LV, left ventricle. View at www.ccu2e.com

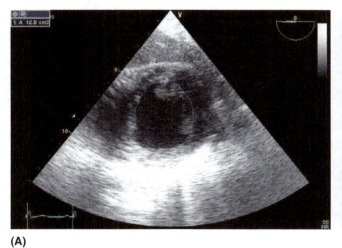

(A)

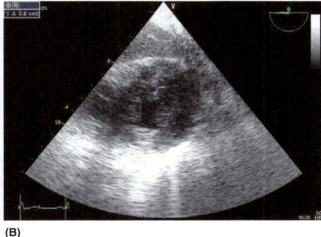

(B)

Figure 10-2 Measurements of left ventricular end-diastolic area (LVEDA) (A) and end-systolic area (LVESA) (B) with transesophageal echocardiography in a short-axis view. The quasi virtual LVESA (3.6 cm^2) is indicative of decreased left ventricular filling pressure.

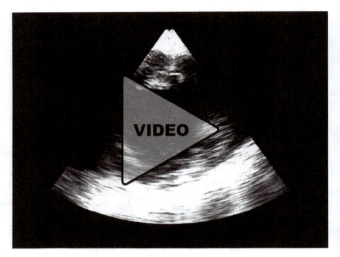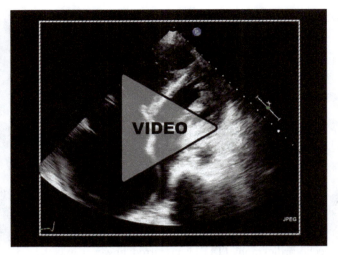

Video 10-4 Same patient as in Video 10.3, but now adequately resuscitated. Notice decrease heart rate, absence of premature contractions, increased LVDA, and increased stroke volume. LVDA, LV diastolic area. View at www.ccu2e.com

Video 10-5 Extreme ACP: note grossly dilated RV and right atrium (RA). LV is obviously compressed by RV resulting in decreased LV diastolic volume and stroke volume and thus hemodynamic instability, left atrium is compressed by the dilated RA further contributing to the lack of LV filling during diastole. This patient died from shock, resulting from hemodynamic consequences of the above, later that day. LV, left ventricle; RV, right ventricle; ACP, acute cor pulmonale. View at www.ccu2e.com

compliance, making the diastolic pressure–volume relationship nonlinear, unpredictable and perhaps subject to change during resuscitation itself. Systolic left ventricular function is also a subject to change in critically ill, both in those, with or without pre-existent cardiac disease. Vieillard–Baron and coauthors demonstrated the development of systolic left ventricular dysfunction in 60% of patient with septic shock. Changing left ventricular function makes it difficult to predict the position of the patient on his/her Frank–Starling curve. It is even difficult to estimate which family of Frank–Starling relationships should utilized to predict fluid responsiveness (Figure 10-1). Furthermore, the development of acute RV failure (ACP), particularly in patients receiving mechanical ventilation with high plateau pressures (>27 cm H_2O) further confounds the issue (see Chapter 11). Unrecognized acute RV failure can mimic hypovolemia hemodynamically but would not respond or even get worse with volume expansion (Video 10-5). Dynamic hemodynamic parameters offer the intensivists the best opportunity of predicting response to fluid resuscitation.

▶ Dynamic Parameters of Volume Responsiveness

Dynamic parameters are used to determine the patients position on his/her Frank–Starling curve (Figure 10-1) and specifically to determine whether the patient is situated **on the ascending portion** of the Frank–Starling curve where an increase of preload results in increase of SV (preload-dependent situation), **or on the plateau** portion where a variation of preload does not alter SV (preload-independent situation). Several approaches can be used to determine on what portion of the preload/SV relationship the ventricle is functioning to establish the diagnosis of preload dependence or independence. Most intensivists use the observation of cardiac responsiveness to either mechanical or spontaneous breathing cycles or more specifically breathing-related variations in intrathoracic pressure. These pressure changes directly effect RV and LV preload and provide a tool to correlate these preload changes to SV.

Alternatively, bedside maneuvers such as passive leg raising (PLR) result in alterations of RV and LV preload can be utilized to establish similar correlations.

Mechanically ventilated versus spontaneously breathing patient

During spontaneous breathing, a contracting (descending) diaphragm creates negative intrathoracic and positive intra-abdominal pressure. This results in a positive pressure gradient and increased blood flow from the abdomen into the chest. By this mechanism, spontaneous breathing significantly increases RV preload and is crucial to maintaining normal hemodynamic status. Mechanical ventilation substantially increases intrathoracic pressure (10-fold if low tidal volume/airway pressure ARDS network guidelines are followed), reducing RV preload and thus has predictably negative hemodynamic consequences. Moreover, it should be noted that traditional positive pressure ventilation also reverses inspiration/expiration phases from a hemodynamic point of view, changing many breathing-related phenomena (i.e., paradoxical pulse) to it's opposite – (reverse pulsus paradoxus). Generally speaking, good correlation exists between IVC diameter and collapsibility and right atrial pressure (RAP). Table 10-1 has been well established and low RAP is virtually predictive of volume responsiveness. On the other hand, elevated RAP may be associated with isolated RV dysfunction and does not entirely exclude possibility of beneficial effect of fluid resuscitation.

TABLE 10-1
Summary of Right Atrial Pressure (RAP) Estimation in Spontaneously Breathing Patient Using Inferior Vena Cava (IVC) Collapse Index

Mean RAP (mmHg)	IVC Diameter (cm)	IVC Collapse (%)
0–5	1.2–2.0	>50
5–10	≥2.0	≥50
10–15	>2.0	<50
≥20	>>2.0	<50

Dynamic echocardiographic parameters in patients on mechanical ventilation

Analysis of the respiratory changes of LV SV during mechanical ventilation provides a dynamic, biventricular evaluation of preload dependence. The respiratory changes of SV can be estimated by Doppler analysis of velocity–time integral (VTI) during TTE or TEE. In clinical studies, maximal ascending aortic flow velocity or VTI variation measured with TEE predict, with high sensitivity and specificity increases in cardiac output after fluid infusion in patients with septic shock. A cutoff value of respiratory cycle changes of 12% for maximal flow velocity variations and 20% for of aortic VTI discriminated responders from nonresponders. Similar information can be obtained from interrogation of ascending aorta with TTE (Figure 10-3) or descending aorta. Another approach to identify volume responsiveness using 2D images. Cannesson assessed LV diastolic area (LVDA) changes by TEE from the short-axis view. They found that a 16% respiratory variation of LVDA predicted fluid responsiveness with a sensitivity of 92% and a specificity of 83%. Utilizing a similar principle, IVC and superior vena cava (SVC) diameter changes during mechanical ventilation can be used to predict fluid responsiveness (Figure 10-4). The IVC diameter by TTE is either

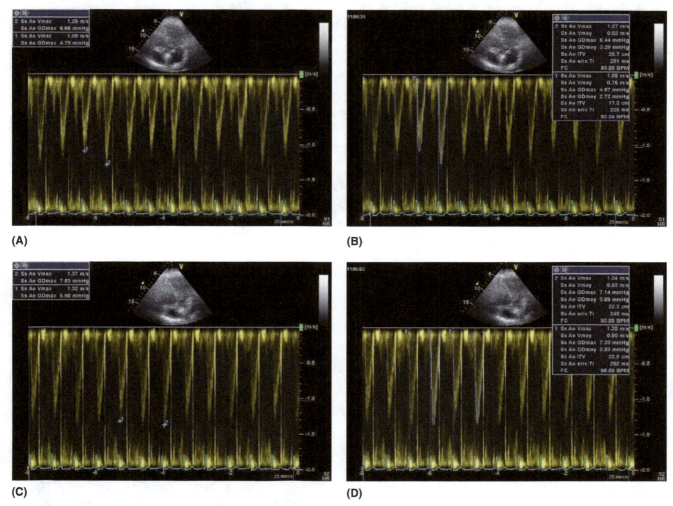

Figure 10-3 Respiratory variations of maximal velocity (V_{max}) (**A** and **C**) and VTI (**B** and **D**) of aortic blood flow recorded with a pulsed Doppler transthoracic echocardiography in a mechanically ventilated patient. (**A** and **C**) Presence of significant respiratory variations of V_{max} ($V_{max} - V_{min}/[V_{max} + V_{min}/2]$; 1.29 − 1.09/1.19 = 17%) and VTI ($VTI_{max} - VTI_{min}/[VTI_{max} + VTI_{min}/2]$; 20.7 − 17.3/19 = 18%). (**B** and **D**) Same patient after volume expansion, regression of the respiratory variations: V_{max} (1.37 − 1.32/1.34 = 4%), VTI (23.5 − 22.3/22.9 = 5%). VTI, velocity–time integral.

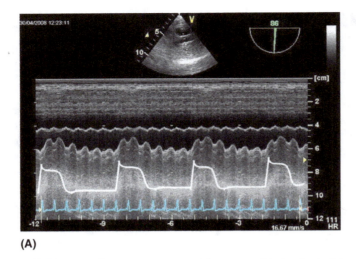

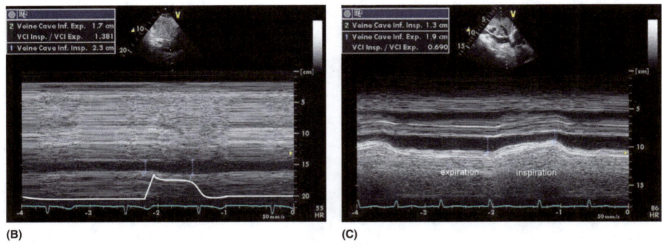

Figure 10-4 Respiratory vena cava variations in different circumstances. (A) Significant superior vena cava collapsibility recorded with transesoephageal echocardiography. (B) Significant inferior vena cava distensibility recorded with transthoracic echocardiography in a mechanically ventilated patient. (C) Significant vena cava collapsibility recorded with transthoracic echocardiography in a spontaneously breathing patient.

assessed directly from 2D images from a subcostal long-axis view or is analyzed from a subcostal long-axis view and recorded by using M-mode (Videos 10-6 and 10-7). Conventionally, a site just proximal to the inflow of the hepatic vein is utilized for the M-mode sampling (Figure 10-5). The SVC diameter is recorded from TEE longitudinal view at 90–100. Cutoff values of 12% [by using (max–min)/mean value)] and 18% [by using (max–min)/min value] for IVC (distensibility index) and 36% for SVC (collapsibility index) were found to accurately (sensitivity 90%, specificity 100%) separate responders and nonresponders. The potential benefit of using SVC is due to the fact that as intrathoracic organ the SVC is subject to greater respiratory variations and intrathoracic pressure resulting from mechanical ventilation. Though SVC collapsibility appears to be the most "reliable index of volume responsiveness," it does require TEE and thus is out of reach of most intensivists in the United States.

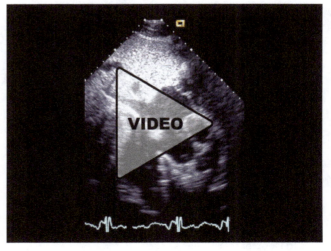

Video 10-6 Subcostal view. Note normal respiratory collapse of the inferior vena cava (IVC). This patient is likely to be a volume responder. View at www.ccu2e.com

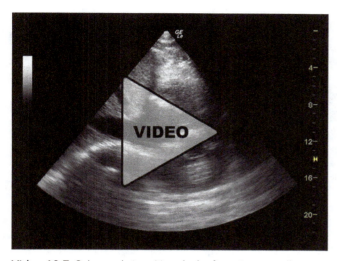

Video 10-7 Subcostal view. Note lack of respiratory collapse and dilated IVC. This patient is unlikely to be a volume responder. IVC, inferior vena cava. View at www.ccu2e.com

However, those methods are not universally applicable. Ventilator induced preload changes as predictors of volume responsiveness have only been evaluated in patients on flow limited, volume cycled ventilation and without patient ventilator dyssynchrony. Furthermore, although the level of positive end expiratory pressure (PEEP) is known to influence venous return and biventricular function the effect of PEEP on echocardiographic assessment of volume responsiveness has not been studied. Other requirements include presence of a normal sinus rhythm, normal intra-abdominal pressure and absence of significant RV dysfunction. Although a positive response to PLR (see below) seems to be predictive of volume responsiveness in mechanically ventilated patients (sensitivity 90% specificity 83%) further studies are necessary to better understand the role of this bedside maneuver in this population of critically ill patients.

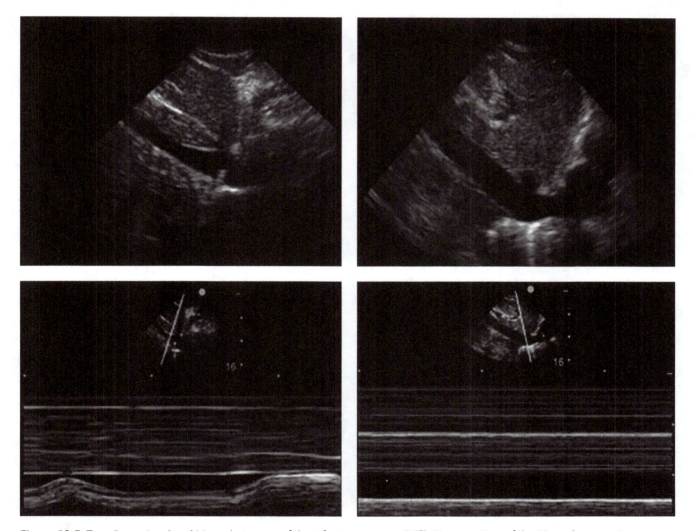

Figure 10-5 Two-dimensional and M-mode images of the inferior vena cava (IVC). Note position of the M-mode curser. Image on the left depicts significant respiratory variations in IVC diameter suggestive of volume responsiveness. Patient on the right is unlikely to positively respond to volume resuscitation.

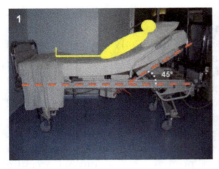
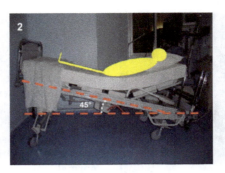
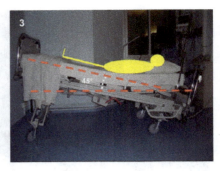

Figure 10-6 The realization of a passive leg raising maneuver in three steps: step 1, at baseline the patient is laying in a semirecumbent position, the trunk of the patient at 45° up to the horizontal; step 2, the entire bed is pivoted to obtain a head down tilt at 45°; and step 3, the head of the bed is adjusted to obtain a strictly horizontal trunk.

Dynamic echocardiographic parameters in spontaneously breathing patients

Response to PLR seems to hold the most promise in assessing volume responsiveness in the wide range of critically ill patients. Several publications have proposed using PLR maneuvers to predict preload responsiveness. This maneuver rapidly mobilizes about 300–500 mL of blood from the lower limbs to the intrathoracic compartment and reproduces the effects of similar volume fluid bolus (Figure 10-1). Being completely reversible this maneuver is devoid of any risks associated with an actual "fluid challenge". The test consists of raising both legs of the supine patient to an angle of 45 in relation to the bed (Figure 10-6 and Video 10-8) while measuring SV and cardiac output before and immediately (sometimes up to 1–3 min) following the PLR maneuver. This may be accomplished by measuring the VTI of the aortic outflow with either TTE (apical five-chamber view) or TEE (deep-gastric view). Monnet et al. demonstrated that when PLR induced an increase of aortic flow of >10%, it was predictive of an increase of aortic flow of >15% in response to volume expansion (sensitivity: 97%; specificity: 94%). Volume expansion was performed with 500 mL of isotonic saline over 10 min. Thirty-seven (52%) of the 71 patients included in this study responded to volume expansion; 22 subjects had spontaneous breathing activity (spontaneous breathing mode with inspiratory assistance). This study also evaluated respiratory cycle induced pulse pressure variations. The authors concluded that respiratory cyclic variations of pulse pressure ≥12% were similarly predictive of an increase of aortic flow by >15% in response to volume expansion in mechanically ventilated patients (sensitivity: 88%; specificity: 93%). However in spontaneously breathing patient's predictive value of respiratory pulse pressure variations was poor. In two other studies aortic VTI, SV and cardiac output were recorded using transthoracic echocardiography in spontaneously breathing patients during a PLR maneuver. Lamia et al. demonstrated a PLR-induced increase in SV of 12.5% or more predicted an increase in SV of 15% or more after volume expansion, with a sensitivity of 77% and a specificity of 100%. In this study, patients were intubated with spontaneous breathing. Static indices of preload such as left ventricular diastolic area and E/e' ratio failed to predict volume responsiveness. Maizel et al. studied 34 spontaneously breathing patients; an increase of cardiac output or SV by >12% during PLR was highly predictive of volume responsiveness. Sensitivity and specificity values were 63% and 89%, respectively. In addition, this study demonstrated that PLR may be used to predict volume responsiveness in patients with atrial fibrillation. Increased intra-abdominal pressure, however, strongly interferes with the ability of PLR to predict fluid responsiveness.

New and intriguing ways of assessing volume responsiveness were recently proposed by our research group. Increases in common carotid artery flow in response to PLR is measured instead of cardiac output. This method combines technical ease with the ability to measure peripheral redistribution of blood flow to vital organs (low resistance bed Chapter 26), which is characteristic of shock in general and septic shock in particular. While increases in cardiac output to PLR may be modest, carotid flow may increase substantially due perhaps to aforementioned flow redistribution, flow mediated arterial dilatation or more likely both (Figure 10-7 and Table 10-2). This new approach may also facilitate the bedside assessment of the severity of shock. Those incapable if

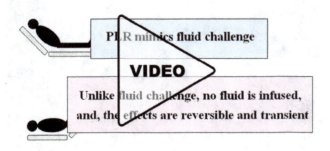

Video 10-8 Physiological explanation (basis) of the passive leg raising (PLR) maneuver. View at www.ccu2e.com

TABLE 10-2
Cardiac Output and Carotid Flow Response to PLR in Volume Responders and Nonresponders

	Responder (n = 17)	Nonresponder (n = 17)	
PLR responders/nonresponder			
Initial SVI (mL/min/M²)	25.2 ± 6.9	31.2 ± 10.2	p = 0.07
Maximal SVI after PLR (mL/min/M²)	33.8 ± 12.3	31.5 ± 10.3	—
% Change in SVI after PLR	29.8 ± 14.0	0.6 ± 4.7	—
	Responder (n = 18)	Nonresponder (n = 16)	
"True" Fluid responders			
Initial SVI (mL/min/M²)	26.2 ± 6.9	31.1 ± 10.1	p = 0.12
Ejection fraction (%)	60 ± 14	45 ± 16	p = 0.02
Stroke volume variation (%)	18.0 ± 5.1	14.8 ± 3.4	p = 0.15
% Change in carotid Doppler flow	79 ± 32	0.1 ± 14	p < 0.0001
Carotid flow* as % CO—baseline	13.1 ± 7.7	12.9 ± 5.7	—
Carotid flow* as % CO—post-PLR	18 ± 27.9	13.1 ± 6.6	—
Change in carotid diameter (mm)—post-PLR	1.1 ± 0.6	0.2 ± 0.3	p = 0.01

PLR = passive leg raising maneuver; SVI = stroke volume index; CO = cardiac output.
*Bilateral carotid blood flow as percentage of cardiac output.

increasing carotid flow may be the patients in whom normal adaptive mechanism of shifting blood to vital organs are no more present (Table 10-2 and Figures 10-8 and 10-9). Additional data need to be collected before recommending carotid artery flow response to PLR to the bedside intensivists.

In conclusion, echocardiography provides the intensivist with several methods to determine volume responsiveness in patients with hemodynamic failure. Dynamic parameters determined by echocardiography are far superior to static (either pressure or echocardiographic) measurements of preload for the determination of volume responsiveness.

The clinician with basic skills in critical care echocardiography may use respiratory variation of the IVC diameter to identify the preload-dependent patient combined with pattern recognition of a small hyperdynamic LV. The intensivist with an advanced TTE skill level may use respiratory variation of SV determined by Doppler echocardiography (VTI) and changes in SV following the PLR maneuver to identify volume responsiveness. Doppler and tissue Doppler

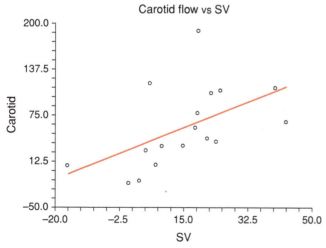

Figure 10-7 General correlation between increase in stroke volume and carotid artery flow in response to passive leg raising. Both parameter predicted positive response to fluid bolus of 1000 mL.

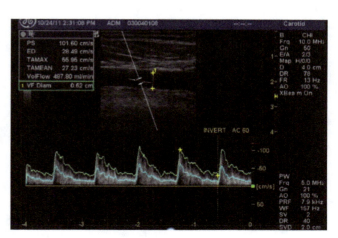

Figure 10-8 Common carotid artery flow prior to PLR in patient with septic shock. PLR, passive leg raising. View at www.ccu2e.com

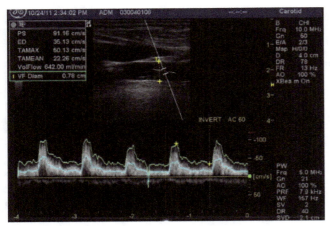

Figure 10-9 Common carotid artery (CCA) flow after PLR in patient with septic shock. Note significant increase in CCA flow. Also note CCA diameter increased, likely due to flow mediated dilatation (FMD). This patient was judged to be a likely candidate to benefit from volume resuscitation and improved hemodynamically after infusion of 1500 mL of lactated ringer solution. FMD is indicative of the relative lack of endothelial dysfunction and thus the ability to respond to neuro-hormonal stimuli redirecting blood to vital organs. View at www.ccu2e.com

measurements may provide additional insights by allowing the estimation of LAP. Intensivists with TEE skills may effectively utilize this modality in patients presenting technical challenges for TTE. The advent of minimally invasive TEE monitoring probes might allow the intensivist to secure views of the SVC that are not available on TTE and real-time LV and RV function monitoring capabilities previously unavailable at bedside. Carotid flow analysis may emerge as new and technically acceptable tools of assessing volume responsiveness and the severity of shock. The widespread use of newer modes of mechanical ventilation (APRV, HFOV) provides new challenges and opportunities for the evaluation of the effects of cardiac performance and volume responsiveness. Further studies are necessary to determine if this increase in physiological insight will translate into improved outcomes for critically ill patients.

SUGGESTED READING

Kircher BJ, Himelman RB, Schiller NB. Noninvasive estimation of right atrial pressure from the inspiratory collapse of the inferior vena cava. *Am J Cardiol.* 1990;66:493–496.

Feissel M, Michard F, Faller JP, et al. The respiratory variation in inferior vena cava diameter as a guide to fluid therapy. *Intensive Care Med.* 2004;30:1834–1837.

Kumar A, Anel R, Bunnell E, et al. Pulmonary artery occlusion pressure and central venous pressure fail to predict ventricular filling volume, cardiac performance, or the response to volume infusion in normal subjects. *Crit Care Med.* 2004;32:691–699.

Marik PE, Monnet X, Teboul JL. Hemodynamic parameters to guide fluid therapy. *Ann Intensive Care.* 2011;1:1.

Michard F, Teboul JL. Predicting fluid responsiveness in ICU patients: a critical analysis of the evidence. *Chest.* 2002;121:2000–2008.

Feissel M, Michard F, Mangin I, et al. Respiratory changes in aortic blood velocity as an indicator of fluid responsiveness in ventilated patients with septic shock. *Chest.* 2001;119:867–873.

Barbier C, Loubières Y, Schmit C, et al. Respiratory changes in inferior vena *cava* diameter are helpful in predicting fluid responsiveness in ventilated septic patients. *Intensive Care Med.* 2004;30:1740–1746.

Vieillard-Baron A, Augarde R, Prin P, et al. Influence of superior vena caval zone condition on cyclic changes in right ventricular outflow during respiratory support. *Anesthesiology.* 2001;95:1083–1088.

Monnet X, Rienzo M, Osman D, et al. Passive leg raising predicts fluid responsiveness in the critically ill. *Crit Care Med.* 2006;34:1402–1407.

Lamia B, Ochagavia A, Monnet X, et al. Echocardiographic prediction of volume responsiveness in critically ill patients with spontaneously breathing activity. *Intensive Care Med.* 2007;33:1125–1132.

Maizel J, Airapetian N, Lorne E, et al. Diagnosis of central hypovolemia by using passive leg raising. *Intensive Care Med.* 2007;33:1133–1138.

Marik PE, Levitov A, et al. The use of NICOM (Bioreatance) and carotid Doppler to determine volume responsiveness and blood flow redistribution following passive leg raising in hemodynamically unstable patients. *Chest.* 2013;143(2):364–370.

ECHOCARDIOGRAPHIC DIAGNOSIS AND MONITORING OF RIGHT VENTRICULAR FUNCTION

Scan QR code or visit www.ccu2e.com for video in this chapter

ADOLFO KAPLAN & PAUL H. MAYO

INTRODUCTION

Right ventricular (RV) dysfunction is common in critically ill patients.[1-3] It is associated with multiple clinical scenarios frequently encountered by the intensivist, including acute cor pulmonale (ACP), acute RV dysfunction of sepsis, and acute RV infarction. In addition, the assessment of RV function is essential for the determination of a patient's preload responsiveness. Echocardiography is the best available method to diagnose and monitor RV function at the bedside, as it provides the intensivist with a prompt, accurate, noninvasive, and serial method to monitor the function of the right heart and its response to different interventions. This chapter describes a variety of echocardiographic methods to assess RV function that are particularly relevant to critical care practice for both the basic and advanced critical care echocardiographer. While the assessment of RV function in the noncritically ill patient is beyond the purview of this chapter, the techniques described here are also applicable to the assessment of RV function in the ambulatory patient.

This chapter is designed to have utility for intensivists with basic critical care echocardiography (CCE) skills. In this case, the examination is limited to the standard two-dimensional (2D) five view approach (see Chapter 6), which focuses on a qualitative visual estimate of RV size and septal dynamics. This approach is a key component of the rapid evaluation of hemodynamic failure.

In addition, this chapter reviews the evaluation of RV function using methods that are relevant only to the intensivist with skill at advanced critical care echocardiography. By definition, these include Doppler-based measurements that are not part of basic CCE. Given the time constraints of bedside scanning in a busy intensive care unit, the discussion will focus on a limited number of methods rather than listing all of the possible methods for evaluation of RV function that are available to the advanced level echocardiographer.

NORMAL RV ANATOMY AND FUNCTION

The RV comprises two anatomically and functionally distinct cavities separated by the crista supraventricularis: an inflow region (the sinus) and an outflow tract (the cone or infundibulum). The tricuspid valve (TV) and its apparatus plus heavily trabeculated myocardium form the sinus. Smooth myocardium and the pulmonic valve form the infundibulum. The sinus generates pressure during systole while the infundibulum modulates this pressure and prolongs its duration. RV contraction occurs serially in three different phases: (a) contraction of the sinus along its longitudinal axis, (b) radial contraction of the RV free wall toward the interventricular septum (IVS), and (c) torsion of the left ventricle (LV) (clockwise rotation of the LV base with counterclockwise rotation of apex) pulling the RV in similar manner. Overall, LV contraction contributes 25% of its own stroke work to the generation of RV stroke work via the IVS.[4]

The normal RV is less muscular than the LV and has a free wall thickness that measures 3–4 mm. As a consequence, it is easily affected by its surroundings and the effects of increased afterload. Unlike the LV, it is able to acutely dilate. Relative to the LV, the RV is a lower pressure chamber, with normal pressures of less than 25/8 mmHg with the patient in the resting state. When afterload increases acutely, the RV is unable to acutely generate higher pressures. However, when subjected to chronic loading conditions, the RV compensates with a hypertrophic response that is suggested by a thickened RV free wall on echocardiography. In this situation, the RV can generate up to systemic-level pressures, such as is seen with advanced pulmonary arterial hypertension.

▶ Acute Cor Pulmonale

ACP is defined as the clinical setting in which the RV experiences a sudden increase in afterload.[5] This may occur in

TABLE 11-1
Causes of Acute Cor Pulmonale
Acute left heart failure (ischemic, myocardial, or valvular origin) Acute pulmonary embolism Acute respiratory distress syndrome (ARDS) Inappropriately adjusted ventilatory support Respiratory and metabolic acidosis[3] Fat emboli Gas emboli Low PaO$_2$

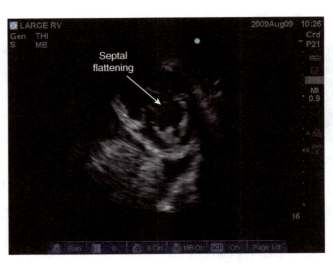

Figure 11-1 This parasternal long-axis view shows a flattened septum. Review of Video 11-1 demonstrates the septal dyskinesia that is associated with this septal flattening.

the context of previously normal RV function or in the RV that is already impaired. Sudden increases in RV afterload occur frequently in critically ill patients (Table 11-1). ACP is synonymous with acute right heart failure. It is characterized by the combination of systolic and diastolic overload, both of which have distinctive echocardiographic features.

Echocardiographic features of RV systolic overload

Dyskinesis is defined as a myocardial segment moving outward during systole. Septal dyskinesia is the echocardiographic hallmark of a sudden elevation of RV systolic afterload and occurs because of ventricular interdependence. When RV afterload is increased, its contraction is prolonged, requiring a longer time for completion than left ventricular systole. Because the RV is still contracting at the end of systole when the LV is beginning to relax, the right intraventricular pressure becomes transiently greater than the left intraventricular pressure, and the IVS is displaced in the direction of the LV cavity.[6] When due to pulmonary vascular processes (e.g., acute respiratory distress syndrome [ARDS] and pulmonary embolism [PE]), septal dyskinesia develops rapidly in the course of disease.

Septal dyskinesia can be assessed qualitatively and quantitatively. The qualitative evaluation consists of observing for paradoxical septal motion by 2D echocardiography. With TTE, septal dyskinesia is well observed from the apical four-chamber and parasternal short-axis views, the latter at the midventricular level papillary muscle level (Figure 11-1 and Video 11-1). Identification of septal dyskinesia is part of the basic CCE examination. M-mode may be used for identification of abnormal septal motion (Figure 11-2).

Quantification of systolic RV overload can also be achieved by measurement of the systolic eccentricity index (EI). To do this, the short-axis view of the mid-LV (when both papillary muscles are displayed) is obtained with transthoracic (TTE) or transesophageal (TEE) echocardiography. At end systole, D1 is measured as the diameter that bisects the papillary muscles and D2 is the orthogonal diameter to D1. The systolic EI = D2/D1. A normal systolic EI is 1. Septal dyskinesia will result in an EI > 1 (Figure 11-3).[7] An atrial septal defect can result in a falsely elevated EI.[8] Therefore, a search for intracardiac shunting should always be considered when the EI is >1.

Systolic RV overload can also be indirectly identified by Doppler assessment of the right ventricular outflow tract (RVOT) or main pulmonary artery (MPA) with both TTE and TEE using pulsed-wave (PW) Doppler. The MPA is imaged in the parasternal short-axis view with TTE and in the great vessel view with TEE. The PW sample volume is placed in the MPA in order to obtain the systolic velocity envelope. The systolic velocity envelope is recorded allowing both qualitative and quantitative assessments of increased pulmonary vascular impedance (Table 11-2). These measurements have methodological problems that include the following:

1. *Poor TTE image quality:* This is problematic in the critically ill patient on ventilator support. The use of TEE obviates this problem.

2. *Misalignment between the ultrasound beam and RVOT jet:* Even with color Doppler guidance, the spectral

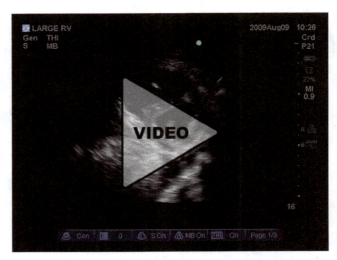

Video 11-1 This parasternal long-axis view shows septal dyskinesia related to right ventricular dysfunction. View at www.ccu2e.com

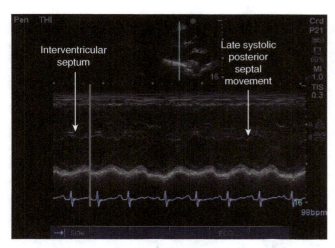

Figure 11-2 This image shows an m-mode tracing with the interrogation line placed at the midventricular level in the parasternal long-axis view. There is late systolic posterior paradoxical movement of the septum consistent with right ventricular pressure overload.

Doppler signal may not reflect the spatial distribution of the pulmonary artery (PA) jet, which is higher along the inner edge of its natural curvature.

3. *Misinterpretation of the spectral Doppler signal:* Only the outer edge of the spectral envelope should be used.
4. *Difficulty in measurement of the short time intervals being measured:* Inter and intraobserver variability is a problem.
5. *The time required to perform the measurements:* The intensivist, having responsibility for image acquisition at the bedside, has limited time to perform a comprehensive examination. Time constraints are a reality in a busy intensive care unit. The intensivist needs to select a limited number of measurements that have utility in defining RV function, as it is unrealistic to perform all possible measurements.

TABLE 11-2
Quantitative RV Output Measurements

	Normal	RV Systolic Overload
Decreased stroke volume	70–100 mL	<70 mL
Decreased RVOT velocity-time integral (VTI)	18 ± 3 cm	<15 cm
Decreased acceleration time	≥120 m/s	<80 m/s
Decreased ejection time	304 ± 23 m/s	<281 m/s
Decreased acceleration time/ ejection time	>0.34^2	<0.34

RV, right ventricular; RVOT, right ventricular outflow tract; VTI, velocity-time integral.

In actual clinical practice and when using TTE, we routinely visualize the MPA through its bifurcation. In the parasternal short axis at the base of the heart, the tri-leaflet aortic valve will be in the center of the screen with the TV on the patient's right and the pulmonic valve on the patients left. In most cases, the anterior leaflet of the pulmonic valve is visualized. With TTE, it may be necessary to tilt the transducer downward and angle it leftward in order to visualize the MPAP (Figure 11-4 and Video 11-2). With TEE, the pulmonic valve, the MPA, and its bifurcation can be readily assessed on the basal short-axis planes, usually with the transducer tip 25–30 cm from the incisors (Figure 11-5 and Video 11-3). We perform Doppler interrogation of the MPAP to obtain a qualitative assessment of its signal, to detect the normal monophasic systolic spectral Doppler contour or the abnormal biphasic pattern that suggests pulmonary hypertension (Figure 11-6). We do not routinely perform comprehensive Doppler analysis beyond measurement of the pulmonary systolic acceleration time which has utility for assessment for pulmonary hypertension (see below).

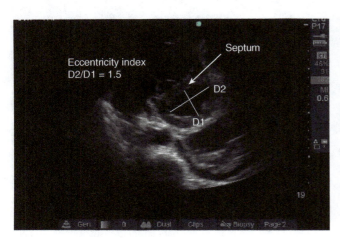

Figure 11-3 This parasternal short-axis view demonstrates measurement of the eccentricity index.

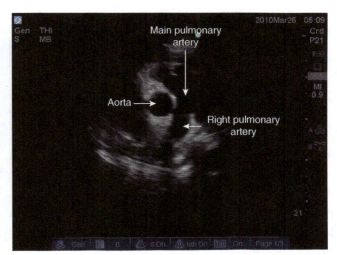

Figure 11-4 This transthoracic parasternal short-axis view shows the main pulmonary artery and its bifurcation.

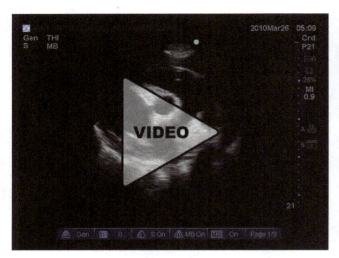

Video 11-2 This transthoracic parasternal short-axis view shows the main pulmonary artery and its bifurcation. View at www.ccu2e.com

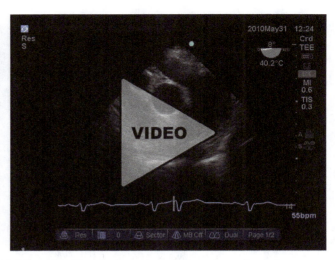

Video 11-3 This transesophageal view shows the main pulmonary artery and its bifurcation. View at www.ccu2e.com

Visualization of the PA with TTE or TEE may occasionally allow diagnosis of a centrally located PE (Video 11-4). This is a key finding in evaluation of the patient with RV failure.

For qualitative assessment of RV systolic function, the intensivist observes the endomyocardial thickening and contraction of the RV free wall and IVS from the apical four-chamber view, in a similar fashion as it is done with the qualitative assessment of the LV function. The contractile function of the RV is graded as normal, mild, moderate, or severely reduced. This approach is dependent upon the skills and experience of the interpreter. There are several quantitative techniques to assess RV contractile function. These include ejection fraction; fractional area of contraction; myocardial performance index; tissue Doppler systolic velocity of the tricuspid annulus; and the measurement of Dp/dt from the tricuspid regurgitation jet. We consider that these measurements are not practical for use by the bedside critical care echocardiographer. A simple measurement of RV systolic function that is easy and reproducible to perform is tricuspid annular plane systolic excursion (TAPSE). Systolic RV failure is associated with reduced TAPSE, which may be measured with M-mode interrogation of the tricuspid annulus. The measurement is made from the apical four-chamber view with the M-mode interrogation line placed through the lateral tricuspid annulus. From a frozen image, the displacement of the annulus during systole is measured using the machine caliper function (Figure 11-7). A TAPSE less than 17 mm indicates RV systolic failure.[9]

Echocardiographic features of RV diastolic overload

RV diastolic overload is synonymous with RV dilation. There are multiple definitions of right heart dilation. It

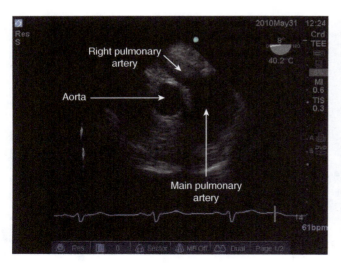

Figure 11-5 This transesophageal view shows the main pulmonary artery and its bifurcation.

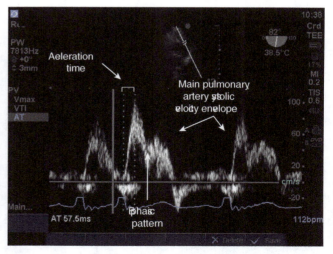

Figure 11-6 This Doppler tracing shows the systolic velocity envelope from the main pulmonary artery (transesophageal view). There is a biphasic contour and the acceleration time is 58 ms; this is consistent with an elevation of pulmonary artery pressure.

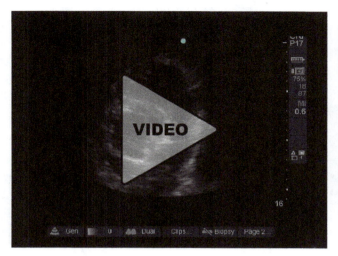

Video 11-4 This short-axis subcostal view shows the main pulmonary artery with a pulmonary embolism. View at www.ccu2e.com

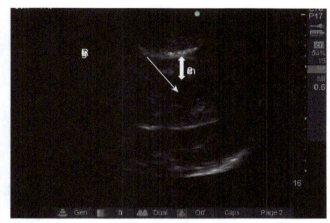

Figure 11-8 This subcostal long-axis view shows an enlarged right ventricle (RV) with a thickened RV free wall. This indicates that the RV has been under load for some period of time.

is difficult to accurately estimate RV volumes with echocardiography because of a failure of geometric models to appropriately reflect the complicated RV anatomy. To circumvent this problem, Jardin and colleagues have proposed a semi-quantitative assessment of right heart diastolic overload.[1] Both ventricular areas were measured at end-diastole by tracing the endomyocardium from the apical four-chamber view. When the endomyocardium was not well visualized, the area was traced to the epicardium. The authors found that the RV end-diastolic area to left ventricular end-diastolic area (RVEDA:LVEDA) ratio correlated well with RV dilation. The normal RVEDA:LVEDA ratio was found to be between 0.36 and 0.6 (0.48 ± 0.12). They defined moderate dilation as a ratio = 0.7–0.9, and severe dilation as a ratio ≥1. Fremont et al. confirmed the prognostic value of end-diastolic area (measured at the beginning of the QRS complex) RVEDA:LVEDA ratio in patients with acute PE.[10] In their registry of 1416 hospitalized patients with acute PE, 31 subjects (3.3%) died. Among patients with systolic blood pressure ≥90 mmHg, the mortality rate was 3.3% for those with a RV/LV ratio ≥0.6, and 1.1% for those with a ratio <0.6. Using mortality receiver operating curves, an RV/LV ratio ≥0.9 had the best sensitivity (72%) and specificity (58%) to discriminate between those patients with the highest risk of dying: 6.6% if the ratio ≥0.9 and 1.9% if <0.9. Chamber size in this study was frequently measured in the parasternal or subcostal views. This is important, as the subcostal view is frequently the best TTE view in critically ill patients on ventilatory support (Figure 11-8 and Video 11-5).

The assessment of RV size in comparison with LV size has many advantages, including its simplicity, avoidance of individual variations in cardiac size, and the reduced interobserver and intraobserver variability introduced by

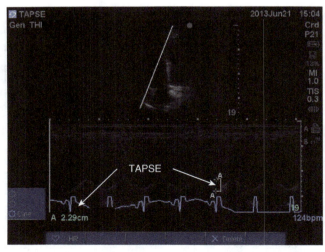

Figure 11-7 This image shows the measurement of tricuspid annular plane systolic excursion using M-mode from an apical four-chamber view.

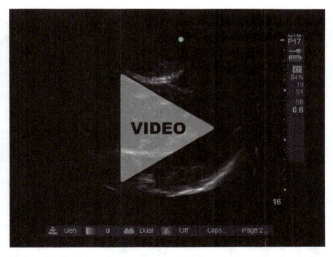

Video 11-5 This subcostal long-axis view shows an enlarged right ventricle (RV) with a thickened RV free wall. This indicates that the RV has been under load for some period of time. View at www.ccu2e.com

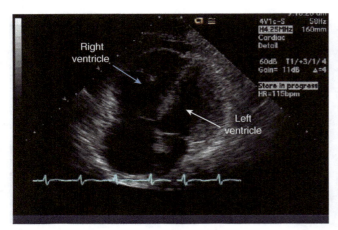

Figure 11-9 This apical four-chamber view shows a large right ventricle.

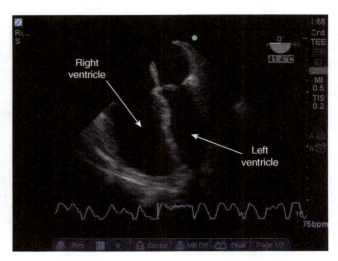

Figure 11-10 This midesophageal four-chamber view shows an enlarged right ventricle.

quantitative methods.[1] Vieillard-Baron et al. evaluated the accuracy of qualitative versus quantitative/semi-quantitative assessments of several echocardiographic parameters by TEE, as performed by intensivist echocardiographers.[11] The authors subjectively classified RV end-diastolic size in comparison with the LV end-diastolic size in the apical four-chamber view as normal, moderately enlarged, and markedly enlarged. The subjective qualitative observation of chamber size correlated well with the quantitative assessment of the RV/LV ratio. The interobserver variability was good ($K = 0.74$, 95%; CI 0.54–0.94). Their results indicate that a trained echocardiographer can readily identify RV diastolic overload with an "eyeball" assessment.

The intensivist with skill at basic CCE can readily assess the presence of RV dilation by comparing its size with the LV. The RV cavity should be smaller than the left. If both ventricular cavities are the same size, the RV is dilated. If the right chamber is larger than the left, it is severely dilated. This is best observed from the apical four-chamber (Figure 11-9 and Video 11-6), the long-axis subcostal views with TTE, and the midesophageal four-chamber view with TEE (Figure 11-10 and Video 11-7).

In addition to enlargement of the RV, an increase in RV diastolic volume will also result in a change of its normal configuration. When enlarged, the RV loses its triangular shape and becomes more rounded in the apical four-chamber view. An oval, instead of half-moon–like, shape is observed both on short- and long-axis views and on parasternal views (Figures 11-11 and 11-12; and Videos 11-8 and 11-9). There are published guidelines on RV chamber quantification by the American Society of Echocardiography (ASE) in conjunction with the European Association of Echocardiography.[12] These measurements have limited clinical utility in critical care practice.

Right heart dilation results in reduced LV filling. Because the pericardium encloses the heart within a relatively stiff envelope, the right heart can only dilate at the expense of the space normally occupied by the larger LV. This leads

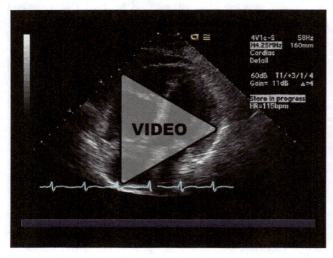

Video 11-6 This apical four-chamber view shows a large right ventricle (RV) as well as apical sparing of RV systolic function (McConnell's Sign). View at www.ccu2e.com

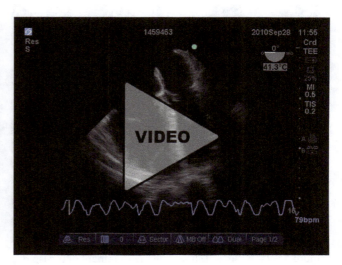

Video 11-7 This midesophageal four-chamber view shows an enlarged right ventricle. View at www.ccu2e.com

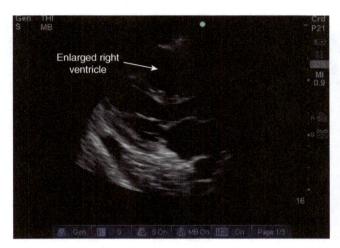

Figure 11-11 This parasternal long-axis view shows a dilated right ventricular outflow track.

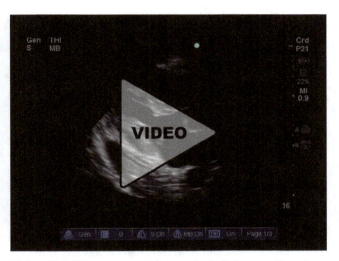

Video 11-8 This parasternal long-axis view shows a dilated right ventricular outflow track with septal dyskinesia. View at www.ccu2e.com

to an impairment of LV filling. PW Doppler interrogation of mitral valve inflow displays a spectral signal consistent with impaired LV filling ($E/A < 1$).[13]

Acute versus subacute/chronic cor pulmonale

There are no definitive criteria to distinguish between ACP and chronic right heart failure. To further complicate this assessment, ACP may occur in a patient with chronic right heart failure. The causes of chronic right heart failure include left heart failure, pulmonary arterial hypertension of any etiology, and a variety of pulmonary processes. The RV wall becomes hypertrophic relatively rapidly if RV outflow impedance is elevated. The RV free wall thickness is best evaluated on the subcostal view at the end of diastole. The normal thickness is 3.3 ± 0.6 mm. After only 48 h of a sudden increase in afterload, the RV free wall thickness may increase to double this width. In chronic cor pulmonale, the RV free wall may thicken to as much as 10 mm. In addition to wall thickening, there may be increased intracavitary muscle trabeculations, and frequently there may be LV hypertrophy.[14] The level of PA pressure calculated by Doppler techniques can also provide a clue that the process is chronic. While the systolic pulmonary arterial pressure (PAPs) in acute conditions is generally <60 mmHg, it can be higher in chronic cor pulmonale. Finally, the confirmation of ACP can be made retrospectively. ACP reverses once the baseline disorder is corrected. The lack of complete reversibility of ACP indicates the presence of chronic cor pulmonale. When faced with a suspected chronic cor pulmonale pattern, the echocardiographer must always rule out left-sided cardiac dysfunction as the primary cause.

▶ Cor Pulmonale and Pulmonary Hypertension

Cor pulmonale is usually associated with an elevation of PAPs. However, if the RV pump function is severely

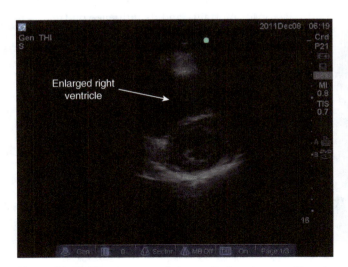

Figure 11-12 This parasternal short-axis view shows a dilated right ventricle.

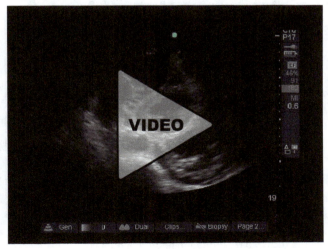

Video 11-9 This parasternal short-axis view shows a dilated right ventricle with septal dyskinesia and septal flattening. View at www.ccu2e.com

impaired, it may not be able to generate significant cardiac output, resulting in pseudo-normalization of PA pressures. Alternatively, the clinician will frequently encounter clinical scenarios where elevated PAPs are present in the absence of ACP. This finding should prompt the physician to rule out intracardiac and intrapulmonary causes of pulmonary arterial hypertension. Intracardiac etiologies include: left-to-right shunts and constrictive pericarditis. Pulmonary etiologies of pulmonary hypertension include PE, including chronic thromboembolic pulmonary hypertension, and lung diseases such as chronic obstructive pulmonary disease and a variety of interstitial lung processes.

▶ Measurements of PAPs

PA systolic, diastolic, and mean pressures can be estimated from the tricuspid and pulmonic regurgitant jets, using the modified Bernouilli equation (Figure 11-13). The tricuspid regurgitant (TR) jet is used to measure PAPs as follows:

$$PAPs = 4 \times (\text{Tricuspid regurgitant jet}_{peak\ velocity})^2 + \text{Right atrial pressure (RAP)}.$$

The TR jet should be interrogated from multiple acoustic windows (apical and parasternal), with transducer angulation to obtain a parallel intercept angle between the ultrasound beam and TR jet (Figure 11-12). Numerous factors can affect the accuracy of the measurement. Technically, it may be difficult to obtain an adequate spectral Doppler envelope or adequate intercept between the ultrasound beam and the TR jet. In this case, a low-intensity TR jet may be augmented by injection of agitated saline contrast. Using estimates of right atrial pressure (RAP) instead of actual measurements can lead to over- or underestimations of PAPs. It is important to use an accurate RAP in the PAPs equation. Inferior vena cava (IVC) size and changes with respi-

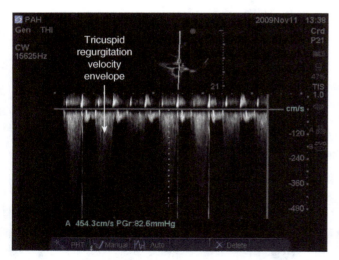

Figure 11-13 This Doppler tracing shows the peak velocity of the tricuspid regurgitation jet from a right ventricular inflow view. The trans-valvular pressure gradient was 83 mmHg. The right atrial pressure was measured at 20 mmHg, giving a pulmonary artery systolic pressure of 103 mmHg.

TABLE 11-3
RAP as Estimated by IVC Size and Dynamic

RAP (mmHg)	IVC Size	IVC Contraction (Inspiration)	Hepatic Vein
0–5	<20 mm	>50%	Normal
10	<20 mm	<50%	Normal
15	>20 mm	<50%	Normal
20	>20 mm	<50%	Dilated

IVC, inferior vena cava; RAP, right atrial pressure.

ratory cycles may be used to estimate RAP (Table 11-3).[14] These measurements are only valid for the spontaneously breathing subject. RAP can also be measured directly, if the patient has a central venous catheter in place.

In addition to PAPs, pulmonary artery diastolic pressure (PAPd) and mean pulmonary artery pressure (PAPm) can be measured from a pulmonic valve regurgitant jet, when present, as follows:

$$PAPd = 4 \times (\text{Pulmonic regurgitant end diastolic velocity})^2 + RAP.$$

A variety of methods to estimate mean PAP have been described.[15] These measurements have limited clinical utility in critical care practice.

CLINICAL SCENARIOS LEADING TO ACUTE COR PULMONALE

▶ Massive PE

PE may be associated with RV dysfunction. Several authors have defined ACP in the context of acute PE using different criteria.[16-18] Because of its simplicity, the RV/LV ratio is the most practical for a bedside application. Using this ratio, Vieillard-Baron et al. reported the incidence of ACP as 61% in 161 subjects with anatomically massive PE.[19] Whether ACP is an independent prognostic factor for mortality and its influence on treatment (e.g., thrombolysis) remains under investigation. Occasionally, a thrombus in transit will be identified in the right heart (Figure 11-14 and Video 11-10). These are typically mobile and may be serpiginous; they are of grave clinical concern. Thrombus may be visible in the main and proximal pulmonary arteries in a parasternal short-axis view with TTE (Figure 11-6 and Video 11-4). The main and proximal PA are readily visualized with TEE, and this is a means of establishing rapid diagnosis of PE in the critically ill patient.[20,21]

Other indirect echocardiographic signs of acute PE include the following:

1. *McConnell sign:* Diffuse hypokinesis of the RV free wall sparing the apex[22] (Video 11-11)
2. *60/60 sign:* RVOT acceleration time <60 m/s in association with PA systolic pressure <60 mmHg (as estimated by TR regurgitant jet)[23]

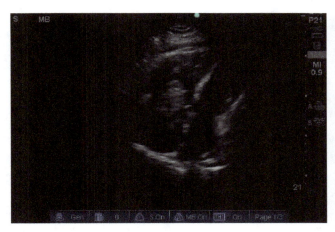

Figure 11-14 This apical four-chamber view shows a thrombus in transit in the right atrium and right ventricle.

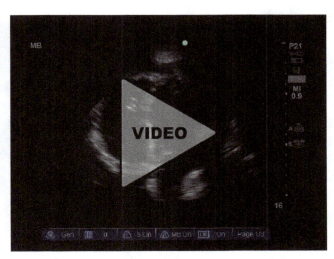

Video 11-11 This apical four-chamber view shows a dilated right ventricle (RV) with diffuse hypokinesis of the RV free wall sparing the apex (McConnell's sign). View at www.ccu2e.com

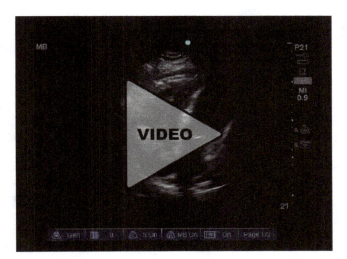

Video 11-10 This apical four-chamber view shows a thrombus in transit in the right atrium and right ventricle. View at www.ccu2e.com

Both of these signs were described retrospectively. When tested in a prospective study of 100 consecutive patients with proven PE, the sensitivity of McConnell and 60/60 signs ranged from 19% to 36%.[23] This was likely due to the subjectivity inherent in determining segmental wall motion abnormality and the high margin of error when measuring the acceleration time. The combination of the two signs increased their sensitivity without compromising their specificity.[23]

▶ Acute Respiratory Distress Syndrome

In patients with ARDS on ventilatory support, the RV can become afterloaded due to factors intrinsic to the disease and factors associated with mechanical ventilation. These include the following:

1. Occlusion of the pulmonary vascular bed (microthrombi, inflammation, interstitial edema, and atelectasis)
2. High transpulmonary pressures that result in pulmonary capillary compression (tidal volume and positive end-expiratory pressure [PEEP] effect)[24,25]
3. Acidosis and hypoxemia with pulmonary vascular constriction[26]
4. Intra-abdominal hypertension[27]

ACP is frequent in ARDS. Vieillard-Baron et al. reported an incidence of 25% in 75 patients with ARDS submitted to protective ventilation, defined as a plateau pressure <30 cm H_2O with a mean PEEP of 6–7 cm H_2O.[28] Mekontso-Dessap et al. described a 22% incidence of ACP in 203 ARDS patients ventilated with mean PEEP of 10 cm H_2O and mean plateau pressure (Pplat) of 23 cm H_2O. Interestingly, there was also a significant increase in shunting through patent foramen ovale (34% vs. 15%), resulting in fewer ventilator-free days at 28 days.[29] Echocardiography can readily identify patterns of ventilatory support that may result in ACP. Serial echocardiography can alert the physician to this possibility and allow adjustment of therapies in a sequential and effective manner.[30,31]

▶ Recruitment Maneuvers

Typically, a recruitment maneuver involves applying a high level of PEEP for a defined period of time. Echocardiography demonstrates inadvertent ACP with significant hemodynamic consequences that can occur during the recruitment maneuver.[32,33] This occurs as a result of acute augmentation of RV afterload due to pulmonary vascular compression from increased transpulmonary pressures and results in reduced cardiac output and hemodynamic instability.

▶ Acute RV Failure of Sepsis

Function of both LV and RV can become depressed in sepsis.[3,34–38] The cardiomyopathy is characterized by its acute onset, reversibility, and the association of a depressed LV systolic function with normal or low LV filling pressures. Vieillard-Baron et al. reported RV dilation in 30% of patients with septic cardiomyopathy using TEE.[39] The RV failure with ACP can become manifest when ventilatory support is applied. By increasing pulmonary vascular resistance, mechanical ventilation can result in ACP in an RV that is already dysfunctional from sepsis. If ACP develops, the clinician should adjust the ventilator settings to minimize alveolar distension, hypoxemia and acidosis, restrict intravenous fluid resuscitation, and add vasoactive therapy to maintain adequate coronary artery perfusion pressure.[5,39]

▶ RV Infarction

RV infarction occurs predominantly due to occlusion of the right coronary artery. In addition to perfusing the RV free wall, this artery also supplies blood to the inferior aspect of the LV and the inferior IVS through the posterior descending artery. As a result, RV infarction is frequently accompanied by LV inferior wall infarction with a corresponding segmental wall abnormality that is detectable with echocardiography. With proximal RCA occlusion, severe acute RV failure may occur. Unlike ACP, PAPs may not be elevated, as the failing RV cannot generate enough cardiac output. A clue to the diagnosis of ischemia is the presence of abnormal endomyocardial thickening and segmental wall motion abnormality of the inferior left ventricular wall and inferior septum. Dilation of the tricuspid annulus secondary to RV dilation can result in acute TR, elevation of RAP, right atrial enlargement, and IVC dilation. Segmental RV wall abnormalities may be detected with echocardiography, and their presence supports the diagnosis of RV infarction. Their detection requires detailed 2D imaging of the RV from multiple views that is not practical for bedside imaging in the intensive care unit.[40] The interested reader is referred to the recent ASE guidelines for the assessment of the right heart in adults for descriptive and graphic representation of RV wall segments and corresponding supplying arteries.[15]

IDENTIFICATION OF PRELOAD RESPONSIVENESS IN PRESENCE OF RIGHT HEART FAILURE

Detection of preload sensitivity is a key part of managing the patient with hemodynamic failure. The presence of RV failure may be a confounder when using dynamic parameters to identify preload sensitivity that utilize stroke volume (SV) variation or a surrogate measurement while the patient is on ventilatory support. Identification of significant respirophasic SV variation (or a surrogate for SV) may predict preload sensitivity, providing the patient is on mechanical ventilatory support while not making any spontaneous breathing effort, is on adequate tidal volume, and has a regular heart rate. However, these dynamic parameters of volume responsiveness should always be evaluated within the context of right heart function. RV failure itself can result in significant pulse pressure variation during tidal positive pressure ventilation, independently of the patient's volume status. The reason for this relates to the effect of the increased intrathoracic pressure on the RV that occurs during the mechanical inspiration. As intrathoracic pressure increases, RV afterload increases. In the presence of RV failure, this results in a reduction in RV SV that is then detected, several cardiac cycles later, as a reduction in LV SV. The clinician may erroneously conclude that the patient is preload sensitive; when, in fact, the respirophasic variation in SV is caused by an adverse RV–ventilator interaction, i.e., if RV function is not evaluated, the "blinded" clinician could erroneously conclude, by relying on dynamic parameters alone, that more volume expansion is necessary. Identification of respirophasic variation of SV requires the intensivist to assess RV function before assuming that the patient is volume responsive. The presence of ACP with septal dyskinesia identifies a potential contraindication to volume resuscitation, even if the dynamic parameters indicate otherwise.

Although the presence of RV failure may contraindicate volume resuscitation in the presence of respirophasic variation of SV, it is also possible that the patient has both RV failure and preload sensitivity simultaneously. Echocardiography can be used to identify this situation. The presence of significant respiratory variation of the IVC (with TTE) or SVC (with TEE) would support coexisting RV failure and preload sensitivity. The SV response to passive leg raising (PLR) can also be used to determine whether volume resuscitation is indicated with the presence of RV failure. Lack of IVC or SVC variation and lack of SV augmentation with PLR with the presence of RV failure would contraindicate volume resuscitation.

CONCLUSION

The intensivist with competence in basic critical care echocardiography has a limited ability to perform Doppler-based assessment of RV function. Basic CCE emphasizes 2D examination of a few key views. Of these, parasternal short, the apical four chambers at the midventricular level, and subcostal long-axis views are the most important for identification of RV dysfunction. A necessary and diagnostic feature of ACP is RV dilation, which can be identified, along with septal dyskinesia, qualitatively by the basic CCE. The finding of a dilated, hypokinetic RV in a patient with shock has major diagnostic implications (e.g., acute PE, inappropriate ventilator settings, and RV infarction). It also has important implications for management because volume resuscitation may have adverse consequences, leading the clinician to favor diuretics and vasoactive medication while simultaneously considering means of reducing RV afterload.

For the advanced echocardiographer, the addition of Doppler examination to standard 2D imaging allows sophisticated assessment of RV hemodynamic function.

Qualitative assessment of the spectral Doppler signal at the level of the MPA and mitral valve inflow permits rapid assessment of RV outflow impedance and LV filling impairment, respectively. An estimate of PA pressures is straightforward. The RV free wall thickness can be measured by 2D or M-mode. If PE is suspected, evaluation for McConnell's combined with the 60/60 sign by TTE and inspection of the MPA and its bifurcation by TTE or TEE is indicated. Respirophasic SV variation may be identified as being caused by RV dysfunction rather than by preload sensitivity. In a busy ICU, it is both impractical and unnecessary to make a very wide range of measurements of RV function. The intensivist will have to decide which are relevant to the clinical situation. Echocardiography should be used not only as a diagnostic tool (e.g., ACP), but to monitor response to interventions. The association between ventilatory settings, such as tidal volume, respiratory rate, intrinsic and extrinsic PEEP, and the level of resultant hypoxemia and acidosis alter RV afterload, and can be manipulated in order to optimize RV function.

REFERENCES

1. Jardin F, Dubourg O, Bourdarias JP. Echocardiographic pattern of acute cor pulmonale. *Chest.* 1997;111:209–217.
2. Ozier Y, Gueret P, Jardin F, Farcot JC, Bourdarias JP, Margairaz A. Two-dimensional echocardiographic demonstration of acute myocardial depression in septic shock. *Crit Care Med.* 1984;12:596–599.
3. Etchecopar-Chevreuil C, François B, Clavel M, Pichon N, Gastinne H, Vignon P. Cardiac morphological and functional changes during early septic shock: a transesophageal echocardiographic study. *Intensive Care Med.* 2008;34:250–256.
4. Hoffman D, Sisto D, Frater RW, Nikolic SD. Left-to-right ventricular interaction with a noncontracting right ventricle. *J Thorac Cardiovasc Surg.* 1994;107:1496–1502.
5. Vieillard-Baron A, Prin S, Chergui K, Dubourg O, Jardin F. Echo-Doppler demonstration of acute cor pulmonale at the bedside in the medical intensive care unit. *Am J Respir Crit Care Med.* 2002;166:1310–1319.
6. Elzinga G, Pienne H, De Jong J. Left and right ventricular pump function and consequences of having two pumps in one heart: a study on isolated cat heart. *Circ Res.* 1980;46:564–574.
7. Ryan T, Petrovic O, Dillon JC, Feigenbaum H, Conley MJ, Armstrong WF. An echocardiographic index for separation of right ventricular volume and pressure overload. *J Am Coll Cardiol.* 1985;5:918–927.
8. Nielsen JC, Kamenir SA, Ko HS, Lai WW, Parness IA. Ventricular septal flattening at end-systole falsely predicts right ventricular hypertension in patients with ostium primum atrial septal defects. *J Am Soc Echocardiogr.* 2002;15:247–252.
9. Tamborini G, Pepi M, Galli CA, et al. Feasibility and accuracy of a routine echocardiographic assessment of right ventricular function. *Int J Cardiol.* 2007;115:86–89.
10. Frémont B, Pacouret G, Jacobi D, et al. Prognostic value of echocardiographic right/left ventricular end-diastolic diameter ratio in patients with acute pulmonary embolism: results from a monocenter registry of 1,416 patients. *Chest.* 2008;133:358–362.
11. Vieillard-Baron A, Charron C, Chergui K, Peyrouset O, Jardin F. Bedside echocardiographic evaluation of hemodynamics in sepsis: is a qualitative evaluation sufficient? *Intensive Care Med.* 2006;32:1547–1552.
12. Lang RM, Bierig M, Devereux RB, et al. Recommendations for chamber quantification: a report from the American Society of Echocardiography's Guidelines and Standards Committee and the Chamber Quantification Writing Group, developed in conjunction with the European Association of Echocardiography, a branch of the European Society of Cardiology. *J Am Soc Echocardiogr.* 2005;18:1440–1463.
13. Menzel T, Wagner S, Kramm T, Mohr-Kahaly S, Mayer E, Braeuninger S, et al. Pathophysiology of impaired right and left ventricular function in chronic embolic pulmonary hypertension: changes after pulmonary thromboendarterectomy. *Chest.* 2000;118:897–903.
14. Jardin F, Gueret P, Prost JF, Farcot JC, Ozier Y, Bourdarias JP. Two-dimensional echocardiographic assessment of left ventricular function in chronic obstructive pulmonary disease. *Am Rev Respir Dis.* 1984;129:135–142.
15. Rudski LG, Wyman WL, Afilalo J, et al. Guidelines for the echocardiographic assessment of the right heart in adults: a report from the American Society of Echocardiography. *J Am Soc Echocardiogr.* 2010;23:685–713.
16. Kasper W, Meinertz T, Kerstin F, Löllgen H, Limbourg P, Hanjörg J. Echocardiography in assessing acute pulmonary hypertension due to pulmonary embolism. *Am J Cardiol.* 1980;45:567–572.
17. Ribeiro A, Lindmaker P, Juhlin-Dannfelt A, Johnsson H, Jorfeldt L. Echocardiography Doppler in pulmonary embolism: right ventricular dysfunction as a predictor of mortality rate. *Am Heart J.* 1997;134:479–487.
18. Goldhaber S, Visani L, De Rosa M. Acute pulmonary embolism: clinical outcomes in the International Cooperative Embolism Registry (ICOPER). *Lancet.* 1999;353:1386–1389.
19. Vieillard-Baron A, Page B, Augarde R, et al. Acute cor pulmonale in massive pulmonary embolism: incidence, echocardiographic pattern, clinical implications and recovery rate. *Intensive Care Med.* 2001;27:1481–1486.
20. Pruszczyk P, Torbicki A, Pacho R, et al. Noninvasive diagnosis of suspected severe pulmonary embolism: transesophageal echocardiography vs spiral CT. *Chest.* 1997;112:722–728.
21. Vieillard-Baron A, Qanadli SD, Antakly Y, et al. Transesophageal echocardiography for the diagnosis of pulmonary embolism with acute cor pulmonale: a comparison with radiological procedures. *Intensive Care Med.* 1998;24:429–433.
22. McConnell MV, Solomon SD, Rayan ME, Come PC, Goldhaber SZ, Lee RT. Regional right ventricular dysfunction detected by echocardiography in acute pulmonary embolism. *Am J Cardiol.* 1996;78:469–473.
23. Kurzyna M, Torbicki A, Pruszczyk P, et al. Disturbed right ventricular ejection pattern as a new Doppler echocardiographic sign of acute pulmonary embolism. *Am J Cardiol.* 2002;90:507–511.
24. Jardin F, Delorme G, Hardy A, Auvert B, Beauchet A, Bourdarais JP. Reevaluation of hemodynamic consequences of positive pressure ventilation: emphasis on cyclic right ventricular afterloading by mechanical lung inflation. *Anesthesiology.* 1990;2:966–970.

25. Howell JB, Permutt S, Proctor DF, Riley RL. Effect of inflation of the lung on different parts of the pulmonary vascular bed. *J Appl Physiol.* 1961;16:71–76.
26. Balanos GM, Talbot NP, Dorrington KL, Robbins PA. Human pulmonary vascular response to 4 h of hypercapnia and hypocapnia measured using Doppler echocardiography. *J Appl Physiol.* 2003;94:1543–1551.
27. Malbrain ML, Cheatham ML, Kirkpatrick A, et al. Results from the international conference of experts of intra-abdominal hypertension and abdominal compartment syndrome. Definitions. *Intensive Care Med.* 2006;32:1722–1732.
28. Vieillard-Baron A, Schmitt JM, Augarde R, et al. Acute cor pulmonale in acute respiratory distress syndrome submitted to protective ventilation: incidence, clinical implications, and prognosis. *Crit Care Med.* 2001;29:1551–1555.
29. Mekontso-Dessap A, Boissier F, Leon R. Prevalence and prognosis of shunting across patent foramen ovale during acute respiratory distress syndrome. *Crit Care Med.* 2010;38:1786–1792.
30. Jardin F, Vieillard-Baron A. Is there a safe plateau pressure in ARDS? The right heart only knows. *Intensive Care Med.* 2007;33:444–447.
31. Bouferrache L, Vieillard-Baron A. Acute respiratory distress syndrome, mechanical ventilation and right ventricular function. *Current opinion in critical care.* 2011;17:30–35.
32. Nielsen J, Østergaard M, Kjaegaaard J, et al. Lung recruitment maneuver depresses central hemodynamics in patients after cardiac surgery. *Intensive Care Med.* 2005;31:1189–1194.
33. Jardin F. Acute leftward septal shift by lung recruitment maneuver. *Intensive Care Med.* 2005;31:1148–1149.
34. Parker MM, McCarthy KE, Ognibene FP, Parrillo JE. Right ventricular dysfunction and dilation, similar to left ventricular changes, characterize the cardiac depression of septic shock in humans. *Chest.* 1990;97:126–131.
35. Jardin F, Brun-Ney D, Auvert B, Beauchet A, Bourdarais JP. Sepsis-related cardiogenic shock. *Crit Care Med.* 1990;18:1055–1060.
36. Vieillard-Baron A, Caille V, Charron C, Belliard G, Page B, Jardin F. Actual incidence of global left ventricular hypokinesia in adult septic shock. *Crit Care Med.* 2008;36:1701–1706.
37. Schneider AJ, Teule GJ, Groeneveld AB, Nauta J, Heidendal GA, Thijs LG. Biventricular performance during volume loading in patients with early septic shock, with emphasis on the right ventricle: a combined hemodynamic and radionuclide study. *Am Heart J.* 1988;116:103–112.
38. Vieillard-Baron A, Schmitt JM, Beauchet A, et al. Early preload adaptation in septic shock? A transesophageal echocardiographic study. *Anesthesiology.* 2001;94:400–406.
39. Vieillard-Baron A, Prin S, Chergui K, Dubourg O, Jardin F. Hemodynamic instability in sepsis: bedside assessment by Doppler echocardiography. *Am J Respir Crit Care Med.* 2003;168:1270–1276.
40. Gemayel CY, Fram DB, Fowler LAA, Kiernan FJ, Kelsey AM, Gillam LD. The importance of using multiple windows for the echocardiographic identification of right ventricular infarction. *JACC.* 2001;37(Suppl 2):1110–1147.

ECHOCARDIOGRAPHIC DIAGNOSIS OF CARDIAC TAMPONADE

MIKHAIL LITINSKI, KEITH GUEVARRA, & ANTHONY D. SLONIM

Scan QR code or visit www.ccu2e.com for video in this chapter

INTRODUCTION

Cardiac tamponade is defined as a decompensated form of cardiac compression caused by the accumulation of pericardial effusion and rising intrapericardial pressure.[1] Cardiac tamponade may complicate any medical condition associated with pericardial effusion, although it is not synonomous with a large pericardial effusion and has its own specific diagnostic criteria based on hemodynamic and echocardiographic signs. Cardiac tamponade causes obstructive shock and should be regarded as a medical emergency. Medical professionals in the disciplines of surgery, internal and emergency medicine should be familiar with the pathophysiology, clinical presentation, and natural progression of cardiac tamponade to avoid delays in the evaluation and management of this life-threatening condition. Echocardiography is an essential tool for the diagnosis of cardiac tamponade and the evacuation of pericardial fluid. Bedside echocardiography is often performed by intensivists as a part of point of care ultrasonography of critically ill patients; therefore, the recognition of the echocardiographic features of cardiac tamponade is essential for the critical care provider.

PATHOPHYSIOLOGY

In a healthy individual, pericardial pressure is lower than atmospheric pressure and essentially equates to negative intrathoracic pressure. While the pericardium expands to accommodate fluid accumulation over a long period of time, the pericardial space remains constant and fixed at any particular moment. Thus, during systole, pericardial pressure becomes more negative due to the rapid reduction in ventricular size. The lower pericardial pressure combined with the forward flow of blood generated by systolic ventricular contraction contribute to increased venous return to the atria. During diastole pericardial pressure increases due to ventricular expansion, which creates a pressure gradient between the atria and ventricles propelling blood forward and defines a rapid filling diastolic phase. Atrial contraction completes ventricular filling during diastole. Cardiac tamponade occurs when pericardial pressure reaches the point at which diastolic pressures in the cardiac chambers equilibrate, atrioventricular and interventricular "competition" for filling volumes occurs and hemodynamic compromise results.[2-4]

First, in late diastole, pericardial pressure exceeds central venous and atrial pressures causing right atrium and caval veins to collapse, thus decreasing right ventricular filling volume. Left atrial collapse is observed in approximately 25% of patients and is a very specific sign of cardiac tamponade.[5] When right ventricular contraction occurs, pericardial pressure decreases and relieves right atrial compression. As pericardial fluid accumulates and the intrapericardial pressure continues to rise, even slight additional pressure increases during early diastole cause the right atrium and ventricle to collapse.[4] The duration of right atrial collapse at >30% of the cardiac cycle and early diastolic RV collapse both have high specificity (>80%) for cardiac tamponade.[6]

Interventricular competition appears more prominent as a function of the respiratory cycle. During inspiration, intrathoracic pressure decreases (becomes more negative), accelerating blood flow to the right-sided cardiac chambers. Because pericardial pressure is substantially elevated in the setting of cardiac tamponade, the right ventricle accommodates additional blood volume by invaginating the interventricular septum (IVS) into the left ventricle (LV) (Figure 12-1). This results in a lower LV stroke volume and a reduction in systemic blood pressure during inspiration. During expiration, when intrathoracic pressure increases (becomes less negative) systemic venous return decreases. The right ventricle expands less because it needs to accommodate less volume, which in turn, allows for the restoration

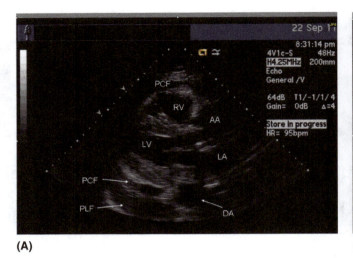 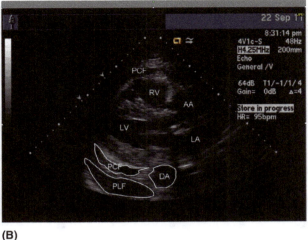

Figure 12-1 (A) Parasternal long-axis view. Spatial relationship between pleural, pericardial effusions, and descending aorta. Pericardial effusion lies anterior to and pleural fluid is posterior to the descending aorta in supine position. (B) White lines indicate approximate borders of pleural, pericardial effusion, and descending aorta. LV, left ventricle; RV, right ventricle; PCF, pericardial effusion; PLF, pleural effusion; DA, descending aorta; AA, ascending aorta; LA, left atrium.

of pulmonary venous return to the left-sided cardiac chambers, now causing the IVS to bulge into the right ventricle. This impedes systemic venous return and causes a "vicious cycle" that leads to hemodynamic compromise.[7]

EPIDEMIOLOGY AND ETIOLOGY

In a recent retrospective review of 50 patients treated for a large pericardial effusion, Kabukcu et al. identified causative factors in 80% of patients.[8] The most common etiology of a large pericardial effusion was cancer (30%) followed up by idiopathic disorders (20%). Other causes included uremia (22%), viral infection (10%), and autoimmune disorders (8%). A small number of cases were attributed to Dressler's syndrome, tuberculosis, purulent pericarditis, and trauma. In another Europian series, which included 322 patients, the most common causes of a large pericardial effusion were the iatrogenic complications of cardiac surgery or endovascular procedures (14%), cancer and myocardial infarction (each 9%), and chronic renal failure (7%). In this series, however, the most common cause of cardiac tamponade, as opposed to just a large pericardial effusion, was acute idiopathic pericarditis (23%) and not an iatrogenic effusion (only 18%).[9] In a retrospective analysis of 4561 patients undergoing open-heart surgery, Joseph et al. found that only 1% of them had moderate to large pleural effusion, with approximately 1/3 of those having features of cardiac tamponade on ultrasound examination.[10] The use of anticoagulants in the preoperative period, female gender and valve surgery were associated with a higher risk for the development of pericardial effusion in this patient population. The prevalence of cardiac tamponade in the general ICU population has not been systematically studied. Most of the studies have focused on the presence of pericardial effusion.

CLINICAL AND LABORATORY INVESTIGATION

Cardiac tamponade is a medical emergency and establishing the diagnosis in a timely manner is of great importance. In many cases, clinicians may identify the underlying disease that led to pericardial fluid accumulation and eventually cardiac tamponade. Soliciting a history of malignancy, recent open-heart surgery or endovascular procedure, uncontrolled hypothyroidism or connective tissue disorder in patients presenting with shock, can help identify important risk factors that contribute to cardiac tamponade. The hemodynamic pattern of cardiac tamponade is obstructive shock. The patient is usually hypotensive and tachycardic with signs of global hypoperfusion, such as an elevated lactate level and end-organ dysfunction. Tachycardia represents a mechanism that allows for the maintenance of cardiac output in the setting of reduced stroke volume. Patients may complain of shortness of breath, chest pain, abdominal discomfort, and dysphagia, likely reflecting visceral congestion.[11] Palpitations may also be present. These features, however, are nonspecific; hence, a broad differential diagnosis should be considered.

Beck's triad was first described in surgical patients who developed acute cardiac tamponade after cardiothoracic procedure by the American surgeon Claude S. Beck in 1935.[12] The classic signs of this triad include arterial hypotension, jugular venous distention, and muffled (or distant) heart sounds. Medical patients who accumulate a pericardial effusion over long periods of time may accommodate large fluid volumes in the pericardial space and exhibit tamponade physiology on ultrasound examination with minimal or no symptoms.[13] Another valuable finding on physical examination, which may direct clinicians to further investigate for cardiac tamponade is pulsus paradoxus (PP).[14] The PP is a reduction of systolic blood pressure (SBP) of

>10 mmHg during inspiration. The underlying mechanism for this excessive reduction in SBP represents impaired LV filling during inspiration due to the bowing of the IVS into the LV space, which results in decreased LV stroke volume. As described above, this process relates to increased systemic venous return to the right cardiac chambers during spontaneous inspiration and an inability of the pericardial space to simultaneously accommodate an expanding RV. The term PP is a misnomer since it is not a "paradox" at all and merely represents an accentuation of the process that takes place in healthy individuals. The measurement of PP is documented by deflating the cuff of the sphygmomanometer until the first Korotkoff tone is auscultated, at which point the examiner should notice the tone's disappearance during inspiration and reappearance during expiration. Then, the cuff is allowed to deflate further until the Korotkoff tone is clearly auscultated during both phases of the respiratory cycle. The difference in SBP between these two points is called the "pulsus paradoxus." Sometimes substantial reductions in pulse intensity on inspiration can be noticed by simply palpating the pulse of the patient, a sign that was first described by Kussmaul in 1873. While PP is most often described in connection with cardiac tamponade, the differential diagnosis of PP includes other potential causes of obstructive shock, such as a massive pulmonary embolism and tension pneumothorax.

Patients with cardiac tamponade may have an audible pericardial rub contrary to the common belief that a pericardial rub is only present in acute pericarditis.[13,15] When larger amounts of fluid accumulate in the pericardial space, the experienced examiner may recognize Ewart's sign, which is bronchial breathing in the base of the left lung due to the left lower lobe bronchus's compression by the large pericardial effusion.

Chest x-rays (CXR) lack the necessary sensitivity needed to establish a diagnosis of cardiac tamponade; however, it is sensitive enough to diagnose a large pericardial effusion. In acute "surgical" tamponade, the rapid accumulation of a small amount of fluid may cause tamponade without any changes on CXR. The cardiac silhouette on CXR usually remains unchanged until at least 200 cc of fluid build up in pericardial space. As the pericardial effusion becomes larger, the cardiac shadow on CXR appears more globular in shape. One of the late and specific signs of a large pericardial effusion on CXR is the "fat pad" sign, best visualized on a lateral view of the CXR. This sign signifies a separation of epicardial and retrosternal adipose tissue by the large pericardial effusion.[16] One meta-analysis found cardiomegaly on CXR to be associated with a sensitivity of >89% for the diagnosis of cardiac tamponade.[17] Pulmonary edema is not a characteristic CXR feature of "medical" cardiac tamponade and should prompt the practitioner to look for alternative explanations.

The electrocardiogram (EKG) should be a part of the critically ill patient's work up. "Electrical alternans" is the term describing the alternating amplitude of one or more complexes on the EKG. It is a very specific sign of a large pericardial effusion and when >2 waves are involved (QRS, P or T waves), it is a pathognomonic feature of pericardial tamponade.[18] Electrical alternans results from alterations of the heart's electrical axis that occur with every beat due to the large cardiac swings in fluid-filled pericardium (Video 12-4). Other commonly cited EKG signs include low QRS voltage and arrhythmias.

ECHOCARDIOGRAPHY IN CARDIAC TAMPONADE

Echocardiography is the primary diagnostic modality for the diagnosis of cardiac tamponade. Over the last few decades, bedside ultrasonography has gained substantial popularity among critical care practitioners as a method that quickly establishes the diagnosis and facilitates a therapeutic intervention.[19]

▶ Pericardial Versus Pleural Effusion

Distinguishing between pleural and pericardial effusions on echocardiogram is important because large pleural effusions can also cause obstructive shock and the management of these two conditions is different.[20] Usually echocardiographic examination starts with obtaining a long parasternal view. The operator should adjust the depth of the ultrasound to optimize visualization of the structures situated around the heart, including lung and/or pleural space. The descending aorta is located posterior to the left atrium. The assessment of the spatial relationship between the descending aorta and fluid surrounding the heart allows the physician to distinguish pericardial fluid from fluid in the pleural space. A large pericardial effusion usually extends between the left atrium and descending aorta, whereas pleural effusion lies posterior to the descending aorta (Figure 12-1 and Video 12-1).

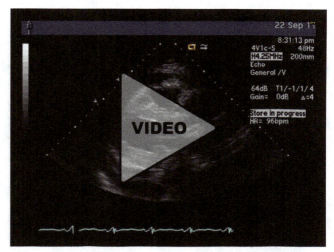

Video 12-1 Parasternal long-axis view. Spatial relationship between pleural, pericardial effusions, and descending aorta. Pericardial effusion lies anterior to and pleural fluid is posterior to the descending aorta in supine position. View at www.ccu2e.com

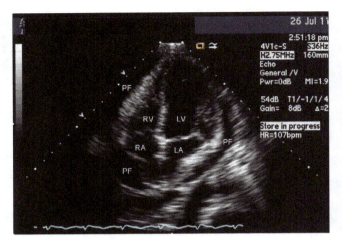

Figure 12-2 Apical four-chamber view. Large pericardial effusion present. Right atrial collapse during diastole. RV, right ventricle; LV, left ventricle; LA, left atrium; RA, right atrium; PF, pericardial effusion.

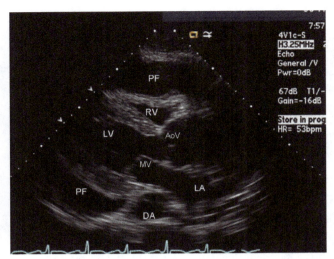

Figure 12-4 Parasternal long-axis view. Large circumferential pericardial effusion is evident. Right ventricle is collapsing during early diastole (mitral valve starts to open and aortic valve is closed). Intraluminal flap in descending aorta, suggesting dissecting aortic aneurism. PF, pericardial fluid; RV, right ventricle; LV, left ventricle; DA, descending aorta; LA, left atrium.

▶ Quantification of Pericardial Effusion

In the supine position, pericardial fluid accumulates around the posterior cardiac wall. The presence of a circumferential pericardial effusion visible in the long parasternal window usually suggests a large pericardial effusion. The short parasternal and four-chamber views (apical and subcostal) may provide a better spatial representation of the cardiac chambers and quantification of pericardial fluid (Figures 12-2 through 12-4 and Videos 12-2 through 12-4). Horowitz and colleagues performed cardiac ultrasonography in 41 patients just prior to cardiac surgery and demonstrated that the M-mode technique is relatively accurate in estimating the volume of pericardial effusion.[21] This finding was later confirmed by the work of Parameswaran and colleagues.[22] However, there was some discrepancy between the amount of pericardial effusion estimated by M-mode ultrasonography and the amount of fluid obtained by direct aspiration. This discrepancy was attributed to the assumption that the pericardial effusion is uniformly distributed in the pericardial sac when, in fact, it is a nonuniform distribution. Recognizing this limitation D'Cruz and Hoffman utilized a formula for the volume of a prolate elipse and applied it to the pericardial sac and cardiac volume, which allowed for fluid assessment in the apical four chamber view of echocardiogram.[23] The pericardial effusion volume was then calculated by subtracting the cardiac volume from that of the pericardial sac. They demonstrated excellent correlation between the actual and estimated volumes of pericardial fluid ($r = 0.97$). These calculations, however, are difficult to perform and rarely used clinically.

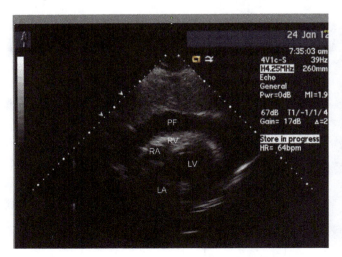

Figure 12-3 Subxiphoid view. Large pericardial effusion present. Right ventricle is completely collapsed during early diastole, sign that is very specific for cardiac tamponade.

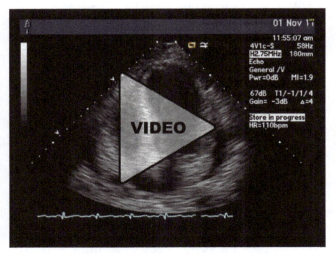

Video 12-2 Apical four-chamber view. Large pericardial effusion present. Right atrial collapse during diastole. View at www.ccu2e.com

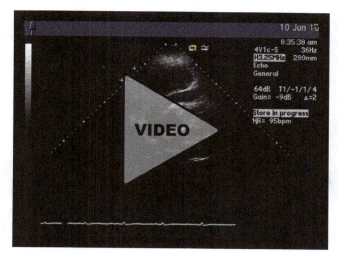

Video 12-3 Subxiphoid view. Large pericardial effusion present. Right ventricle is completely collapsed during early diastole, sign that is very specific for cardiac tamponade. RV, right ventricle; LV, left ventricle; LA, left atrium; RA, right atrium; PF, pericardial effusion. View at www.ccu2e.com

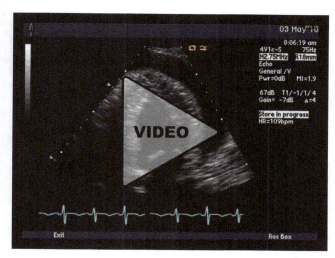

Video 12-4 Apical four-chamber view. Large pericardial effusion, "swinging heart." View at www.ccu2e.com

▶ Two-Dimensional Echocardiographic Features of Cardiac Tamponade

Echocardiographic features of cardiac tamponade reflect the pathophysiologic changes described above. Right-atrial collapse in late diastole is an early sign of tamponade physiology and is 100% sensitive for the diagnosis[24] (Figure 12-2 and Video 12-2). The right atrium is best visualized in the subxiphoid (subcostal) and apical four-chamber views (Figures 12-2 and 12-3; and Videos 12-2 and 12-3). The same views also provide optimal visualization of a large pericardial effusion and "swinging heart" (Video 12-4). As tamponade progresses, the right ventricle demonstrates signs of collapse in early diastole (Figure 12-3; and Videos 12-3 and 12-5). At the same time, bowing of the IVS into the LV during inspiration and into the right ventricle during expiration becomes more apparent (Figure 12-5). It is important to recognize phases of the cardiac cycle while performing and interpreting the echocardiographic study. During late diastole the mitral and tricuspid valves are open and the aortic valve is closed. During systole the atrioventricular valves are closed and the aortic valve is open (Figure 12-4 and Video 12-5). Examining the subxiphoid view also allows the physician to evaluate the inferior vena cava's (IVC) diameter and its respiratory variation. In cardiac tamponade, the IVC is usually enlarged, without a reduction in IVC size during spontaneous inspiration (Figure 12-6, Video 12-6). This is attributed to the fact that the right-sided heart chambers are unable to fully expand during diastole to accommodate the volume of systemic venous return. This results in blood pooling in the IVC.[25]

Clinicians need to be aware of some special circumstances in which the classic echocardiographic signs of cardiac tamponade (e.g. pericardial fluid and compression of

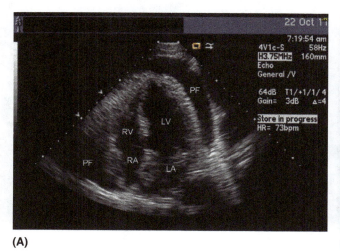

(A)

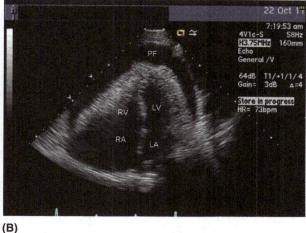

(B)

Figure 12-5 During expiration (**A**), interventricular septum is bowing into the RV and during inspiration to the LV (**B**). PF, pericardial effusion; LV, left ventricle; RV, right ventricle; LA, left atrium; RA, right atrium.

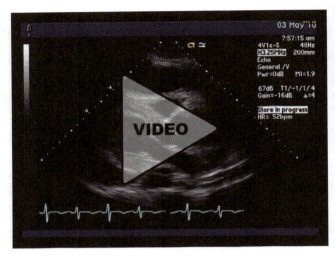

Video 12-5 Long parasternal view. Large pericardial effusion. Right ventricle is nearly collapsing during diastole. View at www.ccu2e.com

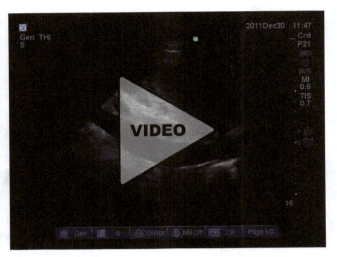

Video 12-6 Plethora of the inferior vena cava (IVC). IVC is enlarged and doesn't show respirophasic changes. IVC plethora is an indicator of elevated right atrial pressure. View at www.ccu2e.com

right-sided cardiac chambers during diastole) are absent. For example, patients may develop a retroatrial hematoma after cardiothoracic surgery, which can be difficult to identify on transthoracic echocardiogram (TTE) and may require transesophageal echocardiography (TEE) to establish the diagnosis.[26] Exclusive compression of the left atrium or ventricle in this situation may lead to pulmonary edema, which is usually not observed when the right-sided chambers are affected. A recent case report by Gollapudi et al. demonstrated that a circumferential pericardial effusion can cause left ventricular tamponade in severe pulmonary hypertension associated with chronic lung disease.[27]

▶ Pulsed Wave Doppler Imaging

Pulsed-wave Doppler imaging allows the physician to evaluate transvalvular flow. In cardiac tamponade, transvalvular flow may be substantially altered and can serve as an indicator that a pericardial effusion is affecting the patient's hemodynamics. An inspiratory increase of transpulmonic and tricuspid valve flow by 40–50% and a reduction in transaortic and mitral valve flow by 20–45% demonstrates hemodynamic instability in this patient population (Figure 12-7). Compromised relaxation of the right atrium and ventricle (diastolic dysfunction) is a marker of cardiac tamponade. An inverse E/A ratio is a characteristic feature of diastolic dysfunction and is observed in cardiac tamponade (Figure 12-8). In the normal condition, most of the right ventricular filling occurs during early diastole (E), which accounts for 80% of right ventricular filling volume. The remaining 20% of right ventricular filling occurs during late diastole (A) as a result of atrial contraction. Thus, the early component of transtricuspid and transmitral flow is seen as a higher spike on Doppler ultrasound than the late

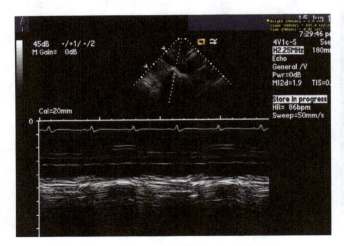

Figure 12-6 Inferior vena cava (IVC) plethora. IVC is large without cyclic changes in diameter during respiration.

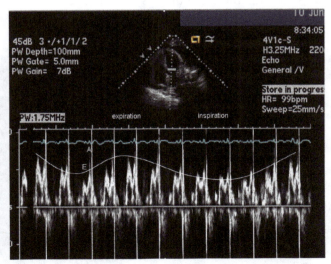

Figure 12-7 Respiratory variation of transmitral flow. Flow increases during expiration and decreases during inspiration. E/A inversed ratio is also observed, signifying left ventricular relaxation impairment.

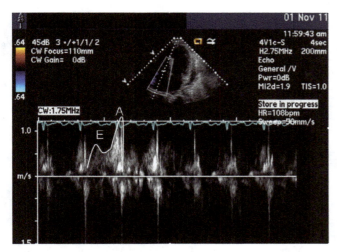

Figure 12-8 Inverted E/A (early to late transvalvular flow) ratio at the tricuspid level, reflecting relaxation impairment of right ventricle.

component. The opposite is observed in cardiac tamponade (Figures 12-7 and 12-8; and Video 12-7).

▶ Treatment of Cardiac Tamponade

The ultimate goal in the treatment of cardiac tamponade is to relieve obstruction of the cardiac chambers caused by pericardial effusion or post-surgical hematoma. This is achieved either by pericardiocentesis or pericardiotomy. While preparing for the procedure, it is important to initiate volume resuscitation to correct latent hypovolemia, which would delay collapse of cardiac chambers.[28] In cardiac tamponade, catecholamines may increase the cardiac index, systemic vascular resistance, and mean arterial blood pressure, but not cerebral or renal blood flow.[29]

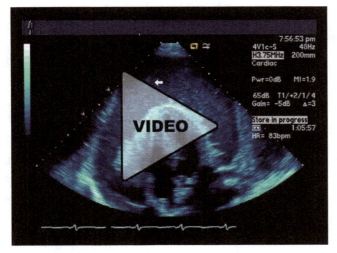

Video 12-7 Ultrasound-guided pericardiocentesis using a subxiphoid approach. After obtaining an adequate subcostal window, needle is inserted between the xiphoid process and the left costal margin. Using real-time echocardiography, the needle is advanced and visualized as it enters the pericardial sac. (Video courtesy of Dr. A. Levitov.) View at www.ccu2e.com

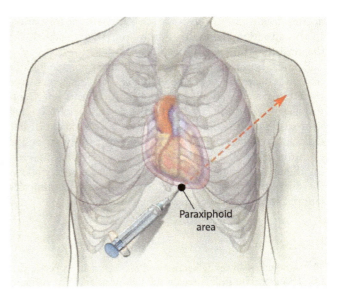

Figure 12-9 Ultrasound-guided pericardiocentesis using a subxiphoid approach. After obtaining an adequate subcostal window, a 16–18 gauge needle is inserted between the xiphoid process and the left costal margin. Using real-time echocardiography, the needle is advanced and visualized as it enters the pericardial sac. (From Spodick DH. Acute cardiac tamponade. *N Engl J Med.* 2003;349:684–690.)

The use of ultrasound during pericardiocentesis allows the operator to identify the area of largest fluid accumulation. It enhances the safety and accuracy of the procedure, provides guidance for the procedure, and confirms appropriate catheter placement in the pericardial space, using contrast ("bubbles") and avoiding traumatic right ventricular puncture. The technical aspects of pericardiocentesis are discussed in detail in Chapter 24. In brief, a 16–18 gauge needle is inserted in the subxiphoid space between the xiphoid process and the left costal margin. The needle can be visualized under ultrasound guidance using a subcostal window as it enters the pericardial sac (Figure 12-9). A catheter can then be inserted to allow for continued drainage of the effusion. It is not unusual that even the removal of a small amount of fluid (50 mL) can restore hemodynamics in a compromised patient. Surgical drainage may be indicated for other types of effusions including malignancies or hematomas. Medical support in the ICU using vasopressors and fluid therapy are important adjuncts while definitive drainage is being undertaken.

SUMMARY

Cardiac tamponade is a life-threatening emergency caused by elevated pericardial pressure and diastolic collapse of the cardiac chambers. A high clinical suspicion based on the recognition of physical findings, EKG and CXR signs should prompt the physician to proceed with echocardiographic examination. Cardiac tamponade after cardiothoracic surgery may occur without substantial fluid accumulation due to postoperative hematoma formation. In this situation, a TEE may be required to establish the diagnosis in a timely manner.

Echocardiographic features of cardiac tamponade include diastolic collapse of the right atrium and ventricle, increased right transvalvular flow during inspiration, and left transvalvular flow during exhalation. Diastolic right or left ventricular dysfunction manifested as a dominance of late diastolic flow over the early diastolic flow through tricuspid or mitral valve (reverse E/A ratio) can also be present. During therapeutic pericardiocentesis, echocardiography allows the operator to confirm catheter placement and minimize complications such as right ventricular puncture.

REFERENCES

1. Guidelines on the Diagnosis and Management of Pericardial Diseases. The Task Force on the Diagnosis and Management of Pericardial Diseases of the European Society of Cardiology. *Eur Heart J.* 2004;25:587–610.
2. Rhee PM, Foy H, Kaufmann C, et al. Penetrating cardiac injuries: a population based study. *J Trauma.* 1998;45:366–370.
3. Reddy PS, Curtis EI, Uretsky BF. Spectrum of hemodynamic changes in cardiac tamponade. *Am J Cardiol.* 1990;66:1487–1491.
4. Beloucif S, Takata M, Shimada M Robotham JL. Influence of pericardial constraint on atrioventricular interactions. *Am J Physiol.* 1992;263:H125–H134.
5. Fusman B, Schwinger ME, Charney R, et al. Isolated collapse of left-sided heart chambers in cardiac tamponade: demonstration by two-dimensional echocardiography. *Am Heart J.* 1991;121:613–616.
6. Gillam LD, Guyer DE Gibson TC, et al. Hydrodynamic compression of right atrium: a new echocardiographic sign of cardiac tamponade. *Circulation.* 1983;68:294–301.
7. Boltwood CM Jr. Ventricular performance related to transmural filling pressure in clinical cardiac tamponade. *Circulation.* 1987;75:941–955.
8. Kabukcu M, Demircioglu F, Yanik E, Basarici I, Ersel F. Pericardial tamponade and large pericardial effusions: casual factors and efficacy of percutaneous catheter drainage in 50 patients. *Tex Heart Inst J.* 2004;31:398–403.
9. Sagrista-Sauleda J, Mercé J, Permanyer-Miralda G, Soler-Soler, J. Clinical clues to the causes of large pericardial effusions. *Am J Med.* 2000;109:95–101.
10. Joseph MX, Disney PJ, Da Costa R, Hutchison SJ. Transthoracic echocardiography to identify or exclude cardiac cause of shock. *Chest.* 2004;126:1592–1597.
11. Spodick DH. Acute cardiac tamponade. *N Engl J Med.* 2003;349:684–690.
12. Beck C. Two cardiac compression triads. *J Am Med Assoc.* 1935;104:714–716.
13. Guberman BA, Fowler NO, Engel PJ, Gueron M, Allen JM. Cardiac tamponade in medical patients. *Circulation.* 1981;64:633–640.
14. Fowler NO. Physiology of cardiac tamponade and pulsus paradoxus, I: mechanisms of pulsus paradoxus in cardiac tamponade. *Mod Concept Cardiovasc Dis.* 1978;47:109–113.
15. Spodick DH. Pericardial rub: prospective multiple observer investigation of pericardial friction in 100 patients. *Am J Cardiol.* 1975;35:357–362.
16. Heinsimer JA, Collins GJ, Burkman MH, Roberts L Jr, Chen JT. Supine cross-table lateral chest roentgenogram for the detection of pericardial effusion. *JAMA.* 1987;257:3266–3268.
17. Roy CL, Minor MA, Brookhart Am, Choudhary NK. Does this patient with pericardial effusion have a cardiac tamponade? *JAMA.* 2007;297:1810–1818.
18. Goldberger AL, Shabetai R, Bhargava V, West BJ, Mandell AJ. Nonlinear dynamics, electrical alternans and pericardial tamponade. *Am Heart J.* 1984;107:1297–1299.
19. Melniker LA, Leibner E, McKenney MG, Lopez P, Briggs WM Mancuso CA. Randomized controlled clinical trial of point-of-care, limited ultrasonography for trauma in the emergency department: the first sonography outcomes assessment program trial. *Ann Emer Med.* 2006;48:227–235.
20. Alam HB, Levitt A, Molyneaux R, Davidosn P, Sample GA. Can pleural effusion cause cardiac tamponade? *Chest.* 1999;116:1820–1822.
21. Horowitz MS, Shultz CS, Stinson EB, Harrison DC, Popp RL. Sensitivity and specificity of echocardiographic diagnosis of pericardial effusion. *Circulation.* 1974;50:239–247.
22. Parameswaran R, Goldberg H. Echocardiographic quantitation of pericardial effusion. *Chest.* 1983;83:767–770.
23. D'Cruz I, Hoffman PK. A new cross sectional Echocardiographic method for estimating the volume of large pericardial effusions. *Br Heart J.* 1991;66:448–451.
24. Gillam LD, et al. Hydrodynamic compression of the right atrium: a new Echocardiographic sign of cardiac tamponade. *J Am Coll Cardiol.* 1988;12:1470–1477.
25. Himelman RB, Kircher B, Rockey DC, Schiller NB. Inferior vena cava plethora with blunted respiratory response: a sensitive Echocardiographic sign of cardiac tamponade. *J Am Coll Cardiol.* 1988;12:1470–1477.
26. Russo AM, O'Connor WH, Waxman HL. Atypical presentation and Echocardiographic findings in patients with cardiac tamponade occurring early and late after cardiac surgery. *Chest.* 1993;104:71–78.
27. Gollapudi RR, Yeager M, Johnson AD. Left ventricular cardiac tamponade in the setting of cor pulmonale and circumferential pericardial effusion. Case report and review of the literature. *Cardiol Rev.* 2005;13:214–217.
28. Gascho JA, Martins JB, Marcus ML, Kerber RE. Effects of volume expansion and vasodilators in acute pericardial tamponade. *Am J Physiol.* 1981;240:H49–H53.
29. Martins JB, Manuel WJ, Marcus ML, Kerber RE. Comparative effects of cathecholamines in cardiac tamponade: experimental and clinical studies. *Am J Cardiol.* 1980;46:59–66.

13

ECHOCARDIOGRAPHIC DIAGNOSIS AND MONITORING OF ACUTE MYOCARDIAL INFARCTION AND ASSOCIATED COMPLICATIONS

Scan QR code or visit www.ccu2e.com for video in this chapter

RODNEY W. SAVAGE

INTRODUCTION

For the patient with acute myocardial infarction (AMI) pressing priorities exist. Symptoms must be ameliorated, lethal arrhythmias identified and treated, arteries opened, and complications identified and managed. In many cases, little is needed beyond a targeted history and physical examination, 12-lead electrocardiogram (ECG), and simple, rapid blood work with prompt thrombolysis or emergency coronary arteriography and balloon angioplasty with or without stenting. In such straightforward cases, point-of-care echocardiography will prove interesting and perhaps helpful if potential complications are identified early. Such study, however, should never delay needed efforts at reperfusion. In other cases, the history and physical examination may be confusing, or ECG and enzymatic data may be conflicting, misleading, or delayed. These situations include (1) typical symptoms but normal or equivocal laboratory studies, (2) atypical symptoms with equivocal or abnormal laboratory studies, (3) pacemaker therapy, (4) left bundle branch block (LBBB) on ECG, (5) presence of new systolic murmur, (6) shock including right ventricular myocardial infarction, (7) late clinical presentation including post-myocardial infarction (MI) pericarditis, (8) large, non-Q-wave MI, (9) true posterior MI, and (10) suspected LV thrombus. In these instances, point-of-care ultrasonography is not only beneficial but also it may be critical for improving the understanding of the patient's condition and selecting appropriate treatment.

TECHNICAL AND ADMINISTRATIVE ISSUES

For point-of-care echocardiography to prove helpful in the acute MI setting, a simple, rapidly activated and portable machine must be present in the proximate clinical area. This machine must provide good-quality two-dimensional and colored Doppler images on a wide variety of challenging patients (chronic obstructive pulmonary disease, obesity). Handheld machines, which are small enough to fit in a laboratory coat pocket, are now available at reasonable cost. In most situations, a full, formal follow-up echocardiogram should be obtained with results correlated to the point-of-care echocardiography findings. Point-of-care operators require training in theory and hands-on techniques plus proctored imaging and interpretation experience. These providers will need to work closely with institutional credentialing bodies to ensure that standards of initial training, ongoing training, and quality assurance are identified and met.

The three standard windows should be interrogated in each patient with and without color-flow Doppler (Figure 13-1A,B). Apical views should be examined first because the two-chamber, four-chamber, and five-chamber views are often readily obtained and identify all left ventricular myocardial segments in addition to the right ventricle (Figure 13-1A). Aortic, mitral, and tricuspid valves are easily identified. Color-flow interrogation in the apical views readily identifies ventricular septal defects and aortic, mitral, and tricuspid insufficiencies. Left parasternal short-axis views should be obtained next with expected good visualization of the mid-left ventricle and left ventricle at base plus aortic and mitral valves en face (Figure 13-1B). The pulmonic valve is often best seen as the aortic valve is brought into view and the transducer rotated slightly to include the right ventricular outflow tract and main pulmonary artery. The left parasternal long-axis views usually miss the left ventricular apex and may provide suboptimal visualization of the inferior and posterior walls even with the gain turned up. The aortic and mitral valves are usually well seen and color-flow Doppler provides good visualization of

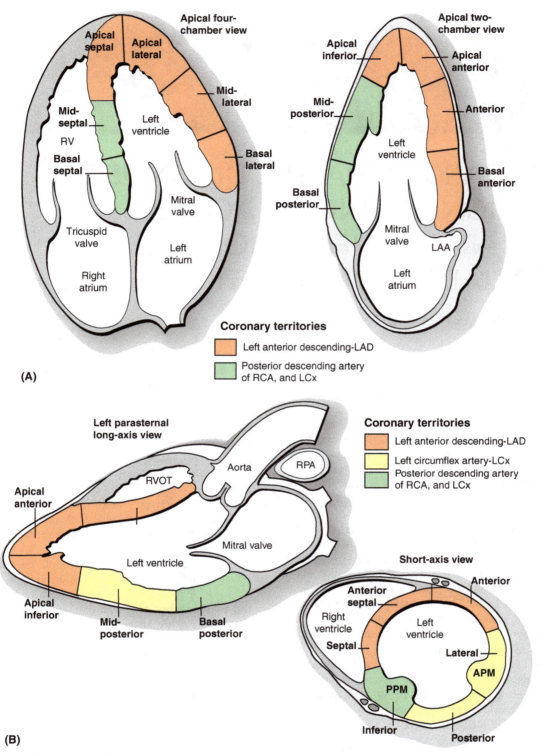

Figure 13-1 Standard views and left ventricular segments. Left ventricular myocardial segments as seen in the standard echocardiographic windows and views with corresponding coronary artery territories. (Reproduced with permission from Yale University Echocardiography laboratory educational website http://www.med.yale.edu/intmed/cardio/echo_atlas/contents/index.html.)

aortic and mitral insufficiencies. Although difficult to obtain in obese patients and in patients with severe chest pain or congestive heart failure, subcostal views prove helpful in visualizing left and right ventricular endocardium in addition to left atrium, right atrium, and aortic, mitral, and tricuspid valves. Sometimes, adequate visualization of the left ventricular apex will only be available in these views. Having the acutely ill, patient bend at the knees will often help in obtaining subcostal views. Sometimes the images are only obtainable after initial medical therapy with oxygen, nitrates, morphine, and diuretics.

During each study, every reasonable effort should be made to identify each major myocardial segment, right ventricular free wall, left atrium, right atrium, aortic, mitral, pulmonic, and tricuspid valves with and without color interrogation. Aortic root, ascending aorta, transverse aorta, and descending aorta should be identified. Pericardial effusion, ventricular septal defect, and left ventricular thrombus should be sought. Structures not adequately visualized cannot be described. If the endocardium is not seen, a wall motion abnormality cannot be identified. After the study, findings must be recorded, even when incomplete or limited, for later correlation and quality assurance. Never make bad decisions based on bad images. The point-of-care echocardiographer must always be ready to obtain assistance from another echocardiographer who may be able to acquire better images, or obtain help from another technology such as cardiac computerized tomography, transesophageal echocardiography, or cardiac catheterization.

TYPICAL SYMPTOMS AND NORMAL/EQUIVOCAL LABORATORIES

Patients may present acutely with typical chest discomfort with symptom onset less than 1 h. The initial ECG may show only peaked T waves or anterior ST-segment depressions. Initial bedside cardiac enzymes may well be negative. With continued ischemia more ST-segment elevations may be seen on subsequent ECGs prompting thrombolysis or emergent catheter-directed intervention. Continued symptoms and positive enzymes might similarly prompt a trip to the catheterization laboratory even without classic ST-segment elevations. During the time between presentation and decision, muscle loss will continue.

When initial diagnostic confusion and uncertainty might lead to costly delays, immediate bedside echocardiography can result in diagnostic clarity and timely reperfusion. In patients presenting very early with acute MI, enzymes will be normal and ECG may show only peaked (hyper acute) T waves. A true posterior MI may show only anterior ST-segment depressions, mirror images of ST-segment elevations. These changes may be unrecognized, subtle, or, in the case of peaked T waves, due to hyperkalemia. Occasionally, similar T waves may occur in young, healthy athletes with or without symptoms. Waiting for ECG evolution or abnormal cardiac enzymes can lead to delay with unnecessary myocardial muscle loss. Bedside echocardiography demonstrating clear segmental wall motion abnormality will prompt earlier decision, treatment, and myocardial salvage.

ATYPICAL SYMPTOMS WITH EQUIVOCAL OR ABNORMAL STUDIES

A minority of patients with acute ischemia lack typical chest discomfort. Atypical presentations include shortness of breath, diaphoresis, nausea, vomiting, abdominal pain, syncope, profound weakness, and feeling of doom. Diabetic and postoperative patients are often asymptomatic or nearly so. Appropriately, emergency department physicians, intensive care physicians, and internal medicine and cardiology consultants cast a broad diagnostic net in these situations. Minor cardiac enzyme abnormalities and nonspecific ECG changes frequently result. Should aggressive treatment await further testing hours down the line? Should the risks of intervention be undertaken in high comorbidity patients without better information? For example, no one likes to take a fresh postoperative patient to the catheterization laboratory for urgent angioplasty with or without stent placement. Immediate echocardiography may show little or no segmental wall motion abnormality. Such a patient should do well with a conservative approach. If a large segmental wall motion abnormality were found, the more aggressive invasive approach might well be worth an increased risk of bleeding in an effort to achieve significant myocardial salvage. Even if catheter-directed intervention did not follow, a large defect might prompt intensive care unit monitoring and more intensive medical therapy.

PACEMAKER THERAPY

Ventricular pacing may certainly mask an acute transmural MI. In the presence of an acute MI, echocardiography will often demonstrate a new segmental wall motion abnormality over and above the expected LBBB contraction timing abnormality seen with right ventricular (RV) pacing (Figure 13-2). A nontransmural event may or may

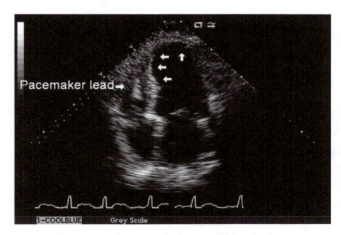

Figure 13-2 Apical four-chamber views in systole showing akinesis of mid and distal anterior septal segments and apex. Note the pacemaker lead in the right heart.

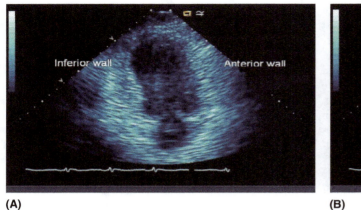 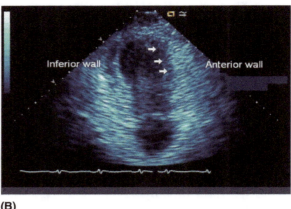

Figure 13-3 Apical two-chamber views in diastole (**A**) and systole (**B**) showing akinesis of anterior myocardial segments. Of special note, there is no myocardial thickening. Similar two-chamber views in diastole (2c) and systole (2d) from a patient with LBBB without MI demonstrate systolic movement and thickening. LBBB, left bundle branch block.

not lead to a noticeable segmental wall motion abnormality. Following a fresh pacemaker lead implantation, a lead tip perforation may cause pericardial irritation with or without a pericardial effusion. Rarely, cardiac tamponade may result. Imaging may avert inappropriate anticoagulation with possible dire consequences, and lead, instead, to pericardiocentesis when cardiac tamponade is present.

LEFT BUNDLE BRANCH BLOCK

Approximately 3.7% of acute MIs present with new or age-undetermined LBBB. Preexisting LBBB does not exclude acute MI in the symptomatic patient. With an early clinical presentation, a normal troponin provides little reassurance and help. Without early revascularization, patients may well suffer large infarctions while waiting for subsequent cardiac enzymes to point the way. Yet, a patient's atypical story may make decision-making tough.

The LBBB causes a contraction timing abnormality of the interventricular septum and anterior wall of left ventricle. The involved myocardium, however, exhibits appropriate thickening when not ischemic or infarcting. LBBB with MI shows the expected segmental wall motion abnormality without myocardial thickening in the infarcting segment (Figure 13-3A,B), making clinical decision much more timely, confident, and straightforward.

MYOCARDIAL INFARCTION AND NEW MURMUR

Myocardial rupture following MI can involve (1) a papillary muscle or papillary muscle head, causing acute mitral regurgitation, (2) the interventricular septum leading to an acute muscular ventricular septal defect, (3) the left ventricular free wall leading rapidly to cardiac tamponade and death, and (4) contained rupture causing pseudoaneurysm. All of these entities, except free wall rupture, include a new systolic murmur. Unidentified and untreated, all carry a poor prognosis that worsens as time passes.

Rupture of a papillary muscle usually occurs 3–5 days after MI. Posteromedial papillary muscle rupture associated with inferior MI (Figure 13-4) occurs more frequently than rupture of the anterolateral papillary muscle associated with anterolateral myocardial infarction. Complete transection leads to rapid hemodynamic deterioration and death due to torrential mitral regurgitation. Rupture of a tip or head of the muscle is more common and usually results in severe, but not overwhelming mitral regurgitation. Treated medically, 90% of patients succumb. However, with a timely diagnosis and surgical intervention, this can be reduced to 40–90%, depending on timing of treatment, severity of left ventricular damage, and severity of shock on presentation.

Rupture of the interventricular septum in MI occurs 3–5 days after the inciting event and causes a new systolic murmur that may include a thrill. Anterior MI (Video 13-1) is more common than inferior MI. Although the diagnosis can be made with an oxygen saturation step-up on right heart catheterization, echocardiography with color Doppler provides more complete and timely diagnosis. With prompt surgical repair, 90% mortality is reduced to 50%.

Survival with free wall rupture occurs rarely only with immediate diagnosis and surgical relief. Only with immediate echocardiography can rapid cardiac tamponade, cardiac arrest, and death be averted by heroic surgical intervention. Most cases occur 3–6 days after initial infarction, usually an anterolateral event. Up to 10% of autopsy series find this situation. Rare case reports of success may become more common, as rapid diagnosis becomes more available. At the other end of the clinical spectrum, post-MI pseudoaneurysm of the left ventricle usually occurs with an inferoposterior event and may be associated with a new

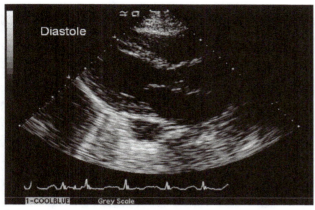
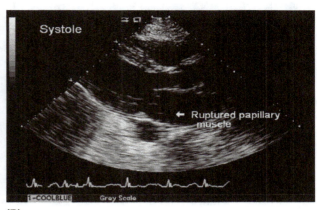
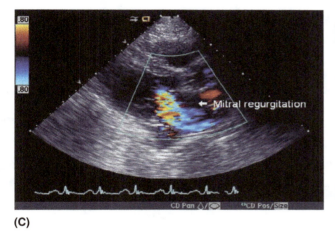

Figure 13-4 Left parasternal long-axis views in diastole (**A**) and systole (**B**) reveal LAD coronary artery distribution akinesis with (using color flow Doppler interrogation [**C**]) severe mitral regurgitation in systole.

systolic murmur, arrhythmia, thromboemboli, and congestive heart failure. Surgical repair is recommended even when asymptomatic, as late rupture presents a real and unpredictable risk.

SHOCK, INCLUDING RIGHT VENTRICULAR MYOCARDIAL INFARCTION

Cardiogenic shock continues to occur in acute MI patients. Usually, large infarctions with late or no reperfusion can be blamed. As noted above, ventricular septal defect, acute mitral regurgitation, and free wall rupture need to be considered. Sometimes, a new infarction of moderate or even small size superimposed on old infarction will lead to shock. With an inferior wall infarction, right ventricular involvement may well lead to shock even with limited left ventricular damage. In such patients, aggressive intravenous fluids, vasopressors, intra-aortic balloon pump support and, rarely, atrioventricular sequential pacing may be needed. Finally, pericardial effusion with cardiac tamponade may lead to a shock state (Figure 13-5). This situation may occur after an inadvertent and unrecognized guide wire micro perforation during attempts at catheter-directed reperfusion. Timely, accurate diagnosis will lead to appropriate lifesaving treatment ranging from emergency angioplasty with or without stenting to coronary artery bypass surgery and ventricular septal defect or mitral regurgitation repair. In the case of cardiac tamponade, anticoagulation must be avoided and drainage promptly undertaken.

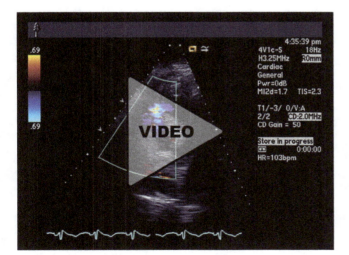

Video 13-1 Modified apical four-chamber view with color Doppler showing distal anterior intraventricular septal and apical akinesis and a focal disruption in the myocardium with left to right shunting typical of an anterior myocardial infarction complicated by a ventricular septal defect. View at www.ccu2e.com

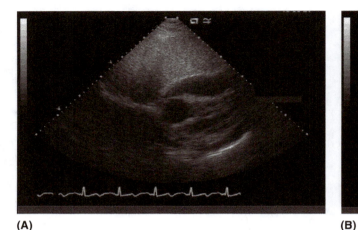
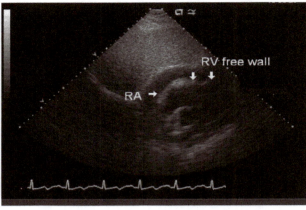
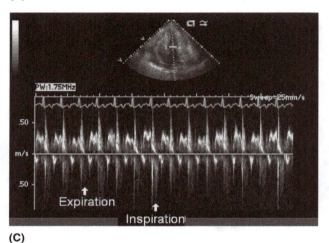

Figure 13-5 Subcostal four-chamber views in diastole (**A**) and systole (**B**) show a moderate pericardial effusion with collapse (arrows) of RV and RA free walls in diastole strongly suggestive of cardiac tamponade. Pulsed Doppler interrogation of LV inflow track with respiration (**C**) shows significant variation in diastolic frequency shift amplitudes inspiration (higher) and expiration (lower), confirming tamponade physiology. Caution must be high when calling wall motion abnormalities in the presence of significant pericardial effusion as both false positive and false negative situations occur. RV, right ventricle; LV, left ventricle; RA, right atrium.

LATE PRESENTATION INCLUDING POSTMYOCARDIAL INFARCTION PERICARDITIS

Patients who present to medical attention late in the course of MI may offer varied and, at times, confusing clinical pictures. Some suffer a stuttering and increasingly severe course. Others experience postinfarction angina, arrhythmia, or congestive heart failure. A well-tolerated infarction may be followed a short time later by a second infarction with increased pain and/or congestive heart failure. Finally, postinfarction pericarditis may cause more pain than the initial infarction, prompting the patient to seek attention. Echocardiography offers immediate assessment of left ventricular function, mechanical complications, and the potential presence of pericardial effusion with or without cardiac tamponade.

LARGE, NON–ST-SEGMENT ELEVATION MYOCARDIAL INFARCTION

Most non–ST-segment elevation MIs can be stabilized medically with coronary arteriography pursued electively, but soon after presentation. Many are small events. In patients who stabilize nicely with limited myocardial damage, a conservative approach can be elected with coronary arteriography pursued later, or reserved for recurrent symptoms, poor left ventricular function on noninvasive evaluation, and/or significant ischemia on stress imaging study. Early in the clinical course, separating small from large events can prove difficult. A bedside echocardiogram may reveal a large segmental wall motion abnormality (Figure 13-6). Even with improving symptoms, a large area of involvement might prompt an aggressive approach with immediate invasive study with anticipated early revascularization.

TRUE POSTERIOR MYOCARDIAL INFARCTION

With true posterior MIs, the ECG may show only anterior ST depressions that, in fact, represent posterior ST elevations. Other potential diagnoses such as acute pulmonary embolism or pleural effusion with pain may lead to delay in correct diagnosis and myocardial loss. Immediately obtained bedside echocardiography

CHAPTER 13 ECHOCARDIOGRAPHIC DIAGNOSIS AND MONITORING OF ACUTE MYOCARDIAL INFARCTION   141

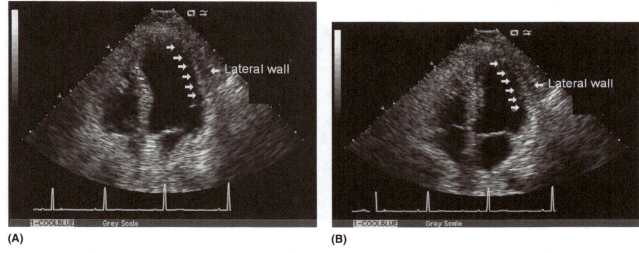

Figure 13-6 Apical four-chamber views in diastole (**A**) and systole (**B**) show akinesis of the lateral segments extending to apex (*arrows*).

(Video 13-2) can readily show posterobasal and inferolateral wall motion abnormalities leading to revascularization. Alternatively, normal wall motion in this setting would point to a pulmonary cause of similar life-threatening potential, but requiring a different therapeutic approach.

LEFT VENTRICULAR THROMBI

Left ventricular thrombi continue to occur after acute MI. These may result in potentially catastrophic emboli to the heart, brain, kidneys, gut, and extremities. Left ventricular thrombi are distinctly more common with an anterior location, large extent, and late presentation and/or revascularization (Figure 13-7). Usually seen in the left ventricular apex, thrombi may be absent with early imaging even in the presence of apical akinesis or dyskinesis, but easily seen 3–5 days later. If full dose anticoagulation is withheld, daily bedside imaging can detect thrombus development and suggest timely change in treatment. In the case of an unexplained thromboembolic event, prompt bedside echocardiography can help lead to an emergency intervention such as thrombolysis or embolectomy.

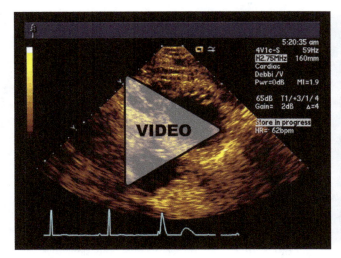
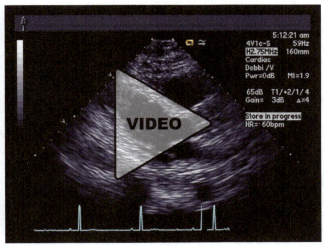

Video 13-2 (**A**) Left parasternal view at the mid-left ventricular level showing inferior and posterior akinesis consistent with a posterior myocardial infarction with R > S in V1 and V2 and ST segment depressions in these leads. (**B**) Left parasternal long-axis view in the same patient showing basal and mid-posterior akinesis. View at www.ccu2e.com

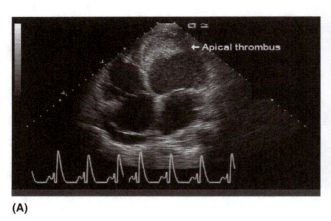 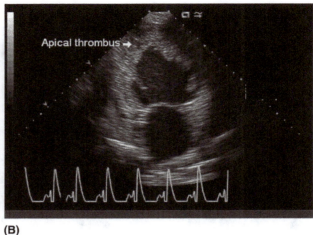

Figure 13-7 Apical four- (**A**) and two- (**B**) chamber views in diastole show a definite apical thrombus.

CONCLUSION

Efficacious treatment of acute MI requires fast, accurate diagnosis and rapid reperfusion. Given the expense and attendant risks of thrombolytic therapy or catheter-directed intervention, overtreatment must be minimized without missing opportunities to save muscle, preserve function, and prolong life. Similarly, major complications require timely diagnosis if surgical intervention, pericardiocentesis, and coronary intervention are to be effective. Echocardiography has long been recognized as helpful in the acute MI environment. Wide deployment of this powerful imaging technology, however, lacked portable equipment and sufficient numbers of adequately trained and experienced operators/interpreters. New, reasonably priced machines provide portability and availability. Emergency department (ED) physicians, ICU physicians, hospitalists, cardiologists, and physician extenders are acquiring the needed training and experience. These professionals will use their skills and expertise with increasing frequency to foster expedited, more accurate diagnosis and, when needed, targeted, aggressive treatment. The above examples serve as a starting point, as providers with readily available bedside imaging will identify new and important applications.

SUGGESTED READING

Peels CH, Visser CA, Kupper AJ, Visser FC, Roos JP. Usefulness of two-dimensional echocardiography for immediate detection of myocardial ischemia in the emergency room. *Am J Cardiol.* 1990;65:687.

Cerqueira MD, Weissman NJ, Dilsizian V, et al. Standardized myocardial segmentation and nomenclature for tomographic imaging of the heart. A statement for healthcare professionals from the Cardiac Imaging Committee of the Council on Clinical Cardiology of the American Heart Association. *Circulation.* 2002;105:539.

Zimetbaum PJ, Josephson ME. Use of the electrocardiogram in acute myocardial infarction. *N Engl J Med.* 2003;348:933.

Romano S, Dagianti A, Penco M, et al. Usefulness of echocardiography in the prognostic evaluation of non-Q-wave myocardial infarction. *Am J Cardiol.* 2000;86:43G.

Shlipak MG, Go AS, Frederick PD, et al. Treatment and outcomes of left bundle branch block patients with myocardial infarction who present without chest pain. *J Am Coll Cardiol.* 2000;36:706.

Birnbaum Y, Chamoun AJ, Conti VR, et al. Mitral regurgitation following acute myocardial infarction. *Coron Artery Dis.* 2002;13:337.

Bias B, Graba J, Siu S, et al. Papillary muscle rupture complicating an acute myocardial infarction. *Can J Cardiol.* 2001;17:722.

Birnbuam Y, Fishbein MC, Blanche C, et al. Ventricular septal rupture after acute myocardial infarction. *N Eng J Med.* 2002;347:1426.

Sugiura T, Nagahama Y, Nakamura S, et al. Left ventricular free wall rupture after reperfusion therapy for acute myocardial infarction. *Am J Cardiol.* 2003;92:282.

Spodick DH. Acute cardiac tamponade. *N Engl J Med.* 2003;349:684.

March KL, Sawada SG, Tarver RD, Kesler KA, Armstrong WF. Current concepts of left ventricular pseudoaneurysm: pathophysiology, therapy, and diagnostic imaging methods. *Clin Cardiol.* 1989;12:531.

Mehta SR, Eikelboom JW, Natarajan MK, et al. Impact of right ventricular involvement on mortality and morbidity in patients with inferior myocardial infarction. *J Am Coll Cardiol.* 2001;37:37.

Pierard LA, Albert A, Henrard L, et al. Incidence and significance of pericardial effusion in acute myocardial infarction as determined by two-dimensional echocardiography. *J Am Coll Cardiol.* 1986;8:517.

Jugdutt BI, Sivaram CA. Prospective two-dimensional echocardiographic evaluation of left ventricular thrombus and embolism after acute myocardial infarction. *J Am Coll Cardiol.* 1989;13:554.

ECHOCARDIOGRAPHIC DIAGNOSIS OF CARDIOMYOPATHIES

NARINDER P. BHALLA, MARGUERITE UNDERWOOD, & ALEXANDER B. LEVITOV

Scan QR code or visit www.ccu2e.com for video in this chapter

INTRODUCTION

In its simplest form, cardiomyopathy (CMP) can be defined as a cardiac disorder involving myocardial dysfunction. Though there are various formal definitions of CMP in the literature, the two major ones are from the World Health Organization (WHO) and from the American Heart Association (AHA). The WHO definition is more clinical, while the AHA definition is more molecular and scientific in its delineation. For the purpose of this chapter, we follow the simpler definition by WHO as it lends itself well to the echocardiographic evaluation of cardiomyopathies.

Cardiomyopathies can also be defined by their etiology, as was done also by the WHO task force in 1995. Since the etiology may not always be obvious, such as in many cases of dilated CMP, this classification is also less useful when discussing the general principles of echocardiographic diagnosis of CMP. The various types of cardiomyopathies, as classified by WHO, are listed in Table 14-1. Each type of CMP can have various etiologies, the discussion of which is beyond the scope of this chapter (see suggested reading list for further information). The various etiologies are nonetheless listed in Table 14-2. Table 14-3 demonstrates the key elements in the echocardiographic evaluation of a patient with a CMP.

As we describe the echocardiographic features of the various cardiomyopathies, we will incorporate the elements described above. The reader should recognize that this chapter assumes familiarity with the basic echocardiographic views and how to obtain those views. It also needs to be emphasized that the two-dimensional image and M-mode interrogations need to be of good quality to make reliable interpretations.

DILATED CMP

Dilated cardiomyopathies have various etiologies, and the dilated state usually represents the response of the myocardium to the various insults. Though the dilated state may represent a common response to multiple types of insults, every effort should be made to identify a potentially remediable cause, as this may significantly influence the prognosis. Dilated cardiomyopathies generally are classified as either ischemic or nonischemic, the latter category being rather broad and inclusive of those caused by valvular diseases (Table 14-2).

Echocardiography is a critical tool in assessing patients with a dilated CMP, and, in some cases, can help elucidate the etiology of the CMP and gauge prognosis and response to treatment. The most common clinical presentation of a patient with a dilated CMP is congestive heart failure, associated with dyspnea and a fluid overload state. Echocardiographic evaluation of a patient presenting with dyspnea, with or without a fluid overload state, should be undertaken early in the course of management if a clear etiology is not evident on presentation, such as symptoms or signs of coronary ischemia, electrocardiograpahic changes suggestive of myocardial ischemia, a history of known CMP, or a recent echocardiogram. If a remediable etiology is suspected, like coronary ischemia and mitral regurgitation (MR), every effort should be made to alleviate the condition. Echocardiography should still be carried out in such a case, and the timing should depend on the availability of the ultrasound equipment and the delay it might cause in treatment. However, the current availability of good-quality portable equipment can expedite such evaluations.

TABLE 14-1
The WHO Classification of Cardiomyopathies

Dilated CMP
Hypertrophic CMP
Restrictive CMP
Arrhythmogenic right ventricular CMP (dysplasia)
Other unclassified cardiomyopathies

CMP, cardiomyopathy; WHO, World Health Organization.

The echocardiographic diagnosis of a dilated CMP rests solely on the demonstration of a dilated, hypofunctional left ventricle. Though various secondary features are frequently evident on the ECG, the diagnosis can only be made by the demonstration of left ventricular (LV) dilatation.

TABLE 14-2
Partial Listing of Etiologies of Cardiomyopathies

Type of CMP	Etiologies (examples)
Dilated CMP	Idiopathic (mostly genetic)
	Familial
	Myocardial ischemia/infarction
	End-stage valvular heart disease
	End-stage hypertensive heart disease
	Infectious (viral myocarditis, Chagas, bacterial, etc.)
	Toxic/metabolic (chemotherapy, alcoholic, cocaine, etc.)
	Tachycardia-induced
	Peripartum
	Rheumatologic (SLE, scleroderma)
	Endocrine disorders (diabetes, thyroid disease, etc.)
	Neuromuscular diseases (Duchenne's, myotonic dystrophy, etc.)
	Electrolyte abnormalities (hypocalcemia, hypophosphatemia, etc.)
	Nutritional deficiencies (thiamine, carnitine, etc.)
	Infiltrative diseases (usually end-stage)
Hypertrophic CMP	Idiopathic/familial (asymmetric)
	Concentric
	Apical
Restrictive CMP	Idiopathic/familial
	Diabetes
	Infiltrative (amyloidosis, sarcoidosis, etc.)
	Storage diseases (hemochromatosis, glycogen storage diseases, etc.)
	Endomyocardial fibrosis
	Rheumatologic (scleroderma)
	Radiation
Unclassified Cardiomyopathies	Isolated LV noncompaction
	LV apical ballooning syndrome
	Endocardial fibroelastosis

CMP, cardiomyopathy; LV, left ventricular; SLE, systemic lupus erythematosus.

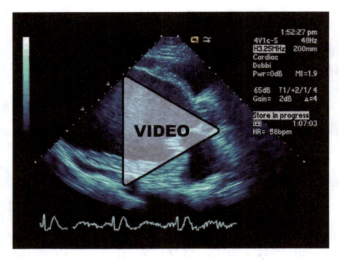

Video 14-1 Parasternal long-axis (PLAX) view of severe Dilative CMP (DCMP). Note left ventricular (LV) dilatation, increase separation of the anterior leaflet of the mitral valve and interventricular septum and presence of the spontaneous LV contrast (poor prognostic sign). Small pericardial effusion is present and is not uncommon with DCMP. View at www.ccu2e.com

▶ Features of Dilated CMP (Videos 14-1 and 14-2)

Left ventricular dilatation (Figure 14-1)

LV dilatation is best evaluated in the parasternal long-axis view (Figure 14-1A). The spherical change in the LV cavity with dilatation is more apparent in this view and is represented by an increasing vertical axis when compared with the horizontal axis (Figure 14-1B). Global dilatation of all four chambers, however, is better appreciated

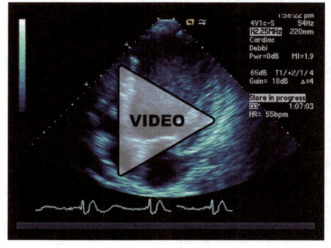

Video 14-2 Apical four-chamber view of severe DCMP note increased LV diastolic volume (LVDV) and poor LV ejection fraction (LVEF). LVEF can be determined by biplane Simpson's method LVEF% = (LVDV − LVSV):LVEDV × 100. LVEDV, left ventricular end diastolic volume. Spontaneous LV contrast is again noted and so is poor separation of the mitral valve leaflets during diastole (likely due to increase LV diastolic pressure). View at www.ccu2e.com

TABLE 14-3	
The Key Elements in the Echocardiographic Evaluation of a Patient with a CMP	
Focused Assessment	**Findings**
Assessment of chamber sizes and mass	Left ventricular and left atrial dilatation Right ventricular dilatation, either primarily or from pulmonary hypertension Increased cardiac mass and hypertrophy
Assessment of valvular function and valve apparatus	Tricuspid regurgitation, usually secondary from pulmonary hypertension Mitral valve regurgitation, either due to primary dysfunction of the valvular apparatus or secondary to annular dilatation A change in the position of the papillary muscles
Assessment of systolic and diastolic function	Doppler flow patterns across the mitral valve Tissue Doppler interrogation Wall motion abnormalities, either segmental or global Grading the systolic and diastolic dysfunction
Assessment of right heart pressures, as this will influence treatment and prognosis	
Assessment of other features	Left atrial or left ventricular thrombus Appearance of the endocardium Assist in the diagnosis of amyloidosis or LV noncompaction, for example

CMP, cardiomyopathy; LV, left ventricular.

in the apical four-chamber view. The LV dilatation may be mild, moderate, or severe, and accurate measurements are important to grade the degree of dilatation. The short-axis view at the level of the papillary muscles is also a good view to assess LV dilatation. If there is difficulty in visualizing the endocardium, echocardiographic contrast can be used; the risk/benefit ratio of the use of such agents should be assessed in each individual patient (we recommend avoiding the agents in acute ischemia and in acute heart failure).

LV wall motion and thickening
(Figure 14-2A–C)

LV wall motion is universally impaired in patients with a dilated CMP (Figure 14-2A,B). The wall motion abnormalities may well be regional in patients with an ischemic etiology. These regional abnormalities correlate well with impairment of vascular supply to the dysfunctional wall. However, basal wall motion may be better preserved than other regions in some patients with a nonischemic, dilated

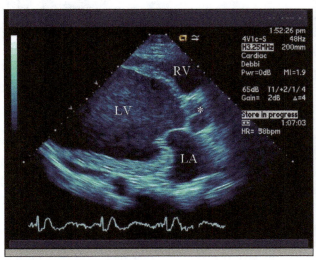

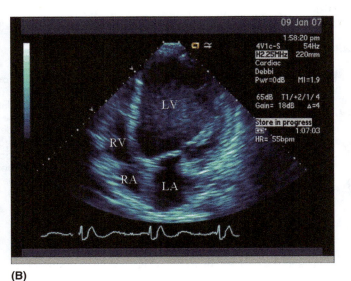

(A)   (B)

Figure 14-1 (A) A two-dimensional image of a parasternal long-axis view in a patient with a dilated cardiomyopathy. Note the dilated LV and the increased long axis of the LV. (B) Two-dimensional image of an apical four-chamber view of a patient with a dilated cardiomyopathy. Note the spherical change in the LV cavity with the dilatation. *Aortic root and aortic valve. LA, left atrium; LV, left ventricle; RA, right atrium; RV, right ventricle.

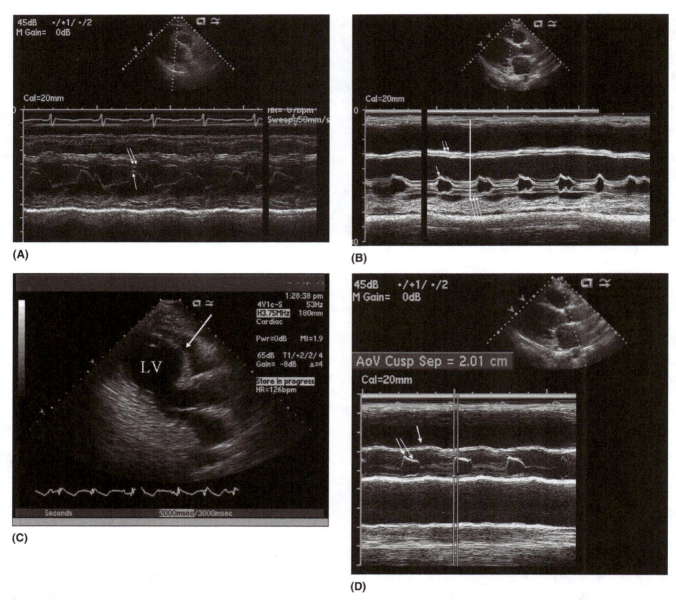

Figure 14-2 (A) M-mode through the mitral valve in a normally contractile heart. Note the close relationship of the mitral E wave (single arrowhead) with the septal M-mode (double arrowheads). This is called the EPSS (E-point septal separation). (B) M-mode recording through the mitral valve in a patient with a dilated cardiomyopathy. Note the significantly abnormal separation between the mitral valve E wave (single arrowhead) and the septal M-mode (double arrowheads). The EPSS is abnormal in this patient. Also note the lack of motion and thickening with systole in the M-mode of the septum and the posterior wall (triple arrowheads). Systole is marked by the vertical solid white line. (C) Two-dimensional imaging in the parasternal long axis in a patient with a previous myocardial infarction. Note the thinned-out septum that is akinetic (arrowhead). The septum bows into the right ventricle with systole. (D) M-mode imaging in the parasternal long-axis view through the aortic root and aortic valve. Note the relatively "flat" motion of the aortic root during the cardiac cycle (single arrowhead) and the "trapezoidal" pattern of aortic valve motion (double arrowheads). See the text for more information.

CMP, leading to occasional confusion with ischemic CMP. This should be kept in mind when trying to distinguish between ischemic and nonischemic etiologies. Another potential issue may arise in patients with a dilated CMP and a left bundle branch block or a dilated CMP and previous cardiac surgery. The bundle branch abnormality may be from the increased mass from the cardiac dilatation or from an ischemic injury in the left anterior descending coronary artery territory. A dyssynchronous septum is seen in such patients and is evident in the parasternal long-axis and the apical four-chamber views. In such cases, one should concentrate on looking at other walls to make the distinction between regional and diffuse wall motion abnormalities. In patients with a previous anterior wall myocardial infarction, other wall motion abnormalities will be apparent, such as apical and/or anterior lateral hypokinesis, akinesis, or dyskinesis. Furthermore, infarcted tissue will appear thinned on two-dimensional imaging (Figure 14-2C).

Though two-dimensional imaging is excellent at assessing wall motion, the importance of M-mode interrogation is often overlooked. M-mode interrogation may allow a better assessment of wall motion than two-dimensional imaging in circumstances where the endocardium is not well visualized by the two-dimensional approach. M-mode imaging is also important in gauging wall thickness. During normal contractility of a myocardial segment, there is motion inward toward the ventricular cavity and associated thickening. M-mode imaging can exhibit the presence or absence of both these phenomena quite well.

▶ **Other Associated Features of Dilated CMP**

Various other features (also called secondary features) may also be evident in patients with a dilated CMP.

Mitral regurgitation (Figure 14-3)

A common secondary feature is MR (also called functional MR). This occurs due to a relative dilatation of the mitral annulus. As the left ventricle dilates and approaches a spherical shape, the mitral valve apparatus is pulled apically. This results in a relative dilatation of the mitral annulus, leading to MR. One has to make an effort, clinically, to sort out whether the MR is a primary phenomenon resulting in the dilated CMP or whether it is the result of the dilated CMP. A transesophageal echocardiogram (TEE) may help in resolving the issue. If the mitral valve apparatus appears structurally normal (absence of leaflet or chordal redundancy, absence of valve thickening, absence of annular calcification, absence of papillary muscle dysfunction), and an ischemic cause of the regurgitation is ruled out, then one should consider the etiology of the regurgitation to be related to the dilated CMP. The best determination of an etiology is important as it may influence the treatment approach and the choice of surgical repair technique for a particular patient. Furthermore, etiology, along with hemodynamic status and LV mechanical status, also influences prognosis with or without surgical treatment. When present secondary to a CMP, the regurgitant jet is usually central (the cause is relative annular dilatation) (Figure 14-3). Various criteria have been established to judge the severity of the regurgitant jet, and though some are better accepted than others, demonstration of flow reversal in the pulmonary veins during systole and a high peak inflow velocity across the mitral valve are good correlates of severe regurgitation. A standard TEE or a three-dimensional study may be superior to standard two-dimensional imaging for determining the severity of the regurgitation. TEE particularly, also helps in deciding the appropriate surgical approach (valve repair/reconstruction vs. replacement).

▶ **M-Mode Features**

In addition to the M-mode features described above, there are other features that should be reviewed when performing an echocardiographic examination of a patient with a dilated CMP.

E-point septal separation (Figure 14-2A,B)

This is best assessed in the parasternal long-axis view with the ultrasound beam through the mitral leaflets. The E point of the mitral valve opening is quite close to the septal wall on M-mode imaging in normal individuals. However, this distance is significantly increased in patients with a dilated CMP (Video 14-1).

Aortic root motion (Figure 14-2D)

In normal circumstances, there is a sinusoidal pattern of motion exhibited by the aortic root with anterior motion during systole. This is best seen in the parasternal long axis, with the ultrasound beam focused through the aortic root at the level of the aortic leaflets. In patients with a dilated CMP, the normal sinusoidal pattern is replaced by a relatively flat pattern of motion.

Changes in aortic valve opening and closing (Figure 14-2D)

The normal pattern of aortic valve opening and closing appears as a rectangular box on M-mode imaging performed in the parasternal long-axis view through the aortic valve. In cases of reduced stroke volume (SV), as is the case in dilated CMP, there is poor opening of the aortic valve and the valve tends to start closing earlier in systole. The pattern changes from that of a rectangular box to a more "trapezoidal" box.

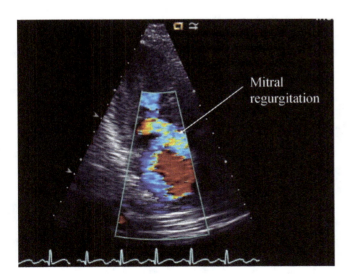

Figure 14-3 Two-dimensional imaging with color-flow showing mitral regurgitation in a patient with dilated cardiomyopathy. Note the central jet location. The mitral regurgitation in these patients is often due to dilatation of the mitral valve annulus.

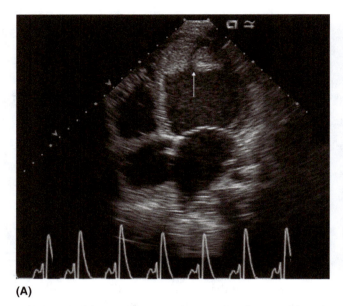 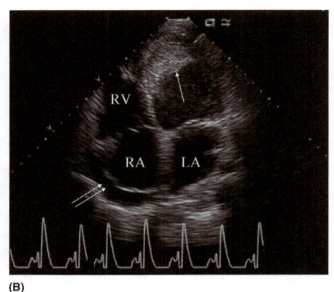

Figure 14-4 (**A**) Two-dimensional imaging in the apical four-chamber view demonstrating a left ventricular thrombus in the apex (arrowhead). (**B**) Apical four-chamber view demonstrating a left ventricular thrombus in the apex (single arrowhead). The thrombus occupies most of the apex. Incidentally, also note the pericardial fluid around the right atrium (double arrowheads). LA, left atrium; RA, right atrium; RV, right ventricle.

▶ LV Thrombus (Figure 14-4)

The presence of a mural thrombus in the LV cavity on two-dimensional imaging can be seen in a dilated CMP. In cases of ischemic CMP, the thrombus is most often seen in an akinetic and/or aneurysmal segment. The presence of thrombus must be distinguished from the endocardium. Though this is usually straightforward, there are helpful techniques that can be utilized if confusion exists. Contrast enhancement can be used to delineate the endocardium. Usually, the contrast will outline the thrombus by circumventing it. Color-flow can also be used in a similar fashion. A color sector focused on the area of concern will outline the thrombus, as color will not go into thrombus. Care should be taken to not have too much gain on the color jet, as this may well obscure the delineation between the thrombus and the endocardium.

▶ Left Atrial Dilatation

Left atrial dilatation is a universally associated finding in dilated CMP. Left atrial size and volume correlate well with the severity and duration of the dilated CMP. The left atrial dilatation is caused by multiple reasons, including the secondary MR, increased diastolic pressures, and potential involvement of the left atrium itself by the myopathic process. Spontaneous echo contrast can be seen commonly in the left atrium because of impaired of blood flow, and may be more prominent if there is associated atrial fibrillation.

▶ Right Heart Findings (Figure 14-5)

There are various right heart-related findings that can be seen in patients with a dilated CMP. These include tricuspid regurgitation, right ventricular (RV) dilatation, and pulmonary hypertension. The RV dilatation is either secondary to pulmonary hypertension, which is commonly seen in such patients, or due to involvement by the myopathic process. The tricuspid regurgitation, in most cases, is a secondary phenomenon from the pulmonary hypertension and RV dilatation, the latter resulting in tricuspid annular dilatation.

▶ Assessment of Systolic and Diastolic Performance

Assessment of systolic and diastolic performance should be done in all patients with a CMP, regardless of type. The relative impairment in these indices is predictive of prognosis and clinical course. Though the evaluation of systolic and diastolic function is described in this section with reference to dilated CMP, similar principles apply with other types of cardiomyopathies.

▶ Doppler Assessment

Doppler interrogation of all patients with a dilated CMP is important, as it can assist with the assessment of systolic and diastolic function, which helps predict prognosis. The most important predictors of survival in dilated CMP are end-diastolic and systolic volumes and ejection fraction.

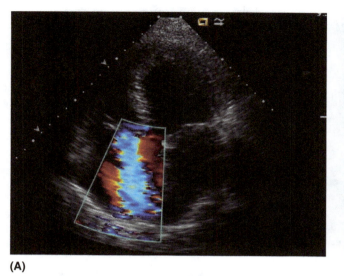 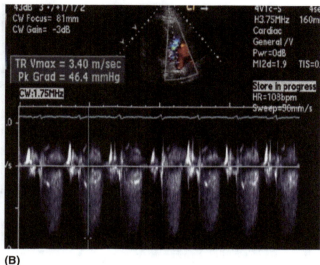

Figure 14-5 (**A**) Apical four-chamber view with color-flow showing tricuspid regurgitation. (**B**) Continuous-wave Doppler recording through the tricuspid valve during systole. There is tricuspid regurgitation present, and the peak gradient across the right ventricle and the right atrium is 46.4 mmHg. If one assumes a right atrial pressure of 10 mmHg and the absence of pulmonic valve stenosis, then the estimated pulmonary artery pressure is 56.4 mmHg, consistent with moderate pulmonary hypertension.

Systolic function assessment

The principles of laminar flow are used in determining the various indices of systolic function. This includes an assessment of SV and cardiac output (CO). The pulsed Doppler can be used to interrogate the flow in the left ventricular outflow tract (LVOT) over a period of time. This generates the time–velocity integral (TVI) (sometimes also referred to as velocity–time integral [VTI]). The mechanical status of the left ventricle is a key component in determining the TVI. Assuming the principles of laminar flow, the SV is a product of the LVOT cross-sectional area (CSA) and the TVI (SV = TVI × LVOT CSA). CO, in turn, is defined as the product of the SV and the heart rate (HR). Because the LVOT CSA can be assumed to be stable for a given patient, and hence a constant, the change in TVI is directly proportional to the change in the LV mechanical status. Hence, an increase in the LVOT TVI can be used as gauge for improvement in LV systolic function when a therapy is undertaken, such as initiation of inotropic support, alleviation of coronary ischemia, treatment of valvular insufficiency with afterload reduction, placement of an intra-aortic balloon pump, or a combination thereof. With appropriate therapy, not only is there an increase in the TVI, but the shape of the envelope also changes from a more parabolic and somewhat blunted one to a more triangular one. Measurements of the acceleration and deceleration times of the mitral regurgitant jet have been identified as predictive of prognosis. These times correlate well with dP/dt (a measurement of LV contractility) obtained at cardiac catheterization in similar patients. An acceleration time (dP/dt) of <600 mmHg/s and a deceleration time (DT) ($-dP/dt$) of <450 mmHg/s identifies a significantly higher risk group, with a decreased event-free survival.

Diastolic function assessment (Figure 14-6)

Doppler assessment of diastolic function relies on interrogation techniques and evaluation of a few key parameters: mitral valve inflow patterns, tissue Doppler interrogation (TDI) techniques, the isovolumic relaxation time (IVRT), mitral flow deceleration time, and pulmonary vein flow patterns. It is important to utilize a combination of the above findings to arrive at a decision regarding the diastolic function of a patient. These parameters tend to be the most predictive with the presence of systolic dysfunction and can be altered by various other clinical issues, such as valvular disease, HRs, and therapeutics. Though a detailed discussion of these parameters is beyond the scope of this chapter, basic principles of the use of Doppler in evaluating diastolic dysfunction are discussed.

Mitral Inflow Pattern. This evaluation should be performed in the apical view with the sample volume placed at the mitral valve tips. The two major components of the inflow pattern are the E wave and the A wave (Figure 14-6A). The rapid early filling phase correlates with the E wave and the latter phase, prompted by the atrial contraction, yields the A wave. In a normal circumstance, the E wave amplitude and velocity and duration are greater than the A wave. Because the E-wave amplitude is greater, in normal individuals the E/A ratio is >1. However, with progressive worsening of diastolic function, there is a change in both the volume and velocity of the E and A waves. The spectrum extends from a mild form (Grade 1), where

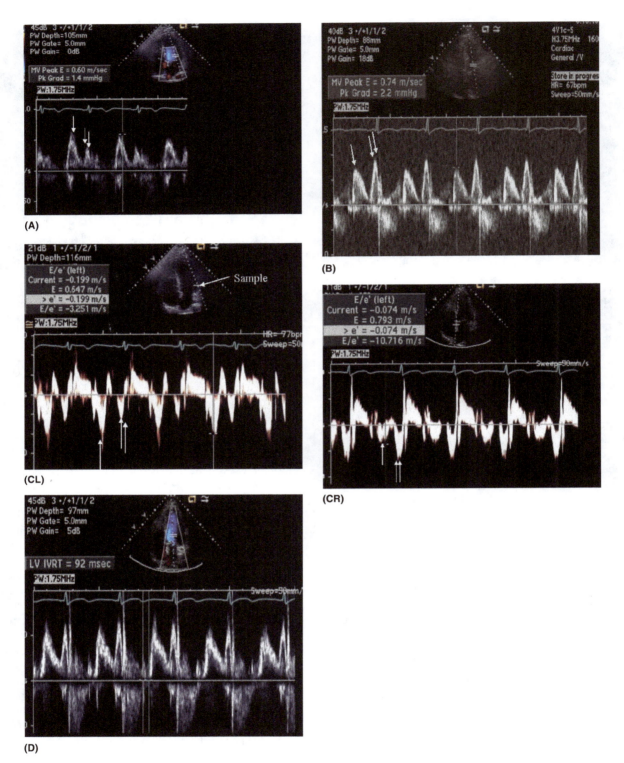

Figure 14-6 (A) The normal pulsed Doppler pattern seen with mitral valve inflow. Note the E/A >1 (E wave: single arrowhead; A wave: double arrowheads). The best flow patterns are recorded with the sample volume placed at the mitral valve tips in the apical four-chamber or apical two-chamber views. (B) Mitral valve inflow recording with pulsed-wave Doppler showing evidence of mild diastolic relaxation abnormality, with E/A < 1 (E wave: single arrowhead; A wave: double arrowheads). (CL) A normal tissue Doppler pattern recorded at the mitral valve leaflet. The E_a/A_a > 1. Note the placement of the sample volume at the lateral aspect of the mitral leaflet (E_a: single arrowhead; A_a: double arrowheads). (CR) Tissue Doppler recording of the mitral valve in a patient demonstrating a diastolic relaxation abnormality. Note the reversal of the E_a/A_a to <1. Because the annular velocity is not volume dependent, obtaining a tissue Doppler avoids the issue with pseudonormalization seen with mitral valve inflow velocity pulsed-wave Doppler measurements in patients with mild diastolic dysfunction (E_a: single arrowhead; A_a: double arrowheads). (D) Normal isovolumic relaxation time (IVRT) is demonstrated here. The IVRT decreases with progressive diastolic dysfunction. (continued)

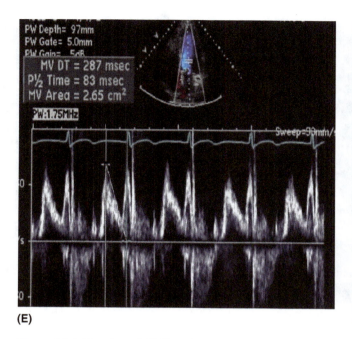
(E)

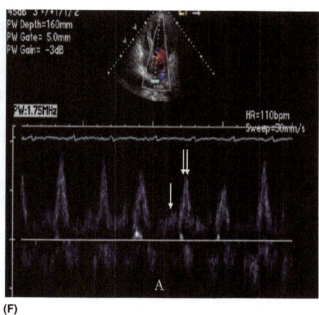
(F)

Figure 14-6 *(Continued)* (**E**) This demonstrates the normal deceleration time (DT) on pulsed-wave Doppler for mitral valve inflow (287 m/s). The deceleration time decreases with progressive diastolic dysfunction, approaching values <140 m/s. (**F**) Pulsed-wave Doppler recording on a transthoracic echocardiogram demonstrating forward flow in the pulmonary veins. Note the predominance of diastolic flow (double arrowheads) over systolic flow (single arrowhead). This demonstrates a significant amount of diastolic dysfunction. Also note the wide pulmonary "a" wave (labeled A).

there is abnormal relaxation, to a severe form (Grade 4), where the compliance is compromised irreversibly.

Grade 1: Abnormal relaxation, with reversal of the E/A ratio and attenuated deceleration of the E wave (Figure 14-6B).

Grade 2: A pseudonormalization pattern, as the ventricle, becomes more noncompliant. Use of the Valsalva maneuver (which decreases preload by diminishing venous return) may help unmask the pathology here by showing a reversed E/A ratio (reminiscent of the pattern in Grade 1).

Grade 3: A markedly increased E/A ratio, with a diminished A wave and an E velocity that almost touches the baseline prior to the A wave.

Grade 4: An irreversible phase, where the E/A ratio is markedly increased and the A wave is diminutive. Furthermore, there is a separation of the E and A waves, with the A wave velocity not always returning to baseline.

Tissue Doppler Interrogation (TDI). This technique has the advantage of not being influenced by atrial rhythm disturbances or by increased HRs. The recommended way is to sample the lateral mitral annulus in the apical view. The velocity of the mitral annulus in diastole correlates with systolic and diastolic function. During diastole, the mitral annulus has two phases: E_a and A_a. These phases are similar to those discussed above in that E_a occurs in early diastole and A_a occurs in late diastole and correlates with the atrial contraction. Similar to the mitral inflow pattern, the E_a is greater than the A_a under normal circumstances. As diastolic abnormalities progress (toward an abnormal relaxation pattern), the early mitral annular velocity decreases, making the E_a/A_a <1. Because the annular velocity is not volume dependent, the potential issue with pseudonormalization (seen with mitral inflow) is avoided, and the ratio remains reversed. As diastolic dysfunction progresses to an irreversible stage, the E_a and A_a waves progressively become lower in amplitude, but the ratio reversal is maintained (Figure 14-6C). A predictor of increasing pulmonary capillary filling pressures is the ratio between the mitral inflow E wave and the E_a wave. An increasing ratio (particularly >15) correlates well with adverse outcomes in both ischemic and nonischemic CMP.

Isovolumic Relaxation Time and Deceleration Time (IVRT and DT) IVRT occurs when systolic flow across the aortic valve ceases (marking the end of systole), but before the mitral valve opens to allow ventricular filling (marking the beginning of diastole). Normal values in adults for IVRT range between 65 and 90 m/s. IVRT will decrease progressively with worsening diastolic function, as the rising left atrial pressure results in earlier opening of the mitral valve. Furthermore, as the left ventricle becomes more noncompliant, it takes on a restrictive filling pattern with a decrease in the DT (<140 m/s), as most of the LV filling occurs in early diastole (Figure 14-6D,E). This gives rise to the S3 gallop in dilated CMP and predicts a higher mortality in patients with symptomatic heart failure. Similar adverse prognosis is seen in patients who have this filling pattern postmyocardial infarction.

Pulmonary Venous Flow Patterns. The left upper pulmonary vein (posteriorly) can be well interrogated by transthoracic echocardiography. This is accomplished in the apical view, and contrast enhancement can be used,

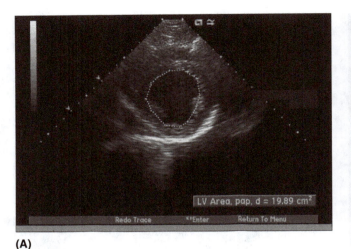 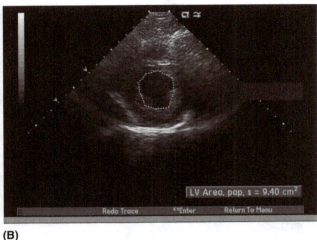

Figure 14-7 Short-axis view demonstrating relative change in ventricular area between systole and diastole.

if necessary. Under normal circumstances, pulmonary venous flow is triphasic. During systole, there is forward flow in the pulmonary veins due to atrial relaxation (the "x" descent) and movement of the base of the heart during the contraction phase. During early diastole, there is a second phase of forward flow through the pulmonary veins due to the open mitral valve (the "y" descent). During late diastole, in sinus rhythm, there is a brief period of reversal of flow in the pulmonary veins because of increasing pressure in the left atrium during atrial systole. When LV dynamics are normal, the amplitude of the systolic phase of pulmonary flow is greater than the amplitude during the diastolic phase. With increasing LV noncompliance, there is incomplete emptying of the left atrium during diastole, raising left atrial pressures. This results in attenuation of pulmonary vein flow during the systolic phase. Conversely, there is an increase in the pulmonary vein flow during diastole, as most of the filling occurs when the mitral valve is open and there is direct emptying into the left ventricle. This increases the amplitude of the diastolic phase of the pulmonary vein flow. In essence, there is a reversal of the systolic and diastolic ratio (Figure 14-6F). Because the left atrial pressure is increased, the flow reversal seen during atrial contraction is more pronounced and lasts longer. There has been some suggestion that if this flow reversal period exceeds the A wave period of the mitral inflow, then the LV end-diastolic pressure exceeds 15 mmHg in the majority of cases.

Myocardial performance index

Myocardial performance index (MPI) is a measurement that is obtained in the apical five-chamber view, as mitral flow and LVOT flow need to be obtained simultaneously (similar to obtaining IVRT). The measurement allows assessment of both systolic and diastolic performance using a single Doppler approach. The concept of MPI relies on interrogating the entire systolic period, which occurs from the closure of the mitral valve of one beat to the opening of the mitral valve of the next beat. This complete systolic period includes in it the isovolumic contraction time (the period between the closure of the mitral valve and the opening of the aortic valve), the ejection period (during which the aortic valve is open and blood is ejected into the aorta), and the IVRT, which has been described earlier. The measurement is given by (IVRT + IVCT)/ET. A normal MPI is 0.40, and increasing values suggest worsening LV function.

▶ **Two-Dimensional and M-Mode Assessment**

Two-dimensional imaging can also be used to assess systolic and diastolic dysfunction.

Assessment of systolic function (Figure 14-7)

Evaluation of systolic function with two-dimensional and M-mode echocardiography uses some of the methods already described earlier, such as wall motion, LV dilatation on linear measurements, and wall thickening. However, two other features for systolic function assessment that use two-dimensional echocardiography are fractional area change (sometimes referred to as fractional shortening) and volume measurements.

Fractional Area Change. Fractional area change looks at the relative change in area, in the short-axis view, between diastole and systole. As mentioned earlier, the decrease in area during systole is due to the inward motion and thickening of the ventricular wall. The formula is given by (area in diastole − area in systole)/area in diastole. The normal values range from 0.35 to 0.60. With significant dilatation and dysfunction of the left ventricle in dilated CMP, values in the 0.15 range can be seen. The limitation with this measurement has to do with regional wall motion abnormalities. For example, in a patient with a LV apical infarction, fractional area change in the midcavity region may well be within the normal range, and will not account for the decrease in ejection fraction from a large akinetic apex. Hence, much like any measurement in echocardiography, the interpreter has to make a conclusion based on multiple measurements and parameters.

Volume Measurements. Volume measurements are usually made using various area and length measurements. Many assumptions go into such measurements regarding the shape of the ventricle, assumed either to be conical or spherical, depending on where the measurement is made and the view used to make the measurement. The most commonly used method for determination of LV volumes is Simpson's rule. In simple terms, this method involves stacking disks with a fixed height along the longitudinal axis of the left ventricle in the apical four-chamber or apical two-chamber view in end-systole and end-diastole. The volume of each disk is calculated and all the volumes are added together to yield the total volume. Care needs to be taken to make sure that the entire ventricular cavity is visualized along its endocardial surface. If there are regional wall motion abnormalities, evaluating volumes in two planes is recommended. Once the end-diastolic and end-systolic volumes have been gained, the difference between the two is the SV. SV multiplied by the HR yields the CO. Recognize that the CO represents the entire flow from the left ventricle when calculated with this technique; hence, it will include the regurgitant volume if mitral or aortic regurgitation is present, and may not necessarily represent the true output into the aorta. Ejection fraction can also be calculated using Simpson's rule as (end-diastolic volume − end-systolic volume)/end-diastolic volume (Video 14-2).

HYPERTROPHIC CMP

Though the disease pattern of hypertrophic CMP was described over a century ago, the true characterization of the disease was not realized until the 1950s. Various features have been described in association with the disease, but the only consistent finding is that of inappropriate LV hypertrophy with relation to the hemodynamic load. Hypertrophic CMP has a familial predilection, and various genetic mutations in 1 of 14 sacromeric genes (14q11), resulting in myocardial fiber disarray have been associated with this autosomal dominant pattern of inheritance. There is, however, varied penetrance, leading to different types of phenotypic expression of the disease. The various forms of primary hypertrophic CMP include, hypertrophic CMP (with or without obstruction), apical hypertrophic CMP, and hypertrophic CMP of the elderly. Secondary hypertrophic CMP, the hallmark of which is a pattern of concentric hypertrophy, is usually a late result of hypertension and characterizes hypertensive heart disease. Echocardiography is extremely important in characterizing the various forms of hypertrophic cardiomyopathies, and this is discussed below with reference to each of the above entities. The most common imaging views that are used for discerning the type of hypertrophic CMP include parasternal long axis, short axis, and apical four chambers. All interrogation modalities are important, though M-mode is probably the least utilized.

▶ Hypertrophic CMP (with or without Obstruction)

This particular entity has had various names associated with it, including idiopathic hypertrophic subaortic stenosis and muscular subaortic stenosis. Because obstruction may not always be present, hypertrophic CMP is a more appropriate term. Clinically speaking, timely diagnosis of this disorder in the critical care setting can be potentially lifesaving by avoiding critical treatment errors. An example is a 44-year-old male patient who presents with precordial discomfort and dyspnea. The chest discomfort description has some typical anginal features, and the patient has dyslipidemia and a family history of sudden death and premature cardiovascular disease. The discomfort is ongoing and on examination a systolic murmur is identified at the base of the heart. The remainder of the examination is relatively unremarkable, and the ECG shows T wave inversions in the precordial leads. A diagnosis of unstable angina or acute coronary syndrome and its treatment could be potentially problematic in such a patient. This patient may well have hypertrophic CMP with an obstructive gradient. Administering nitroglycerine to control the chest discomfort may have the paradoxical effect of worsening the discomfort and precipitating hypotension and heart failure by worsening the obstructive gradient and MR. Hence, a good history and examination along with echocardiography may well avoid such pitfalls in management.

M-mode and two-dimensional assessment (Figure 14-8)

M-mode findings were the original way of diagnosing hypertrophic CMP, and used a septal wall–to–posterior wall thickness ratio at the end of diastole of greater than 1.3. This finding can be seen in other scenarios as well, such as RV hypertrophy with pulmonary hypertension. Two-dimensional echocardiography has aided in solidifying the diagnosis by

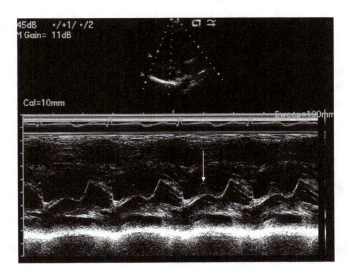

Figure 14-8 M-mode recording in a patient with hypertrophic cardiomyopathy. Note the systolic anterior motion of the mitral valve (*arrowhead*).

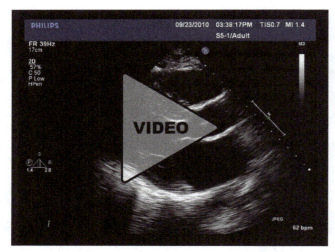

Video 14-3 Parasternal long-axis (PLAX) view of the patient with hypertrophic CMP/HOCM. Note increased thickness of the interventricular septum and small LVEDV. CMP, cardiomyopathy. View at www.ccu2e.com

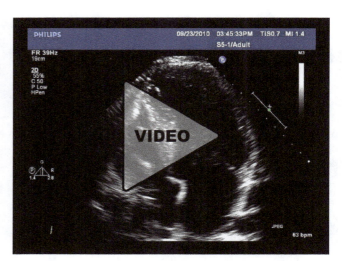

Video 14-4 Patient with hypertrophic CMP/HOCM. Position of the transducer is Apical 4 chamber view but it seems to be tilted some upwards. Note thick interventricular septum, elongated anterior (left on the screen) leaflet of the mitral valve with anterior motion during systole (SAM). CMP, cardiomyopathy; SAM. View at www.ccu2e.com

eliminating confusion, and the septal thickness is usually at least 15 millimeters (mm) (Video 14-3). The asymmetrical septal hypertrophy is most prominent in the midportion between the base and the apex in the parasternal long-axis view, and a variety of thicknesses can be seen from mild hypertrophy to massive hypertrophy (septal thickness of 60 mm). In a recent study, the septal hypertrophy pattern on echocardiography was used to predict the potential for myofilament mutations. The midseptal thickness pattern (also termed the reverse septal pattern) was significantly associated with an abnormal genetic pattern in 79% of those who had this septal morphology. Left ventricular outflow tract obstruction is another important finding in this type of hypertrophic CMP (though it does not have to be present to make the diagnosis). The thickened septum and an elongated anterior mitral leaflet create the outflow tract obstruction. This abnormal geometry also leads to mitral valve regurgitation and systolic anterior motion (SAM) of the mitral valve (Videos 14-4 and 14-5). The degree of MR is directly related to the degree of the outflow tract obstruction and the anterior displacement of the mitral valve. Other two-dimensional features include a small LV cavity, normal or increased motion of the posterior wall, with abnormal motion of the septum, and fluttering of the aortic valve due to turbulent flow in the outflow tract in systole. All of these features can occur to varying degrees, and may be made more apparent by various provocative maneuvers (see Section "Doppler assessment").

Doppler assessment (Figure 14-9)

Doppler assessment, both with color and spectral analysis, is critical to the diagnosis of hypertrophic CMP. Colored Doppler assessment is important for characterizing the degree of mitral valve regurgitation. The MR jet is usually central and late peaking, coinciding with the greatest anterior motion during systole. The later peak of the mitral valve regurgitation in patients with outflow tract gradients distinguishes it from cases of structural mitral valve regurgitation. Hence, the MR is not holosystolic in patients with dynamic outflow tract gradients. Furthermore, there can often be confusion when interrogating the MR and the outflow tract velocity on continuous-wave Doppler. The onset of the MR signal is usually later than that of the outflow tract signal. The

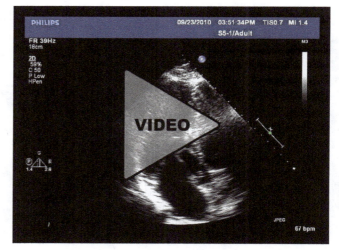

Video 14-5 Patient with hypertrophic CMP/HOCM. Apical three-chamber (long-axis) view and obvious SAM of the anterior leaflet of the mitral valve with LV outflow obstruction visualized. Note thick interventricular septum, elongated anterior (right on the screen towards the noncoronary cusp of the aortic valve) leaflet of the mitral valve. Also note during systole (when aortic valve is opened) anterior leaflet of the mitral valve is moving forward, touching thickened interventricular septum (SAM), which result in additional outflow obstruction. CMP, cardiomyopathy; SAM, systolic anterior motion. View at www.ccu2e.com

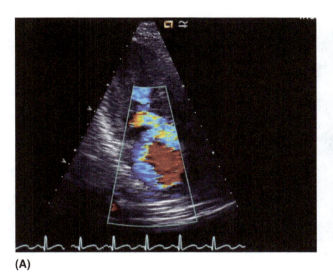 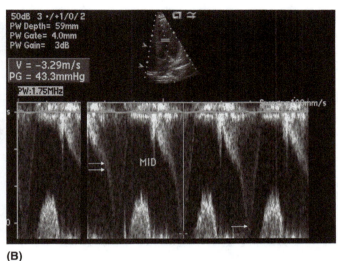

Figure 14-9 (**A**) Color-flow Doppler recording in a patient with hypertrophic cardiomyopathy demonstrating severe mitral regurgitation. The regurgitant jet is usually central and peaks later in systole. (**B**) Pulsed-wave Doppler recording during systole in the left ventricular outflow tract in a patient with hypertrophic cardiomyopathy. Note the late peaking pattern (*single arrowhead*) and the jagged knifelike pattern (*double arrowheads*).

shape of the outflow tract signal is also different, usually in the shape of a dagger, because of the late-peaking velocity. Spectral analysis during systole and diastole provides information on the severity of the outflow tract obstruction and the degree of diastolic dysfunction. Provocative maneuvers include any physiologic (such as a Valsalva maneuver) or pharmacologic manipulation (such as amyl nitrate) that result in decreased LV volume, or increased contractility. In the critical care setting, use of inotropes, volume depletion, tachycardia, and use of nitrates can all serve as provocative maneuvers, and can worsen the outflow tract gradient. Certain inhalation anesthetics and regional anesthetic agents can also worsen the outflow gradient, and should be avoided in patients with hypertrophic CMP. Doppler interrogation of the outflow tract velocity can be used to measure the therapeutic effect of an intervention, whether pharmacologic (use of negatively chronotropic calcium channel blockers or beta blockers) or invasive (ablative therapy of the first septal perforator). A change in the degree of mitral valve regurgitation on color Doppler can also be used to assess response to therapy. Diastolic dysfunction is present in the majority of the patients with hypertrophic CMP, and it does not have to be associated with an outflow tract obstruction. Furthermore, the degree of diastolic dysfunction does not always correlate with the degree of hypertrophy.

▶ Apical Hypertrophic CMP

This disorder is seen mostly in the Japanese population, and accounts for up to 25% of Japanese patients with hypertrophic CMP. It is distinctly uncommon in the Western world. Angiography usually defines the typical features of the disease with a spade-shaped ventricle on LV injection. The ECG reveals deeply inverted precordial T waves.

The usual course is benign in such patients, and they tend to be minimally symptomatic. On echocardiography, there is no outflow tract pressure gradient. On two-dimensional imaging, the base of the heart has normal thickness, and there is an increase in wall thickness toward the apex. This essentially reduces the size of the apical cavity. Contrast enhancement during the echocardiographic study can help define the endocardial border at the apex. Care should be taken to visualize the apex in its full longitudinal view, as foreshortening can mimic the hypertrophy. Occasional diastolic dysfunction can be seen in these patients, particularly with changes in volume status. Atrial fibrillation is the most common clinical complication in such patients.

▶ Hypertrophic CMP of the Elderly (Figure 14-10)

This is usually seen in patients who have been hypertensive; however, the hypertrophy tends to be eccentric rather than concentric. The septum tends to hypertrophy to a greater degree, and this, coupled with the change in angulation of the septum accompanied with aging, results in an outflow tract gradient. Systolic anterior motion of the mitral valve is also seen and can result in mitral valve regurgitation. Genetic abnormalities distinct from those seen in patients with the early onset familial form of hypertrophic CMP (described above) have been defined in such patients. The echocardiographic features are similar to those described above in the hypertrophic CMP section, and outflow tract obstructive gradients can achieve a severity seen in the familial forms.

▶ Secondary Hypertrophic CMP (Table 14-4)

The most common etiologies include hypertension and aortic stenosis. There is usually concentric hypertrophy

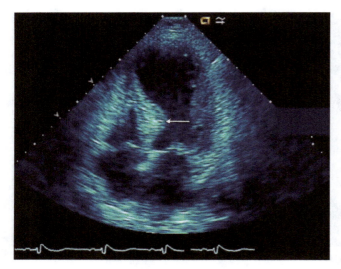

Figure 14-10 Two-dimensional image of the apical four-chamber view in an elderly patient with eccentric hypertrophic cardiomyopathy. Note the hypertrophied septum represented as a septal "knuckle" (*arrowhead*).

of the left ventricle. Systolic function tends to be normal, but if these disorders progress untreated, the final result is a dilated CMP with all its attendant features and clinical prognosis. Diastolic dysfunction is common in these patients and a depleted volume status can potentially provoke midcavitary obstruction of the left ventricle with a gradient. Echocardiography can be used to measure and index the LV mass in such patients, and there are defined criteria for the same (Table 14-4). The emphasis in treating these patients should be on the underlying disease state and keeping them euvolemic. Hemodynamics of hypertrophic CMP can also be seen in patients who have a history of hypertension and have hyperdynamic LV wall motion because of volume depletion. This situation is further augmented in the critical care setting when such a patient is hypotensive and is put on inotropic support. A dynamic outflow tract obstruction is created, and MR can occur due to the systolic anterior motion of the mitral valve. Repletion of volume and weaning of the inotropic support will usually return the hemodynamics toward normal.

TABLE 14-4				
American Society of Echocardiography Criteria for Grading Left Ventricular Hypertrophy (LVH)			
	Mild LVH	Moderate LVH	Severe LVH
Male	103–116 g/m²	117–130 g/m²	>130 g/m²
Female	89–100 g/m²	101–112 g/m²	>112 g/m²

Modified from: Lang RM, Bierig M, Devereux RB, et al. Recommendations for chamber quantification: a report from the American Society of Echocardiography's Guidelines and Standards Committee and the Chamber Quantification Writing Group, developed in conjunction with the European Association of Echocardiography, a branch of the European Society of Cardiology. *J Am Soc Echocardiogr*. 2005;18:1440–1463.

▶ Athlete's Heart

Steady endurance and strength training results in physiologic and electrical changes in the cardiovascular system. These changes are also accompanied by changes in LV volume, wall thickness, and mass. Such changes need to be distinguished from pathological changes, as they are reversible on cessation of the training, and usually do not alter prognosis (unless accompanied by other cardiac pathology or with use of pharmacologic agents, such as anabolic steroids). Echocardiography can help in distinguishing the two subsets. The LV hypertrophy is usually symmetric in athletes, and the wall thickness is usually less than or equal to 12 mm. Though series looking at trained athletes have described wall thicknesses of up to 16 mm, they are typically less than 16 mm. A wall thickness of greater than 16 mm should prompt an investigation to rule out a primary hypertrophic CMP. The LV diastolic dimension is typically greater than 50 mm in trained athletes, while it is less than that in hypertrophic CMP (usually <45 mm). On Doppler evaluation of diastolic function, the patterns are normal in the athletic heart, as is the left atrial dimension on two-dimensional imaging.

RESTRICTIVE CMP

Restrictive CMP is characterized by normal ventricular chamber sizes with impaired filling during diastole. Though hypertrophy of the ventricles is typically absent, certain acquired forms, such as amyloidosis, can cause LV wall thickening. Amyloidosis remains the classic association with infiltrative restrictive CMP, though it is uncommon as a disease entity (Videos 14-6 and 14-7). Because

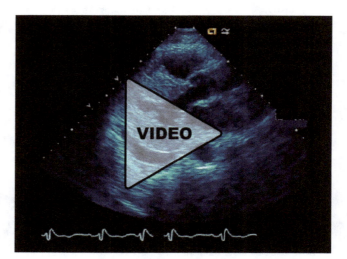

Video 14-6 Patient with restrictive CMP due to amyloidosis. Parasternal long-axis (PLAX) view. Note thick interventricular septum and inferior wall of the LV with shimmering speckled pattern of the myocardium specific of this illness. Small pericardial effusion and dilated coronary sinus (due to increased right ventricular pressure) are also visible and common for restrictive CMP. Restrictive diastolic filling result in exceedingly low LVDV, and thus stroke volume and cardiac output, with normal or elevated LVEF. CMP, cardiomyopathy; LVDV, LV diastolic volume; LVEF, LV ejection fraction. View at www.ccu2e.com

CHAPTER 14 ECHOCARDIOGRAPHIC DIAGNOSIS OF CARDIOMYOPATHIES 157

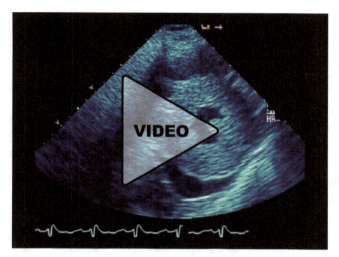

Video 14-7 Patient with restrictive CMP due to Amyloidosis. Parasternal short-axis (PSAX) view. Note thick interventricular septum all wall segments of the free LV with shimmering speckled pattern of the myocardium specific of this illness. Anterolateral papillary muscle is clearly visible secondary to its increased thickness. Hemodynamic consequences of this are obvious and described in 14-6. Pericardial effusion is again present, best visible on the bottom of the screen adjacent to the inferior wall (due to accumulation in the dependent position). CMP, cardiomyopathy. View at www.ccu2e.com

hemochromatosis are examples of storage diseases that lead to a restrictive CMP. Various other important causes include radiation therapy, endomyocardial fibrosis (particularly in tropical regions), anthracycline toxicity, and metastatic cancers. Restrictive physiology can be confused at times with constrictive physiology. This issue can usually be resolved with careful history taking, a good echocardiographic study, and evaluation of the pericardium. On some occasions, an endomyocardial biopsy may be necessary to sort the issue. Because the main feature of restrictive CMP is diastolic dysfunction, a careful Doppler analysis of diastolic function is important in these patients. The Doppler principles of diastolic function assessment have been discussed earlier in this chapter, and aspects will be highlighted below. Increased LV noncompliance results in substantially elevated left atrial pressures, and significant atrial dilatation is the rule in patients with restrictive CMP. Needless to say, atrial arrhythmias can be quite common in these patients, particularly atrial fibrillation. Pulmonary venous pressures are also increased, giving rise to the symptoms of heart failure. Secondary pulmonary hypertension is commonly seen in these patients.

▶ **Two-Dimensional and M-Mode Assessment (Figure 14-11)**

The major findings on two-dimensional imaging and M-mode imaging include normal ventricular chamber size and preserved systolic function. As the disease progresses, the left ventricle may develop some systolic dysfunction, although initially, this is without dilation. Though LV hypertrophy is absent in the idiopathic form, it is commonly seen in infiltrative diseases such as amyloidosis and in chronic hypertension. Biatrial enlargement is also seen (Videos 14-6 and 14-7).

the cause of heart failure in restrictive CMP is impaired diastolic filling and progressive diastolic dysfunction, various other forms of heart disease can result in a "restrictive physiology." These include hypertrophic CMP (discussed earlier), concentric hypertrophy from long-standing hypertension, hypertrophic heart disease of the elderly, and idiopathic restrictive CMP. Glycogen storage diseases and

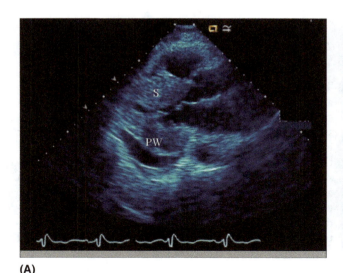

(A)

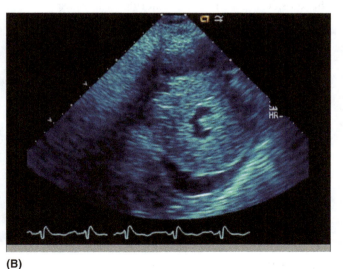

(B)

Figure 14-11 (**A**) Two-dimensional imaging in parasternal long axis of a patient with amyloidosis. Note the thickened septum (S) and posterior wall (PW). Although this is a systolic frame, there is severe hypertrophy present. (**B**) Two-dimensional imaging in the short-axis view of the same patient represented in (A). Note the severe concentric hypertrophy with a somewhat refractile myocardium, typical of amyloidosis.

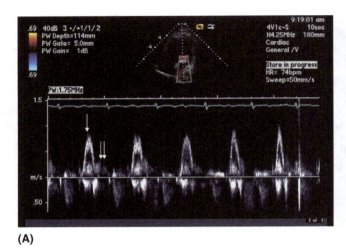 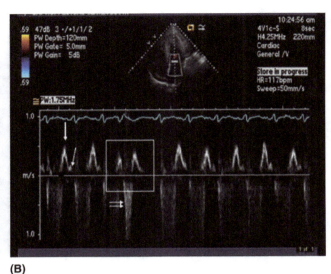

Figure 14-12 (A) Mitral valve inflow Doppler pattern showing a restrictive filling pattern. Note the predominant E wave (single arrowhead) and the lack of any significant A wave (double arrowheads). (B) Mitral valve inflow Doppler pattern showing a severely restrictive filling pattern. The diastolic filling occurs almost entirely during the E wave (thick arrowhead). The A wave is quite diminutive (thin arrowhead). There is an incidental finding of a ventricular premature beat during the recording (rectangle). Note the interruption of the diastolic filling by the premature beat and the occurrence of "diastolic mitral regurgitation" seen below the baseline (double arrowheads).

▶ Doppler Assessment (Figure 14-12)

Doppler assessment remains the hallmark in diagnosing the diastolic dysfunction accompanying restrictive CMP. Mitral valve inflow velocities, mitral annular tissue Doppler interrogation, and assessment of the pulmonary venous flow patterns should be performed routinely in such patients. Since restrictive CMP is a global process, there is simultaneous involvement of the right ventricle. This can be used to an advantage from the standpoint of echocardiographic diagnosis. Similar patterns, as seen on the left side, are seen on the right side with tricuspid valve inflow velocities and hepatic vein flows.

As mentioned earlier in this section, it may become necessary to distinguish restrictive physiology from constrictive physiology in some patients. Echocardiographic features can be used to distinguish between the two scenarios. The left atrial size is normal in constriction, but is enlarged as a rule in restriction. The septal motion is abnormal in constriction and normal in restriction. The septum becomes a physiologic part of the right ventricle in constriction (particularly in constrictive effusive physiology). Hence, the septal position varies with respiration in constriction, with increased right-sided inflow during inspiration pushing the septum into the left ventricle and compromising diastolic filling of the left ventricle. Evaluation of transmitral inflow reveals a significant respiratory variation in the E-wave velocity (usually ≥25%). The E-wave velocity of the transmitral flow is impaired during inspiration and increases greatly during expiration. This is contrasted by a lack of such variation in restriction. Though the E/A ratio is increased in both constriction and restriction (usually ≥2), the A wave is relatively well preserved in constrictive effusive physiology. Much of the diastolic filling in constrictive effusive states occurs during the atrial contraction. Hence, a patient who is hemodynamically compromised from such physiology may experience complete cardiovascular collapse if the rhythm changes to atrial fibrillation, particularly with a rapid ventricular response. Another Doppler feature distinguishing constriction from restriction is the respiratory variation in IVRT that occurs in constriction and is unchanged (albeit decreased) in restriction. On tissue Doppler investigation of the lateral mitral annulus, the E-wave velocity is normal in constriction and diminished in restriction.

ARRHYTHMOGENIC RIGHT VENTRICULAR DYSPLASIA

This is a somewhat rare entity and is characterized by abnormal morphology of the right ventricle. Though echocardiography has been used extensively for the diagnosis of this disorder, cardiac magnetic resonance imaging is also becoming an important tool. The myocardium of the RV free wall is replaced with fibrous and/or fatty tissue. Malignant ventricular arrhythmias and sudden death are the major concerns in patients with this disorder. The echocardiographic diagnosis is based primarily on two-dimensional and M-mode imaging. Echocardiographic features include hypokinesis of the RV free wall, occasional aneurysmal dilatation of the RV free wall, and increased echogenicity of the RV free wall from the deposition of collagen and/or adipose tissue. Though the disease has been linked with RV issues, progressive LV dysfunction has been described. In one pathologic study, 76% of the hearts with arrhythmogenic right ventricular dysplasia (ARVD) had LV involvement. The involvement in this study was more pronounced, with a longer history of the disease, and was associated with more significant cardiomegaly, inflammatory infiltrates, and heart failure. The LV abnormalities were also linked to clinical arrhythmias.

UNCLASSIFIED CARDIOMYOPATHIES

Three major syndromes will be discussed in this section. These include endocardial fibroelastosis, left ventricular noncompaction (LVNC), and the transient LV apical ballooning syndrome (also called broken heart syndrome, stress-induced CMP, or Takotsubo CMP in Japan). Though these syndromes have features of dilated CMP or restrictive CMP, they do not neatly fall into the respective categories.

▶ Endocardial Fibroelastosis

This disease is seen primarily in infants and fetuses. It is characterized by deposition of collagen and elastin in the ventricular walls. It is associated with hypertrophy and endocardial thickening. The disease has an association with viral infections, autoimmune diseases, and congenital left-sided obstructive lesions. In late stages, it presents as a dilated CMP with restrictive physiology. Treatment is usually unsuccessful in infants with the primary form of the disease, and transplantation offers the only recourse.

▶ Left Ventricular Noncompaction (Figure 14-13)

This is a rare disorder associated with heart failure, thromboembolism, and ventricular arrhythmias. It is caused by

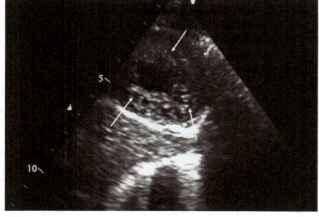
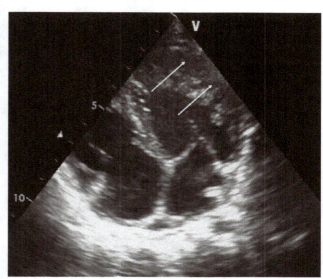
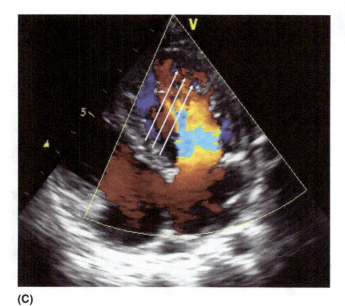

Figure 14-13 (**A**) A cross-sectional view of the left ventricle in a patient with LV noncompaction. Note the "sinusoids" (*arrowheads*) that make up the noncompacted layer. (**B**) An apical four-chamber view demonstrating LV noncompaction. The arrowheads point to the noncompacted layer. (**C**) An apical four-chamber view of a noncompacted left ventricle with color-flow into the noncompacted areas (*arrowheads*). The color-flow signifies blood flow into the noncompacted "sinusoids." LV indicates left ventricular.

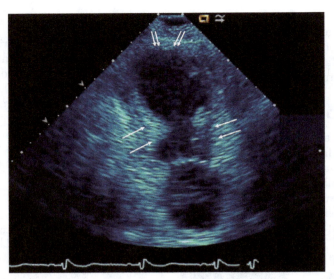

Figure 14-14 An apical two-chamber view of the left ventricle from a patient with transient apical ballooning syndrome. This systolic frame demonstrates normal inward motion and thickening of the inferior base and the anterior base (*single arrowheads*) and the lack of motion and ballooning of the apex (*double arrowheads*).

a developmental arrest of compaction of the LV myocardial trabecular network. This results in sinusoidal recesses that communicate with the endocardium and are filled with blood. There is, however, no communication to the epicardium. Echocardiographic diagnosis is based primarily on two-dimensional and colored Doppler imaging. On two-dimensional imaging, particularly in the apical views, there is a distinction between the compacted and the noncompacted portion of the myocardium, appearing as two layers. A ratio of noncompacted to compacted layer of ≥2:1 in end-systole is considered diagnostic of noncompaction. The myocardium in most of the noncompacted segments is hypokinetic, and is seen in the apical, midinferior and midlateral regions. On color-flow Doppler, blood flow can be seen into the sinusoidal recesses. Other associated echocardiographic features include LV dilatation, Doppler evidence of diastolic dysfunction, LV thrombus, and abnormal papillary muscle structure.

▶ **Transient LV Apical Ballooning Syndrome**
(Figure 14-14; Videos 14-8 and 14-9)

This syndrome was first described in Japan (called Takotsubo CMP there), but it has since been seen in other populations, including the United States. It presents with signs and symptoms of a myocardial infarction, and is associated with ST-segment elevation and apical wall motion abnormalities but without evidence of obstructive coronary artery disease on coronary angiography. The onset is triggered by either significant emotional or physical stress (sudden loss of a family member, sudden life-threatening accident, medical illness, physical abuse). A recent study looked prospectively at patients admitted to the intensive care unit (ICU) with serial echocardiography to see how many developed the apical ballooning. Of 92 patients, 26 had the pathology on echocardiography with a mean ejection fraction of 33 ± 8%. Compared with the patients without the pathology, those with apical ballooning more frequently had sepsis as the admission diagnosis for the ICU (62% vs. 14%), a higher incidence of developing hypotension on admission and use of inotropes, and higher frequency of cardiomegaly and pulmonary congestion. Sepsis was the only associated feature with the cardiac pathology. The findings resolved in 20 of the 26 patients (77%) within 2–25 days (mean 7.4 ± 5.6 days). The two-month survival was lower in the group with apical ballooning compared with those without the pathology (52% vs. 71%, respectively). The echocardiographic features include apical akinesis or dyskinesis (Video 14-8)

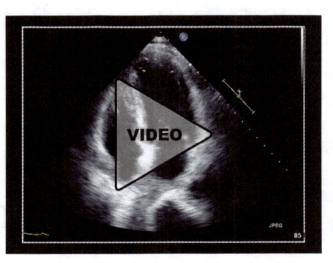

Video 14-8 Apical four-chamber view of the patient with apical ballooning (Takotsubo) syndrome. Note classical apical (dyskinesis) ballooning with preservation or even hyperkinesis of other ventricular segments. View at www.ccu2e.com

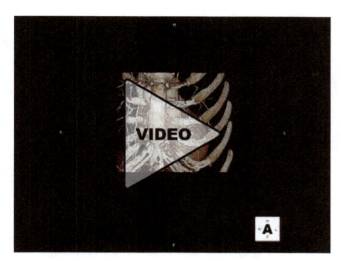

Video 14-9 Computerized tomography angiogram (CTA) of the patient with apical ballooning (Takotsubo) syndrome. Note classical apical ballooning with preservation of other ventricular segments. Also of great importance the lack of the coronary artery disease with widely patent coronary arteries (note), since left anterior descending artery occlusion will result in similar echocardiographic and CTA picture and should be ruled out. View at www.ccu2e.com

on two-dimensional imaging; presence of LV thrombus has been seen resulting in a cerebrovascular accident; the basal wall may exhibit hyperkinesis and generate an LVOT gradient similar to that seen in hypertrophic CMP, with resultant MR. Systolic anterior leaflet of the mitral valve can be also present. The ejection fraction is reduced, though not always severely (mostly because of hyperkinesis of other ventricular segments). Mortality is uncommon and is the result of arrhythmias or mechanical complications.

SUGGESTED READING

Abergel E, Chatellier G, Hagege AA, et al. Serial left ventricular adaptations in world-class professional cyclists: implications for disease screening and follow-up. *J Am Coll Cardiol*. 2004;44:144–149.

Aurigemma GP, Gottdeiner JS. Predictive value of systolic and diastolic function for incident congestive heart failure in the elderly: the Cardiovascular Health Study. *J Am Coll Cardiol*. 2001;37:1042–1048.

Binder J, Ommen SR, Gersh BJ, et al. Echocardiography-guided genetic testing in hypertrophic CMP: septal morphological features predict the presence of myofilament mutations. *Mayo Clin Proc*. 2006;81:459–467.

Braunwald E, Seidman CE, Sigwart U. Contemporary evaluation and management of hypertrophic CMP. *Circulation*. 2002;106:1312–1316.

Chen C, Rodriguez L, Lethor JP, et al. Continuous wave Doppler echocardiography for noninvasive assessment of left ventricular dP/dt and relaxation time constant from mitral regurgitant spectra in patients. *J Am Coll Cardiol*. 1994;23:970–976.

Corrado D, Fontaine G, Marcus FI, et al. Arrhythmogenic right ventricular dysplasia/CMP: need for an international registry. *Circulation*. 2000;101:e101–e106.

Dec GW. Recognition of the apical ballooning syndrome in the United States. *Circulation*. 2005;111:388–390.

Devereux RB, Roman MJ, Paranicas M, et al. A population-based assessment of left ventricular systolic dysfunction in middle-aged and older adults: the Strong Heart Study. *Am Heart J*. 2001;141:439–446.

Dujardin KS, Tei C, Yeo TC, et al. Prognostic value of Doppler index combining systolic and diastolic performance in idiopathic dilated CMP. *Am J of Cardiol*. 1998;82:1071–1076.

Fans R, Coats AJ, Henein MY. Echocardiography derived variables predict outcome in patients with non-ischemic dilated CMP with or without a restrictive filling pattern. *Am Heart J*. 2002;144:343–350.

Feigenbaum H, Armstrong WF, Ryan T. *Feigenbaum's Echocardiography*. 6th ed. Philadelphia, PA: Lippincott Williams & Wilkins; 2004.

Felker GM, Thompson RE, Hare JM, et al. Underlying causes and long-term survival in patients with initially unexplained CMP. *N Engl J Med*. 2000;342:1077–1084.

Frischknecht BS, Jost CH, Oechslin EN, et al. Validation of non-compaction criteria in dilated CMP, and valvular and hypertensive heart disease. *J Am Soc Echocardiogr*. 2005;18:865–872.

Garcia MJ, Thomas JD, Klein AL. New Doppler echocardiographic applications for the study of diastolic function. *J Am Coll Cardiol*. 1998;32:865–875.

Gemayel C, Pelliccia A, Thompson PD. Arrhythmogenic right ventricular dysplasia. *J Am Coll Cardiol*. 2001;38:1773–1781.

Groote P, Millaire A, Foucher-Hossein C, et al. Right ventricular ejection fraction is an independent predictor of survival in patients with moderate heart failure. *J Am Coll Cardiol*. 1998;32:948–954.

Kjaergaard J, Hastrup Svendsen J, Sogaard P, et al. Advanced quantitative echocardiography in arrhythmogenic right ventricular CMP. *J Am Soc Echocardiogr*. 2007;20:27–35.

Koelling TM, Aaronson KD, Cody RJ, et al. Prognostic significance of MR and tricuspid regurgitation in patients with left ventricular systolic dysfunction. *Am Heart J*. 2002;144:524–529.

Kolias TJ, Aaronson KD, Armstrong WF. Doppler-derived dP/dt and –dP/dt predict survival in congestive heart failure. *J Am Coll Cardiol*. 2000;36:1594–1599.

Kushwaha SS, Fallon JT, Fuster V. Restrictive CMP. *N Eng J Med*. 1997;336:267–276.

Lang RM, Bierig M, Devereux RB, et al. Recommendations for chamber quantification: a report from the American Society of Echocardiography's Guidelines and Standards Committee and the Chamber Quantification Writing Group, developed in conjunction with the European Association of Echocardiography, a branch of the European Society of Cardiology. *J Am Soc Echocardiogr*. 2005;18:1440–1463.

Maddukuri PV, Vieira ML, DeCastro S, et al. What is the best approach for the assessment of left atrial size? Comparison of various unidimensional and 2-dimensional parameters with three-dimensional echocardiographically determined left atrial volume. *J Am Soc Echocardiogr*. 2006;19:1026–1032.

Maron BJ, Gardin JM, Flack JM, et al. Prevalence of hypertrophic CMP in a general population of young adults. Echocardiographic analysis of 4111 subjects in the CARDIA Study. Coronary Artery Risk Development in (Young) Adults. *Circulation*. 1995;92:785–789.

Maron BJ, Towbin JA, Thiene G, et al. Contemporary definitions and classification of the cardiomyopathies: an American Heart Association Scientific Statement from the Council on Clinical Cardiology, Heart Failure and Transplantation Committee; Quality of Care and Outcomes Research and Functional Genomics and Translational Biology Interdisciplinary Working Groups; and Council on Epidemiology and Prevention. *Circulation*. 2006;113:1807–1816.

Maron MS, Olivotto I, Betocchi S, et al. Effect of left ventricular outflow tract obstruction on clinical outcome in hypertrophic CMP. *N Engl J Med*. 2003;348:295–303.

Niimura H, Patton KK, McKenna WJ, et al. Sarcomere protein gene mutations in hypertrophic CMP of the elderly. *Circulation*. 2002;105:446–451.

Oechslin EN, Jost CHA, Rojas JR, et al. Long-term follow-up of 34 adults with isolated left ventricular noncompaction: a distinct CMP with poor prognosis. *J Am Coll Cardiol*. 2000;36:493–500.

Palka P, Lange A, Donnelly JE, Nihoyannopoulos P. Differentiation between restrictive CMP and constrictive pericarditis by early diastolic Doppler myocardial velocity gradient at the posterior wall. *Circulation*. 2000;102:655–662.

Pelliccia A, Maron BJ, Spataro A, et al. The upper limit of physiologic cardiac hypertrophy in highly trained elite athletes. *N Engl J Med*. 1991;324:295–301.

Richardson P, McKenna W, Bristow M, et al. Report of the 1995 World Health Organization/International Society and Federation of Cardiology Task Force on the Definition and Classification of Cardiomyopathies. *Circulation*. 1996;93:841–842.

Rihal CS, Nishimura RA, Hatle LK, Bailey KR, Tajik AJ. Systolic and diastolic dysfunction in patients with clinical diagnosis of dilated CMP. Relation to symptoms and prognosis. *Circulation*. 1994;90:2772–2779.

Sakamoto T. Apical Hypertrophic CMP (apical hypertrophy): an overview. *J Cardiol*. 2001;37(suppl 1):161.

Shapiro LM, McKenna WJ. Distribution of left ventricular hypertrophy in hypertrophic CMP: a two dimensional echocardiographic study. *J Am Coll Cardiol*. 1983;2:437–444.

Sharkey SW, Lesser JR, Zenovich AG, et al. Acute and reversible CMP provoked by stress in women from the United States. *Circulation*. 2005;111:472–479.

Siqueira-Filho AG, Cunha CL, Tajik AJ, et al. M-mode and 2-dimensional echocardiographic features in cardiac amyloidosis. *Circulation*. 1981;63:188–196.

Sun JP, James KB, Yang XS, et al. Comparison of mortality rates and progression of left ventricular dysfunction in patients with idiopathic dilated CMP and dilated versus non-dilated right ventricular cavities. *Am J Cardiol*. 1997;80:1583–1587.

Tabata T, Thomas JD, Klein AL. Pulmonary venous flow by Doppler echocardiography: revisited 12 years later. *J Am Coll Cardiol*. 2003;41:1243–1250.

Temporelli PL, Corra U, Imparato A, et al. Reversible restrictive left ventricular diastolic filling with optimized oral therapy predicts a more favorable prognosis in patients with chronic heart failure. *J Am Coll Cardiol*. 1998;31:1591–1597.

Ward RP, Weinert L, Spencer KT, et al. Quantitative diagnosis of apical CMP using contrast echocardiography. *J Am Soc Echocardiogr*. 2002;15:316–322.

Zipes DP, ed. *Braunwald's Heart Disease: A Textbook of Cardiovascular Medicine*. 7th ed. Philadelphia, PA: Elsevier Health Sciences; 2004.

ECHOCARDIOGRAPHIC EVALUATION OF VALVE FUNCTION AND ENDOCARDITIS

ROBERT ARNTFIELD & PAUL H. MAYO

Scan QR code or visit www.ccu2e.com for video in this chapter

INTRODUCTION

Echocardiography is an effective means of assessing cardiac valve function. It is useful for a rapid qualitative assessment or a more comprehensive assessment for all forms of valve function using transthoracic echocardiography (TTE) and transesophageal echocardiography (TEE). Doppler assessment allows an accurate quantitative measurement of the severity of stenotic and regurgitant lesions. The extent to which the critical care echocardiographer applies the sophisticated tools of the cardiologist to assess valvular heart disease is highly variable. By training, background, and interest, cardiologists often take the lead in this aspect of echocardiography. However, the intensivist who performs echocardiography should have some fundamental competence in assessing valve function, as many patients in the intensive care unit (ICU) may have valve dysfunction that adversely impacts their cardiopulmonary status.

In general, the intensivist will be interested primarily in the identification of catastrophic valve failure or valve dysfunction that is sufficiently severe to impact the hemodynamic functioning of the patient. Conversely, the identification of lesser degrees of valve disease or normal valve function are also of interest, as the intensivist may then determine that valve failure is not a contributing factor to the patient's critical illness. This chapter will review the echocardiographic assessment of valve function from the perspective of the bedside intensivist.

LEVEL OF TRAINING

Intensivists who perform critical care echocardiography (CCE) will typically demonstrate competence in basic CCE (several standard two-dimensional [2-D] views without comprehensive training in Doppler), but may also have competence in advanced CCE (see also Chapter 4). The latter is equivalent to level 2 training by standard cardiology criteria.[1] Intensivists who have basic training in echocardiography have a limited ability to assess valve function. Without training in quantitative spectral Doppler measurements, the basic-level examiner can identify obvious mechanical failure of the mitral valve (MV; e.g., a flail leaflet, ruptured chordae, or ruptured papillary muscle) or obvious aortic valve (AV) disruption. Severe stenosis of these valves may also be apparent. By definition, intensivists with training in basic echocardiography do not have comprehensive Doppler training and lack the ability to perform quantitative measurements of valve function.

The qualitative assessment of valve function is, however, in the domain of the basic critical care echocardiographer and may be carried out using color Doppler. This is not to suggest that the use of color Doppler is straightforward and without nuance. The pitfalls of color Doppler include gain settings, wall jet effects,[2] angle effects, and shadowing by surrounding structures, such as prosthetic valve apparatus or a calcified annulus, and are not intuitively obvious. Of particular concern with these pitfalls is that the echocardiographer may miss a severe valvular lesion due to misinterpretation of the color Doppler image. Thus, a key cognitive skill for the basic critical care echocardiographer is to recognize when to call for a consultation from a more experienced echocardiographer. If there is the possibility of significant valve dysfunction, a comprehensive study should be performed by an echocardiographer with advanced training.

Intensivists with proficiency in advanced CCE have, by definition, the capability to assess valve function that is similar to that of a fully trained cardiology echocardiographer. This proficiency may be particularly useful when immediate cardiology echocardiography services are not available. The advanced intensivist echocardiographer who is directly involved at the patient's bedside is also able to immediately perform the study. Patients with severe valve failure may have life-threatening hemodynamic failure requiring prompt intervention, such as vasoactive medication, mechanical assist devices, or valve replacement. This cannot wait for the convenience of a delayed echocardiogram.

A common indication for bedside echocardiography in the ICU is to identify a cause for cardiopulmonary failure. The assessment of valve function is a key part of the bedside examination for several reasons. First, severe valve failure may be the primary cause of the shock state or respiratory failure. Early recognition of severe valve failure may allow for lifesaving interventions. Second, significant valve dysfunction may combine with another disease process to worsen cardiopulmonary failure. It is essential that the coexisting valve lesion be identified, as this may have a major influence on management. Finally, the absence of significant valvular dysfunction is useful information in a patient with hemodynamic failure.

The focus here is on the identification and quantification of major valve failure, as this is the most immediate concern of the bedside critical care clinician. Comprehensive assessment of valve function requires training in Doppler analysis, so some of the following discussion assumes interest or prior knowledge in advanced CCE.

TRICUSPID VALVE (TV)

The evaluation of the TV focuses on the assessment of tricuspid regurgitation (TR), as tricuspid stenosis is an uncommon lesion. The echocardiographic examination of the TV starts with 2-D analysis of the valve and support structures. A flail leaflet, lack of coaptation, vegetation or mass, right ventricular or right atrial (RA) dilation, tricuspid annular calcification, or the presence of hardware (pacer wire, valve repair/replacement), all suggest the possibility of significant TR. The 2-D study includes examination of the valve from multiple sites: parasternal long- and short-axis, apical four-chamber, and subcostal. The severity of TR by color Doppler is classed as mild, moderate, and severe. It is important to properly set the color gain and to interrogate the jet at multiple angles. The severity of TR may be measured semiquantitatively by measuring the color jet area.[3] Minimal TR may often be detected in normal individuals.[4] A simple "eyeball" method of judging severity is to consider that TR is severe when the jet hits the back wall of the RA or occupies the entire RA (Figure 15-1 and Video 15-1). Severe TR is often associated with volume overload of the right ventricle; although this finding is not specific to TR. Spectral Doppler of the TR jet may provide additional information of severity. If the intensity of the continuous-wave (CW) Doppler TR signal is greater than that of the inflow signal, or if the CW TR jet has a truncated downslope, the TR is likely to be severe. Measurement of the CW jet velocity permits estimation of pulmonary arterial systolic pressure (PASP). However, PASP does not necessarily correlate with the severity of TR. In theory, the severity of TR is amenable to quantitative measurements using the continuity principle or proximal isovelocity surface area (PISA) method. In practice, this is seldom performed or required in the ICU setting.

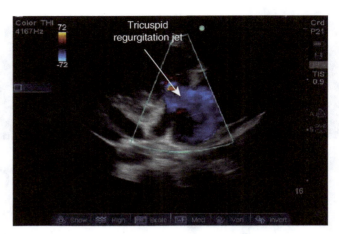

Figure 15-1 This right ventricular inflow view shows severe tricuspid regurgitation.

PULMONIC VALVE (PV)

The evaluation of the PV generally focuses on assessment for pulmonic valve regurgitation (PR), as PV stenosis is uncommon. Trace PR is often detected in normal individuals. More severe PR may be seen with endocarditis or pulmonary hypertension. The echocardiographic examination of the PV starts with 2-D imaging of the valve. Rarely, a vegetation may involve the valve, or a leaflet prolapse may be identified. The PV is difficult to image with 2-D technique and is usually limited to the parasternal short-axis view and a short-axis view from the subcostal region. Color Doppler is the primary means of detecting PR (Figure 15-2 and Video 15-2). The subcostal approach is frequently a superior angle for Doppler analysis because the interrogation

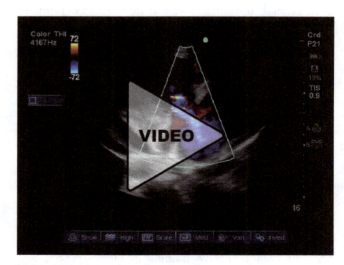

Video 15-1 This right ventricular inflow view shows severe tricuspid regurgitation. View at www.ccu2e.com

CHAPTER 15 ECHOCARDIOGRAPHIC EVALUATION OF VALVE FUNCTION AND ENDOCARDITIS 165

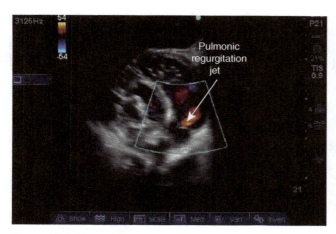

Figure 15-2 This subcostal short-axis view shows mild pulmonic regurgitation.

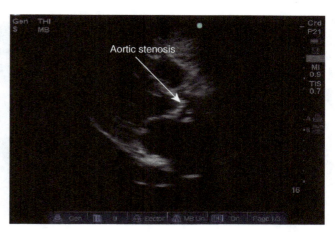

Figure 15-3 This parasternal long-axis view shows a calcified aortic valve that has reduced mobility on the video clip consistent with severe aortic stenosis (AS). While the 2-D image suggests severe AS, quantification of the severity of AS requires Doppler-based measurements.

line may be placed parallel with the blood flow through the PV and proximal pulmonary artery. Regurgitation is detected by color Doppler and is classed as trace, mild, moderate, or severe.[3] Because PR usually has minimal hemodynamic consequence, clinical echocardiographers often use an "eyeball" approach to grading the severity of PR. Spectral Doppler analysis of valve function is not generally used to assess the severity of PR. However, spectral Doppler of the PV area is important for other reasons, such as the measurement of cardiac shunts, pulmonary artery diastolic pressure, and indirect evidence for pulmonary arterial hypertension.

AV: AORTIC STENOSIS (AS)

Aortic stenosis is a common valvular lesion in the critical care unit. When it is severe, it has major hemodynamic consequences. When it coexists with other causes of shock, such as distributive shock, it complicates hemodynamic management. Many patients come to the ICU with the diagnosis already established. However, in others, it is unknown at the time of presentation. The intensivist with basic-level echocardiography training may suspect the diagnosis by 2-D scanning. The stenotic valve is often hyperechoic or heavily calcified with obviously reduced movement (Figure 15-3 and Video 15-3).

Advanced level training is required for a complete assessment of the AV. This begins with 2-D study to rule out sub- or supravalular stenosis or a stenotic bicuspid valve, which lack the characteristic 2-D features of typical AS. However, these entities have the same physiological consequence. Included in the 2-D examination is planimetry of the valve area in short axis both by TTE or TEE.[5]

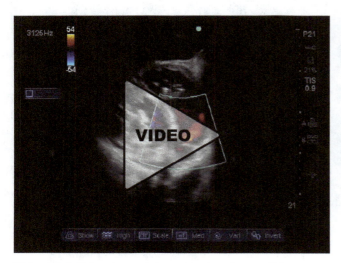

Video 15-2 This subcostal short-axis view shows mild pulmonic regurgitation. View at www.ccu2e.com

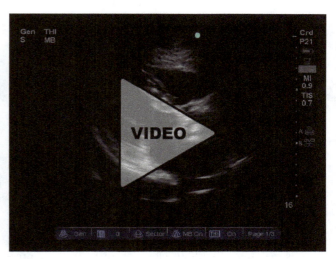

Video 15-3 This parasternal long-axis view shows a calcified thickened aortic valve that has reduced mobility on the video clip consistent with severe aortic stenosis (AS). While the 2-D image suggests severe AS, quantification of the severity of AS requires Doppler-based measurements. View at www.ccu2e.com

Three methods for identifying severe AS exist. Spectral Doppler analysis is the most reliable method of identifying severe AS. As the AV area narrows, the velocity of blood flow through it rises. The peak velocity across the valve is measured with CW Doppler and reliably reflects the pressure gradient across the valve according to the modified Bernoulli equation.[6] A second method for quantification of AS is the continuity equation.[7] This is based on the principle that the stroke volume measured at one point in the heart should equal the stroke volume at another point in the heart (barring shunt or valvular regurgitation). A final method compares the velocity (or velocity time integral [VTI]) of the left ventricular outflow tract (LVOT) to that of the AV.[8]

Commonly accepted values indicating severe AS include[9]:

1. Peak AV velocity >4.5 m/s.
2. Mean pressure gradient across the AV >50 mm Hg.
3. AV area <0.75 cm^2
4. LVOT VTI/aortic VTI <0.25.

Accurate assessment of AS requires skill in advanced echocardiography. Common pitfalls include underestimation of the peak velocity and mean pressure gradient due to poor CW Doppler interrogation angle. The AS jet may also be eccentric; therefore, the examiner must use multiple points of measurement, including the suprasternal and right parasternal sites. This may require the use of a small, non-imaging CW transducer. Further, assessing AS is frequently more difficult using TEE, compared to TTE which may provide more parallel alignment with blood flow through the valve. Accurate measurement of the LVOT diameter is required, as any error is squared in the calculation of the LVOT area. The LVOT VTI may be overestimated if the pulsed wave (PW) sample volume is placed too close to the AV with resulting measurement of flow acceleration near the valve orifice. Patients with poor LV function and AS may have pseudosevere AS that improves when the measurements are made during dobutamine infusion.[10]

AV: AORTIC REGURGITATION (AR)

Trace or mild clinically inconsequential AR by color Doppler analysis is a common finding of CCE. On the other hand, acute severe AR may be immediately life threatening because the LV has no time to adapt to the sudden volume overload, resulting in fulminant pulmonary edema compounded by a low-flow state. The aortic balloon pump is specifically contraindicated with severe AR, and urgent valve replacement may be life saving. Chronic severe AR is often well tolerated because the LV has had time to dilate; and, with the maintenance of good LV function, forward flow is maintained without elevation of hydrostatic pressure in the lung. However, chronic severe AR may eventually lead to hemodynamic failure. When it coexists with other causes of shock, it may complicate hemodynamic management. The degree of regurgitation is afterload

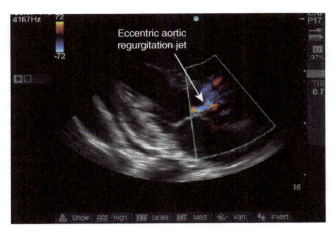

Figure 15-4 This parasternal long-axis view shows an eccentric aortic regurgitation jet, a pericardial effusion, and a dilated aortic root. A dissection flap is visible in the descending aorta. The dissection also involved the proximal aorta.

sensitive, so that the identification of significant AR has an important influence on acute hemodynamic management.

The evaluation for AR begins with the 2-D examination. Dilation of the aortic root, proximal aortic dissection (Figure 15-4 and Video 15-4), abnormal valve architecture, noncoaptation or prolapse of valve leaflets (Figure 15-5 and Video 15-5), or vegetation (Figure 15-6 and Video 15-6), all suggest the possibility of significant AR. M-mode findings of severe AR include anterior MV diastolic fluttering, early closure of the MV, and the presence of a B-wave on M-mode of the MV. AR may occur due to dilation of the aortic ring with valvular incompetence from nonapposition of the leaflets. Valve anatomy may be normal in this situation. Alternatively, AR may occur due to structural failure of the valve itself from such factors as endocarditis, rheumatic heart disease, Marfan's syndrome, congenitally abnormal

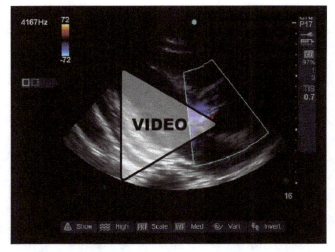

Video 15-4 This parasternal long-axis view shows an eccentric aortic regurgitation jet, a pericardial effusion, and a dilated aortic root. A dissection flap is visible in the descending aorta. The dissection also involved the proximal aorta. View at www.ccu2e.com

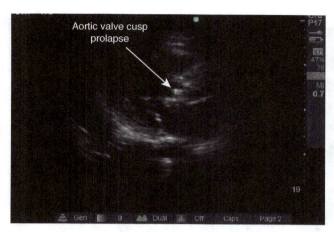

Figure 15-5 This parasternal long-axis view shows an aortic valve leaflet (noncoronary cusp) prolapsing into the left ventricular outflow tract. The valve failure occurred due to endocarditis.

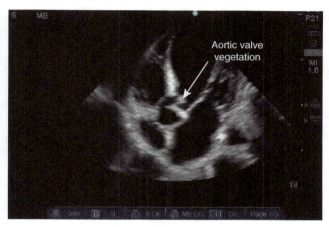

Figure 15-6 This apical five chamber view shows a vegetation on the aortic valve.

valves, degenerative calcific changes, or aortic dissection. None of these anatomic abnormalities allow determination of the severity of AR.

Doppler studies allow several methods to determine the severity of AR. Color Doppler performed preferentially in the parasternal long- and short-axis view with TTE (or equivalent views with TEE) is one method of determining the severity of AR (Figure 15-7 and Video 15-7).

The length of the regurgitant jet does not correlate well with severity. The jet area in a short-axis view, relative to the LVOT area, or the width of the jet at its origin, relative to the LVOT width in long axis, is considered a good index of severity.[3] The width of the vena contracta,[11] the smallest width of the jet below flow convergence, is another index of severity that relies on color Doppler. The pressure half time (PHT) of the AV regurgitant jet measured with CW Doppler falls in proportion to the severity of the AR, although the PHT is load dependent. Severe AR results in a high mitral E-wave velocity as well as diastolic retrograde flow in the descending aorta.[12]

The continuity principle and PISA method[13] may be used to quantify the severity of AR. These methods are laborious, so the bedside echocardiographer frequently relies on color Doppler and PHT.

Commonly accepted values indicating severe AR are as follows[3]:

1. Regurgitant jet width/LVOT diameter ratio >65%.
2. Regurgitant jet area/LVOT area ratio >60%.
3. Vena contracta width >6 mm.
4. PHT <200 m/s.
5. Holodiastolic flow reversal in the descending aorta.
6. Effective regurgitant orifice >0.30 cm^2.
7. Regurgitant volume >60 mL.
8. Regurgitant fraction >50%.

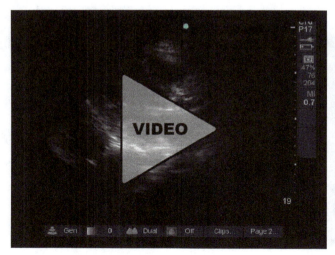

Video 15-5 This parasternal long-axis view shows an aortic valve leaflet (noncoronary cusp) prolapsing into the left ventricular outflow track. The valve failure occurred due to endocarditis. View at www.ccu2e.com

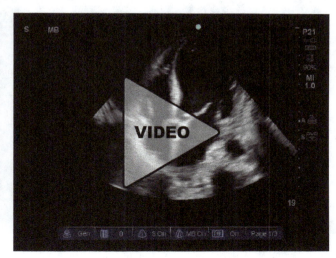

Video 15-6 This apical five chamber view shows a vegetation on the aortic valve. View at www.ccu2e.com

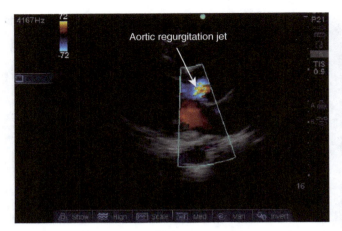

Figure 15-7 This parasternal long-axis view shows aortic regurgitation (AR) with the jet diameter occupying greater than 65% of the left ventricular outflow tract diameter. This is consistent with severe AR.

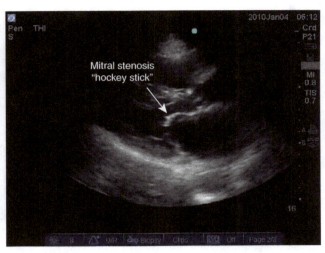

Figure 15-8 This parasternal long-axis view image shows a "hockey stick" configuration of the anterior leaflet of the mitral valve. This is consistent with mitral stenosis (MS). Determination of the severity of the MS requires Doppler-based measurements.

MV: MITRAL STENOSIS (MS)

Compared with AS, MS is uncommon in the ICU. When it is severe, it has major hemodynamic consequences. When it coexists with other causes of shock, it complicates hemodynamic management. For example, tachycardia has an adverse effect in patients with MS, so the prompt identification of severe MS allows the intensivist to intervene to reduce heart rate. Most patients with MS arrive in the ICU with the diagnosis already established. However, in others, it will be unknown at the time of presentation. Most cases are caused by rheumatic heart disease, although severe mitral annular calcification may also cause the condition. In addition to the typical immobility of the valve tips ("hockey stick configuration"; Figure 15-8

and Video 15-8), 2-D imaging may demonstrate calcified leaflets and subvalvular structures, immobility of the posterior MV leaflet, and "fish mouth" valve orifice in short axis. Planimetry of the MV area is possible from the parasternal short-axis view. Heavy calcification and poor gain settings may result in inaccurate planimetry results.

Diagnosis of severe MS requires Doppler measurements. Severity of MS may be estimated from the mean diastolic pressure gradient across the valve using CW Doppler from an apical view (Figure 15-9). This Doppler envelope is also used to measure the PHT of the diastolic inflow to apply the following formula:

MV area (MVA) cm^2 = 220/PHT (Figure 15-10).

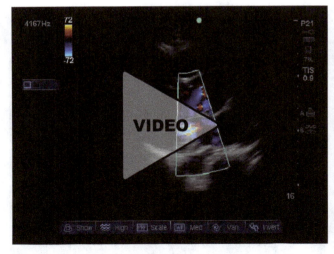

Video 15-7 This parasternal long-axis view shows aortic regurgitation (AR) with the jet diameter occupying greater than 60% of the left ventricular outflow track diameter. This is consistent with severe AR. There is mitral regurgitation (MR) with a left atrial wall jet that makes it difficult to estimate the severity of the MR. View at www.ccu2e.com

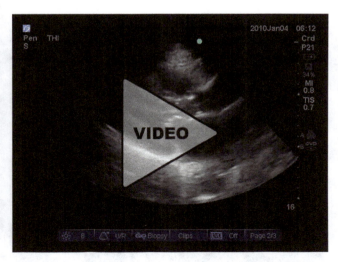

Video 15-8 This parasternal long-axis view shows a "hockey stick" configuration of the anterior leaflet of the mitral valve. This is consistent with mitral stenosis. Determination of the severity of the MS requires Doppler-based measurements. View at www.ccu2e.com

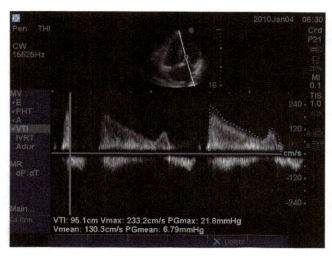

Figure 15-9 This image shows the continuous-wave Doppler signal of the mitral valve inflow from Figure 15-8. The mean pressure gradient is 6.8 mmHg, indicating that the mitral stenosis is not severe.

PHT is load dependent. It may be prolonged by factors independent of the MV area, such as abnormal LV relaxation, decreased LV compliance, elevated LV diastolic pressures, coexisting mitral regurgitation (MR), or low cardiac output. The MVA may also be measured using the continuity principle and PISA. Atrial fibrillation is common with MS. This complicates quantitative measurements of MS using Doppler techniques because 5–10 cardiac cycles must be measured, making the process very laborious.

Commonly accepted values indicating severe MS are as follows[14]:

1. Resting mean pressure gradient >10 mm Hg.
2. MVA <1.0 cm^2.
3. PHT >220 m/s.

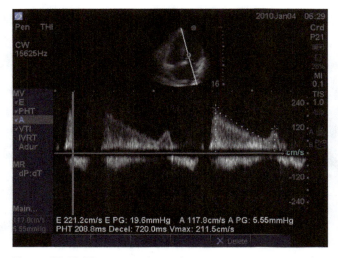

Figure 15-10 This image shows the continuous-wave Doppler signal of the mitral valve inflow from Figure 15-8. The pressure half time is 208 ms indicating that the mitral stenosis is not severe.

MV: MITRAL REGURGITATION

Mitral regurgitation is common in the ICU. Functional MR refers to MR that is caused by LV remodeling without structural abnormalities of the valve itself. Conceptually, the annulus of the valve is enlarged so that valve closure is incomplete. On 2-D echocardiography, the valve leaflets appear normal. The MR is only detectable by Doppler analysis. Structural abnormalities of the valve apparatus may also cause MR. These include MV prolapse, rheumatic heart disease, mitral annular calcification, endocarditis, flail leaflet, ischemic papillary muscle dysfunction, and ruptured chordae. Acute failure of the valve apparatus may cause life-threatening cardiopulmonary failure, while chronic severe MR may complicate hemodynamic management of the critically ill. The advanced critical care echocardiographer should be able to perform a comprehensive evaluation of MV function to identify patients with severe MR.

The 2-D examination serves to identify structural abnormalities associated with MR. The basic-level critical care echocardiographer may be able to identify flail chordae (Figure 15-11 and Video 15-9), noncoapting valves, or valve destruction by endocarditis (Figure 15-12 and Video 15-10), but Doppler analysis is required for a definitive assessment of severity. Color Doppler is a practical means of assessing severity of MR. The area of the color-flow jet of MR relative to the left atrial (LA) size is a simple means of assessing severity of MR (Figure 15-13 and Video 15-11).

However, as discussed previously, the assessment of MR by color Doppler has limitations that may not be obvious to the basic-level echocardiographer. Spectral Doppler may demonstrate characteristics suggesting severe MR. The CW Doppler MR jet has increased intensity with severe MR. Severe MR may cause reversal of systolic flow in the pulmonary vein. The width of the vena contracta is also an index of severity, as a width >7 mm is associated with severe MR (Figure 15-14). When vena contracta

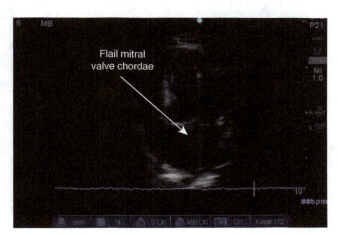

Figure 15-11 This apical four chamber view shows thickened mitral leaflets and ruptured chordae.

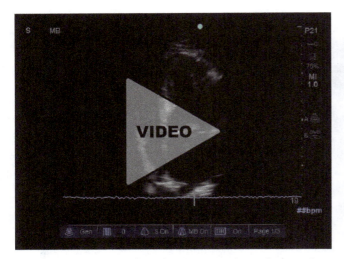

Video 15-9 This apical four chamber view shows thickened mitral leaflets and a ruptured chordae. View at www.ccu2e.com

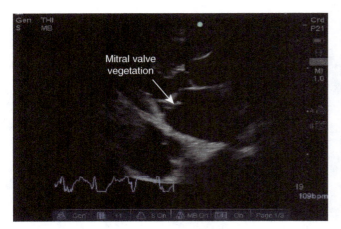

Figure 15-12 This parasternal long-axis view shows a vegetation on the mitral valve.

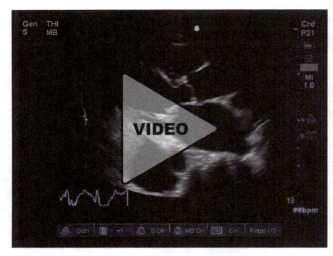

Video 15-10 This parasternal long-axis view shows a vegetation on the mitral valve. View at www.ccu2e.com

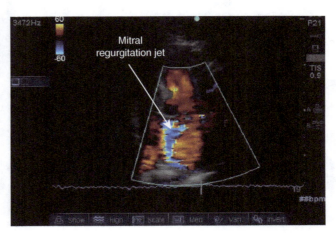

Figure 15-13 This image is similar to that in Figure 15-11, but with the addition of color Doppler. There is severe mitral regurgitation.

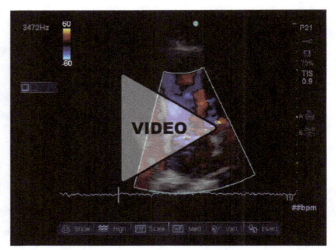

Video 15-11 This image is similar to that in Video 15-10, but with the addition of color Doppler. There is severe mitral regurgitation. View at www.ccu2e.com

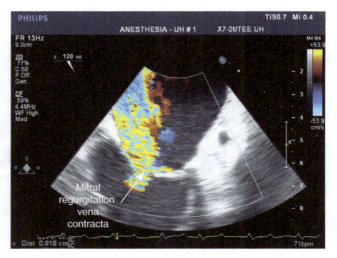

Figure 15-14 This image of the mitral valve using transesophageal echocardiography, shows an eccentric mitral regurgitation (MR) jet with a vena contracta of 8 mm. This is consistent with severe MR.

measurement and Doppler color-flow signal yield ambiguous results, the continuity principle or PISA allow quantitative measurement of MR. The PISA method is effective for a central MR jet, while the continuity method is required for an eccentric jet.

Commonly accepted values indicating severe MR are as follows[6]:

1. 2-D evidence of severe MV apparatus failure.
2. Effective regurgitant orifice >0.40 cm^2.
3. Regurgitant volume >60 mL.
4. Regurgitant fraction >50%.
5. Vena contracta >7 mm.
6. Pulmonary vein systolic flow reversal.
7. MR color Doppler jet >10 cm^2 or occupying >40% of the LA area.

MR is load dependent. For example, a patient with hypertension in association with cardiogenic pulmonary edema may have severe MR on initial echocardiographic examination. Following afterload reduction, the MR may be much improved. MR in association with cardiac chamber enlargement may show improvement following diuresis, as the mitral annulus becomes smaller in size, the MV leaflets can coapt more effectively.

THE ROLE OF TEE IN THE EVALUATION OF VALVE FUNCTION

TTE is very effective in evaluating valve function in the ICU. However, if image quality is poor, TEE may be necessary to fully evaluate valve function. TEE is particularly effective for imaging the MV and performing Doppler evaluation of the MV. The AV is also well situated for 2-D imaging and color Doppler evaluation with TEE, but is not well oriented for use of spectral Doppler. The PV and TV are often not well seen for 2-D imaging, and reliable Doppler analysis of these valves is difficult with TEE. TEE has special utility in the evaluation of prosthetic valve function, as discussed below.

EVALUATION OF PROSTHETIC VALVE FUNCTION

Evaluation of prosthetic valve function is a demanding part of echocardiography. Without special commitment that includes performance of a high volume of prosthetic valve echocardiographic cases, it is unlikely that the intensivist will be able maintain a high degree of competence in the field. For a definitive evaluation of prosthetic valve function, the intensivist will serve patients well by requesting cardiology consultation. If there is a delay in performing the definitive study, the intensivist should perform a screening echocardiogram, particularly if the patient is hemodynamically unstable. Generally, the evaluation of a mechanical prosthetic AV and MV requires TEE for adequate visualization. The AV may be difficult to completely visualize with TTE, if a mechanical valve is in the aortic position. A mechanical valve in the aortic position frequently blocks the view of the LA and MV when using the parasternal approach, while an MV prosthesis will block adequate visualization of the LA from both the parasternal and apical approaches. In this situation, the use of TEE will allow better visualization of posterior structures. The screening 2-D examination includes a search for valve instability, thrombus, vegetation, and paravalvular abscess or regurgitation. If visualized by a screening study, they may require urgent intervention.

EVALUATION FOR INFECTIVE ENDOCARDITIS

The intensivist with basic CCE skill may identify a vegetation on 2-D imaging. However, if there is clinical suspicion of endocarditis, to definitively rule out endocarditis requires an advanced critical care echocardiographer or cardiologist to be involved. Typical echocardiographic findings of infective endocarditis are as follows[15]:

1. The presence of an oscillating intracardiac mass on a valve or valve support structure, on a foreign device in the heart, or in the path of a regurgitant jet.
2. New valvular regurgitation.
3. New dehiscence of a mechanical valve.
4. Cardiac abscess.

Typically, infected vegetations occur on the upstream side of the valve (e.g., atrial side for TV or MV and LVOT side for AV). TV vegetations are generally larger than left-sided lesions. PV endocarditis is rare. It has been associated with the use of the pulmonary artery catheter. The intensivist with basic-level training may be able to recognize obvious vegetations (Figure 15-15 and Video 15-12; Figure 15-16 and Video 15-13).

However, smaller vegetations may be difficult to recognize, other valves may be affected to a subtle extent, and there may be significant failure of valve or perivalvular

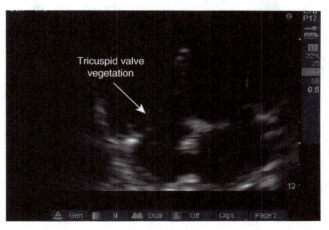

Figure 15-15 This apical four chamber view shows a tricuspid valve vegetation.

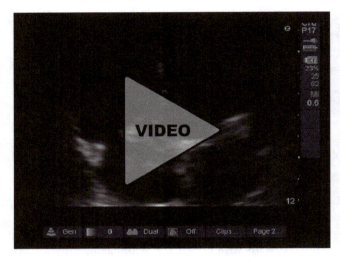

Video 15-12 This apical four chamber view shows a tricuspid valve vegetation. View at www.ccu2e.com

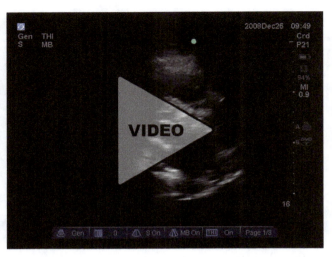

Video 15-13 This parasternal long-axis view shows a vegetation associated with the posterior mitral valve leaflet and a thickened hyperechoic immobile aortic valve consistent with aortic stenosis. View at www.ccu2e.com

function that will not be apparent to the basic-level echocardiographer. If the intensivist with basic skill identifies vegetations, it is advisable to proceed with a comprehensive study. Clinical suspicion combined with nondiagnostic screening studies mandates a comprehensive examination by an echocardiographer with advanced training. In general, echocardiography to evaluate for the possibility of native valve endocarditis should be performed by a skilled echocardiographer because the findings may be subtle. Fully trained echocardiographers with a background in TEE are qualified for this level of evaluation. Evaluation for prosthetic valve endocarditis presents a difficult challenge. In the case of a nondiagnostic study of a prosthetic valve, the intensivist should seek consultation with a cardiology echocardiographer with specific experience in the field.

Findings consistent with endocarditis are major criteria for the diagnosis of the disease; however, the diagnosis depends on the clinical context. The patient with positive blood cultures for *Staphylococcus aureus* and a large vegetation on the MV is not subtle. However, the difficulty arises when the pretest probability is low, yet there are findings consistent with endocarditis on echocardiography, particularly if the findings are minimal. This may occur when an abnormality that might be consistent with endocarditis is detected as an incidental finding in a patient with critical illness and other explanation for signs of infection.

False-positive findings for endocarditis include the following:

1. Persistent abnormality of the valve from previously treated infective endocarditis, such as a persistent vegetation or scarring of the valve. One hint that the process is no longer active is that, as the vegetation "ages," it may become more echo dense, or even calcify. The presence of a vegetation does not necessarily mean that there is an active infection at that site. Clinical correlation is required.

2. Nonbacterial thrombotic endocarditis. Platelet fibrin deposition on damaged valve endothelium may cause nonbacterial thrombotic vegetations that have the appearance of infective endocarditis on echocardiography. The basal portion of the MV is most often affected, but the process may extend to the chordae and papillary muscles. The cause is unknown, but the disease is associated with antiphospholipid syndrome, systemic lupus erythematosus, and malignancy (marantic endocarditis).

3. Other mimickers. Lambl's excrescences are an incidental finding that may resemble small vegetations. They are idiopathic linear mobile structures that are found most commonly on the upstream side of the AV. Papillary fibroelastoma is a small benign tumor that occurs on

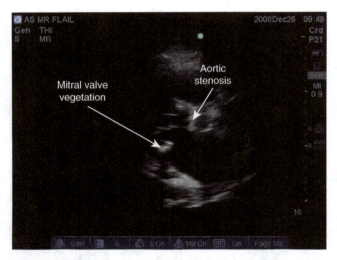

Figure 15-16 This parasternal long-axis view shows a vegetation associated with the posterior mitral valve leaflet and a thickened hyperechoic aortic valve consistent with aortic stenosis.

either surface of the AV or MV and occasionally on the other valves or endomyocardial surface. They may have a "sea anemone" appearance with mobile finger-like projections. Rarely, metastatic tumors may adhere to heart valves, and mimic infective endocarditis. Sterile thrombus may adhere to intracardiac devices, such as pacemaker wires or on the endomyocardium of the RA or RV, and have the appearance of infected vegetation.

It is not always possible to distinguish an infected vegetation from one of these abnormalities based on the morphologic pattern alone. Combining clinical assessment with the echocardiographic results is essential for establishing the diagnosis of infective endocarditis. Formal criteria for the diagnosis of infective endocarditis are available.[15] Echocardiography plays a major role in establishing the diagnosis, but other criteria are also important.

Good image quality is particularly important when the echocardiographic examination is being performed for possible infective endocarditis. TEE has superior resolution when compared to TTE. This image quality difference may be particularly evident in the ICU where obesity, edema, dressings, and hyperinflated lungs may commonly degrade TTE images. TEE is more sensitive than TTE in detecting vegetations and the complications of infective endocarditis, such as involvement of periaortic structures, annular abscess, or disruption of the MV apparatus.

When should the intensivist use TEE in evaluation for endocarditis? A reasonable approach is to use TEE when the TTE is nondiagnostic and the clinical suspicion of infective endocarditis is high. Suspicion of infective endocarditis involving a prosthetic valve is a strong indication for TEE. Echocardiography of prosthetic valve endocarditis may require an echocardiographer with specific expertise in that application.

Echocardiography has major application in the identification and stratification of complications of endocarditis. Echocardiography is the primary imaging modality used to identify anatomic complications of infective endocarditis. These include valve leaflet failure, perforation of valve leaflet or adjacent structure, abscess, aneurysm, fistula, and prosthetic valve dehiscence, all of which may lead to life-threatening hemodynamic failure. Serial echocardiography may demonstrate progression of anatomic complications predictive of catastrophic valve failure. The echocardiographer should work in close cooperation with the cardiac surgeon to determine the timing and type of surgical intervention that may be required for progressive valve failure.

Embolic events are another major complication of infective endocarditis. Echocardiography is useful in determining risk of embolism because the risk is largely determined by the size of the vegetation. Vegetations >10 mm in size have substantial risk of embolism.

▶ Practical Application in the ICU

Ultimately, the mark of the competent critical care sonographer is to not only identify valvular disease when present, but to appropriately integrate the importance of the findings in to the care pathway of the patient in front of them. The cardiologist's approach to assessment of valve function will necessarily be different than the intensivist. The cardiologist is an expert at the quantitative analysis of valve function, and has special expertise in decisions regarding the long-term management of valvulopathy, such as medical treatment and the timing of valve repair or replacement. The intensivist with skill at basic CCE lacks the ability to make advanced Doppler-based measurements of valve function. Their primary role is to screen the patient for catastrophic or severe valve failure with 2-D imaging supplemented with color Doppler. If any question remains, they must ask for consultation from a colleague who has advanced echocardiography training.

The intensivist with skill at advanced CCE has the ability to perform measurements that are typical of cardiology-type valve assessment (i.e., continuity calculation, PISA, vena contracta, or volumetric measurements). These may not be practical at the bedside of the patient with severe cardiopulmonary failure, but are applicable in the patient who is stable. In assessing the patient with acute hemodynamic failure, the advanced critical care echocardiographer is advised to use a rapid approach to assessing valve function. Detailed assessment of valve may wait until the patient is stable and may be performed by the cardiologist or intensivist who is competent in advanced CCE. In the context of critical illness, valvular lesions may be broadly classified into three distinct groups:

1. Devastating valvular lesion capable of causing acute severe cardiorespiratory failure.
2. Important valvular lesion complicating the management of critical illness but that is not the primary cause of the cardiorespiratory failure.
3. Incidental valvular lesion suitable for routine follow-up.

CONCLUSION

For the intensivist, echocardiographic assessment of valve function is useful to answer **three key questions**:

1. Is there valvular failure that is catastrophic and that requires urgent surgical consultation?
2. Is there severe but noncatastrophic valve failure that requires specific medical therapy or that will complicate management of coexisting critical illness?
3. Is there mild or moderate valve dysfunction that is only incidental to the primary critical illness?

The intensivist with basic critical care echocardiography skills can identify valvular abnormalities on 2-D imaging, particularly if they are severe, but otherwise has limited capability to assess valvular function. The use of color Doppler to assess the severity of valvular abnormality is sufficiently challenging that the basic-level echocardiographer may need consultation to assist with diagnosis. The basic-level echocardiographer may screen for major valve failure, but will need a definitive study if the clinical situation suggests the possibility of significant valve failure. The intensivist with advanced critical care echocardiography skills is able to fully evaluate valve function using 2-D examination and Doppler measurements in a manner identical to cardiology-based echocardiography. The identification and quantification of severe valvular stenosis or regurgitation is especially important, as it may have a major influence on the management of the patient with hemodynamic failure.

REFERENCES

1. Quinones MA, Douglas PS, Foster E, et al. ACC/AHA clinical competence statement on echocardiography. *J Am Coll Cardiol*. 2003;41:687–708.
2. Cape EG, Yoganathan AP, Weyman AE, Levine RA. Adjacent solid boundaries alter the size of regurgitant jets on Doppler color flow maps. *J Am Coll Cardiol*. 1991;17:1094–1102.
3. Zoghbi WA, Enriquez-Sarano M, Foster E, et al. American Society of Echocardiography. Recommendations for evaluation of the severity of native valvular regurgitation with two-dimensional and Doppler echocardiography. *J Am Soc Echocardiogr*. 2003;16:777–802.
4. Klein AL, Burstow DJ, Tajik AJ, et al. Age-related prevalence of valvular regurgitation in normal subjects: a comprehensive color flow examination of 118 volunteers. *J Am Soc Echocardiogr*. 1990;3:54–63.
5. Cormier B, Iung B, Porte JM, Barbant S, Vahanian A. Value of multiplane transesophageal echocardiography in determining aortic valve area in aortic stenosis. *Am J Cardiol*. 1996;77:882–885.
6. Currie PJ, Seward JB, Reeder GS, et al. Continuous-wave Doppler echocardiographic assessment of severity of calcific aortic stenosis: a simultaneous Doppler-catheter correlative study in 100 patients. *Circulation*. 1985;71:1162–1169.
7. Zoghbi WA, Farmer KL, Soto JG, Nelson JG, Quinones MA. Accurate noninvasive quantification of stenotic aortic valve area by Doppler echocardiography. *Circulation*. 1986;73:452–459.
8. Otto CM. Valvular stenosis. In: Otto CM, ed. *Textbook of Clinical Echocardiography*. 3rd ed. Philadelphia, PA: WB Saunders Co; 2004:287.
9. Oh JK, Seward JB, Tajik JA. Valvular heart disease. In: Oh JK, Seward JB, Tajik JA, eds. *The Echo Manual*. 3rd ed. Philadelphia, PA: Lippincott Williams & Wilkins; 2007:191.
10. deFilippi CR, Willett DL, Brickner ME, et al. Usefulness of dobutamine echocardiography in distinguishing severe from nonsevere valvular aortic stenosis in patients with depressed left ventricular function and low transvalvular gradients. *Am J Cardiol*. 1995;75:191–194.
11. Roberts BJ, Grayburn PA. Color flow imaging of the vena contracta in mitral regurgitation: technical considerations. *J Am Soc Echocardiogr*. 2003;16:1002–1006.
12. Takenaka K, Dabestani A, Gardin JM, et al. A simple Doppler echocardiographic method for estimating severity of aortic regurgitation. *Am J Cardiol*. 1986;57:1340–1343.
13. Tribouilloy CM, Enriquez-Sarano M, Fett SL, Bailey KR, Seward JB, Tajik AJ. Application of the proximal flow convergence method to calculate the effective regurgitant orifice area in aortic regurgitation. *J Am Coll Cardiol*. 1998;32:1032–1039.
14. Oh JK, Seward JB, Tajik JA. Valvular heart disease. In: Oh JK, Seward JB, Tajik JA, eds. *The Echo Manual*. 3rd ed. Philadelphia, PA: Lippincott Williams & Wilkins; 2007:204.
15. Li JS, Sexton DJ, Mick N, et al. Proposed modifications to the Duke criteria for the diagnosis of infective endocarditis. *Clin Infect Dis*. 2000;30:633–638.

ECHOCARDIOGRAPHIC EVALUATION OF CARDIAC TRAUMA

KEITH GUEVARRA, MIKHAIL LITINSKI, & ANTHONY D. SLONIM

INTRODUCTION

Traumatic injuries to the chest wall can arise from blunt or penetrating forces. Blunt cardiac injury occurs commonly in thoracic injury approximately 20–76% of the time and is often overlooked.[1] The range of presentations from an asymptomatic cardiac bruise to a severe cardiac rupture necessitates early recognition. Furthermore, the consequences can be quite serious and potentially fatal for unrecognized cardiac injuries; hence, early assessment and aggressive management can lead to improved outcomes. Ultrasound provides a useful method of evaluating cardiac trauma because it is readily available at the bedside, provides good image quality, and can be used serially to monitor the effects of interventions.

UTILITY OF TRANSTHORACIC ECHOCARDIOGRAPHY IN TRAUMA PATIENTS

The patient history, including an understanding of the mechanism of injury, and the physical examination remain primary methods of gathering objective information for the trauma victim. Although there are limited data to support the use of ultrasound in blunt cardiac injury, cardiac ultrasound complements the history and physical examination particularly if there is concern for anatomical irregularities, pericardial effusion, apical thrombi, or structural damage, such as cardiac contusions, concussion, muscle rupture, or valvular disruption, that would be difficult to identify through physical examination alone. Cardiac ultrasound can also help to assess hemodynamic profiles, volume status, and the cardiac index. Transthoracic echocardiogram (TTE) is warranted as a component of the focused assessment with sonography in trauma (FAST) examination and when questionable signs are encountered on the physical examination or when symptoms manifest after a traumatic injury. Table 16-1 provides a summary of the indications for echocardiography in trauma patients.[2]

One of the important contributions of cardiac ultrasound is that it has portability and is noninvasive. It can be used serially to monitor a patient over time. This is highly relevant for the hemodynamic assessment of trauma patients. In a study by Gunst et al., transthoracic ultrasonographic measures were well correlated with cardiac index and central venous pressure measurements obtained by a pulmonary artery catheter.[3]

SEQUELA AFTER BLUNT CARDIAC INJURY

Blunt cardiac trauma can lead to myocardial injury and manifest as wall motion abnormality on echocardiogram without evidence of transmural myocardial infarction on electrocardiogram. The most common form of this condition is a cardiac contusion. The mechanism of injury results from direct pressure to the heart as it makes contact between the sternum and the spine. This results in an acceleration/deceleration type of injury with the heart hitting the internal sternum. Upward pressure transmitted from increased intraabdominal pressure may also worsen the effect.[4] While there is currently no gold standard for diagnosis, there are some common features of the condition, including an impact on the right ventricle, tricuspid valve, and the left ascending coronary artery, most due to their location in proximity to the chest wall.

Patients with blunt cardiac injury may have a wide variety of manifestations. First, minor electrocardiogram changes or mild cardiac enzyme elevation may occur. Therefore, it is important to start surveillance by obtaining a baseline electrocardiogram and trending cardiac enzyme levels prior to obtaining an echocardiogram. Second, complex arrhythmias that can range from ST segment changes, heart blocks, or ventricular arrhythmias. Third, pump

> **TABLE 16-1**
> Summary of Indications for Cardiac Ultrasonography in Traumatic Injury[2]
>
> - History of chest trauma: Penetrating or blunt trauma to the chest
>   - Including mechanically ventilated patients with multiple trauma, especially chest trauma
>   - Follow-up study after blunt or penetrating injury
>   - Hemodynamically stable patients with suspicion of myocardial contusion
> - Cardiac/aortic/valvular injury: Possibility of cardiac or aortic injury from crush or deceleration injury
>   - Patients with widened mediastinum or suspicion of aortic damage
>   - Suspicion of valvular or myocardial dysfunction history in trauma patients
>   - Patient with suspected aortic dissection via transesophageal echocardiogram (TEE)
> - Hemodynamic monitoring
>   - Hemodynamically unstable patients with history of chest trauma
>   - Reevaluation of hemodynamically stable patients

failure may arise either from direct injury to the myocardium or conduction abnormalities. In addition to these common manifestations, several important complications need to be kept in mind including:

- Coronary artery laceration, which can lead to hemopericardium or cardiac tamponade
- Septal rupture, which can present as valvular dysfunction with or without concomitant heart failure
- Ventricular dilatation
- Intracardiac shunt and thrombosis
- Free wall rupture, which often leads to instantaneous death

In stable asymptomatic patients with a normal electrocardiogram after blunt cardiac injury, cardiac ultrasonography may not be helpful. However, echocardiogram may demonstrate wall motion abnormalities after trauma to the chest even if the patient is asymptomatic. Since many patients may not have a prior echocardiogram, the difficulty rests in determining whether the abnormalities were preexistent or a result of the injury.

An electrocardiogram has mixed results in terms of its diagnostic value in trauma patients. In a study by Weiss et al., an electrocardiogram was nondiagnostic in 73% of patients with a cardiac contusion.[5] If the electrocardiogram changes are new, evolving, or result from the trauma event, this may be suggestive of a cardiac contusion.[6] Despite these findings, an electrocardiogram is recommended as a primary surveillance in patients with suspected blunt cardiac trauma.

The use of cardiac enzymes in blunt cardiac trauma is of questionable value. Ferjani et al. have demonstrated that, in general, troponin levels, particularly troponin I or troponin T, have more diagnostic value than creatine kinase MB fraction; nonetheless, their clinical value in myocardial contusion is limited.[7] It has been suggested that when troponin I and T levels are normal, blunt cardiac trauma is quite rare. One important caveat to this statement is that the optimal timing of these markers is important in realizing their diagnostic value. Troponin levels can peak in 4–6 hours and last for 4–6 days after cardiac trauma. Echocardiogram may be a helpful adjunct if performed within the 4–6 hours of trauma but may have less utility if the cardiac enzymes are normal after the 4–6 hours.

Other potential causes of hemodynamic compromise may occur after chest trauma and have similar manifestations to blunt cardiac trauma, such as hemothorax, pneumothorax, massive active hemorrhage, and pericardial effusion. A shock state that is unresponsive to blood or fluid resuscitation with a finding of hemothorax, could possibly be due to myocardial rupture. Therefore, hemodynamically unstable patients require immediate cardiac ultrasound to help rule out these other causes of instability.

Myocardial perfusion scintigraphy still has limited diagnostic value in blunt cardiac trauma. Large transmural defects are necessary to visualize evidence of cardiac injury using this test. In addition, the right ventricle is also poorly visualized and right ventricular injury can be missed.

SEPTAL AND VALVULAR INJURY

Septal and valvular injury can also occur either individually or together after traumatic injury to the chest wall but they are rare occurrences. The cardiac septum can experience a small tear or a significant rupture depending on the force of the injury. The most commonly injured cardiac valve is the aortic valve followed by the mitral and then the tricuspid valve. The patient may present with a new murmur, widened pulse pressure, flash pulmonary edema, or heart failure often due to a disruption of a valvular leaflet, chordae tendineae, or papillary muscle tear.

A septal tear can also lead to an intracardiac shunt. There are also reports of right to left shunt through the patent foramen ovale after a tricuspid valve regurgitation. The most common site of a septal tear is at the apex of the intraventricular septum (Figure 16-1). Color Doppler in a four-chamber view can be performed with TTE. A bedside bubble study can also help to identify an intracardiac shunt when "air bubbles" can be seen moving within 1–2 cardiac cycles between parallel chambers. However, there are instances where TTE images are suboptimal and TEE images may be required for better visualization of the cardiac valves (Figure 16-2).

PENETRATING CARDIAC INJURY

A penetrating cardiac injury is highly fatal, with a probability of survival <20% when it occurs. The most common site of injury is the right ventricle because of its anterior location in the chest.[8] The left ventricle can also be injured, especially with high-velocity projectiles, and is associated with a higher mortality than a right ventricular injury. Hemorrhagic shock is a common cause of death in these

CHAPTER 16 ECHOCARDIOGRAPHIC EVALUATION OF CARDIAC TRAUMA

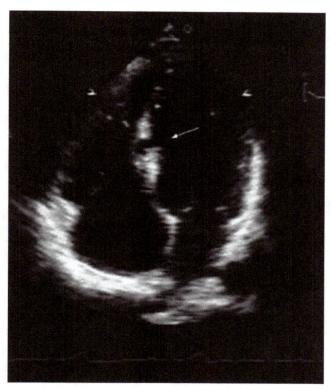

Figure 16-1 Transthoracic echocardiogram apical four-chamber view demonstrating incomplete transverse tear (*arrow*) of the interventricular septum. This image was obtained from a 50-year-old man involved in a 40 mph motor vehicle crash into a tree. (Image courtesy of Lisa Motavalli, M.D., retrieved from http://cme.mcgill.ca/php/pre.php?id=597 and hosted by the McGill Faculty of Medicine.)

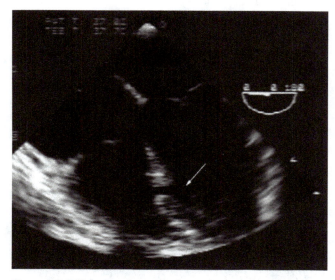

Figure 16-2 Transesophageal echocardiogram four-chamber view from a 50-year-old man involved in a 40 mph motor vehicle crash into a tree (same patient as in Figure 16-1), demonstrating incomplete septal tear (*arrow*). Only a thin membrane in the area of the rupture separates the two ventricles. (Image courtesy of Lisa Motavalli, M.D., retrieved from http://cme.mcgill.ca/php/pre.php?id=597 and hosted by the McGill Faculty of Medicine.)

patients and as little as 50 mL of blood in the pericardium is enough to cause hemodynamically significant cardiac tamponade.[1] The atrial chambers of the heart can also be injured with penetrating trauma and multiple cardiac chambers can be injured depending on the mechanism of injury. The coronary arteries are also susceptible to laceration because of their location.

Plummer et al. demonstrated that the patients with penetrating cardiac injury, who had echocardiography performed, had earlier diagnosis, disposition, and survival as compared to patients that had no echocardiogram.[9] The purpose of ultrasonography is often to determine the need for an urgent or emergent procedure/surgery (i.e., pericardial window, tube placement) to alter a potentially fatal outcome. A subcostal (subxiphoid) ultrasound view may provide the best image of the pericardium and it may need to be done immediately even prior to a chest X-ray to avoid delay for an emergent thoracotomy.

Rozycki performed a prospective trial of bedside echocardiogram in 261 patients and demonstrated that ultrasound had a sensitivity of 100% and accuracy of 97.3% on patients with possible penetrating cardiac injury. The mean time from echocardiogram to surgical intervention was 12.1 minutes.[10] These findings support the use of bedside cardiac ultrasound as an initial modality for the evaluation of patients with penetrating precordial wounds. If feasible, TEE may provide better images and potentially better diagnostic capabilities for blunt myocardial injury.[11]

AORTIC INJURY

Injury to the aorta can occur from either blunt injury of the chest, penetrating injury, or even from rapid deceleration. It can range from a complete transection of the aorta, where the patient may die at the accident scene, to a partial or full aortic intimal injury that can present as hemodynamically stable. Fifty percent of aortic ruptures can occur in the first 24 hours and 80% within the first week after trauma if not repaired.[12] Unfortunately, transthoracic ultrasonography has a limited role in assessing aortic injuries. TEE may provide better images. Other indications for TEE include suboptimal images that occur with TTE in hemodynamically unstable patients, hemodynamically unstable patients that are on mechanical ventilatory support, and postoperative trauma patients that cannot be adequately positioned for TTE. Patients who require TEE may require endotracheal intubation for airway protection prior to performing this procedure. Angiography or aortogram remains the gold standard for diagnosis, although TEE has good sensitivity and specificity in identifying aortic injuries. These tests can be time consuming and may not be feasible in hemodynamically unstable patients, who cannot tolerate transfer.

Certain findings can be seen clearly with TEE that may indicate trauma-related injury. These are:

- Intramural aortic hematoma
- Intimal and medial flap with pseudoaneurysm
- Intimal tear

- Intimal mural thrombus
- Dilated aortic isthmus
- Mediastinal hematoma

Smith et al. were able to demonstrate that TEE had a sensitivity of 100% and specificity of 98% in identifying traumatic aortic injury near the isthmus. The study also demonstrated no complications associated with TEE. The study further concluded that TEE should be an initial test in suspected traumatic aortic injury because of its accuracy, safety, and portability.[6] Goarin had similar results with respect to the sensitivity and specificity of TEE for diagnosing aortic injury in blunt trauma patients. In addition, the authors found that TEE was able to detect small aortic intimal injuries that a CT or angiography could not detect.[13] The main concern with TEE is that concomitant esophageal injuries or compromised airway may represent important contraindications to the procedure. TEE also requires more expertise in performing and attaining views.

PERICARDIAL EFFUSION

Cardiac tamponade is a clinical diagnosis that may often accompany penetrating chest trauma, but may not manifest itself during physical examination, especially if the pericardial effusion is small or insignificant. Ultrasonographic evidence of right ventricular and atrial collapse during diastole is specific for cardiac tamponade, but may also occur in patients with preexisting right ventricular hypertrophy and preexisting effusion. Using TTE, the image is better visualized in a four-chamber view (Figure 16-3).

The presence of pericardial fluid, clot, or thrombi should be ruled out in trauma patients. This image can be obtained with transthoracic subxiphoid or transthoracic parasternal long-axis view (Figures 16-3 and 16-6). Once found, a patient can be immediately taken for a lifesaving sternotomy or pericardiocentesis. Bedside echocardiogram would be helpful to detect the effusion. Lack of evidence of such can also help avoid unnecessary procedure/testing for the patient.

Cardiac tamponade resulting from trauma is due to blood accumulation within the nonelastic pericardium. Tamponade can develop slowly even with minute rate of hemorrhage. If there is concurrent bleeding that occurs in other organs, the right ventricle is vulnerable to early collapse both from decrease preload volume and constrictive physiology caused by the pericardial blood and this can be life threatening. On the contrary, there have been reports of tamponade having a protective effect. In the setting of a small pericardial tear, pericardial tamponade can limit exsanguination into the hemithorax unless the increasing amounts of pericardial blood cause a rise in the intrapericardial pressure. If the intrapericardial pressure overwhelms the diastolic pressure of the right ventricle, cardiovascular collapse can occur unless the pericardium is decompressed.

Pericardial fluid can be distinguished from pleural effusion when the hypoechoic fluid posterior to the left atrium tapers anteriorly the descending aorta as seen in the parasternal long-axis view (Figures 16-4 and 16-5). Pericardial fluid initially settles in the posterior aspect of the left ventricle and as the fluid continues to accumulate, it can eventually be seen in the anterior part of the heart. Pleural effusion, on the other hand, will appear as an anechoic fluid posterior of the descending aorta.

A pericardial window is an invasive method for the diagnosis of a pericardial effusion. Freshman showed that cardiac ultrasonography is less expensive and less invasive than either a subxiphoid pericardial window or thoracotomy.[14] When comparing the diagnostic value of the two,

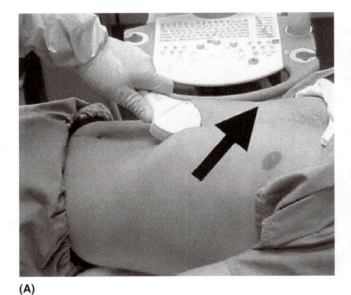
(A)

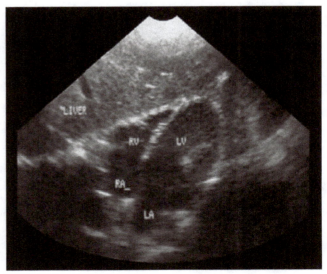
(B)

Figure 16-3 The FAST examination in the pericardial window view. (**A**) Location of the transducer to obtain cardiac views. (**B**) Normal cardiac anatomy and liver. LA, left atrium; LV, left ventricle; RA, right atrium; RV, right ventricle. (Reproduced with permission from Dr. RA Jones.)

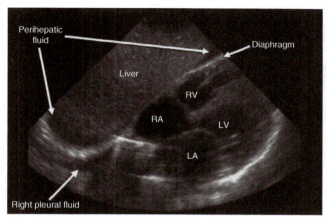

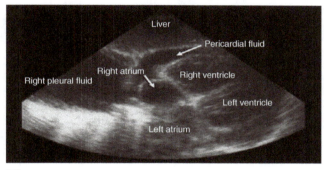

Figure 16-4 The FAST examination in the pericardial window view. (**A**) Cardiac window and presence of a right pleural effusion as well as perihepatic fluid. (**B**) Cardiac window with both pericardial and pleural effusions. (Reproduced with permission from Dr. RA Jones.)

Meyer et al. showed that subxiphoid exploration was more sensitive than echocardiogram (sensitivity, 100% vs. 56%; specificity, 92% vs. 93%; and accuracy, 92% vs. 90%, respectively).[15] When there is no evidence of hemothorax, echocardiogram had a sensitivity (100% vs. 100%), specificity

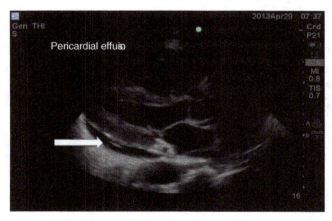

Figure 16-5 Parasternal long-axis view of the heart with a pericardial effusion (*white arrow*). The anechoic fluid is located above the descending aorta, which would make this a pericardial effusion versus a pleural effusion.

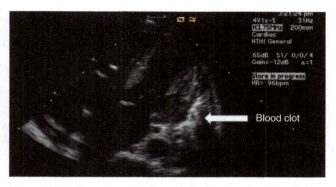

Figure 16-6 Four-chamber view of the heart with a blood clot (*white arrow*) within a pericardial effusion.

(89% vs. 91%), and accuracy (90% vs. 91%). The sensitivity is significantly reduced to 56% when a hemothorax is found and this is possibly due to a tear in the pericardium that allows pericardial fluid to drain to the hemithorax, ultimately reducing the size of the pericardial fluid. Mandavia et al. were able to show in a prospective study that emergency department physicians can reliably examine the pericardium for pericardial effusion 97.5% of the time.[12]

Bedside ultrasound can also be useful in guiding a pericardiocentesis. Injecting agitated saline through the pericardial catheter or pericardial window and visualizing this fluid within the cardiac sac can determine the proper placement for the catheter or needle.[16] The ultrasound can also help to reassess the size of the pericardial effusion after a pericardiocentesis is performed and monitor for reaccumulation.

Hemopericardium cannot be easily identified with bedside cardiac ultrasound since it may not appear fully anechoic. The presence of a clot within the pericardium can be visualized with parasternal long axis, subxiphoid view, or four-chamber view depending on the clot size (Figure 16-6).

ELECTRICAL AND HEAT STROKE-RELATED CARDIAC INJURY

There have been reports of echocardiographic findings related to acute electrical injury[17] and severe heat stroke. Electrical shock causes myocardial injury due to the transcardiac passage of current directed to the heart. In addition, arrhythmia-induced hypotension causes ischemic injury. There are associated EKG changes and an elevation of cardiac enzymes due to direct injury. Ultrasound may demonstrate severe global left ventricular hypokinesis and even biventricular hypokinesis depending on the degree of injury. The hypokinesis often resolves on follow-up echocardiogram, but there may be some persistence of wall motion abnormality.[17]

Severe heat stroke appears as a diffuse hypokinesis on echocardiogram. It is also associated with EKG changes, such as T-wave inversion and ST segment elevation, and with elevation of cardiac enzymes. Cardiac injury is possibly due to diffuse vasospasm and cathecholamine toxicity causing myocardial ischemia. Heat stroke-related cardiac dysfunction often returns to baseline as the temperature is treated.[18]

LIMITATIONS OF ECHOCARDIOGRAPHY

Although transthoracic echocardiography has several important benefits, there are also some notable limitations for obtaining good quality images (Table 16-2). Often, the ability to change a trauma patient's position during ultrasound scanning for cardiac views is limited (i.e., left lateral decubitus with left arm placed toward the head) or restricted based on the nature of the injury (i.e., concomitant neck injury, lower extremity fractures). A more experienced operator may be able to assist with image acquisition. In addition, TTE has limited view of the right ventricular outflow tract due to near-field artifact.[5] Therefore, a transesophageal echocardiography may provide better image acquisition but is again limited by the operator's experience and the patient's ability to tolerate a more invasive procedure.

CONCLUSION

Bedside cardiac ultrasonography has an important role in the assessment of cardiac injury related to trauma because it complements the physical examination at the point of patient care. This diagnostic technique provides the trauma patient with early access to critical and potentially lifesaving therapeutic interventions for the hemodynamically unstable patient Because of its portability, it can be used serially to reassess and monitor improvement from therapy or monitor for complications. Figure 16-7 is a summary on how to approach cardiac trauma.

TABLE 16-2

Limitations to Cardiac Ultrasound Image Acquisition

1. Pathologic hyperinflated lungs (i.e., chronic obstructive pulmonary disease or emphysema) or from positive pressure ventilation
2. Postoperative subcutaneous emphysema
3. Morbid obesity
4. Severe cachexia
5. Surgical incisions, drains, or bandages on open wounds on the chest
6. Chest tubes
7. Subcutaneous air
8. Pneumopericardium
9. Pain at probe site
10. Inadequate patient positioning
11. Severe abdominal distension
12. Uncooperative patient

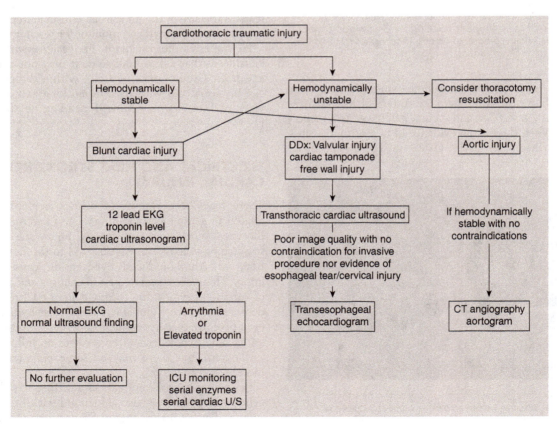

Figure 16-7 Diagnostic approach to cardiac trauma.[19]

REFERENCES

1. Bernardin B, Troquet JM. Initial management and resuscitation of severe chest trauma. *Emerg Med Clin North Am.* 2012;30:377–400.
2. Kohli-Seth R, Neuman T, Sinha R, Bassily-Marcus A. Use of echocardiography and modalities of patient monitoring of trauma patients. *Curr Opin Anaesthesiol.* 2010;23:239–245. Review.
3. Gunst M, Ghaemmaghami V, Sperry J, et al. Accuracy of cardiac function and volume status estimates using the bedside echocardiographic assessment in trauma/critical care. *J Trauma.* 2008;65:509–516.
4. Sybrandy KC, Cramer MJ, Burgersdijk C. Diagnosing cardiac contusion: old wisdom and new insights. *Heart.* 2003;89:485–489. Review.
5. Weiss RL, Brier J, O'Connor W, Ross S, Brathwaite C. The usefulness of transesophageal echocardiography in diagnosing cardiac contusions. *Chest.* 1996;109:73–77.
6. Smith MD, Cassidy JM, Souther S, et al. Transesophageal echocardiography in the diagnosis of traumatic rupture of the aorta [comments]. *N Engl J Med.* 1995;332:356–362.
7. Ferjani M, Droc G, Dreux S, et al. Circulating cardiac troponin T in myocardial contusion. *Chest.* 1997;111:427–433.
8. Pasquale M, Nagy K, Clarke J. Practice management guideline for screening of blunt cardiac injury. *J Trauma.* 1998;44:941–956.
9. Plummer D, Brunette D, Asinger R, et al. Emergency Department Echocardiography Improves Outcome in Penetrating Cardiac Injury. *Ann Emerg Med.* 1992;21:709–712.
10. Rozycki GS, Feliciano DV, Ochsner MG, et al. The role of ultrasound in patients with possible penetrating cardiac wounds: a prospective multicenter study. *J Trauma.* 1999;46:543–551.
11. Josephs SA. The use of current hemodynamic monitors and echocardiography in resuscitation of the critically ill or injured patient. *Int Anesthesiol Clinics.* 2007;45:31–59.
12. Mandavia D, Aragona J, Chan L, et al. Ultrasound training for emergency physicians—a prospective study. *Acad Emerg Med.* 2000;7:1008–1014
13. Goarin JP, Cluzel P, Gosgnach M, et al. Evaluation of transesophageal echocardiography for diagnosis of traumatic aortic injury. *Anesthesiology.* 2000;93:1373–1377.
14. Freshman SP, Wisner DH, Weber CJ. 2-D echocardiography: emergent use in the evaluation of penetrating precordial trauma [comments]. *J Trauma.* 1991;31:902–905 [discussion: 905–906].
15. Meyer DM, Jessen ME, Grayburn PA. Use of echocardiography to detect occult cardiac injury after penetrating thoracic trauma: a prospective study. *J Trauma.* 1995;39:902–907.
16. Chiang HT, Lin M. Pericardiocentesis guided by two-dimensional contrast echocardiography. *Echocardiography.* 1993;10:465–469.
17. Homma S, Gillam LD, Weyman AE. Echocardiographic observations in survivors of acute electrical injury. *Chest.* 1990;97:103–105.
18. Wakino S, Hori S, Mimura T, Miyatake S, Fujishima S, Aikawa N. A case of severe heat stroke with abnormal cardiac findings. *Int Heart J.* 2005;46:543–550.
19. Salehian O, Teoh K, Mulji A. Blunt and penetrating cardiac trauma: a review. *Can J Cardiol.* 2003;19:1054–1059.

SECTION III

Ultrasound Evaluation of the Neck, Trunk, and Extremities

ULTRASOUND EVALUATION OF THE NECK AND UPPER RESPIRATORY SYSTEM

CHRISTIAN H. BUTCHER

Scan QR code or visit www.ccu2e.com for video in this chapter

INTRODUCTION

Ultrasound of the neck and upper respiratory system has many potentially useful clinical applications.[1] Aside from vascular access (see Chapter 27), some of these indications include confirmation of satisfactory endotracheal tube (ETT) placement, evaluation of the larynx, guidance for percutaneous tracheostomy, evaluation of the paranasal sinuses, and assessment of vocal cord disorders. The data demonstrating improved outcomes by using ultrasound for imaging the upper airway remain scarce. However, there are important opportunities to improve care for the intensive care unit (ICU) patient that can be derived from its use.

PARANASAL SINUSES

Ultrasound use for the evaluation of the paranasal sinuses was recognized in Europe as technically feasible to confirm the presence of sinus disease as early as the 1960s.[2] However, widespread clinical application emerged only recently with the development of low-cost, high-quality bedside ultrasound imaging technology. Earlier studies established ultrasound as an alternative to computed tomography (CT) for the diagnosis of maxillary sinus disease and described the typical findings associated with sinusitis.[3,4] With improvements in imaging, more recent reports focused on improving the diagnostic accuracy of ultrasound by performing postural maneuvers.[5] In 2006, Vargas et al. investigated the role of ultrasound for performing transnasal puncture of the maxillary sinus in intubated ICU patients. In patients suspected of having sinusitis, they found ultrasonographic evidence of maxillary sinusitis in 70% of patients, and of these, 93% had positive results from transnasal puncture, demonstrating the comparability of ultrasound to CT for the diagnosis and transnasal puncture of sinusitis.[6] More recent studies investigated the characterization, or "staging," of sinus fluid collections by noting the presence or absence of acoustic streaming in a model of sinusitis. More viscous collections (pus) are less likely to undergo acoustic streaming than less viscous collections.[7]

There are no studies that describe an improvement in ICU outcomes by using ultrasound instead of standard CT, even though a CT scan has more radiation, is more expensive, and requires the transportation of critically ill patients to and from the radiology department as well as the use of valuable critical care nursing time. There are important roles, however, for CT imaging of the sinuses that cannot be duplicated with ultrasonography. These include any planned surgical procedure involving the sinuses, suspected sinus trauma, and suspected malignant disease. This discussion focuses on the use of ultrasound for the evaluation of paranasal sinusitis.

Sinus disease is important to recognize in critically ill patients because it is a source of fever, which leads to costly diagnostic workups and empiric therapeutic regimens.[8,9] In addition, maxillary sinus disease is an independent risk factor for the development of nosocomial lung infections.[10] Although not studied in any systematic fashion, it is also conceivable that undiagnosed sinusitis may lead to significant pain and agitation, resulting in the increased use of sedatives and analgesics, which could then delay extubation.

▶ Technique

The anatomy of the paranasal sinuses is shown in Figure 17-1. The sinuses most amenable to ultrasonographic examination are the maxillary and frontal sinuses; however, most studies have been performed on the maxillary sinus. The maxillary sinus is contained within the maxilla, and is bordered by the orbital floor superiorly, the hard palate inferiorly, the nasal wall medially, and the zygoma laterally.

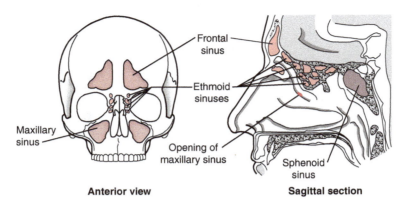

Figure 17-1 Anatomy of the paranasal sinuses. (*Source:* http://www.merck.com/mmpe/sec08/ch089/ch089a.html [in public domain].)

In the normal state, the sinus is air filled, thus impairing the transmission of ultrasound energy. In this case, what is seen is the anterior wall only, with some artifact known as "acoustic shadowing" (Figure 17-2), which obscures all underlying structures; this is considered a negative study. When filled with fluid, ultrasound penetrates the anterior wall, "travels" through the fluid, and strikes the posterior or lateral walls and "reflects" back to the transducer, resulting in an image of the sinus cavity in its entirety (Figure 17-3). This is known as a "sinusogram," which is a positive study. A partial sinusogram, where only the posterior wall or a side wall is seen, can occur due to the presence of an air–fluid level in the sinus or mucosal thickening. The patient's position influences the appearance of the fluid in a partial sinusogram. In the supine position, fluid can "layer out" away from the anterior wall, resulting in either acoustic shadowing or a partial sinusogram. However, when placed in a semirecumbent or upright position, the fluid (if present) will follow gravity and cover the floor of the sinus, coming in contact with the anterior wall. When imaged, this results in either a partial or complete sinusogram, depending on how much fluid is present and on the transducer orientation or angulation (Figure 17-4).

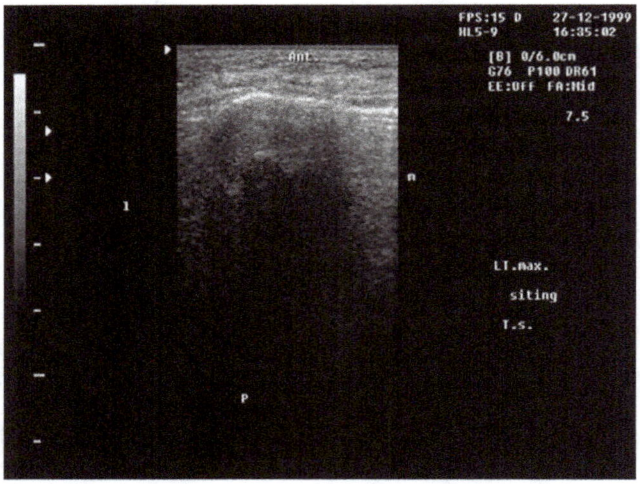

For a sinus ultrasound, patients can be placed in a semirecumbent position. A 3–5 MHz cardiac probe with a small footprint is used. Proper transducer position is demonstrated in Figure 17-5. The horizontal plane is scanned first, angulating the probe cephalad (toward the orbital floor) and caudally (toward the floor of the sinus); this is followed by turning the transducer 90° and scanning from the medial to the lateral wall. The technique is then repeated on the alternate side. A complete ultrasound maxillary sinus scan, in contrast to CT scanning, can be performed in <60 seconds. If a complete sinusogram is seen, no further evaluation is necessary and the patient should be treated for sinusitis. If a partial sinusogram is obtained, postural maneuvers may help elucidate the cause: sinusitis versus

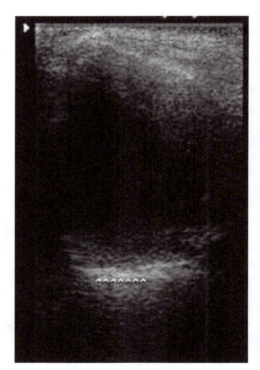

Figure 17-3 Abnormal, fluid-filled maxillary sinus showing anterior and posterior walls.

Figure 17-2 Normal maxillary sinus showing anterior wall only.

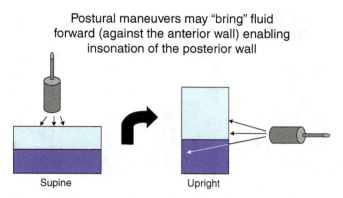

Figure 17-4 Diagram showing the effect of changing patient position from supine to upright. Note that in the supine position, fluid (dark blue) does not contact the anterior wall, thus the ultrasound beam cannot "penetrate." However, in the upright position, the fluid layers out inferiorly with gravity, and comes into contact with the anterior wall. The ultrasound then penetrates to the posterior wall, resulting in either a partial sinusogram (if imaged vertically) or a complete sinusogram (if imaged horizontally).

mucosal thickening. Until proficiency with the ultrasound technique is mastered, bedside ultrasound can be correlated with CT scan.

VOCAL CORDS

Ultrasonography has recently been shown to be helpful in the in vivo analysis of vocal cord function. Clinical utility of this technique includes the pre- and/or postsurgical evaluation of vocal cord function at the time of thyroid or complex thoracic surgery,[11] assessment for the presence/absence of vocal cord paralysis,[12] or identification of vocal cord dysfunction syndrome. One recent study shows a reasonable correlation between findings of ultrasonography when compared to laryngoscopy in cases of vocal cord paresis.[13] In addition, ultrasound has been shown to be a useful adjunct to endoscopy in vocal cord injection procedures, typically performed to improve phonation in cases of unilateral vocal cord paralysis.[14]

The technique of vocal cord visualization is fairly straightforward, but the operator should expect a learning curve. Using a high-resolution linear array transducer (6–13 mHz) usually works best. Position the patient supine with the neck slightly extended. Palpate the external anatomy, including thyroid and cricoids cartilages. Place the transducer transversely over the midportion of the thyroid cartilage perpendicular to the axis of the trachea. Move the transducer axially along the thyroid cartilage until the glottis structures are visualized; identifying the arytenoids first, which are bright structures and, therefore, usually easy to identify, helps orient the operator. Slight angulation of the probe cranially or caudally may improve visualization. Once the cords are visualized, have the patient "hum" to assess cord function in real time (Video 17-1).

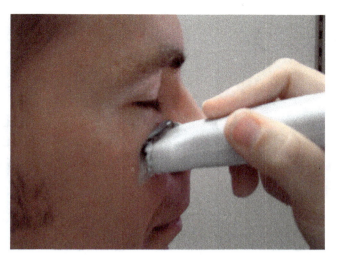
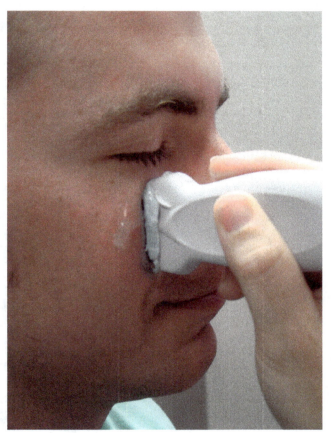

Figure 17-5 Proper transducer position. Top, horizontal; bottom, vertical.

LARNYX/ENDOTRACHEAL INTUBATION

In 1987, Raphael and Conard used B-mode 2D transtracheal ultrasound to assess the capability of ultrasound to visualize and confirm ETT placement.[15] In this study, the investigators were primarily interested in verifying the intratracheal placement in patients already known to have successful tracheal intubations. The study was not

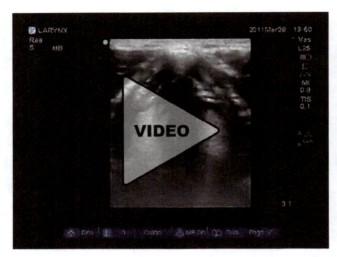

Video 17-1 Vocal chord (VC) ultrasound. Short-axis view of the VC with patient "humming" demonstrating intact VC function bilaterally. View at www.ccu2e.com

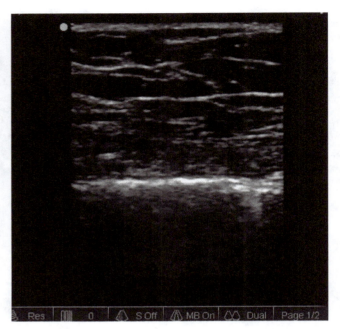

Figure 17-6 Visceral–parietal pleural interface (VPPI). Normal appearance of the pleural surfaces. The white line "shimmers" during respiration.

attempting to identify esophageal intubation or any other malposition. The authors suggested that ETT cuffs be filled with saline to reduce the acoustic impedance of the air-filled ETT balloon, which would improve ultrasound transmission (similar to having a full bladder during abdominal ultrasonography). The contrast between the air-filled trachea and saline-filled balloon allows the position of the ETT to be identified more easily. It was also suggested that a longitudinal view, combined with a slight to-and-fro motion, could improve visualization. They concluded that this technique was beneficial for certain patient populations like pregnant women or patients receiving frequent chest radiographs to monitor ETT position. Building on this data, a recent study demonstrated that novice sonographers, after only a 50-minute training session, could accurately identify the intratracheal position of a saline-filled ETT cuff,[16] underscoring the relative accessibility of these techniques to most practitioners.

A blinded, prospective study of 40 patients undergoing elective surgery was performed to identify esophageal intubation using 2D ultrasound.[17] The authors identified esophageal intubations with a sensitivity of 100% and correctly identified all five esophageal intubations, and 34 out of 35 tracheal intubations. Two additional studies, using both live patients and cadavers, confirmed the high sensitivity and specificity of 2D ultrasound to evaluate ETT position.[18,19] In addition, improved sensitivity and specificity could be achieved by using a dynamic approach (visualization of the tube during placement) as compared with a static approach (confirmation of placement after the fact).[19] Multiple studies have also concluded that tracheal ultrasound is as effective as traditional capnography for determining ETT position, and that the technique is faster than auscultation/capnography, even in obese patients.[20]

Endotracheal tube malposition in the right mainstem bronchus can also be identified by using bilateral pleural ultrasound.[21–24] The parietal–visceral pleural interface can be easily identified with a high-frequency probe (Figure 17-6). This interface, known as the visceral–parietal pleural interface (VPPI), has a characteristic "shimmering" appearance during lung ventilation. The two pleural surfaces can be seen to slide past one another, which is responsible for producing the shimmering effect. If the ETT is positioned in a mainstem bronchus, the sliding or shimmering will either be greatly reduced or absent on the contralateral side. This assumes that there is no anatomic airway obstruction, such as an obstructing tumor, causing the reduced or absent pleural shimmer, which could lead to a false-positive test and inappropriate repositioning of the ETT. This approach was confirmed by Weaver et al. using cadavers.[25] The sensitivity for identifying esophageal intubation was 95–100% and the sensitivity for a right mainstem intubation versus a tracheal intubation was lower, at 70–75%, using the sliding lung sign.

Other applications for upper airway ultrasound, aside from verification of ETT position, include appropriate ETT size selection, confirmation of laryngeal mask airways, the prediction of a difficult airway, and the prediction of postextubation stridor. Lakhal et al. studied whether or not appropriate selection of ETT size could be informed by using translaryngeal ultrasound. After measuring the diameter of the airway in the subglottic region by translaryngeal ultrasound, the investigators then compared their measurement to those obtained by using magnetic resonance imaging and found a strong correlation between the two measurements. The authors suggested that ultrasound could accurately gauge the diameter of the subglottic airway and could guide selection of an appropriately sized ETT.[26] Gupta et al. published a study comparing ultrasound evaluation of laryngeal mask airway (LMA) position compared to endoscopy in patients undergoing elective intubation for same-day surgery procedures. The authors concluded that ultrasound accurately assessed LMA position, and that this technique could potentially replace endoscopy in this patient population.[27]

Pretracheal soft tissue (PST) swelling is identified as a risk factor for difficult laryngoscopy and can be identified using ultrasound.[28] Patients were clinically classified as either "difficult" or not, followed by ultrasonographic quantification of PST. Difficult patients had PST measurements of 28 ± 2.7 mm, compared with 17.5 ± 1.8 mm for nondifficult laryngoscopy. These findings were refuted by Komatsu, who concluded that ultrasound quantification was unable to predict subsequent difficult laryngoscopy in a cohort of obese patients.[29] A more recent study by Wojtczak showed that ultrasound could easily measure the hyo-mental distance in obese and morbidly obese patients, and that this measurement may be predictive of difficult intubation.[30] A study by Lahav et al. investigated the association between ultrasonographic measurements of tongue base width and severity of obstructive sleep apnea (OSA).[31] The results showed a strong association between tongue base width and the severity of sleep-disordered breathing on polysomnography, and the authors implied that this technique could be a useful screening test for OSA. However, other measurements, such as anterior neck fat tissue thickness or umbilical fat tissue thickness, failed to establish an association between these ultrasound-derived measurements and disease severity in patients with diagnosed OSA.[32] Having a noninvasive tool to assist with predicting difficult laryngoscopy and difficult-to-intubate patients, as well as predicting those at highest risk for OSA would be desirable; however, the data currently available are equivocal for these indications.

Ding et al. studied whether translaryngeal ultrasound measurements of airway column width around the ETT could predict postextubation stridor. A preextubation air leak test and ultrasonographic measurements of air column widths were obtained on intubated patients. The air column width was measured with the balloon inflated and deflated. The patients who developed stridor had an air leak at 25 cc compared with 300 cc in the nonstridor group. The air column width in the normal group was 6.4 mm, compared with 4.5 mm in the stridor group. The authors concluded that preextubation translaryngeal quantification of the air column width could help identify patients at risk for postextubation stridor.[33] There are several limitations to this study, including the effect of ETT size on air column width and the presence of secretions, which would decrease air column width measurements. Although inconclusive, this represents an exciting opportunity for further investigation.

▶ Technique

Endotracheal malposition is a common problem in the ICU. Accordingly, most of the data on the use of ultrasound for airway management focus on the verification of ETT position. Two basic techniques are available for this purpose: translaryngeal ultrasound to evaluate the proximal trachea

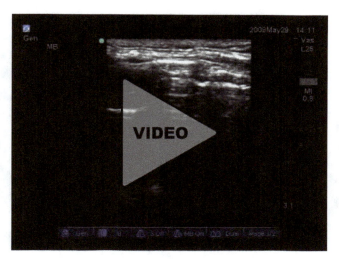

Video 17-2 Long-axis view of the trachea during endotracheal intubation. Note ETT coming from the left (patient's head) below tracheal rings. View at www.ccu2e.com

and evaluate for proximal malposition, and pleural ultrasound to evaluate for distal malposition of the ETT.

Translaryngeal 2D ultrasound for visualization of the ETT is best performed longitudinally during ETT placement, so-called "dynamic guidance." This requires that the ultrasound equipment be readily available during intubation. A midline longitudinal view, using a 5–7 MHz linear array (vascular) probe, through the larynx at the level of the cricoid cartilage is optimal. The "depth" of the image should be set deep enough to visualize the tracheal lumen and not just the anterior tracheal wall. Remember that air produces significant artifact due to its high acoustic impedance and structures lying deeper to air will generally not be seen. However, with careful examination and practice, the presence of the ETT can be seen with this view as an echogenic stripe lying deep to the anterior tracheal wall (Videos 17-2 and 17-3). While this may initially be considered

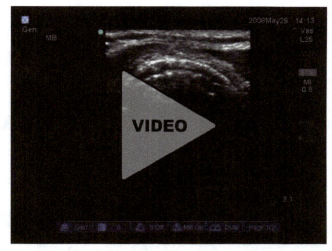

Video 17-3 Short-axis view of the trachea during endotracheal intubation. Note ETT appearing in the plane below tracheal rings. View at www.ccu2e.com

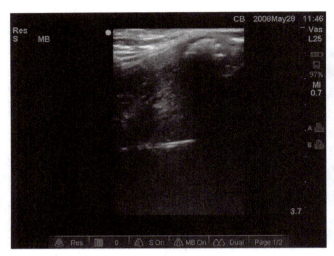

Figure 17-7 Longitudinal view through the trachea showing the distal tip of the ETT (bright white line).

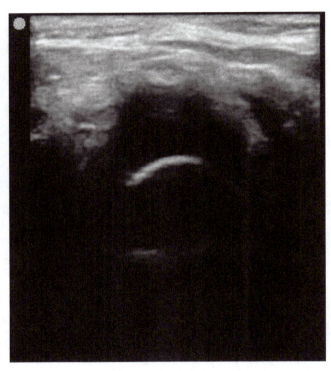

Figure 17-9 Transverse view through the trachea showing the anterior surface of the ETT (bright white, curvilinear structure).

a reverberation artifact from the tracheal wall itself, with further practice, the anterior surface of the ETT can be appreciated, particularly in the setting of a "high," or subglottic intubation. In this case, the echogenic stripe does not continue the entire length of the image (Figure 17-7). Angulation of the probe under the manubrium is sometimes necessary to visualize the tip of the ETT (Figure 17-8). In cases of a relatively low intubation, the tip will not be seen. To enhance this technique, a transverse ultrasound examination looking for the curved, echogenic contour of the anterior ETT may be helpful (Figure 17-9). Again, angulation under the manubrium may be required. In general, if the tip of the tube is seen without significant angulation under the manubrium in either the longitudinal or transverse view, it is likely to be within the proximal trachea and may require advancement.

Pleural ultrasound (see Chapter 18), is an extremely useful tool to evaluate for esophageal intubation, confirm tracheal intubation, and determine mainstem intubation in most patients. Conveniently, the same probe used for translaryngeal ultrasound (linear array, 5–7 MHz) can also be used to evaluate the VPPI. As discussed above, in cases of satisfactory tracheal intubation, and in the absence of unilateral airway obstruction from a tumor or foreign body, there will be bilateral and equal pleural sliding during respiration (Video 17-4). In cases of esophageal intubation, there will be minimal or no pleural sliding (caused by the cardiac cycle, known as the lung pulse). This would

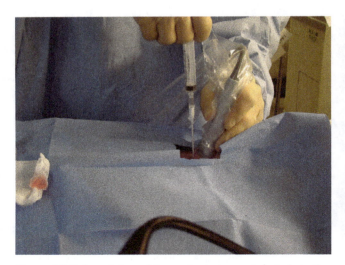

Figure 17-8 Angulation of the probe to image inferiorly to the manubrium.

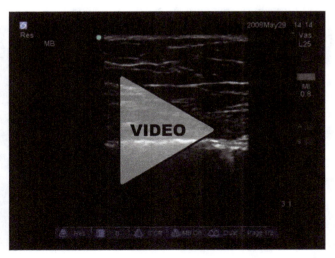

Video 17-4 Intact "pleural sliding" producing shimmering effect sometimes described as the "ants crawling" at the interphase between parietal and visceral pleura. View at www.ccu2e.com

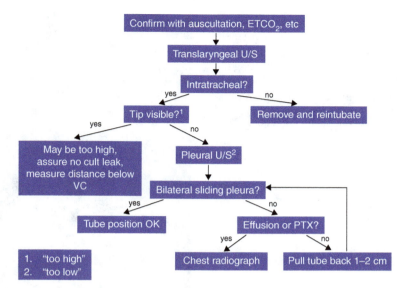

Figure 17-10 Algorithm for determining satisfactory ETT placement.

be associated with desaturation, reduced breath sounds, epigastric gurgling with bagging, and an undetectable end-tidal CO_2 prompting immediate tube removal and tracheal reintubation. In cases of distal malposition, such as a right mainstem intubation, there would be vigorous pleural sliding on the right, with diminished or absent sliding on the left. There is importance in comparing one side of the chest to the other, similar to techniques of lung auscultation learned in medical school. A combined approach of translaryngeal ultrasound to identify proximal malposition of the ETT, paired with pleural ultrasound to identify distal malposition, may be a viable alternative to chest radiography to verify tube position. Figure 17-10 demonstrates an algorithm that we use for this purpose. This same basic technique can be applied to other situations, such as confirming proper double-lumen ETT placement.[1] The limitations of using lung sliding to verify ETT position include the presence of any process that causes loss of lung sliding, such as pneumothorax, pleural scarring, or severe parenchymal lung disease, that prevents lung inflation (e.g., severe adult respiratory distress syndrome (ARDS) or pneumonia).

PERCUTANEOUS TRACHEOSTOMY

Percutaneous dilatational tracheostomy (PDT) has become the procedure of choice for providing long-term airway access in many institutions. Once considered only for "ideal" candidates, the procedure is now being performed safely in the morbidly obese and in those with prior neck surgery or coagulopathy. Recently, there has been significant attention to studying the application of ultrasound to PDT to reduce complications, especially in patients belonging to high-risk groups.

Examination of the anterior neck prior to surgical tracheostomy was first described by Bertram et al. in 1995,[34] in a study in which 50 patients underwent an ultrasound evaluation of the neck prior to the operation. This study established the feasibility of performing a targeted ultrasound examination to identify anatomic variations that may complicate the procedure. Sustic et al. first reported on the use of ultrasound guidance for percutaneous tracheostomy,[35] and the clinical utility of this technique has been confirmed in several other reports.[36-39] These studies demonstrate the benefits of ultrasound for both the selection of an insertion site and an appropriately sized tracheostomy tube,[40] in addition to allowing visualization of aberrant anatomy.

Although safe, PDT can be associated with life-threatening complications, such as severe bleeding and malposition. Most bleeding events are delayed two to three weeks after placement, and are due to erosion of the brachiocephalic artery caused by the high-pressure tracheostomy tube cuff. However, bleeding can also occur at the time of tracheostomy placement. A recent case of fatal hemorrhage following PDT was reported.[41] In this case, the authors cited the cause of hemorrhage as an aberrant right subclavian artery, following thyroid surgery that coursed high in the neck at the level of the cricoid cartilage before turning toward the extremity. In a follow-up letter, Gwilym and Cooney[42] reported their experience with hemorrhage caused by injury to the lowest thyroid artery during PDT. Ultrasound mapping of the neck was not performed in either case, although the latter group now uses ultrasound regularly. In addition, Muhammad et al. published their series of 497 cases in which bleeding occurred in 5%, usually due to an inferior thyroid vein, brachiocephalic vein, or high communicating anterior jugular vein.[43] Clearly, aberrant vascular anatomy exists and should be screened for.

Malposition is another complication of PDT. However, the selection of an appropriate insertion site minimizes risk. Proximal malposition could cause damage to the vocal cords at the time of insertion (immediate damage), or could cause the tracheostomy tube to lie directly underneath the vocal cords and damage them over time, resulting in permanent vocal cord dysfunction and hoarseness. Distal malposition could result in the tip of the tracheostomy tube abutting the carina during neck flexion or lying in a mainstem bronchus. Contact with the carina results in cough, patient-ventilator dyssynchrony, difficult suctioning, suction trauma, and bleeding. Using ultrasound, the tracheal cartilages can be counted and the appropriate site marked on the skin, usually between the second and third tracheal cartilage, which can easily eliminate proximal malposition. Careful ultrasound examination to identify the insertion site reduces the incidence of cranial malposition from 33% to 0%.[44] In addition, the distance from the carina to the subglottic area can be measured by bronchoscopy, providing a rough estimate of tracheal length, which minimizes the risk of distal malposition. Therefore, using these two techniques, malposition of any kind can be virtually eliminated.

Another potential complication of PDT, as commonly performed, is hypercarbia. Most procedures are endoscopically guided, which is associated with hypercarbia when compared to surgical tracheostomy or tracheostomy with ultrasound guidance alone (without bronchoscopy). In one study comparing pCO_2 levels in patients undergoing endoscopically guided PDT, ultrasound-guided PDT, or surgical tracheostomy, the pCO_2 increased up to 24 mm Hg in the bronchoscopy group, compared with 8 mm Hg in the ultrasound group and 3 mm Hg in the operative group.[45] This has implications for patients in whom hypercarbia is undesirable, such as neurotrauma patients or patients with elevated intracranial pressure.

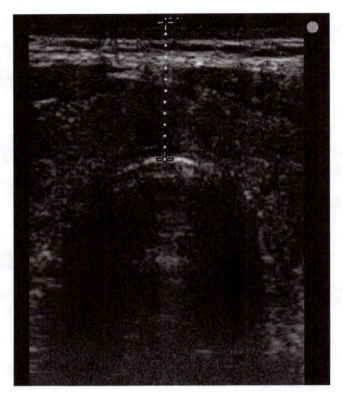

Figure 17-11 Measuring the pretracheal soft tissue to help with proper tracheostomy tube selection. Distances much greater than 2.5 cm may require a proximal long tracheostomy type.

▶ Technique

Selection of an appropriately sized tracheostomy tube can be aided by ultrasound in several ways. A B-mode scan of the PSTs, utilizing a 7 MHz linear array probe, allows an estimation of the distance from the skin to the anterior tracheal wall. Based on this information, the operator can choose either a standard tube for small distances or one with a proximal long segment for longer distances. This measurement can be performed in either a longitudinal or transverse orientation (Figure 17-11) and is best performed at the proposed insertion site. Also, the diameter of the trachea can be easily estimated by a transverse measurement of the tracheal lumen, again at the level of the proposed insertion site. This measurement guides the selection of a tube with a compatible diameter (Figure 17-12).

Selection of an insertion site is easily accomplished with a midline, longitudinal view of the trachea from cricoid cartilage to sternal notch (Figure 17-13). The tracheal cartilages can be counted, and the appropriate site can be marked on the skin, usually between the second and third tracheal cartilage. This, of course, requires that the patient be sedated enough that there is no movement of the head or neck between skin marking and tracheostomy insertion. If movement occurs during this window, the area needs to be rescanned to confirm that the skin mark is still appropriate.

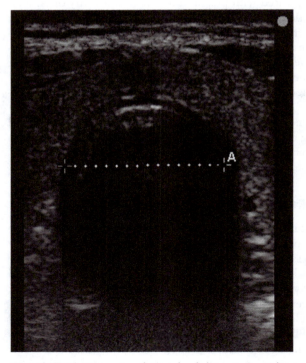

Figure 17-12 Measuring the tracheal diameter to aid proper tracheostomy tube selection.

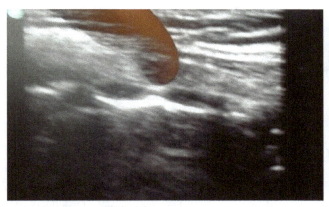

Figure 17-13 Midline longitudinal view of trachea, showing the tracheal rings. Superior is to the left, inferior to the right. The ring furthest to the left is the fist tracheal ring. The thumb indicates the desired insertion site.

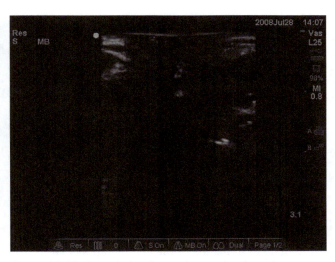

Figure 17-15 Cannulating the trachea under dynamic guidance utilizing a longitudinal ultrasound view.

After selection of an insertion site, a scan of the overlying tissues with color-flow Doppler should be performed to identify any vascular structures at risk for damage during the procedure. This is performed in both a longitudinal and transverse orientation to look for "bridging" jugular veins, high brachiocephalic vessels, or thyroid veins or arteries. When examining the trachea transversely, the thyroid gland, including both lobes, the isthmus, and the location of the carotid arteries and jugular veins, especially in patients with prior neck surgery, should be examined (Figure 17-14).

Cannulation of the trachea can be visualized under dynamic guidance. To achieve this, a longitudinal view just lateral to the midline is obtained. The cannulation needle is then applied to the skin in the midline; the needle causes an indentation of the subcutaneous tissue (Figure 17-15), which approximates the needle tract. The needle position can be adjusted either caudally or cranially, until this indentation overlies the desired puncture site. This is called longitudinal positioning. Once the desired longitudinal position is achieved, the probe can be rotated 90° to guide the transverse position of the needle (Figure 17-8). Transverse position is less important than longitudinal position, as the puncture site is somewhat anterior. The ultrasonographic view is seen in Figure 17-16. When the needle is

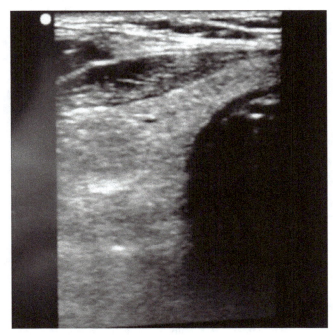

Figure 17-14 Transverse view through the trachea, showing the right lobe of the thyroid gland as well as the thyroid isthmus.

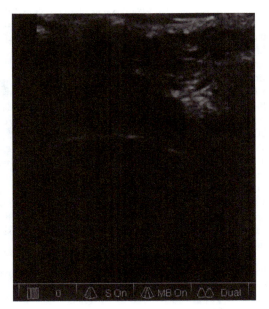

Figure 17-16 Transverse view through the trachea showing cannulation in the midline. The needle position can be adjusted under ultrasound guidance to assure a midline puncture. The acoustic shadow can be seen as two-angled vertical lines overlying the midportion of the tracheal ring.

in the desired position, cannulation can occur in the conventional manner. After tube placement, especially if bronchoscopy is not used to verify tube position, remember to scan the anterior chest bilaterally for sliding pleura; this confirms an intratracheal placement that is not too low.

In our practice, ultrasonography has not replaced bronchoscopy in the guidance of PDT. Bronchoscopy retains certain advantages, including the direct visualization of the position of the ETT during withdrawal and visualization of the posterior tracheal wall during needle cannulation and dilation. In addition, in cases of overzealous ETT tube withdrawal, one can easily reintubate the trachea over the bronchoscope.

SUMMARY

Ultrasound examination of the neck and upper airway has many useful clinical applications in the ICU. Maxillary sinusitis is commonly overlooked, yet easily identifiable with ultrasound, sometimes obviating the need for CT. Confirmation of ETT placement, probably the most common indication for "STAT" portable chest radiographs in the ICU, can be achieved with a high degree of confidence by using ultrasound. Percutaneous tracheostomy can be made even safer by performing a few simple scans to identify aberrant anatomy and to locate an appropriate insertion site. Utilization of this technology can help provide timely, cost-effective, and safe care for patients.

REFERENCES

1. Sustic A. Role of ultrasound in the airway management of critically ill patients. *Crit Care Med.* 2007;35:S173–S177.
2. Abdurasulov DM, Amilova AA, Fazylov AA, et al. On the use of ultrasonics in the diagnosis of diseases of the maxillary sinuses. *Nov Med Priborostr.* 1964;24:30–33.
3. Lichtenstein D, Biderman P, Meziere G, et al. The sinusogram, a real-time ultrasound sign of maxillary sinusitis. *Intensive Care Med.* 1998;24:1057–1061.
4. Hilbert G, Vargas F, Valentino R, et al. Comparison of B-mode ultrasound and CT in the diagnosis of maxillary sinusitis in mechanically ventilated patients. *Crit Care Med.* 2001;29:1337–1342.
5. Vargas F, Boyer A, Bui HN, et al. A postural change test improves the prediction of a radiological maxillary sinusitis by ultrasonography in mechanically ventilated patients. *Intensive Care Med.* 2007;33:1474–1478.
6. Vargas F, Bui HN, Boyer A, et al. Transnasal puncture based on echographic sinusitis evidence in mechanically ventilated patients with suspicion of nosocomial maxillary sinusitis. *Intensive Care Med.* 2006;32:858–866.
7. Jönsson P, Sahlstrand-Johnson P, Holmer NG, et al. Feasibility of measuring acoustic streaming for improved diagnosis of rhinosinusitis. *Ultrasound Med Biol.* 2008;34(2):228–238.
8. Holzapfel L, Chastang C, Demingeon G, et al. A randomized study assessing the systematic search for maxillary sinusitis in nasotracheally mechanically ventilated patients. *Am J Respir Crit Care Med.* 1999;159:695–701.
9. Marik PE. Fever in the ICU. *Chest.* 2000;117:855–869.
10. Rouby JJ, Laurent P, Gosnach M, et al. Risk factors and clinical relevance of nosocomial maxillary sinusitis in the critically ill. *Am J Respir Crit Care Med.* 1994;150: 776–783.
11. Kundra P, Kumar K, Allampalli V, et al. Use of ultrasound to assess superior and recurrent laryngeal nerve function immediately after thyroid surgery. *Anaesthesia.* 2012;67: 301–302.
12. Wang CP, Chen TC, Lou PJ, et al. Neck ultrasonography for the evaluation of the etiology of adult unilateral vocal fold paralysis. *Head Neck.* 2012;34(5):643–648.
13. Amis RJ, Gupta D, Dowdall JR, et al. Ultrasound assessment of vocal fold paresis: a correlation case series with flexible fiberoptic laryngoscopy and adding the third dimension (3-D) to vocal fold mobility assessment. *Middle East J Anesthesiol.* 2012:21(4):493–498.
14. Ng SK, Yuen HY, van Hasselt CA, et al. Combined ultrasound-endoscopy-assisted vocal fold injection for unilateral vocal cord paralysis: a case series. *Eur Radiol.* 2012;22(5):1110–1113.
15. Raphael DT, Conard FU 3rd. Ultrasound confirmation of endotracheal tube placement. *J Clin Ultrasound.* 1987;15:459–462.
16. Uya A, Spear D, Patel K, et al. Can novice sonographers accurately locate an endotracheal tube with a saline-filled cuff in a cadaver model? A pilot study. *Acad Emerg Med.* 2012;19(3):361–364.
17. Milling TJ, Jones M, Khan T, et al. Transtracheal 2-D ultrasound for identification of esophageal intubation. *J Emerg Med.* 2007;32:409–414.
18. Werner SL, Smith CE, Goldstein JR, et al. Pilot study to evaluate the accuracy of ultrasonography in confirming endotracheal tube placement. *Ann Emerg Med.* 2007;49: 75–80.
19. Ma G, Davis DP, Schmitt J, et al. The sensitivity and specificity of transcricothyroid ultrasonography to confirm endotracheal tube placement in a cadaver model. *J Emerg Med.* 2007;32:405–407.
20. Pfieffer P, Bache S, Isbye DL, et al. Verification of endotracheal intubation in obese patients—temporal comparison of ultrasound vs. auscultation and capnography. *Acta Anaesthsiol Scand.* 2012;56(5):571–576.
21. Chun R, Kirkpatrick AW, Sirois M, et al. Where's the tube? Evaluation of hand-held ultrasound in confirming endotracheal tube placement. *Prehosp Disaster Med.* 2004;19:366–369.
22. Pfieffer P, Rudolph SS, Borglum J, Isbye DL. Temporal comparison of ultrasound vs. auscultation and capnography in verification of endotracheal tube placement. *Acta Anaesthsiol Scand.* 2011;55(10):1190–1195.
23. Brun PM, Bessereau J, Cazes N, et al. Lung ultrasound associated to capnography to verify correct endotracheal tube positioning in prehospital. *Am J Emerg Med.* 2012;30(9):2080-e5–6.
24. Sim SS, Lien WC, Chou HC, et al. Ultrasonographic lung sliding sign in confirming proper endotracheal intubation during emergency intubation. *Resuscitation.* 2012;83(3):307–312.
25. Weaver B, Lyon M, Blaivas M. Confirmation of endotracheal tube placement after intubation using the sliding lung sign. *Acad Emerg Med.* 2006;13:239–244.

26. Lakhal K, Delplace X, Cottier JP, et al. The feasibility of ultrasound to assess subglottic diameter. *Anaesth Analg*. 2007;104:611–614.
27. Gupta D, Srirajakalidindi A, Hable N, Haber H. Ultrasound confirmation of laryngeal mask airway placement correlates with fiberoptic laryngoscope findings. *Middle East J Anesthesiol*. 2011;21(2):283–287.
28. Ezri T, Gewurtz G, Sessler DI, et al. Prediction of difficult laryngoscopy in obese patients by ultrasound quantification of anterior neck soft tissue. *Anaesthesia*. 2003;58:1111–1114.
29. Komatsu R, Sengupta P, Wadhwa A, et al. Ultrasound quantification of anterior soft tissue thickness fails to predict difficult laryngoscopy in obese patients. *Anaesth Intensive Care*. 2007;35:32–37.
30. Wojtczak JA. Submandibular sonography: assessment of hyomental distances and ratio, tongue size, and floor of the mouth musculature using portable sonography. *J Ultrasound Med*. 2012;31(4):523–528.
31. Lahav Y, Rosenzweig E, Heyman Z, et al. Tongue base ultrasound: a diagnostic tool for predicting obstructive sleep apnea. *Ann Oto Rhinol Laryngol*. 2009;118(3):179–184.
32. Ugur KS, Ark N, Kurtaran H, et al. Subcutaneous fat tissue thickness of the anterior neck and umbilicus in patients with obstructive sleep apnea. *Otolaryngol Head Neck Surg*. 2011;145(3):505–510.
33. Ding LW, Wang HC, Wu HD, et al. Laryngeal ultrasound: a useful method in predicting post-extubation stridor. A pilot study. *Eur Resp J*. 2006;27:384–389.
34. Bertram S, Emshoff R, Norer B. Ultrasonographic anatomy of the anterior neck: implications for tracheostomy. *J Oral Maxillofac Surg*. 1995;53:1420–1424.
35. Sustic A, Zupan Z. Ultrasound guided tracheal puncture for non-surgical tracheostomy. *Intensive Care Med*. 1998;24:92–98.
36. Bonde J, Norgaard N, Antonsen K, et al. Implementation of percutaneous dilation tracheotomy-value of preincisional ultrasonic examination? *Acta Anaesthesiol Scand*. 1999;43:163–166.
37. Hatfield A, Bodenham A. Portable ultrasonic scanning of the anterior neck before percutaneous dilational tracheostomy. *Anaesthesia*. 1999;54:660–663.
38. Muhammad JK, Patton DW, Evans RM, et al. Percutaneous dilational tracheostomy under ultrasound guidance. *Br J Oral Maxillofac Surg*. 1999;37:309–311.
39. Sustic A, Zupan Z, Eskinja N, et al. Ultrasonographically guided percutaneous dilational tracheostomy after anterior cervical spine fixation. *Act Anaesthesiol Scand*. 1999;43:1078–1080.
40. Muhammad JK, Major E, Patton DW. Evaluating the neck for percutaneous dilational tracheostomy. *J Craniomaxillofac Surg*. 2000;28:336–342.
41. Shlugman D, Satya-Krishna R, Loh L. Acute fatal haemorrhage during percutaneous tracheostomy. *Br J Anaesth*. 2003;90:517–520.
42. Gwilym S, Cooney A. Acute fatal haemorrhage during percutaneous trachestomy. *Br J Anaesth*. 2004;92:298.
43. Muhammad JK, Major E, Wood A, et al. Percutaneous tracheostomy: hemorrhagic complications and the vascular anatomy of the anterior neck. A review based on 497 cases. *Int J Oral Maxillofac Surg*. 2000;29:217–222.
44. Sustic A, Kovac D, Zgaljardic Z, et al. Ultrasound guided percutaneous dilational tracheostomy: a safe method to avoid cranial misplacement of the tracheostomy tube. *Intensive Care Med*. 2000;26:1379–1381.
45. Reilly PM, Sing RF, Giberson FA, et al. Hypercarbia during tracheostomy: a comparison of percutaneous endoscopic, percutaneous Doppler, and standard surgical tracheostomy. *Intensive Care Med*. 1997;23:859–864.

ULTRASOUND EVALUATION OF THE PLEURA

LEWIS EISEN, PETER DOELKEN, & SAHAR AHMAD

Scan QR code or visit www.ccu2e.com for video in this chapter

INTRODUCTION

As early as 1967, it was apparent that ultrasound was ideally suited for the detection of pleural effusions.[1] In addition, thoracic ultrasonography can also detect less common pleural pathology, guide thoracentesis, and other pleural procedures. As a result, its role for critical care physicians has become increasingly important.

GENERAL CONSIDERATIONS IN PLEURAL ULTRASOUND

Ultrasound examination of the pleura is influenced by the surrounding structures. The ribs block ultrasound waves and prevent deeper structures from being visualized. In contrast, air reflects ultrasound. The surface of aerated lung will reflect most of the ultrasound waves. The point of reflection is immediately below the pleura. However, if the lung is consolidated or atelectatic, it can be readily visualized.

In addition to the artifacts seen in other aspects of medical ultrasonography, there are specific artifacts, such as rib shadowing, that are found commonly in pleural ultrasound. Air reverberation artifacts, which originate below the pleura, are another artifact type that can be commonly observed by clinicians (see Chapter 19). Translational artifacts, due to patient breathing or mechanical ventilation, may also confuse the examiner.[2]

Obesity and subcutaneous edema can degrade image quality. Significant edema may also present problems in judging the depth for procedures. The presence of subcutaneous air will make visualization of deeper structures problematic. The use of firm pressure on the skin and the use of a coupling medium will reduce some artifacts. Artifacts are often visible in only one scanning plane, so changing the probe angle may cause artifacts to disappear. Further, artifacts usually will not move with the respiratory cycle. The observation of an image throughout several respiratory cycles often helps to clarify the issue.

ULTRASOUND MACHINE REQUIREMENTS AND MACHINE CONTROL

Pleural ultrasonography can be performed with many different types of two-dimensional ultrasound machines. Doppler capability is not needed. A probe with a small "footprint" to easily fit between rib spaces should be used. The preferred ultrasound probe is a phased array transducer with a frequency of 2–5 MHz (typically 3.5 MHz) that may also be used for cardiac ultrasonography. Probes with higher frequencies can visualize the pleural surface, but lack adequate penetration for clinical applications that require visualization of deeper thoracic structures.

In order to standardize image interpretation, the use of uniform probe orientation and a screen marker is required. The machine should be set up, so that the image marker on the screen is in the upper left corner of the screen. When using the longitudinal scanning plane, the probe should be oriented with the probe marker positioned cephalad. If this orientation is maintained, the cephalad direction will always be to the left of the screen.

The gain and depth should be adjusted so that the chest wall, pleural surfaces, and deeper structures, such as the liver or spleen, with overlying diaphragm are well visualized. It is recommended that the depth setting first be set to near-maximum depth, which allows for an overview of deep structures; and then can be adjusted so that the relevant target is in the center of the screen. When better visualization of the pleural surface and superficial structures is required, the depth setting can be adjusted to allow for examination of near-field structures. Alternatively, a higher frequency transducer may be used to improve resolution of near-field structures, though with resulting reduction in penetration.

NORMAL PLEURAL EXAMINATION

The pleural ultrasound examination should be performed in a systematic fashion. With the probe applied in a rib interspace using a longitudinal scanning plane, the pleural surface appears as a bright line between the chest wall and the air artifact of the lung or the pleural effusion. By sliding the probe longitudinally along the chest wall, adjacent interspaces can be examined. After completing an entire scan line, the probe can be moved medially or laterally and another scan line can be obtained. In this way, a near-complete mapping of the pleura can be obtained.

The diaphragmatic pleura can be viewed through a transhepatic approach. On the patient's left side, in the absence of pleural fluid, the full length of the diaphragmatic pleura may be difficult to identify due to the presence of aerated lung that blocks ultrasonographic visualization of the structure. The mediastinal pleura generally cannot be visualized with a transthoracic probe. The visceral subcostal pleura may be obscured by rib shadowing. Changing the probe angle or altering the patient's position can overcome this problem.

The normal pleura is 0.2–0.4 mm thick.[3] Although the frequency of the probe used for general ultrasonography does not allow for resolution of the individual parietal and visceral pleura, this does not have clinical relevance for the intensivist. A complete ultrasound examination of the pleura in the ambulatory patient is usually performed with the patient in an upright position. This poses particular problems for the intensivist, because patients are often in the supine position while mechanically ventilated and sedated. Fortunately, many pleural abnormalities can be detected via an anterior and lateral thoracic examination of a supine patient. If the posterior chest must be examined, the supine patient may be placed in a lateral decubitus position. If a major change in a patient's position is required to perform pleural ultrasonogaphy, the intensivist must pay careful attention to support lines and tubes to avoid unplanned device removal.

PLEURAL EFFUSION

Pleural effusion is a common problem in the intensive care unit (ICU). Mattison et al. reported a prevalence of 62% in medical ICU patients.[4] The most common causes were heart failure, atelectasis, parapneumonic effusion, and hepatic hydrothorax. Malignancy accounted for 3.2% and empyema accounted for 1.6%. Compared with patients without effusions, patients with effusions are sicker and have longer ICU stays and longer durations of mechanical ventilation.

Ultrasonography is well suited for the identification and evaluation of fluid, because fluid is less echogenic than soft tissue. Many studies have demonstrated the usefulness of ultrasound for this indication. Pleural effusions as small as 3–5 mm can be detected ultrasonographically.[5] Clinical examination is neither sensitive nor specific for the detection of pleural effusion.[6] Pleural ultrasonography is superior to standard chest radiography in detecting the presence of pleural effusions and in distinguishing pleural effusions from atelectasis or pleural thickening.[5,7] Compared with the reference standard of chest computerized tomography (CT) scan, pleural ultrasound has 93% sensitivity and specificity for pleural effusions.[8] When a patient has complete opacification of a hemithorax, ultrasound has 95% sensitivity for pleural effusion.[9]

The supine chest radiograph in patients in the ICU has poor performance characteristics for the detection of pleural fluid. ICU radiographs suffer from problems with penetration, rotation, and magnification. In the supine patient, pleural effusions accumulate in dependent areas. Thoracic opacities in a supine chest radiograph may be caused by a pleural effusion, a parenchymal process, such as consolidation, or by a combination of these processes. Pleural ultrasound outperforms chest radiography when compared with chest CT for identification of pleuropulmonary abnormalities.[8] Intensive care unit radiographs often cannot distinguish between pleural and parenchymal abnormalities.[10–12] In a series of ICU patients, supine radiographs detected only 61.4% of pleural effusions when compared with those detected by ultrasound.[13]

Free-flowing pleural effusions layer posteriorly in the thorax of the supine patient. Patients with multiple lines or a compromised hemodynamic and oxygenation status are difficult to position sitting upright in bed. If the patient is supine, the bed mattress may prevent the easy visualization of small pleural effusions. One option is for the examiner to place the transducer in the posterior axillary line while angling the probe up toward the center of the body to visualize smaller effusions. In unstable patients, who have effusions that are difficult to visualize, positioning the patient in a lateral decubitus position may be helpful. The examiner should always identify three findings (Figure 18-1) indicating the presence of a pleural effusion:

1. Anatomic boundaries: This requires definitive identification of the diaphragm and subdiaphragmatic organs (liver and spleen, depending on the side), the heart

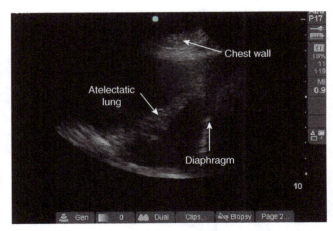

Figure 18-1 This image shows the typical anatomic boundaries that surround a hypoechoic pleural effusion. The image is obtained using a transducer. The 3.5 MHz transducer is in longitudinal orientation and placed perpendicular to the chest wall to scan through the 8th intercostal space in the right mid-axillary line.

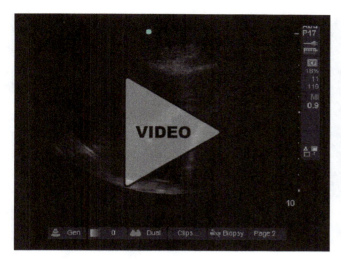

Video 18-1 This video shows the typical anatomic boundaries that surround a hypoechoic pleural effusion. The 3.5 MHz transducer is in longitudinal orientation and placed perpendicular to the chest wall to scan through the 8th intercostal space in the right mid-axillary line. View at www.ccu2e.com

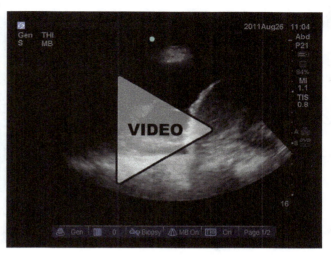

Video 18-2 This video shows the typical anatomic boundaries that surround a hypoechoic pleural effusion. The 3.5 MHz transducer is in longitudinal orientation and placed perpendicular to the chest wall to scan through the 8th intercostal space in the right mid-axillary line. View at www.ccu2e.com

(on the left side), the chest wall, and the surface of the lung (Figure 18-1 and Video 18-1).

2. Hypoechoic space: This requires definitive identification of a relatively echo-free space surrounded by the typical anatomic boundaries that is the pleural effusion (Figure 18-2 and Video 18-2).

3. Dynamic changes: This requires definitive identification of dynamic changes that are characteristic of a pleural effusion (Videos 18-3 and 18-4).

Definitive identification of the diaphragm is essential in order to localize a pleural effusion. This is required for safe thoracentesis, as inadvertent subdiaphragmatic device insertion is a potentially catastrophic complication of thoracentesis. By scanning in the mid to posterior axillary line, the diaphragm is identified as a curvilinear structure above the liver or spleen that has respirophasic movement (Figure 18-3 and Video 18-5). An occasional error of the inexperienced scanner is to mistake the hepatorenal or splenorenal space for the diaphragm and the overlying liver or spleen as an echo dense pleural effusion. Careful attention to ultrasonographic anatomy is required to avoid this dangerous pitfall.

Generally, pleural fluid is less echogenic than the adjacent liver or spleen. A complex pleural effusion may have

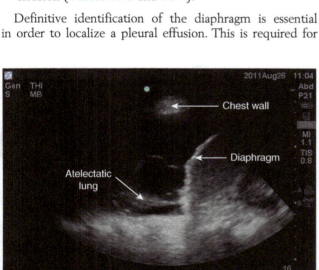

Figure 18-2 This image shows a relatively hypoechoic space surrounded by typical anatomic boundaries: the chest wall, the surface of the lung, and the diaphragm. The 3.5 MHz transducer is in longitudinal orientation and placed perpendicular to the chest wall to scan through the 8th intercostal space in the right mid-axillary line.

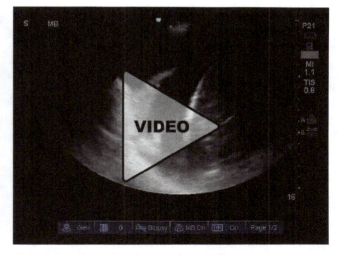

Video 18-3 This video shows a pleural effusion with respirophasic and cardiophasic movement of atelectatic lung. The 3.5 MHz transducer is in longitudinal orientation and placed perpendicular to the chest wall to scan through the 7th intercostal space in the right mid-axillary line. View at www.ccu2e.com

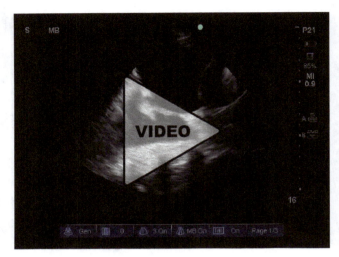

Video 18-4 This video shows a pleural effusion with respirophasic and cardiophasic movement of echogenic elements within the effusion. The 3.5 MHz transducer is in longitudinal orientation and placed perpendicular to the chest wall to scan through the 6th intercostal space in the left mid-axillary line. View at www.ccu2e.com

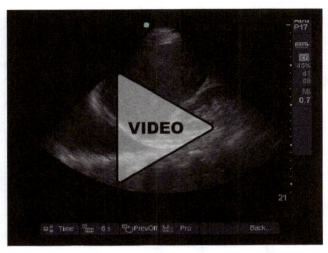

Video 18-5 This video shows a pleural effusion, the diaphragm, and liver and the kidney. Definitive identification of the diaphragm is essential in order to localize a pleural effusion. This is required for safe thoracentesis, as inadvertent subdiaphragmatic device insertion is a potentially catastrophic complication of thoracentesis. The 3.5 MHz transducer is in longitudinal orientation and placed perpendicular to the chest wall to scan through the 9th intercostal space in the right mid-axillary line. View at www.ccu2e.com

echogenicity similar to these organs. The inside of the chest wall, because it is a stationary structure, should not undergo dynamic changes with respiration. Lung tissue will generally become atelectatic when it is compressed by the neighboring pleural effusion and appears as a tissue density structure on ultrasonographic examination (Figure 18-4 and Video 18-6). This is termed sonographic hepatization of lung, as sonographically, atelectatic lung has the same echodensity as liver. The compressed lung can be visualized floating in the pleural fluid. This has been termed lung flapping or the jellyfish sign (Video 18-7). Aerated lung may move into the scanning field during the respiratory cycle. Interposition of aerated lung into the scanning plane will block visualization of deeper structures. This has been termed the curtain sign (Video 18-8). If the operator is familiar with M-mode ultrasound, examination of the pleural surface generally will show a sinusoid sign, indicating dynamic movement of the pleural surface within a fluid-filled space (Figure 18-5).[14]

Other findings characteristic of pleural effusions include the plankton sign, which is caused by swirling debris agitated by cardiac or respiratory motion in a pleural effusion (Video 18-9). Fibrin strands may be seen moving in synchronization with cardiac pulsations or respiratory motion (Video 18-10). These strands may be visibly connected to

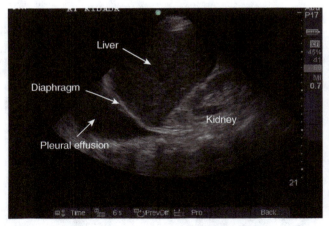

Figure 18-3 This image shows a pleural effusion above the diaphragm, the liver, the hepatorenal space, and the kidney. These structures must be positively identified before thoracentesis in order to avoid inadvertent subdiaphragmatic device insertion. The 3.5 MHz transducer is in longitudinal orientation and placed perpendicular to the chest wall to scan through the 9th intercostal space in the right mid-axillary line.

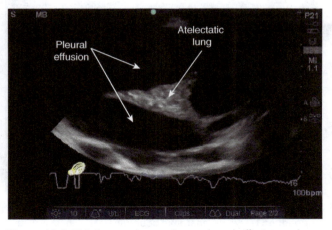

Figure 18-4 This image shows a large pleural effusion and atelectatic lung. The 3.5 MHz transducer is in longitudinal orientation and placed perpendicular to the chest wall to scan through the 6th intercostal space in the left mid-axillary line.

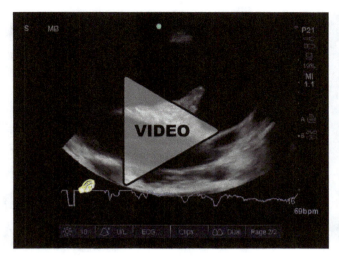

Video 18-6 This video shows a large pleural effusion and atelectatic lung. The 3.5 MHz transducer is in longitudinal orientation and placed perpendicular to the chest wall to scan through the 6th intercostal space in the right mid-axillary line. View at www.ccu2e.com

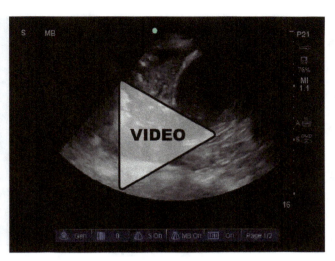

Video 18-8 This video shows a small pleural effusion and adjacent alveolar consolidation of the lung. With each inspiration, aerated lung is interposed into the imaging window with loss of visualization of the underlying structures. This is termed the curtain sign. The 3.5 MHz transducer is in longitudinal orientation and placed perpendicular to the chest wall to scan through the 8th intercostal space in the left mid-axillary line. View at www.ccu2e.com

one or more of the pleural surfaces. The hematocrit sign may be observed in cases of cellular pleural effusions of different etiologies. The effusion is layered into two phases of different echogenicity by gravitational effect (Video 18-11).

In addition to the identification of a pleural effusion, the examiner should seek to characterize the fluid and quantify its amount. Several authors have developed rules to quantify the amount of fluid in the pleural space with reasonable accuracy.[15–18] In most circumstances, it is sufficient to qualitatively judge a pleural effusion as small, moderate, or large. Semiquantitative measures based on the degree of extension of the anechoic space from the costophrenic angle have been used to identify outpatients with varying degrees of worsening heart failure. In a prospective analysis, the finding of pleural effusion by ultrasound was strongly associated with worsened heart failure status, including serum B-type natriuretic peptide elevation above baseline, with semiquantitative volume being larger in symptomatic patients.[19]

The echogenicity of the fluid should be characterized. Transudates are almost always anechoic.[20] However, they may also have a complex nonseptated pattern.[21] They do not have a homogenous hyperechoic or septated pattern. Highly cellular exudates may be homogenously echogenic. Echogenic swirling patterns are suggestive of

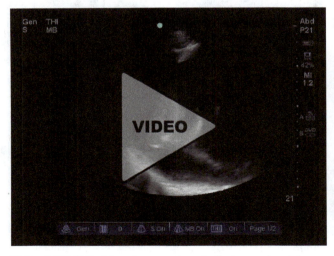

Video 18-7 This video shows a pleural effusion and mobile atelectatic lung. This is termed lung flapping or the jellyfish sign. The 3.5 MHz transducer is in longitudinal orientation and placed perpendicular to the chest wall to scan through the 7th intercostal space in the right mid-axillary line. View at www.ccu2e.com

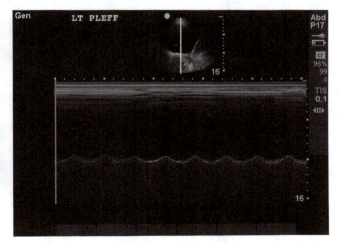

Figure 18-5 This image shows an M-mode of a pleural effusion demonstrating respirophasic movement of the lung. This is a convenient method of documenting the presence of a pleural effusion without the need for a video clip.

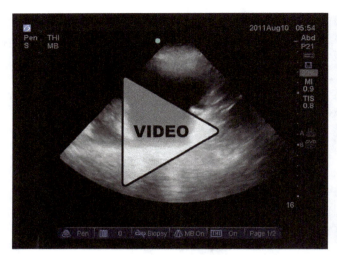

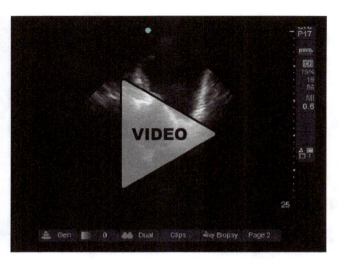

Video 18-9 This video shows a pleural effusion with respirophasic and cardiophasic movement of echogenic elements within the effusion. This is termed the plankton sign. The 3.5 MHz transducer is in longitudinal orientation and placed perpendicular to the chest wall to scan through the 7th intercostal space in the right mid-axillary line. View at www.ccu2e.com

Video 18-11 This video shows a pleural effusion with well-demarcated interface between an echogenic-dependent layer and an anechoic nondependent layer. This is termed the hematocrit sign, and is caused by gravitational effect on cellular components of the fluid. The 3.5 MHz transducer is in longitudinal orientation and placed perpendicular to the chest wall to scan through the 6th intercostal space in the left mid-axillary line. View at www.ccu2e.com

exudates (particularly malignant effusion; Videos 18-12 and 18-13); however, this pattern can also be seen occasionally in transudative effusions.[22] Exudative effusions may have an echogenic pattern that is not homogenous. Debris, strands, or septations may be visible. In the case of parapneumonic effusions, these structures indicate either a complicated parapneumonic effusion or an empyema.[23] Patients with septated effusions visible on ultrasonography require longer hospital stays, longer chest tube drainage, and more often require fibrinolytic therapy or surgery for

adequate drainage (Figures 18-6 and 18-7; Videos 18-14 and 18-15).[21] Pleural ultrasound is superior to CT scan in visualizing septations within a pleural effusion.[24]

The most complicated effusions are loculated. Loculated effusions characteristically occur in a nondependent position and do not move with changes in body position. Loculated effusions often appear as thick-walled circular fluid collections. A complete pleural ultrasound is required to identify the presence of a loculated effusion because its position may be nondependent.

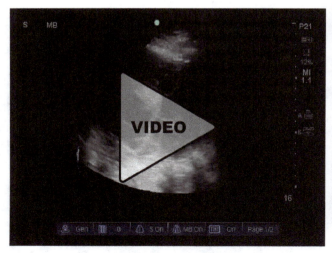

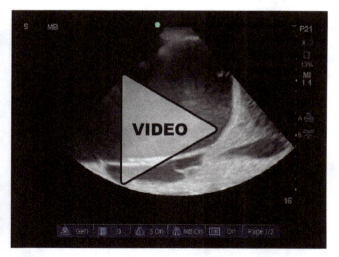

Video 18-10 This video shows a pleural effusion with respirophasic and cardiophasic movement of echogenic strands within the effusion. The 3.5 MHz transducer is in longitudinal orientation and placed perpendicular to the chest wall to scan through the 6th intercostal space in the left posterior axillary line. View at www.ccu2e.com

Video 18-12 This video shows a swirling echogenic pleural effusion that is typical of an acute hemothorax. The diaphragm has a reverse curvature and there is a defect in the descending aorta consistent with traumatic laceration. The 3.5 MHz transducer is in longitudinal orientation and placed perpendicular to the chest wall to scan through the 8th intercostal space in the left posterior axillary line. View at www.ccu2e.com

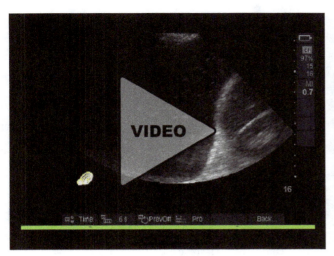

Video 18-13 This video shows a pleural effusion in which are multiple punctate echogenic foci that represent bubbles within the effusion. This was caused by an esophageal perforation. The 3.5 MHz transducer is in longitudinal orientation and placed perpendicular to the chest wall to scan through the 8th intercostal space in the left mid-axillary line. View at www.ccu2e.com

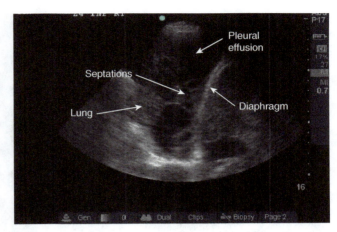

Figure 18-7 This image shows a multiseptated pleural effusion in a subpulmonic position. This pattern is consistent with a complex parapneumonic effusion or empyema that will require fibrinolytic treatment or surgical drainage The 3.5 MHz transducer is in longitudinal orientation and placed perpendicular to the chest wall to scan through the 7th intercostal space in the left mid-axillary line.

Once a pleural fluid has been characterized by ultrasound, the intensivist is left with the question of whether a thoracentesis should be performed. Thoracentesis is a safe procedure in the ICU, even in mechanically ventilated patients.[13,25–29] For a particular patient, the intensivist should assess the risk and benefits of thoracentesis. The intensivist should observe multiple respiratory cycles to avoid interposition of any vital structure.[30]

When the feasibility is assured, thoracentesis may be performed for diagnostic or therapeutic reasons (see Chapter 24). Tu et al. studied 94 febrile ICU patients with pleural effusions. A total of 61.7% had infectious exudates of which 15/95 (16.0%) were empyemas. Subgroup analysis of those patients with empyema showed that all of the patients with empyema had either a complex hyperechoic pattern, a complex septated pattern, or a homogenously echogenic pattern. They concluded that in the febrile patient, nonechoic and hypoechoic effusions do not require immediate thoracentesis because they are unlikely to represent empyemas.[23] Fartoukh et al. studied routine thoracentesis of pleural effusions in the ICU. They concluded that of the 82 patients without contraindication to thoracentesis,

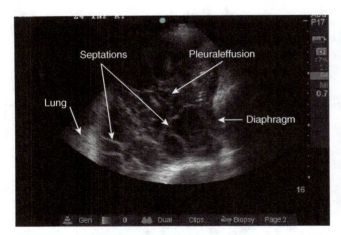

Figure 18-6 This image shows a multiseptated pleural effusion. This pattern is consistent with a complex parapneumonic effusion or empyema that will require fibrinolytic treatment or surgical drainage The 3.5 MHz transducer is in longitudinal orientation and placed perpendicular to the chest wall to scan through the 8th intercostal space in the left mid-axillary line.

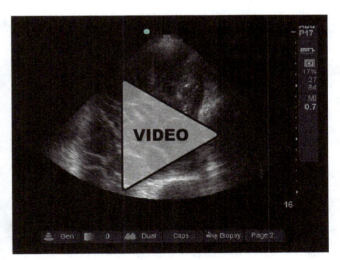

Video 18-14 This video shows a multiseptated pleural effusion. This pattern is consistent with a complex parapneumonic effusion or empyema that will require fibrinolytic treatment or surgical drainage The 3.5 MHz transducer is in longitudinal orientation and placed perpendicular to the chest wall to scan through the 8th intercostal space in the left mid-axillary line. View at www.ccu2e.com

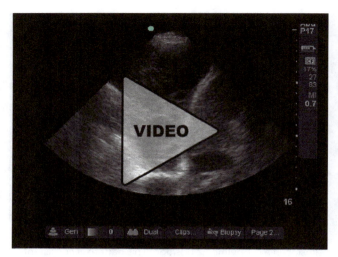

Video 18-15 This video shows a multiseptated pleural effusion. This pattern is consistent with a complex parapneumonic effusion or empyema that will require fibrinolytic treatment or surgical drainage. The 3.5 MHz transducer is in longitudinal orientation and placed perpendicular to the chest wall to scan through the 7th intercostal space in the left mid-axillary line. View at www.ccu2e.com

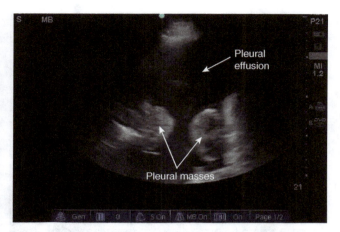

Figure 18-8 This image shows a pleural effusion with pleural masses caused by metastatic breast cancer. The 3.5 MHz transducer is in longitudinal orientation and placed perpendicular to the chest wall to scan through the 7th intercostal space in the left mid-axillary line.

the presumptive diagnosis was changed in 45.1% of the patients and treatment was changed in 35.4%.[25] This evidence indicates that, in an ICU patient meeting standard indications, thoracentesis should be performed.

The benefits of therapeutic thoracentesis have been harder to prove. Ahmed et al. performed thoracentesis on 22 ventilated patients in the surgical ICU. The mean fluid removed was 1262 mL. Drainage of pleural effusions resulted in increased oxygen delivery and consumption. There was a reduction in pulmonary capillary wedge pressure, and the pulmonary arteriovenous shunt decreased.[31] Chen et al. described an oxygenation benefit to US-guided thoracentesis in a population of mechanically ventilated medical ICU patients with heart failure. The greatest improvement in paO_2 and PaO_2/FiO_2 after therapeutic thoracentesis was seen in patients with normal pleural elastance, smaller change in pleural pressures, and larger volume of pleural fluid evacuated.[32] Doelken et al. demonstrated a reduction in the work of breathing after thoracentesis in eight patients receiving mechanical ventilation; however, no change in respiratory system resistance, compliance, intrinsic positive end-expiratory pressure, or gas exchange was evident.[33] Kupfer et al. found that US-guided positioning of small bore chest tube drainage of pleural effusion expedited liberation from mechanical ventilation. While this was a retrospective nonrandomized analysis, safety for the procedure under US guidance was established.[34] Because all of these individual measurements offered only a limited assessment of a complex system, the clinician should weigh the risks and benefits of thoracentesis in each patient. In our opinion, thoracentesis of large pleural effusions helps liberate patients from mechanical ventilation; however, more research in this area is required.

SOLID PLEURAL ABNORMALITIES

A variety of solid pleural abnormalities may be visualized as echogenic structures within the pleural space (Figure 18-8 and Video 18-16). Benign pleural tumors, such as benign mesothelioma, lipomas, or chondromas, may be seen. They will be surrounded by a distinct capsule and will not invade tissue planes. A complementary imaging modality may be required for confirmation. Pleural ultrasound has utility in the diagnosis of pleural malignancy. Sonographic findings which hold a 73% sensitivity and 100% specificity for malignant disease at the pleura include pleural thickening to greater than 10 mm, diaphragmatic thickening to greater than 7 mm, and pleural nodularity.[35] Malignant

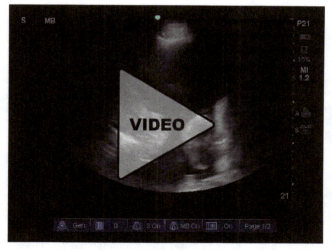

Video 18-16 This video shows a pleural effusion with pleural masses caused by metastatic breast cancer. The 3.5 MHz transducer is in longitudinal orientation and placed perpendicular to the chest wall to scan through the 7th intercostal space in the left mid-axillary line. View at www.ccu2e.com

mesothelioma will have hypoechoic thickening of the pleural surface with irregular or indistinct borders. Malignant mesothelioma may invade the diaphragm or chest wall. It may also be nodular in character. Pleural metastatic disease will often be accompanied by a pleural effusion. Metastatic lesions are frequently multiple. Their echogenicity is variable. Chest wall and diaphragmatic invasion will be apparent. Two case series demonstrated the value and accuracy of ultrasound for detecting chest wall invasion by lung cancer.[36,37] Pleural fibrosis is the end-result of multiple types of pleural injury. Pleural thickening will be evident. Respiratory movement will be diminished or absent at this location.[38] In addition to helping to characterize lesions, pleural ultrasonography is ideally suited for guiding biopsy.

CONCLUSION

Pleural ultrasonography allows the intensivist to identify, characterize, and access pleural effusions. Ultrasonographic diagnosis of a pleural effusion requires the identification of a relatively hypoechoic space surrounded by typical anatomic boundaries (the diaphragm and underlying liver or spleen, the heart on the left side, the chest wall, and the surface of the lung) in association with characteristic dynamic changes.

REFERENCES

1. Joyner CR Jr, Herman RJ, Reid JM. Reflected ultrasound in the detection and localization of pleural effusion. *JAMA*. 1967;200:399–402.
2. Schuler A. Image artifacts and pitfalls. In: Mathis G, Lessnau KD, eds. *Atlas of Chest Sonography*. Berlin, Germany: Springer-Verlag; 2003:137–145.
3. Reuss J. The pleura. In: Mathis G, Lessnau KD, eds. *Atlas of Chest Sonography*. Berlin, Germany: Springer-Verlag; 2003:17–35.
4. Mattison LE, Coppage L, Alderman DF, et al. Pleural effusions in the medical ICU: prevalence causes and clinical implications. *Chest*. 1997;111:1018–1023.
5. Gryminski J, Krakowka P, Lypaceqicq G. The diagnosis of pleural effusion by ultrasonic and radiologic techniques. *Chest*. 1976;70:33–37.
6. Diacon AH, Brutsche MH, Soler M. Accuracy of pleural puncture site: a prospective comparison of clinical examination with ultrasound. *Chest*. 2003;123:436–441.
7. Kelbel C, Borner N, Schadmand S, et al. Diagnosis of pleural effusions and atelectasis: sonography and radiology compared. *Rofo*. 1991;154:159–163.
8. Lichtenstein D, Goldstein I, Mourgeon E, et al. Comparative diagnostic performances of auscultation, chest radiography, and lung ultrasonography in acute respiratory distress syndrome. *Anesthesiology*. 2004;100:9–15.
9. Yu C, Yang P, Chang D, et al. Diagnostic and therapeutic use of chest sonography: value in critically ill patients. *AJR*. 1992;159:695–701.
10. Mirvis SE, Tobin KD, Kostrubiak I, et al. Thoracic CT in detecting occult disease in critically ill patients. *AJR*. 1987;148:685–689.
11. Overfors C, Hedgecock MW. Intensive care unit radiology: problems of interpretation. *Radiol Clin North Am*. 1978;16:407–409.
12. Yu CJ, Yang PC, Wu HD, et al. Ultrasound study in unilateral hemithorax opacification: image comparison with computed tomography. *Am Rev Respir Dis*. 1993;147:430–434.
13. Lichtenstein DA, Hulot JS, Rabiller A, et al. Feasibility and safety of ultrasound-aided thoracentesis in mechanically ventilated patients. *Intensive Care Med*. 1999;25:955–958.
14. Lichtenstein DA. Pleural effusion and introduction to lung ultrasound. In: Lichtenstein DA, ed. *General Ultrasound in the Critically Ill*. Berlin, Germany: Springer-Verlag; 2005;96-104.
15. Balik M, Plasil P, Waldauf P, et al. Ultrasound estimation of volume of pleural fluid in mechanically ventilated patients. *Intensive Care Med*. 2006;32:318–321.
16. Eibenberger KL, Dock WI, Ammann ME, et al. Quantification of pleural effusions: sonography versus radiography. *Radiology*. 1994;191:681–684.
17. Roch AMD, Bojan M, Michelet P, et al. Usefulness of ultrasonography in predicting pleural effusions >500 ml in patients receiving mechanical ventilation. *Chest*. 2005;127:224–232.
18. Vignon P, Castagner C, Berkane V, et al. Quantitative assessment of pleural effusion in critically ill patients by means of ultrasonography. *Crit Care Med*. 2005;33:1757–1763.
19. Kataoka H. Ultrasound pleural effusion sign as a useful marker for identifying heart failure worsening in established heart failure patients during follow-up. *Congest Heart Fail*. 2012;18(5):272–277.
20. Yang PC, Luh KT, Chang DB, et al. Value of sonography in determining the nature of pleural effusion: analysis of 320 cases. *AJR Am J Roentgenol*. 1992;159:29–33.
21. Chen HJ, Tu CY, Ling SJ. Sonographic appearances in transudative pleural effusions: not always an anechoic pattern. *Ultrasound Med Biol*. 2008;34:362–369.
22. Chian CF, Su WL, Soh LH, et al. Echogenic swirling pattern as a predictor of malignant pleural effusions in patients with malignancies. *Chest*. 2004;126:129–134.
23. Tu CY, Hsu WH, Hsia TC, et al. Pleural effusions in febrile medical ICU patients chest ultrasound study. *Chest*. 2004;126:1274–1280.
24. McLoud TC, Flower CD. Imaging the pleura: sonography, CT, and MR imaging. *Am J Roentgenol*. 1991;156:1145–1153.
25. Fartoukh M, Azoulay E, Galliot R, et al. Clinically documented pleural effusions in medical ICU patients: how useful is routine thoracentesis? *Chest*. 2002;121:178–184.
26. Gervais DA, Petersein A, Lee MJ, et al. US-guided thoracentesis: requirement for postprocedure chest radiography in patients who receive mechanical ventilation versus patients who breathe spontaneously. *Radiology*. 1997;204:503–506.
27. Godwin JE, Sahn SA. Thoracentesis: a safe procedure in mechanically ventilated patients. *Ann Intern Med*. 1990;113:800–802.
28. Mayo PH, Goltz HR, Tafreshi M, et al. Safety of ultrasound-guided thoracentesis in patients receiving mechanical ventilation. *Chest*. 2004;125:1059–1062.
29. McCartney JP, Adams JW, Hazard PB. Safety of thoracentesis in mechanically ventilated patients. *Chest*. 1993;103:1920–1921.
30. Lichtenstein DA. Ultrasound in the management of thoracic disease. *Crit Care Med*. 2007;735:S250–S261.

31. Ahmed SH, Ouzounian SP, Dirusso S, et al. Hemodynamic and pulmonary changes after drainage of significant pleural effusions in critically ill, mechanically ventilated surgical patients. *J Trauma*. 2004;57:1184–1188.
32. Chen WL, Chung CL, Hsiao SH, Chang SC. Pleural space elastance and changes in oxygenation after therapeutic thoracentesis in ventilated patients with heart failure and transudative pleural effusions. *Respirology*. 2010;15(6):1001–1008.
33. Doelken P, Abreu R, Sahn S, et al. Effect of thoracentesis on respiratory mechanics and gas exchange in the patient receiving mechanical ventilation. *Chest*. 2006;130:1354–1361.
34. Kupfer Y, Seneviratne C, Chawla K, Ramachandran K, Tessler S. Chest tube drainage of transudative pleural effusions hastens liberation from mechanical ventilation. *Chest*. 2011;139(3):519–523.
35. Qureshi NR, Rahm an NM, Gleeson FV. Thoracic ultrasound in the diagnosis of malignant pleural effusion. *Thorax*. 2009;64:139–143.
36. Suzuki N, Siatoh T, Kitamura S. Tumor invasion of the chest wall in lung cancer: diagnosis with US. *Radiology*. 1993;187:39–42.
37. Sugama Y, Tamaki S, Kitamura S, et al. Ultrasonographic evaluation of pleural and chest wall invasion of lung cancer. *Chest*. 1988;93:275–279.
38. Mayo PH, Doelken P. Pleural ultrasonography. *Clin Chest Med*. 2006;27:215–227.

ULTRASOUND EVALUATION OF THE LUNG

PIERRE KORY & PAUL H. MAYO

Scan QR code or visit www.ccu2e.com for video in this chapter

INTRODUCTION

Lung ultrasonography is easy to learn, simple to perform, and has strong clinical utility for the critical care clinician. Interestingly, radiologists have not been instrumental in developing critical care applications of lung ultrasonography. Perhaps because lung ultrasonography in the intensive care unit (ICU) is a purely bedside technique, it required a frontline ICU clinician to develop the field. Dr. Daniel Lichtenstein is responsible for developing critical care lung ultrasonography. In the 1990s, he established the principles of the field and developed the semiology of lung ultrasonography that is in current use.[1] Based on his original and continued work, in the past few years there have been numerous published studies from other groups, which have served to validate and expand the field. This section will review critical care applications of lung ultrasonography.

BASIC PRINCIPLES OF LUNG ULTRASONOGRAPHY

Air is the enemy of the ultrasonographer. There is a large difference in the acoustic impedance and velocity of ultrasound between tissue and air. This leads to complete reflection of the ultrasound wave at the first air–tissue interface. When combined with the unfavorable attenuation coefficient of air, this leads to a pattern of repeating horizontal lines consistent with a reverberation artifact or a homogeneous amorphic grayness that occupies the ultrasound screen deep to the tissue–air interface. This frustrates any attempt to scan through air to deeper body structures.

The alveolar lung parenchyma is normally filled with air; so well-aerated lung is not visible as a discreet structural entity with ultrasonography, as the ultrasound waves are blocked and reflected by air. When a disease process reduces the amount of air within the lung, ultrasound findings change in a predictable fashion. Atelectatic lung is airless so it appears as a discrete structure with tissue echogenicity. Likewise, lung that is consolidated from pneumonia appears as a well-defined hyperechoic structure. Lung that is edematous, though still aerated, has ultrasonographic findings that are different from normally aerated lung. One of the limitations of lung ultrasonography is that abnormalities that do not involve the pleural surface cannot be visualized, such as focal lesions surrounded by aerated lung. Fortunately, most lung processes that are of interest to the intensivist (e.g., pneumonia, hydrostatic pulmonary edema, lesional edema) extend to the periphery of the lung.

MACHINE REQUIREMENTS

Lung ultrasonography may be performed with a wide variety of ultrasound machines with two-dimensional (2D) scanning capability. It was fully described using a machine manufactured in 1990. A 3.5–5.0 MHz transducer of convex sector design works well. Vascular transducers of higher frequency may also yield serviceable images, although the examination may be limited by a lack of penetration in the larger patient. A microconvex transducer has the advantage that it fits well between rib interspaces. As lung ultrasonography will generally be performed in the context of a whole body approach, many groups use a phased array cardiac transducer for general critical care ultrasonography (lung, pleura, abdominal) to reduce cost. The small footprint of the cardiac transducer permits scanning between rib interspaces. Some machines allow the phased array cardiac transducer to be quickly configured with settings that are optimized for abdominal and thoracic imaging. Transducers of linear design may be used, but these are difficult to use in a longitudinal scanning orientation in the thin individual. Paradoxically, high-end, recent generation ultrasound machines may yield inferior lung ultrasound images compared with machines from the 1990s. Complex image smoothing technology that is appropriate for advanced cardiac imaging may provide suboptimal results for lung ultrasonography.

PERFORMANCE OF LUNG ULTRASONOGRAPHY

By convention, lung ultrasonography is generally performed in a longitudinal scanning plane with the transducer held perpendicular to the skin surface. Multiple sites on the chest are scanned in sequence. It is advisable to scan the thorax using a standard section approach, as results can then be reported in reference to a particular area. Many patients who are critically ill are in a supine position. This presents a challenge to the ultrasonographer, as the posterior thorax may be difficult to image by virtue of being blocked by the surface of the bed. For the purpose of scanning an ICU patient, the chest may be divided into anterior, lateral, and posterior areas. The anterior area is bordered by the sternum and the anterior axillary line, while the posterior axillary line borders the lateral and posterior areas. The posterior thorax is an important area to image because the majority of pleural effusions and consolidations are found in the dependent thorax. To image these areas, the transducer must be pressed into the mattress with the probe face angled anteriorly. Alternatively, the patient may be rolled to a lateral decubitus position to fully expose the posterior thorax. Lung ultrasonography is then performed, as with the lateral and anterior exam, by applying the transducer at multiple interspaces on the back. The optimal manner of scanning the thorax is to move the transducer across the chest wall in a series of scan lines examining each interspace and underlying lung in sequence. This allows the examiner to construct a three-dimensional (3D) image of the thorax from multiple 2D images gathered in organized scan-line sequences.

A pitfall to avoid is the failure to place the probe posteriorly enough on a supine patient, thus missing dependant consolidations and pleural effusions not seen more anteriorly or laterally along the diaphragm. Thoracic ultrasonography of the patient who is able to sit up with arms abducted allows much easier scanning of the entire thorax with the multiple scan-line technique, but this is not usually feasible in the critically ill patient.

KEY FINDINGS OF LUNG ULTRASONOGRAPHY

Lung ultrasonography is superior to standard supine radiography and similar to chest computerized tomography (CT) in detecting pneumothorax, normal aeration patterns, alveolar–interstitial fluid accumulation, lung consolidation, and pleural fluid.[2] Novice lung ultrasonographers are often challenged by the lack of visually familiar anatomical correlates that are seen when scanning other organs, such as the heart or kidney, whose boundaries can be well delineated. Many of the lung images are not "intuitive" to the novice, given that the lung is represented most often by artifactual linear echogenic patterns deep to the pleural line. Fortunately, these patterns are few, discrete, and easy to master. The key findings of lung ultrasonography for critical care applications are as follows.

▶ Lung Sliding

With the transducer in a longitudinal orientation, perpendicular to the skin surface, and centered between two adjacent ribs, a typical lung ultrasound image with the depth adjusted to examine the pleural interface can be displayed (Figure 19-1). The transducer should be situated so that the two rib shadows are located to the sides of the image, with the hyperechoic horizontally orientated pleural line appearing in the center of the image approximately 0.5 cm deep to the edge of the rib shadows. The pleural

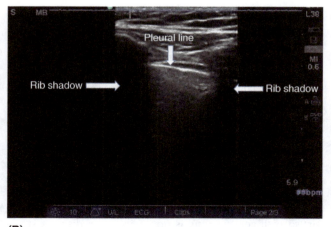

Figure 19-1 (A) The image is obtained using a 3.5 MHz transducer. The transducer is in longitudinal orientation and placed perpendicular to the chest wall to scan through the second intercostal space. The pleural line, the rib shadows, and A lines are identified. (B) The image is obtained using a 7.5 MHz transducer held in an identical fashion as in (A).

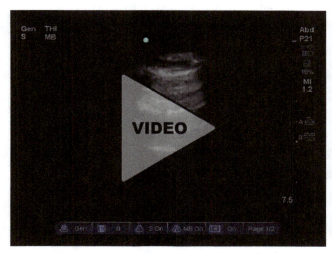

Video 19-1 The rib pleural line, the rib shadows, and A lines and lung sliding are present. The image is obtained using a 3.5 MHz transducer. The transducer is in longitudinal orientation and placed perpendicular to the chest wall to scan through the second intercostal space in the mid-clavicular line. View at www.ccu2e.com

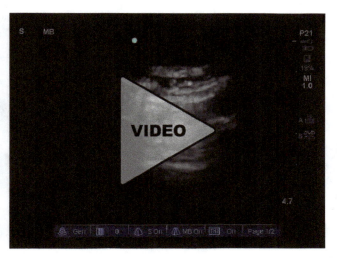

Video 19-3 Lung pulse is present. The image is obtained using a 3.5 MHz transducer. The transducer is in longitudinal orientation and placed perpendicular to the chest wall to scan through the second intercostal space in the mid-clavicular line. View at www.ccu2e.com

line represents the apposition of the visceral and parietal pleural surfaces. In the normal examination, the pleural surfaces move against each other during the respiratory cycle. This causes the finding of lung sliding, which is a shimmering mobile pleural line that moves in synchrony with the respiratory cycle (Videos 19-1 and 19-2). A related finding is lung pulse. With lung pulse, the pleural line moves synchronously with cardiac pulsation, as the force of cardiac pulsation is sufficient to cause movement of the lung and overlying visceral pleura (Video 19-3). Sliding lung and lung pulse are dynamic findings that

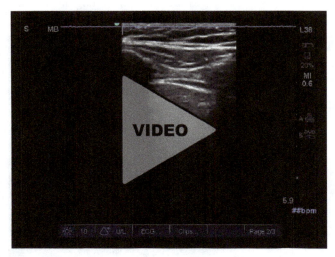

Video 19-2 Lung sliding is present. The image is obtained using a 7.5 MHz transducer. The transducer is in longitudinal orientation and placed perpendicular to the chest wall to scan through the second intercostal space in the mid-clavicular line. The higher frequency 7.5 MHz probe results in better resolution of the pleural interface, compared to that obtained with the 3.5 MHz probe, although with less depth of penetration. View at www.ccu2e.com

require real-time 2D scanning. For convenience, they may be recorded with M-mode for purposes of easy documentation (Figure 19-2).

The findings of lung sliding and lung pulse have major significance because they exclude the presence of a pneumothorax at the site of transducer application with a high level of certainty.[3] Lung sliding and pulse can only be seen when the ultrasound waves propagate to the deeper visceral pleura. When pleural air is interposed between the pleural surfaces, as occurs with pneumothorax, the air acts as a barrier to ultrasound; so lung sliding is lost.

Since air within the pleural space distributes to the anterior thorax in the supine patient, the critically ill patient is ideally positioned for the examination. Multiple anterior rib interspaces sites may be easily examined for sliding lung over both hemithoraces so that the intensivist can promptly and confidently rule out pneumothorax. Several groups have reported on the superiority of ultrasonography to rule out pneumothorax when compared with supine chest radiography.[4–7]

Although the presence of lung sliding effectively rules out the presence of pneumothorax at the site being examined, the absence of lung sliding is not as useful (Videos 19-4 and 19-5); as loss of lung sliding may occur in conditions other than pneumothorax. Any process that greatly reduces the movement of air into the lung will reduce or eliminate lung sliding. Mainstem bronchial intubation or occlusion (e.g., mucous plug, blood clot, foreign body, and tumor) will ablate lung sliding on the side of the blockage. Similarly, any process that impairs lung inflation, such as severe pneumonia, apnea, or adult respiratory distress syndrome (ARDS), will result in an absence of lung sliding. Processes which lead to pleural symphysis (inflammatory, neoplastic, therapeutic, cicatricial) cause loss of lung sliding. Apnea causes loss of lung sliding, though necessarily of

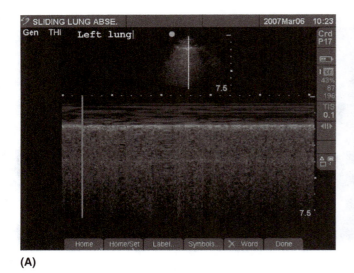
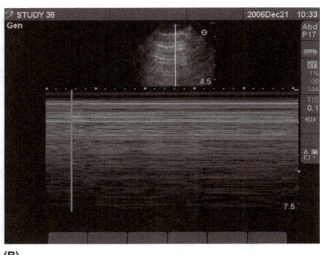

Figure 19-2 M-mode ultrasound image demonstrating "seashore sign": (**A**) consistent with sliding lung and "stratosphere" sign and (**B**) consistent with the absence of sliding lung.

short duration. In summary, the *presence* of lung sliding is a powerful sign because it rules out the possibility of a pneumothorax being present. The *absence* of lung sliding is less useful.[8]

▶ Lung Pulse

In certain situations, a lung pulse may be observed in the absence of lung sliding. This is a to-and-fro movement along the pleural line caused by transmission of cardiac pulsations. For example, with a unilateral mainstem bronchial block, lung sliding will be lost ipsilateral to the block due to the lack of air entry into the affected lung but a lung pulse can be seen, providing strong alternative evidence of the lack of pneumothorax.[9]

▶ Lung Point

Although absence of lung sliding is not specific for pneumothorax, the presence of a lung point can provide definitive evidence of a pneumothorax. The lung point is found where partially collapsed lung moves in and out of the pneumothorax space in phase with the respiratory cycle. Some pneumothoraces are total, that is, the lung is completely collapsed; but most are partial with some remaining apposition of the visceral and parietal pleura at some point along the thorax, usually lateral or posterior depending on the size of the pneumothorax. A lung point is described as the sudden appearance of lung sliding from the edge of the screen, arriving in an area where an A line pattern (see below) and lack of lung sliding are initially

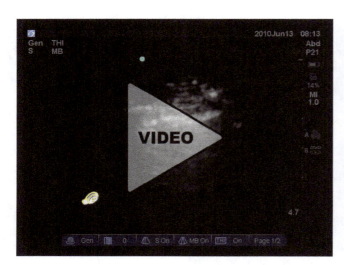

Video 19-4 There is absent lung sliding. The image is obtained using a 3.5 MHz transducer. The transducer is in longitudinal orientation and placed perpendicular to the chest wall to scan through the second intercostal space in the mid-clavicular line. View at www.ccu2e.com

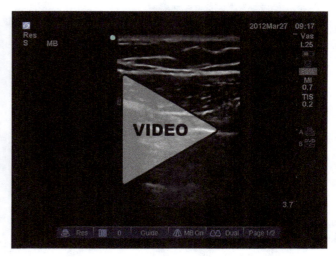

Video 19-5 There is absent lung sliding. The image is obtained using a 7.5 MHz transducer. The transducer is in longitudinal orientation and placed perpendicular to the chest wall to scan through the second intercostal space in the mid-clavicular line. View at www.ccu2e.com

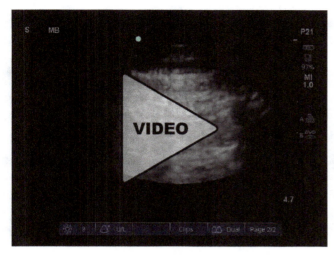

Video 19-6 A lung point is present. The partially deflated lung moves into the pneumothorax space in respirophasic pattern. Identification of a lung point is diagnostic for a pneumothorax. The image is obtained using a 3.5 MHz transducer. The transducer is in longitudinal orientation and placed perpendicular to the chest wall to scan through the 6th intercostal space in the anterior axillary line. View at www.ccu2e.com

noted. The lung sliding appears and disappears because the partially collapsed lung inflates to touch the chest wall and deflates away from the chest wall in synchrony with the respiratory cycle. Designated as the lung point, this finding is diagnostic of pneumothorax (Videos 19-6 and 19-7).[10] Unfortunately, while 100% specific for pneumothorax, lung point has only a moderate sensitivity for detection of pneumothorax. The low sensitivity is, in part, related to operator experience. The detection of lung sliding is an entry-level skill, while finding a lung point requires more experience. A high-frequency linear vascular transducer is useful in finding a lung point, as it has superior resolution when compared to the phased array transducer that is more commonly used. The search for a lung point is one circumstance where the examiner may routinely use transverse or oblique scanning planes to better examine the long axis of the rib interspaces. The finding of absent lung sliding should cause the examiner to promptly search for a lung point. Absent lung sliding suggests the possibility of pneumothorax; identification of an associated lung point, if present, confirms the diagnosis.

▶ A Lines

Using standard scanning technique with a scanning depth set to examine deeper structures, normally aerated lung yields characteristic air artifacts called "A lines." An A line is a horizontally orientated line, similar in appearance to the pleural line but seen below it (Figure 19-1 and Video 19-1) at a depth equal to the distance between the skin surface and the pleural line. The reason for this is that the A lines are reverberations of the pleural line, caused by echoes which reflect off the air just deep to the pleural line which then reflects off the probe face which then reflects off the air just deep to the pleura line. When this later reflection returns to the probe, it is interpreted as a deeper tissue plane similar to the pleural line, but twice as far away. This is known as a reverberation artifact and occurs when there is an air interface deep to the probe. A lines can appear singly or multiply, but are always separated by the same distance. In the presence of sliding lung, A lines indicate normally aerated lung. When present without sliding lung, they suggest either air between the visceral and parietal pleura, for example, a pneumothorax or simply pleurodesis of the two surfaces from inflammation or intervention. A lines with lung sliding are strongly correlated with a normal aeration pattern on CT scan.[2]

▶ B Lines

Using standard scanning technique with depth set to examine deeper structures, lung may yield a characteristic pattern of air artifact termed B lines. B lines have several distinct characteristics (Figure 19-3 and Videos 19-8 and 19-9):

B lines:

- are vertical in orientation and may occur as one or more per field (sometimes termed comet tails or lung rockets),
- originate at the pleural interface,
- extend ray-like to the bottom of the screen,
- efface A lines where the two intersect, and
- move in synchrony with lung sliding. However, they are not necessarily mobile, as in the case of B lines in the absence of lung sliding.

The appearance of B lines thus excludes the presence of pneumothorax.[11] B lines are characteristic of lung edema or any process that infiltrates the interstitium of the lung,

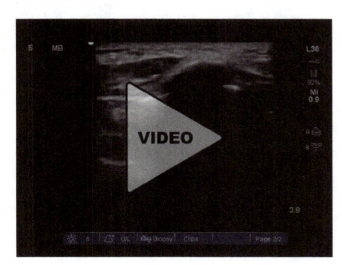

Video 19-7 A lung point is present. The partially deflated lung is seen to move underneath a rib into the pneumothorax space in respirophasic pattern. Identification of a lung point is diagnostic for a pneumothorax. The image is obtained using a 7.5 MHz transducer. The transducer is in longitudinal orientation and placed perpendicular to the chest wall to scan through the 5th intercostal space in the anterior axillary line. View at www.ccu2e.com

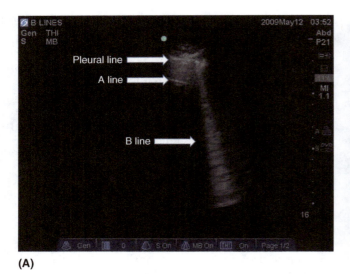
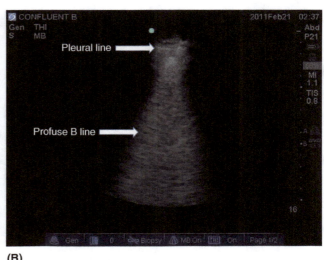

Figure 19-3 (**A**) A single B line is present. The image is obtained using a 3.5 MHz transducer in longitudinal orientation scanning through an intercostal space. (**B**) Profuse B lines are present so that individual B lines cannot be identified. The image is obtained using a 3.5 MHz transducer held in an identical fashion as in (**A**).

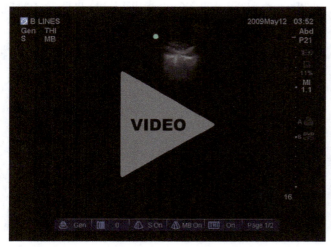
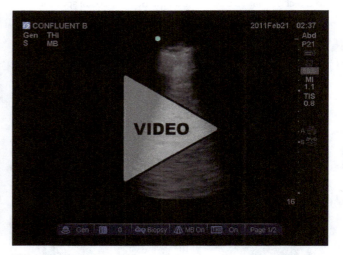

Video 19-8 A single B line is present. The image is obtained using a 3.5 MHz transducer. The transducer is in longitudinal orientation and placed perpendicular to the chest wall to scan through the 8th intercostal space in the mid-axillary line. A few B lines are commonly encountered in this region as a normal finding. View at www.ccu2e.com

Video 19-9 Profuse B lines are present to the extent that individual B lines cannot be identified. The image is obtained using a 3.5 MHz transducer. The transducer is in longitudinal orientation and placed perpendicular to the chest wall to scan through the 3rd intercostal space in the mid-clavicular line. View at www.ccu2e.com

such as inflammation, neoplasm, or scarring.[12-16] The presence of B lines is strongly correlated with alveolar or interstitial pattern abnormalities on CT scan (ground glass or reticular pattern abnormality).[2] Depending on the disease process that is causing the B lines; they may be focal, scattered, or profuse in distribution. Like any radiographic abnormality on standard chest radiograph or chest CT, clinical correlation is required to determine the cause of the B lines. For example, normal individuals may have several B lines on examination of the lateral lower lung interspaces that are of no clinical consequence. Pneumonia may manifest with focal B lines detected in the segment or lobe that is involved. Cardiogenic pulmonary edema (CPE) is associated with profuse bilateral B lines, whereas idiopathic pulmonary fibrosis results in scattered B lines. More than two B lines in a single field are considered significant.

▶ **Consolidation**

Using standard scanning techniques with a scanning depth set to examine deeper structures, consolidated lung yields a characteristic ultrasound pattern (Figure 19-4 and Videos 19-10 and 19-11). Consolidated lung is tissue density.[17] It has similar echogenicity as the liver; so it is referred to as sonographic hepatization of lung. If the bronchial structures that supply the affected consolidated lung are patent, the consolidated lung may have sonographic air bronchograms within it. These appear as hyperechoic foci that

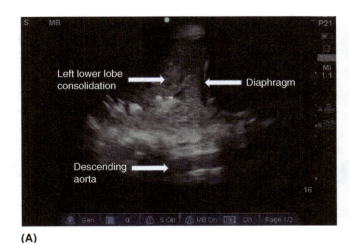 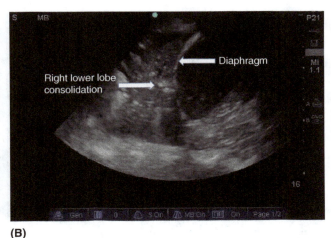

Figure 19-4 (A) There is alveolar consolidation of the left lower lobe. The diaphragm and descending aorta are identified. The image is obtained using a 3.5 MHz transducer in longitudinal orientation scanning through 6th intercostal space in the mid-axillary line on the left. (B) There is alveolar consolidation of the right lower lobe. The diaphragm is identified. The image is obtained using a 3.5 MHz transducer in longitudinal orientation scanning through 6th intercostal space in the mid-axillary line on the right.

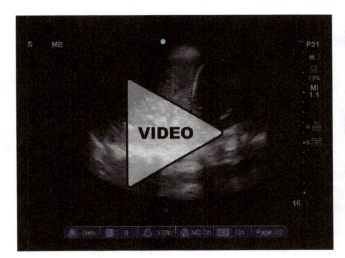 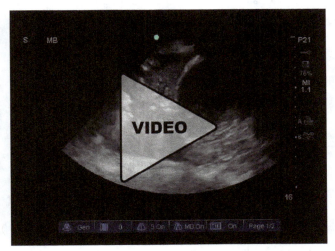

Video 19-10 There is alveolar consolidation of the left lower lobe. The diaphragm and descending aorta are identified. The transducer is in longitudinal orientation and placed perpendicular to the chest wall to scan through the 6th interspace in the mid-axillary line. View at www.ccu2e.com

Video 19-11 There is alveolar consolidation of the right lower lobe. During inspiration, the aerated lung moves into the scanning plane and blocks visualization of the consolidated lung (curtain sign). There is a small pleural effusion. The transducer is in longitudinal orientation and placed perpendicular to the chest wall to scan through the 6th intercostal space in the mid-axillary line. View at www.ccu2e.com

represent small amounts of air in the bronchi. They may be mobile, reflecting movement of air within the bronchus due to respiratory activity (Video 19-12). The examiner may easily localize consolidation to a specific lobe or segment of the lung. The finding of consolidation with lung ultrasonography is strongly correlated with results of chest CT.[2] The finding of consolidation on lung ultrasonography is purely descriptive, and similar to the finding of consolidation on chest radiography or chest CT. Any process that renders the alveolar compartment airless will demonstrate consolidation on lung ultrasonography or with other radiographic techniques. All causes of airless lung, such atelectasis (compressive, resorptive, or cicatricial), infiltrative processes (tumor, purulent material as in pneumonia), or severe pulmonary edema with complete filling of the alveolar compartment, will yield the ultrasonographic finding of lung consolidation. Lung ultrasonography identifies the consolidation; the clinician determines its cause.

▶ **Pleural Effusion**

Pleural effusion may be observed when performing lung ultrasonography. Knowledge of lung ultrasonography is essential for proficiency in pleural ultrasonography. A complete discussion of pleural ultrasonography is found in Chapter 18.

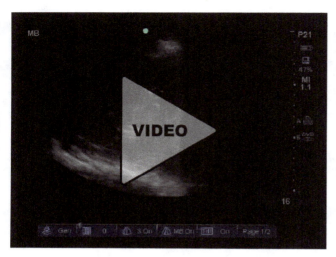

Video 19-12 There is alveolar consolidation of the right lower lobe with mobile air bronchograms represented by punctate hyperechoic foci within the consolidated lung that move in respirophasic manner. These represent intrabronchial air, and their mobility indicates that the bronchus supplying area is patent. The transducer is in longitudinal orientation and placed perpendicular to the chest wall to scan through the 6th intercostal space in the mid-axillary line. The gain is reduced in order to better visualize the air collections. View at www.ccu2e.com

CLINICAL APPLICATIONS OF LUNG ULTRASONOGRAPHY

▶ Rapid Evaluation of Acute Respiratory Failure

The critical care clinician frequently evaluates the patient with acute respiratory failure. The limitations of standard chest radiography have already been discussed and include, in the acute situation, an element of time delay. Chest CT has time delay, risk of transport of the unstable patient, and major radiation exposure.[18] The intensivist who is equipped with a portable ultrasound unit brings to the bedside a device that is superior to the standard chest radiography, and that is as accurate as chest CT for applications that are relevant to critical care medicine.

A useful method for diagnosing the underlying cause of acute respiratory failure using lung ultrasonography is the "BLUE" protocol described by Lichtenstein using four anatomic scan points on each hemithorax.[19] The overall pattern of findings from these four points can be used to diagnose the predominant disease process leading to respiratory failure. This diagnostic approach has excellent sensitivity and specificity for the diagnosis of pneumonia, pulmonary edema, pulmonary embolism, and chronic obstructive pulmonary disease, respectively (using vascular compression ultrasonography to differentiate the final two diagnoses). Using this algorithmic approach, lung ultrasonography allows rapid identification of the cause for acute respiratory failure in rapid-response-team events, the emergency department, and at the bedside of the acutely decompensating patient in the ICU.

In similar fashion, lung ultrasonography is useful in evaluating the patient on mechanical ventilatory support with acute desaturation, where the intensivist needs immediate diagnosis of a potentially life-threatening event. Barring obvious causes (e.g., mechanical failure of the ventilator/endotracheal tube system, unplanned extubation, severe patient/ventilator dyssynchrony, etc.), the intensivist may use ultrasonography to rule out pneumothorax and mainstem bronchial block (endotracheal tube movement or mucous plugging) and evaluate for acute pulmonary edema or embolism. Lung ultrasonography is readily combined with basic echocardiography and leg study for deep venous thrombosis to yield maximal diagnostic information in the emergency evaluation of severe cardiopulmonary failure.

▶ Clarification of the Ambiguous Chest Radiograph

Chest radiography in the supine critically ill patient on ventilator support is frequently difficult to interpret. A complex 3D structure is viewed in two dimensions. The problem is compounded by the common occurrence of rotation, penetration, and projection artifact. The resultant radiograph shows nonspecific radiodensity, where the clinician cannot discern between normal lung, alveolar or interstitial abnormalities, consolidation, or pleural effusion. Lung ultrasonography is an excellent means of clarifying the results of an ambiguous chest radiograph in the ICU. It is possible that lung ultrasonography could largely replace standard chest radiography in the ICU.[20,21]

▶ Evaluation for Pneumothorax

Lung ultrasonography is very effective for rapidly ruling out pneumothorax. In patients on mechanical ventilatory support, a pneumothorax is particularly dangerous because it may be under the threat of tension. The supine chest radiography has been shown to be unreliable in ruling out pneumothorax. Lung ultrasonography may be used to rule out pneumothorax with minimal time delay and a high degree of accuracy in the ICU. In addition, it is useful in the emergency evaluation of pneumothorax in cases of thoracic trauma.[6,7] Lung ultrasonography may be used to evaluate for postprocedure pneumothorax (following thoracentesis or subclavian/internal venous access). It is a straightforward exercise to identify sliding lung *before* the planned procedure. Following the procedure, the continued presence of sliding lung rules out procedure-related pneumothorax, whereas the new absence of sliding lung where it was previously present is strong evidence for a procedure-related pneumothorax.

▶ Lung Point

It is a simple matter to rule out a pneumothorax. Definitive diagnosis of the presence of a pneumothorax is more difficult and requires the identification of a lung point. When pneumothorax is suspected due to the absence of detectable lung sliding, the diagnosis can be confirmed with 100% specificity when a lung point is found.[10] The lung point is the edge of the pneumothorax and is usually found over the lateral chest. It is seen during inspiration, when a portion of the visceral pleural surface that has been pushed away from the parietal pleura by pleural air is now inflated sufficiently to again contact the parietal pleura, causing the sudden appearance of lung sliding. During expiration, the lung retracts out of the scanning plane. Lung point represents the appearance and disappearance of lung sliding and must occur within an area of A lines.

▶ Advanced Applications of Lung Ultrasonography

Lung ultrasonography has been used to address some clinical questions of interest to the intensivist and pulmonologist.

Differentiating acute respiratory distress syndrome from CPE

Copetti et al. demonstrated the ability of lung ultrasound to discriminate between ARDS and CPE.[22] The most specific sign for ARDS was the finding of areas of normal aeration (sparing) within a hemithorax scan showing predominant interstitial syndrome findings (B lines). These spared areas were found in 100% of ARDS patients and 0% of CPE patients. Similarly, pleural line abnormalities, such as thickening >2 mm, coarse, irregular appearance, or subpleural consolidations were found in 100% of ARDS patients and only 25% of CPE patients. The finding of profuse B lines bilaterally with a smooth pleural surface was highly suggestive of CPE.

Predicting extubation failure

Soummer et al. devised a lung ultrasound scoring (LUS) system which highly correlated with the severity of lung edema or loss of aeration.[23] In this system, a value of 0 is assigned to any interspace examined which reveals "dry lung," that is, A lines with lung sliding pattern. The value of 1 is assigned to areas with regularly spaced B lines consistent with interlobular septal thickening. A value of 2 is assigned to interspaces with confluent B lines filling the visualized interspace that is consistent with interstitial and alveolar edema, and a value of 3 is assigned to areas of consolidation whereby the lung is completely airless or filled with fluid. Using a standard protocol examining six interspaces over each hemithorax leads to a maximum possible LUS score of 36. Performing LUS scores before and after a 30-minute spontaneous breathing trial (SBT), a loss of aeration (increase in LUS score >4 points)-predicted extubation failure. An end-SBT LUS score >17 also predicted extubation failure.

Measurement of lung recruitment

Bouhemad et al, reported on the utility of the LUS score to predict the effects of postive end expiratory pressure (PEEP) in ARDS patients.[24] Performing LUS exams at PEEP = 0 and PEEP = 15, they found that a decrease of LUS score of 8 using the higher PEEP resulted in an average increase of lung volume >600 mL. If the LUS score increased by 4 or less, the volume increased by an average of 75–450 mL. One limitation of this application is that although it can predict increases in lung volume with higher PEEP, this method cannot distinguish between lung hyperinflation with PEEP and physiologically beneficial lung recruitment.

Other applications of lung ultrasonography

Lung ultrasonography may be used to guide transthoracic needle or device insertion for purposes of biopsy of a lesion that is adjacent to the pleural surface.[25] Intraparenchymal lesions are not visible because the surrounding lung is aerated and blocks ultrasonographic visualization of the lesion. An exception is lung abscess, where the surrounding lung is generally consolidated thereby permitting visualization of the abscess.[26] Lung ultrasonography can be used for the targeted insertion of a drainage catheter into a lung abscess, if clinically indicated. Lung ultrasonography may be used to confirm successful endotracheal tube placement[27] and to rule out a right mainstem bronchial intubation. Lung ultrasonography has utility in the diagnosis of high-altitude pulmonary edema in remote locations[28] and for the identification of lung contusion.[29] It may be useful for the diagnosis of pulmonary embolism.[30]

LIMITATIONS OF LUNG ULTRASONOGRAPHY

▶ Operator-Related

Lung ultrasonography requires that the intensivist has specific training in image acquisition, image interpretation, and integration of the results into an effective management strategy. Lung ultrasonography is performed by the frontline intensivist without input from the radiologist or ultrasound technician. A bedside technique, its clinical utility is completely dependent on the skill of the intensivist–ultrasonographer. Adequate training in the field is a requirement.

▶ Machine-Related

Not all ultrasound machines can produce adequate image quality for lung ultrasonography. In particular, extensive image processing may degrade the image quality required for lung ultrasonography. Near-field clutter and lack of resolution of the pleural interface are problems with some recent-generation machines.

▶ Documentation-Related

Critical care lung ultrasonography is frequently performed on an emergency basis in the ICU. The intensivist may be handling multiple tasks, and there may be insufficient time to label and save images that are being quickly obtained from multiple sites on the thorax or to issue a complete written report of all findings. Chest radiography and chest CT scans result in durable reviewable hard copies that are read and documented by well-organized radiology services. The same may not be said for lung ultrasonography.

Difficulty with documentation can lead to problems. First, lack of documentation is a medical–legal concern. Second, the lack of documentation also impacts on the need to know what previous lung ultrasound results showed in a particular patient. In a busy ICU, the ICU team might perform numerous rapid lung scans each day and use the results for important immediate management decisions. Deficient documentation and a limited ability to retrieve ephemeral images for review may prevent the clinician from comparing today's result with those of yesterday.

▶ Miscellaneous

Lung ultrasonography cannot resolve lesions that are surrounded by aerated lung. Chest wall dressings and massive edema or obesity may preclude adequate imaging of the lung. Subcutaneous air prohibits lung ultrasonography at the site of the air collection.

CONCLUSION

Lung ultrasonography has strong utility for the frontline intensivist. It can identify pneumothorax, alveolar/interstitial changes, consolidation, and pleural effusion. It is superior to supine radiography in the ICU. Proficiency in lung ultrasonography will help the intensivist clarify the ambiguous chest radiograph, promptly recognize postprocedure pneumothorax, and rapidly evaluate the patient with acute respiratory failure.

REFERENCES

1. Lichtenstein DA. *Whole Body Ultrasonography in the Critically Ill*. Berlin, Germany: Springer-Verlag; 2010: 117-208.
2. Lichtenstein D, Goldstein I, Mourgeon E, Cluzel P, Grenier P, Rouby JJ. Comparative diagnostic performances of auscultation, chest radiography, and lung ultrasonography in acute respiratory distress syndrome. *Anesthesiology*. 2004;100:9-15.
3. Lichtenstein DA, Menu Y. A bedside ultrasound sign ruling out pneumothorax in the critically ill. Lung sliding. *Chest*. 1995;108:1345-1348.
4. Lichtenstein DA, Mezière G, Lascols N, et al. Ultrasound diagnosis of occult pneumothorax. *Crit Care Med*. 2005;33:1231-1238.
5. Soldati G, Testa A, Sher S, Pignataro G, La Sala M, Silveri NG. Occult traumatic pneumothorax: diagnostic accuracy of lung ultrasonography in the emergency department. *Chest*. 2008;133:204-211.
6. Blaivas M, Lyon M, Duggal SA. Prospective comparison of supine chest radiography and bedside ultrasound for the diagnosis of traumatic pneumothorax. *Acad Emerg Med*. 2005;12:844-849.
7. Kirkpatrick AW, Sirois M, Laupland KB, et al. Hand-held thoracic sonography for detecting post-traumatic pneumothoraces: the Extended Focused Assessment with Sonography for Trauma (EFAST). *J Trauma*. 2004;57: 288-295.
8. Lichtenstein DA, Meziere GA. Relevance of lung ultrasound in the diagnosis of acute respiratory failure: the BLUE protocol. *Chest*. 2008;134:117-125.
9. Lichtenstein DA, Lascols N, Prin S, Mezière G. The "lung pulse": an early ultrasound sign of complete atelectasis. *Intensive Care Med*. 2003;29:2187-2192.
10. Lichtenstein D, Mezière G, Biderman P, Gepner A. The "lung point": an ultrasound sign specific to pneumothorax. *Intensive Care Med*. 2000;26:1434-1440.
11. Lichtenstein D, Mezière G, Biderman P, Gepner A. The comet-tail artifact: an ultrasound sign ruling out pneumothorax. *Intensive Care Med*. 1999;25:383-388.
12. Lichtenstein D, Mezière G. A lung ultrasound sign allowing bedside distinction between pulmonary edema and COPD: the comet-tail artifact. *Intensive Care Med*. 1998;24: 1331-1334.
13. Lichtenstein D, Mézière G, Biderman P, Gepner A, Barré O. The comet-tail artifact. An ultrasound sign of alveolar-interstitial syndrome. *Am J Respir Crit Care Med*. 1997;156:1640-1646.
14. Agricola E, Bove T, Oppizzi M, et al. "Ultrasound comet-tail images": a marker of pulmonary edema: a comparative study with wedge pressure and extravascular lung water. *Chest*. 2005;127:1690-1695.
15. Agricola E, Picano E, Oppizzi M, et al. Assessment of stress-induced pulmonary interstitial edema by chest ultrasound during exercise echocardiography and its correlation with left ventricular function. *J Am Soc Echocardiogr*. 2006;19:457-463.
16. Jambrik Z, Monti S, Coppola V, et al. Usefulness of ultrasound lung comets as a nonradiologic sign of extravascular lung water. *Am J Cardiol*. 2004;93:1265-1270.
17. Lichtenstein DA, Lascols N, Mezière G, Gepner A. Ultrasound diagnosis of alveolar consolidation in the critically ill. *Intensive Care Med*. 2004;30:276-281.
18. Brenner DJ, Hall EJ. Computed tomography—an increasing source of radiation exposure. *N Engl J Med*. 357:2277-2284.
19. Lichtenstein DA, Meziere GA. Relevance of lung ultrasound in the diagnosis of acute respiratory failure. *Crit Care Med*. 2008;134:117-125.
20. Zanobetti M, Poggioni C, Pini R. Can chest ultrasonography replace standard chest radiography for evaluation of acute dyspnea in the ED? *Chest*. 2011;139:1140-1147.
21. Ioos V, Galbois A, Chalumeau-Lemoine L, Guidet B, Maury E, Hejblum G. An integrated approach for prescribing fewer chest x-rays in the ICU. *Ann Intensive Care*. 2011;1(1):4.
22. Copetti R, Soldati G, Copetti P. Chest sonography: a useful tool to differentiate acute cardiogenic pulmonary edema from acute respiratory distress syndrome. *Cardiovasc Ultrasound*. 2008;6:1-10.
23. Soummer A, Perbet S, Brisson H, et al., and the Lung Ultrasound Study Group. Ultrasound assessment of lung aeration loss during a successful spontaneous breathing trial predicts postextubation distress. *Crit Care Med*. 2012;40:2064-2072.
24. Bouhemad B, Bresson H, Le-Guen M, Arbelot C, Lu Q, Rouby JJ. Bedside ultrasound assessment of positive end-expiratory pressure-induced lung recruitment. *Am J Resp Crit Care Med*. 2011;183:341-347.
25. Sheth S, Hamper UM, Stanley DB, Wheeler JH, Smith PA. US guidance for thoracic biopsy: a valuable alternative to CT. *Radiology*. 1999;210:721-726.
26. Lichtenstein D, Peyrouset O. Is lung ultrasound superior to CT? The example of a CT occult necrotizing pneumonia. *Intensive Care Med*. 2006;32:334-335.

27. Weaver B, Lyon M, Blaivas M. Confirmation of endotracheal tube placement after intubation using the ultra-sound sliding lung sign. *Acad Emerg Med.* 2006;13:239–244.
28. Fagenholz PJ, Gutman JA, Murray AF, Noble E, Thomas SH, Harris NS. Chest ultrasonography for the diagnosis and monitoring of high-altitude pulmonary edema. *Chest.* 2007;131:1013–1018.
29. Soldati G, Testa AR, Silva F, Carbone L, Grazia P, Nicolò GS. Ultrasonography in lung contusion. *Chest.* 2006;130:533–538.
30. Mathis G, Blank W, Reissig A, et al. Thoracic ultrasound for diagnosing pulmonary embolism: a prospective multicenter study of 352 patients. *Chest.* 2005;128:1531–1538.

ULTRASOUND EVALUATION OF THE ABDOMEN

SARAH C. SHAVES & HEIDI L. FRANKEL

Scan QR code or visit www.ccu2e.com for video in this chapter

INTRODUCTION

The intensivist caring for the critically ill patient may often consider abdominal pathology when assessing for the causes of the patient's ill health. Patient symptoms, vital signs, and laboratory tests together with physical examination may leave the clinician with a broad differential diagnosis. Imaging is a frequent tool used to refine the differential diagnosis. Plain film of the abdomen can show obstructive bowel gas pattern or free air, mass effect from organomegaly or ascites, but gives limited information about solid organs. Computerized tomography (CT) is a better test for retroperitoneum, bowel, or for solid organ injury, but is neither portable nor obtained as quickly as bedside ultrasound. Magnetic resonance imaging generally is a relatively lengthy examination, is contraindicated in patients with pacemakers or some other implantable devices, and is often not readily available. Focused ultrasound, however, is quickly available and can often help to identify the problem or exclude diagnoses and assist with therapy.

The American Institute of Ultrasound in Medicine (AIUM) lists 13 indications for abdominal ultrasound (Table 20-1). Many of these indications may be the leading cause of a patient's illness; all can complicate other medical conditions. Causes of pain, for instance, may be assessed by ultrasound. Pain due to acute cholecystitis or ureteral obstruction, peritonitis due to abscess, or vascular occlusions may be detected. The cause of biliary obstruction or explanation for a rapid drop in hematocrit may be identified. Palpable abnormalities can be confirmed. Obstructive uropathy can be evident as a cause of renal insufficiency. Ascitic fluid can be followed by serial examinations. Liver metastases may be the etiology of elevated liver function tests or explain the increased risk for pulmonary embolism. Bladder distension can be assessed in the neurogenic bladder of a patient with spina bifida. A focused examination for free fluid in the trauma patient may affect operative decisions. The transplant organ can be evaluated for early complications. Ultrasound guidance can also decrease the risk associated with vascular and body interventions. For the critically ill, a point-of-care ultrasound examination that combines an evaluation of abdominal organs, vascular structures, and the peritoneal spaces for fluid may focus the physicians' attention to the most likely causes of a patient's ill health.

TRANSDUCER SELECTION AND SUPPLIES

▶ Transducer Selection

Two probes form the basis for evaluation of the abdomen. The low frequency curved 5.2 MHz transducer provides excellent penetration and a large far-field for abdominal organs and peritoneal spaces. A small footprint-phased array transducer (microconvex 4.2 MHz probe) is useful for intercostal spaces, in the obese, and in the area of bandages and other tight areas. A linear probe is useful for identifying the pleura or other small parts like the scrotum that are only a few centimeters or less from the probe. It will not provide the many centimeters of penetration needed to visualize through the liver.

▶ Ultrasound Coupling Agent

Ultrasound gel applied to the probe or patient's body will provide a clear acoustic window. It may be used in conjunction with a probe cover if contamination is likely. Probe sheaths in varying sizes are commercially available. First, apply gel generously to the footprint of the probe, cover the probe with the sheath, and then apply another layer of gel to the outside of the probe. Whenever sheathing, care should be taken to avoid air bubbles between the probe and sheath that will cause reflective artifact in the image. If they occur, they can be manually milked aside.

TABLE 20-1
AIUM Indications for Abdominal and/or Retroperitoneal Ultrasonography

A. Abdominal, flank, and/or back pain.
B. Signs or symptoms referred from the abdominal and/or retroperitoneal regions, such as jaundice or hematuria.
C. Palpable abnormalities, such as an abdominal mass or organomegaly.
D. Abnormal lab values or abnormal findings on other imaging examinations suggestive of abdominal and/or retroperitoneal pathology.
E. Follow-up of known or suspected abnormalities in the abdomen and/or retroperitoneum.
F. Search for metastatic disease or an occult primary neoplasm.
G. Evaluation of suspected congenital abnormalities.
H. Abdominal trauma.
I. Pre- and posttransplantation evaluation.
J. Planning for and guiding an invasive procedure.
K. Search for the presence of free or loculated peritoneal and/or retroperitoneal fluid.
L. Suspicion of hypertrophic pyloric stenosis or intussusceptions.
M. Evaluation of a urinary tract infection.

AIUM = American Institute of Ultrasound in Medicine.
Source: http://www.aium.org/resources/guidelines.aspx. © 2012 by the American Institute of Ultrasound in Medicine. Used with permission.

▶ Cleaning Transabdominal Transducers

Transducers must be cleaned before use and between patients according to guidelines described for ultrasound transducers. The AIUM recommends that after each use probes should be cleaned with soap and water, quaternary ammonium sprays or wipes as directed by the manufacturer in the operating manual. Heavy contamination with blood or enteric contents may warrant additional cleaning. Probes should be sheathed if contamination is likely. The probe including the cord must still be cleaned after use even if sheathed because of reported leakage rates. Strict adherence to cleaning guidelines must be followed to prevent spread of infection from one patient to another and to ensure equipment longevity.

Base unit

The ideal ICU ultrasound unit should be portable, easy to use, highly reliable, relatively indestructible, and inexpensive. Ultra-small units, although intuitively attractive, particularly in locations with limited space, may be taken from the ICU and then be unavailable when needed. Their image resolution remains limited. Even larger ultrasound units, particularly if easy to use and with good resolution, can be easily removed from the ICU. In our ICU, we resolved this problem by assigning the less expensive equipment to simpler tasks (i.e., vascular access) and leaving the more sophisticated machines for torso imaging. Most focused ICU abdominal ultrasound examinations do not rely on the use of Doppler imaging. The addition of reliable Doppler capability to the ultrasound unit may complicate the issues of size, expense, and require additional training.

Data capture

Portable printers can be added to ICU ultrasound units to capture selected images for documentation purposes. Images and videos can be captured through video cards. Digital information can alternatively be stored through the use of a cloud-based electronic health record or picture archiving system without the need for physical records that can be easily lost or destroyed.

IMAGE ORIENTATION AND ANATOMIC CORRELATION

Scanning in a focused ICU abdominal ultrasound assessment is performed in transverse and longitudinal planes. By convention, in a transverse plane, the indicator on the probe is pointing to the patient's right side and this corresponds to the left side of the display screen just like the convention used with CT scanning. In a longitudinal plane, the indicator on the probe is pointed toward the patient's head and corresponds to the left side of the display screen with the toes oriented toward the right. In actual practice, off-axis imaging where the probe is oriented in a transverse or longitudinal plane relative to the structure being imaged (and not necessarily lined up with the sagittal sinus or true transverse plane through the patient) is frequently used when locating the common bile duct or evaluating the kidneys in long axis. The patient is typically positioned supine and the sonographer stands at the patient's right side, scanning with his or her right hand. The room lights should be dimmed to improve the visualization of the screen.

TERMINOLOGY

Abdominal structures are described in terms of echotexture. A black or anechoic appearance can represent simple fluid, such as ascites, bile, or urine. A long artifact from a shadow behind a rib or stone can also be anechoic. Blood or pus will be hypoechoic, or darker than the surrounding structures, due to fluid but with cellular material causing low level echoes; sludge in the gallbladder or debris in the urinary bladder can also cause low level echoes. The liver and spleen are generally described as having medium echotexture. The kidneys are normally lower in echotexture than the liver. Fat such as in the retroperitoneum or portal triads will be echogenic, or brighter echotexture than surrounding structures, but will not shadow. Highly sound-absorptive structures, like the ribs, kidney stones or gallstones, will appear brightly echogenic and behind them the sound will be attenuated causing a shadowing artifact; gas in the bowel is reflective and shows "dirty shadowing" due to a mix of fluid, which transmits sound waves and gas and leads to streaky shadows.

▶ Focused Assessment with Sonography for Trauma (FAST) Examination

The FAST protocol originated as a limited ultrasound examination to rapidly assess for abdominal free fluid or pericardial effusion as a noninvasive alternative to diagnostic peritoneal lavage (originally the Focused Abdominal Sonography in Trauma). This highly sensitive test has expanded to include an evaluation of the pleural space as the extended FAST exam, or eFAST, for pneumothorax. In addition to making these important findings, the eFAST can reduce the time to necessary interventions, such as thoracostomy tube or emergent surgical exploration.

The eFAST protocol is classically performed with the patient supine. Ultrasonography practiced in this fashion has high sensitivity for the detection of free fluid; as little as 100 cc of fluid (and likely less with machines of higher quality) may be detected. Changes in patient position may shift expected findings and Trendelenburg position increases the sensitivity of the test for the detection of abdominal free fluid.

A high-frequency linear probe is used first to evaluate the pleural space in the midclavicular lines (or the highest point in the chest if the patient is not supine) to evaluate for pneumothorax with the probe marker directed toward the head. The low-frequency probe can be used if it is more expedient. Begin with the probe in the second interspace and slide caudally viewing the interspaces between ribs. Normally, the visceral pleura is visible sliding past the parietal pleura beneath the probe with occasional comet tails (reverberation artifact from pleura). With a pneumothorax, there is a loss of normal pleural sliding (see Chapter 19).

The low-frequency probe is then placed in the subxiphoid position with the probe marker positioned toward the patient's right side (Figure 20-1). Using the liver as an

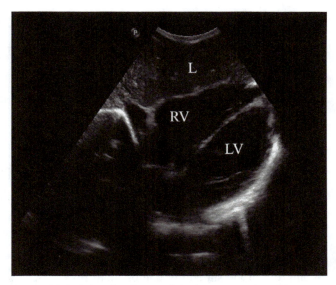

Figure 20-2 Subxiphoid view of the heart using liver (L) as acoustic window. RV, right ventricle; LV, left ventricle.

acoustic window, the probe is angled superiorly to interrogate the heart for a pericardial effusion (Figure 20-2). Fluid will appear as anechoic or a hypoechoic stripe between echogenic pericardium closer to the probe and medium echotexture and beating myocardium further away from the probe (see Chapter 10).

The low-frequency probe is then turned with the probe marker directed toward the head to begin an evaluation of the abdomen. The hepatorenal space (Morison's pouch) is evaluated for fluid between the liver and right kidney in the longitudinal plane in the anterior axillary line at the 7th to 9th ribs, the most dependent part of the peritoneal cavity in the supine position. Fluid will appear anechoic, separating the liver from right kidney (Figure 20-3).

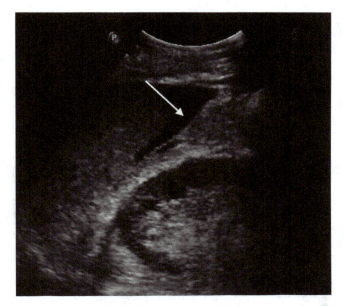

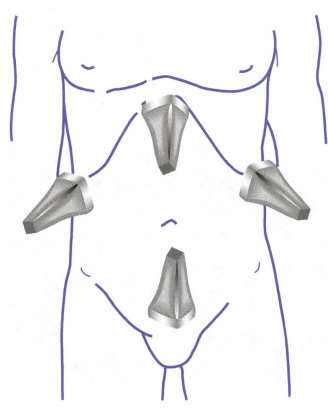

Figure 20-1 Probe position for four standard FAST views.

Figure 20-3 Fluid (arrow) in hepatorenal space between liver and right kidney.

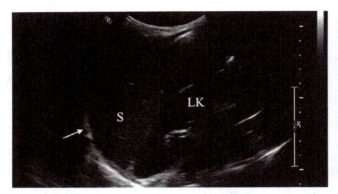

Figure 20-4 Left upper quadrant showing splenorenal space between spleen (S) and left kidney (LK); diaphragm (*arrow*) cephalad to the spleen.

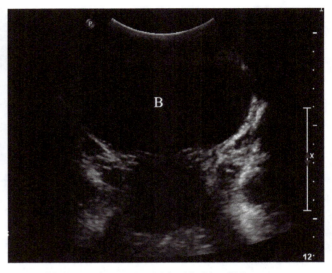

Figure 20-6 Anechoic urine in the bladder (B) in transverse plane.

Sliding the probe superiorly one or more rib interspaces will identify the thick echogenic diaphragm and allow for evaluation of pleural effusion above the liver and beneath the more echogenic and shadowing lung. The probe may need to be moved to avoid shadowing ribs.

Additional longitudinal imaging is then made in left upper quadrant evaluating the splenorenal space between the left kidney and spleen in the mid or posterior axillary line (e.g., in more of a coronal plane) between the 10th and 11th ribs to detect fluid (Figures 20-4 and 20-5). A more posterior approach is necessary on the left to avoid shadowing gas in the stomach. Once again sliding cephalad one or more rib interspaces will identify the echogenic diaphragm and allow for an evaluation of the left pleural space for effusion.

Finally, attention is turned to the most dependent portion of the pelvis, the rectovesicular space and anterior vesicouterine space in females. The probe is placed above the pubic bone and pelvis interrogated in transverse and longitudinal planes (Figure 20-6). Fluid in the urinary bladder will provide an acoustic window to evaluate for the presence of anechoic or hypoechoic free fluid in the peritoneal spaces (Figure 20-7).

A pneumoperitoneum can also be identified by focused FAST ultrasound. Analogous to the lack of pleural sliding with pneumothorax, there is a lack of peritoneal sliding with pneumoperitoneum. A massive pneumoperitoneum may even be associated with an inability to obtain the traditional FAST views.

The eFAST exam can be readily repeated if negative or if the patient deteriorates. It should not replace CT as a more sensitive test for the detection of solid organ injury or for the evaluation of the retroperitoneum, which is not well evaluated due to shadowing from bowel gas. It should also not delay surgical intervention if emergent abdominal exploration is indicated. In addition, imaging can be

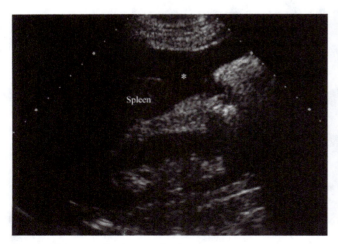

Figure 20-5 Free fluid around spleen (*).

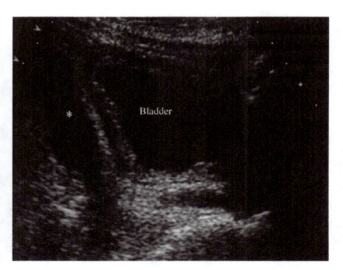

Figure 20-7 Hypoechoic fluid (*) above urinary bladder in sagittal plane.

CHAPTER 20 ULTRASOUND EVALUATION OF THE ABDOMEN 223

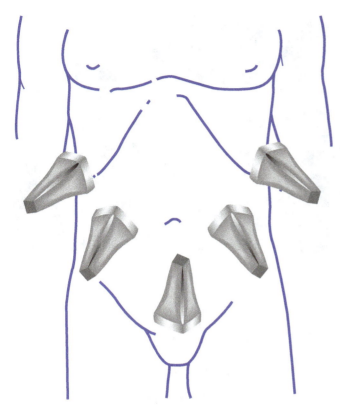

Figure 20-8 Five abdominal exam views.

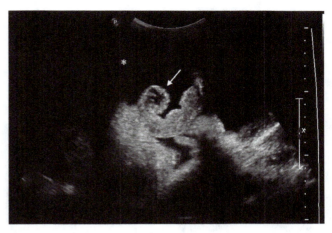

Figure 20-9 Fluid (*) around bowel (arrow).

suboptimal in certain patients, such as the morbidly obese, uncooperative patients, in patients with subcutaneous emphysema, or dressings that limit visualization. In these patients, CT may be indicated instead of the eFAST. The inability of FAST to distinguish fresh blood from ascites makes the use of focused abdominal ultrasound less helpful in the ICU patient. In addition to the abdominal views, the gutters should also be assessed for fluid in the ICU (Figure 20-8).

The amount of fluid present in the peritoneal cavity has been described by several scoring systems. These are valuable in the emergency department to judge the eventual need for therapeutic laparotomy even in the face of hemodynamic normality. These scoring systems are less useful in the ICU setting. In addition, some major abdominal pathologies, such as colonic or duodenal perforation, pancreatitis, acute mesenteric arterial thrombosis, or ruptured aneurysm, may have little if any significant associated free fluid.

The nature of free fluid in the ICU patient may provide clues to its origin and significance. Simple anechoic fluid may be visualized in a patient with right heart failure or cirrhosis. A large volume of fluid may completely surround the liver and bowel, particularly if a chronic disease state is present (Figure 20-9).

Simple fluid can also be seen with aggressive overhydration and with fresh blood. Echoes within the fluid suggest an exudative process. This may be due to organizing clots, most commonly near the site of origin of the bleeding, or with peritonitis and may have internal septations or loculations in addition to low-level echoes. A new loculated fluid collection in a patient with peritoneal signs may be due to perforated bowel. Fluid loculations may complicate the drainage from peritoneal dialysis catheters or ventriculoperitoneal shunts (Figure 20-10). When ultrasound is used to guide fluid sampling, paracentesis should be performed where the maximum amount of fluid is located, with the safest path by the needle to the target (Figure 20-11; see Chapter 25).

There are multiple limitations to performing abdominal ultrasound in the ICU patient. Rib shadows may make visualization of the liver and spleen more difficult. Bowel gas may obscure the ability to obtain quality images of the pancreas and great vessels. Obese patients are more challenging to evaluate as the ultrasound energy is attenuated by fat tissue. Extensive dressings in burn or postop patients may prevent imaging in optimal windows for evaluation of abdominal structures. Patients may not be able to breath-hold or may

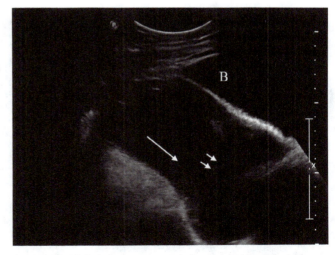

Figure 20-10 Pelvic abscess posterior to bladder (B) with debris (long arrow) and septations (double arrow).

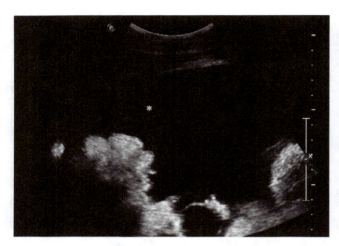

Figure 20-11 Large pocket of free fluid (*) in the left lower quadrant.

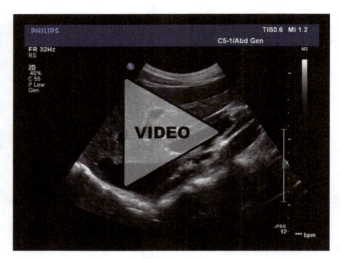

Video 20-2 Cine clip of right lobe liver, transverse plane. View at www.ccu2e.com

be mechanically ventilated making imaging more difficult. The physician performing ultrasound must be able to be patient and flexible, looking between ribs instead or from a subcostal approach, waiting for end-inspiration in a patient on a ventilator, rolling the patient to get a better view of the spleen from a more posterior position.

LIVER ULTRASOUND

Focused liver ultrasound may assist the intensivist in identifying diffuse liver disease, such as cirrhosis or steatosis, liver masses or abscess, ductal dilatation, portal gas, and perfusion in a transplanted liver. More detailed analysis of the liver will rarely impact therapy in the ICU.

The liver is imaged at end-inspiration in longitudinal and oblique transverse planes following the subcostal margin (Videos 20-1 and 20-2). In some patients, the liver is best seen via an intercostal approach because of its relatively superior position, or if the patient cannot follow directions for breath holding. The liver parenchyma is of medium echotexture with a smooth capsule. Hepatic veins are anechoic tubular structures draining the liver superiorly to the inferior vena cava (IVC; Video 20-3). The normal long length of the right lobe in the midclavicular line is 15 cm or less (Figure 20-12).

The main portal veins and portal triads are notable for surrounding echogenic fat with the portal veins being the largest structures in the portal triad. The hepatic veins and portal veins divide the liver into surgical segments. The normal intrahepatic ducts are barely visible at the portal triads. The hepatic artery branches are typically not resolved. The main portal vein enters the midportion of the liver at the porta hepatis and divides into left and right branches. The main portal vein, the common bile duct, and the hepatic artery in the hepatoduodenal ligament are imaged at the porta hepatis with the portal vein

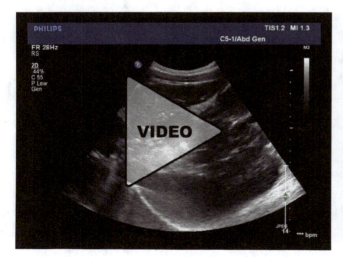

Video 20-1 Cine clip of left lobe liver, sagittal plane. View at www.ccu2e.com

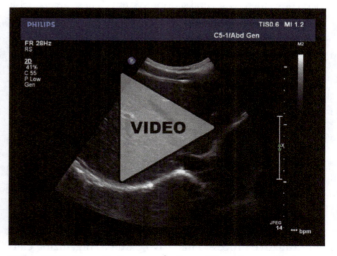

Video 20-3 Cine clip transverse view of liver demonstrating hepatic veins draining to IVC. View at www.ccu2e.com

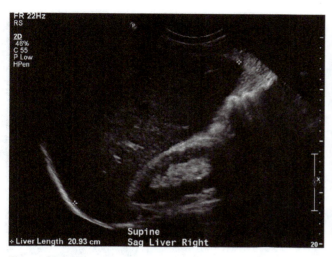

Figure 20-12 Hepatomegaly (cursors).

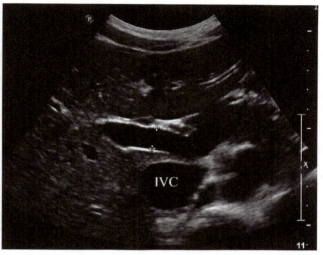

Figure 20-14 Measuring main portal vein (cursors), located anterior to inferior vena cava (IVC).

being the largest of the three and posterior to duct and artery (Figure 20-13).

The main portal vein in most patients measures 12 mm or less and has continuous low-velocity flow toward the liver. Flow is hepatopetal (waveform above the baseline) and may demonstrate phasicity with respirations (Figures 20-14 and 20-15). Hepatic arterial flow is generally biphasic low resistance with high-diastolic flow. In general, flow in the hepatic veins and IVC is bidirectional and impacted by the cardiac cycle and respiratory phase (Video 20-4).

A small liver with a nodular capsule and heterogeneously increased echotexture may be seen in a patient with end-stage cirrhosis (Figure 20-16). Ascitic fluid and splenomegaly may be present indicating portal hypertension. There may be reversal of portal venous flow away from the liver (Figure 20-17). Diffusely enlarged echogenic liver due to

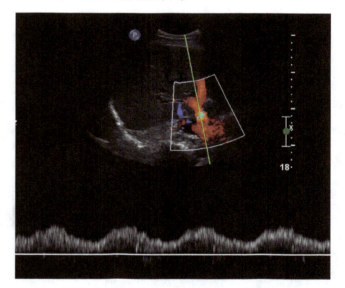

Figure 20-15 Main portal vein demonstrating hepatopetal Doppler flow (above the baseline) with phasicity.

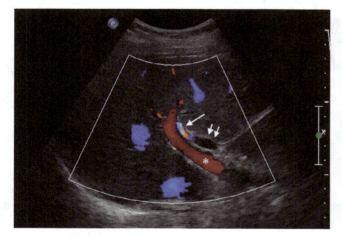

Figure 20-13 Color Doppler image at porta hepatis demonstrating hepatopetal flow in main portal vein (*), smaller hepatic artery (arrow), and anechoic common bile duct (double arrows).

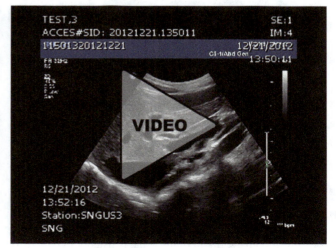

Video 20-4 Cine clip of inferior vena cava posteriorly at the liver demonstrating phasicity with respirations. View at www.ccu2e.com

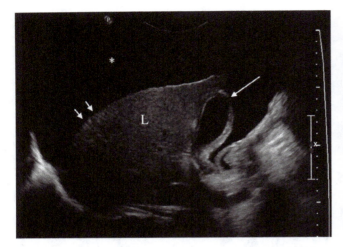

Figure 20-16 Cirrhotic liver (L) with nodular contour (*double arrows*), thickened gallbladder wall (*arrow*), and ascites fluid (*) indicating portal hypertension.

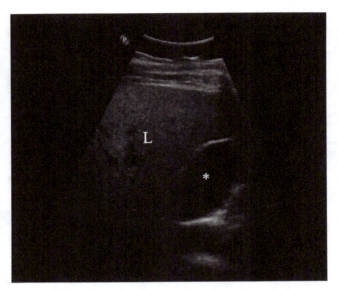

Figure 20-18 Echogenic liver (L) in patient with steatosis. Gallbladder (*).

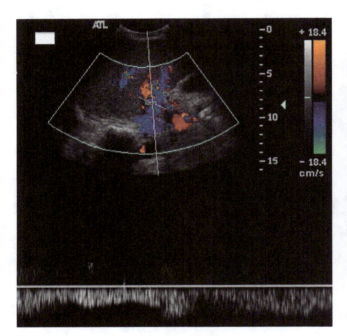

Figure 20-17 Hepatofugal Doppler flow (below the baseline) in patient with cirrhosis.

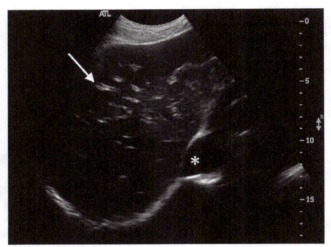

Figure 20-19 Echogenic portal triads (*arrow*) in patient with hepatic congestion. IVC (*).

steatosis is more common (Figure 20-18). Penetration of the ultrasound beam may be attenuated, thereby decreasing resolution of the intrahepatic structures.

Hepatic congestion such as may be seen with hepatitis or right heart failure will be seen as echogenic portal triads standing out more prominently against a background of edematous decreased echotexture liver (the "starry night" pattern); there may also be hepatic vein and IVC enlargement (Figure 20-19). Liver tumors are more commonly hypoechoic than hyperechoic, although the most common benign liver mass, the hemangioma, is usually hyperechoic as is hepatocellular carcinoma (Figures 20-20 and 20-21).

A liver abscess may appear as a hypoechoic or heterogeneous mass due to the presence of pus or phlegmonous liver and may not have enhanced through transmission (Video 20-5). Although CT is a much more sensitive test for the evaluation of liver injury, a discrete hyperechoic pattern may indicate acute liver laceration in the trauma patient; later with hemolysis, hypoechoic hematomas may be seen (Video 20-6).

Portal venous air is uncommonly seen, but appears as echogenic foci moving with blood flow to the periphery of the liver, where it is seen as echogenic branching structures. Finally, arterial and venous flow into and from a transplanted liver may be evaluated with Doppler technology, although not a routine feature of the intensivist's focused examination.

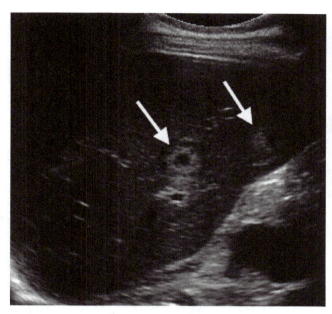

Figure 20-20 Hyperechoic metastases from prostate cancer (*arrows*).

SPLENIC ULTRASOUND

The spleen is homogeneous in echotexture and in the adult less than 12–14 cm in sagittal long length (Figure 20-22). A focused splenic ultrasound will not commonly provide significant clinical guidance to the intensivist. However, splenomegaly may explain thrombocytopenia, demonstrate metastatic disease, or confirm suspicion of underlying portal

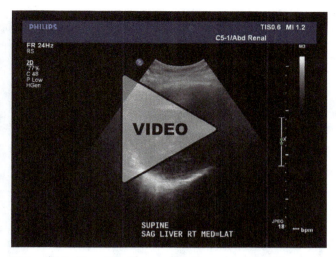

Video 20-5 Cine clip of hypoechoic liver abscesses. View at www.ccu2e.com

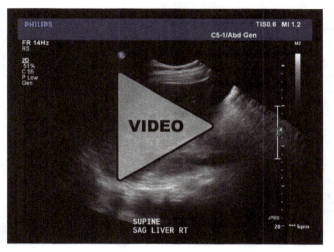

Video 20-6 Cine clip of hematoma due to liver laceration. View at www.ccu2e.com

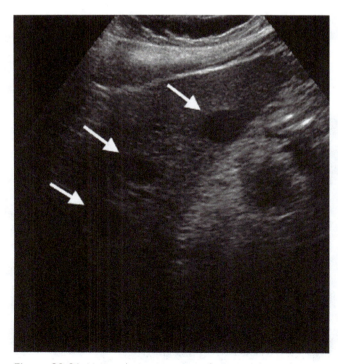

Figure 20-21 Hypoechoic metastases from esophageal carcinoma (*arrows*).

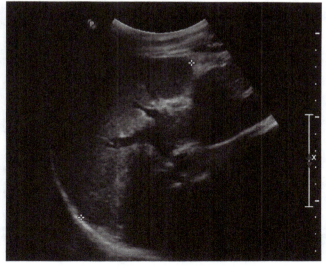

Figure 20-22 Measuring long length of spleen (calipers).

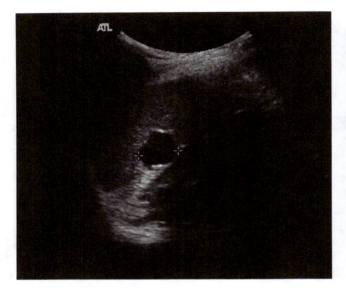

Figure 20-23 Anechoic splenic cyst (calipers).

hypertension. A splenic abscess or pseudocyst may be seen as a hypoechoic lesion in otherwise usually homogeneous medium echotexture organ (Figure 20-23). Metastases in the spleen are less common than in the liver, but they are also typically hypoechoic. The CT is a more sensitive test for the detection of splenic trauma and normal ultrasound appearance does not exclude the possibility of laceration. Localization of the spleen can also prevent injury when performing paracentesis.

GALLBLADDER, BILIARY ULTRASOUND, AND PANCREAS

Ultrasound interrogation of the biliary tree may provide the intensivist with answers to questions of the etiology of right upper quadrant pain or jaundice. The gallbladder is imaged in longitudinal and transverse sweeps (Video 20-7).

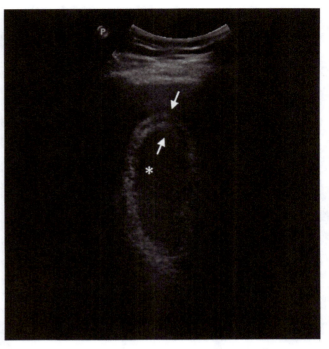

Figure 20-24 Acute cholecystitis with sludge (*) and gallbladder wall thickening (arrows).

The gallbladder contains anechoic fluid and the wall thickness is no greater than 3 mm. Gallbladder interrogation can detect nonshadowing sludge, echogenic shadowing stones, gallbladder wall thickening and distension, or pericholecystic fluid (Figure 20-24 and Video 20-8). Gallbladder wall thickening measuring >3 mm and pericholecystic fluid are secondary signs of acute cholecystitis but not specific. Wall thickening can also be seen with multiple etiologies, such as hepatitis or cirrhosis, right heart failure, cytomegalovirus infection in AIDS patients (Video 20-9).

The patient should be evaluated for pain as the gallbladder passes beneath the probe, the sonographic Murphy

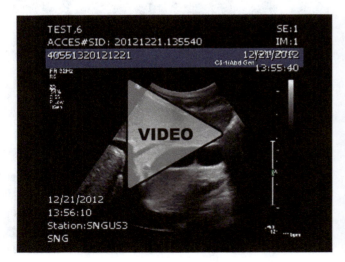

Video 20-7 Cine clip of normal gallbladder. View at www.ccu2e.com

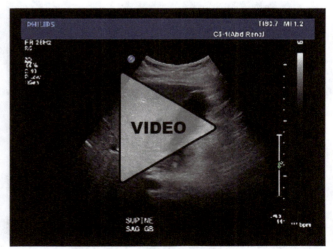

Video 20-8 Cine clip of gallbladder with shadowing stones. View at www.ccu2e.com

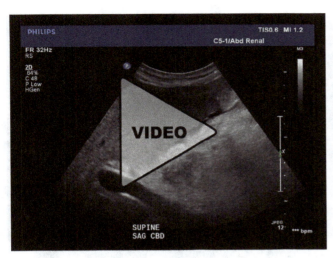

Video 20-9 Cine clip of gallbladder wall thickening in cirrhosis. View at www.ccu2e.com

sign. Sometimes the gallbladder is so filled with shadowing stones, no anechoic bile is seen. The gallbladder in these cases is identified by the wall-echo-shadow complex (wall-stones-posterior shadow) or WES sign (Figure 20-25). The combination of gallstones with a sonographic Murphy sign has positive predictive value of 92% for acute cholecystitis. The gallbladder is generally distended due to impacted stone in the neck or cystic duct, so in the absence of gallbladder distension, other causes for pain should be considered.

Acalculous cholecystitis is most commonly seen in ICU patients who develop gallbladder ischemia due to predisposing vascular insufficiency, diabetes, trauma or burns, or a prolonged fasting state. Sonographic findings may be nonspecific, but percutaneous drainage of a distended gall-

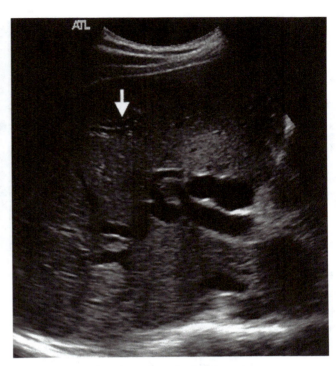

Figure 20-26 Dilated intrahepatic duct (arrow).

bladder may be indicated if there is a suspicion for acalculus cholecystitis.

The intrahepatic ducts paralleling the portal veins are considered dilated if they are greater than 2 mm or more than 40% of the size of adjacent vein in the portal triad (Figure 20-26). Right and left hepatic ducts measure no more than 6 mm. Color flow can confirm that the parallel tubular structures represent ducts without flow. The common bile duct is ≤6 mm under the age of 60, but increases minimally with age afterwards (roughly 1 mm per decade over 60 years). It may also be larger in a patient who has had a cholecystectomy. The common bile duct is to the left of the artery (Figure 20-27). The causes for biliary duct

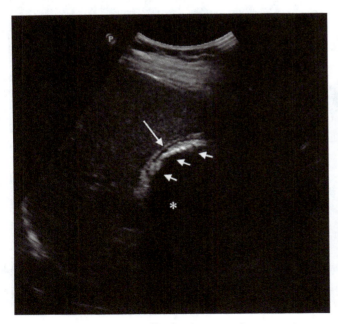

Figure 20-25 Gallbladder filled with stones demonstrating wall-echo-shadow (WES) sign. Gallbladder wall (long arrow), gallstones (short arrows), shadow (*).

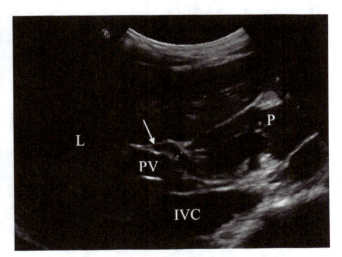

Figure 20-27 Common bile duct (calipers) anterior to larger portal vein (PV) and to the left of the hepatic artery (arrow). L, liver; P, pancreas; IVC, inferior vena cava.

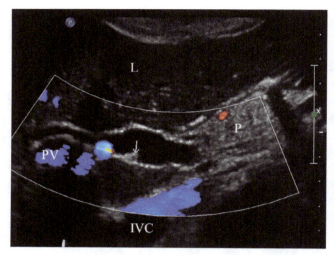

Figure 20-28 Dilated common duct containing sludge (*arrow*) anterior to portal vein (PV). IVC, inferior vena cava; P, pancreas; L, liver.

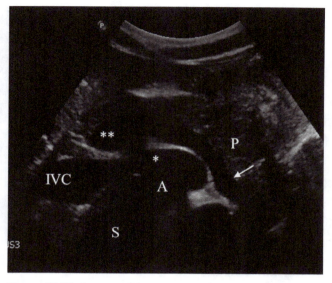

Figure 20-30 Pancreas (P) anterior to splenic vein (*arrow*) and portal confluence (**). Superior mesenteric artery (*) between splenic vein and aorta (A). Inferior vena cava (IVC) to the right of the aorta and spine (S) posterior and to the right of the aorta.

obstruction in a patient with dilated ducts or abnormal serum bilirubin should be sought either within the liver, at the porta hepatis or at pancreas (i.e., stone, stricture, mass), although ultrasound may not detect common bile duct stones or other lesions due to artifact from gas in duodenum (Figure 20-28). Biliary air appears as echogenic streaks following portal triads, typically centrally located and static with occasional branching (Figure 20-29). Post-transplant or postoperative biliary complications, such as bilomas, may also be assessed.

The pancreas may be difficult to identify, particularly in a patient with ileus, due to overlying bowel gas. A normal pancreatic parenchyma is homogeneous in echotexture and the duct should be no more than 4 mm in diameter (Figure 20-30). Pancreatitis may result in an enlarged gland with hypoechoic areas, but this is not universal; peripancreatic edema or pseudocysts may also be visualized (Figure 20-31). Chronic calcific pancreatitis may

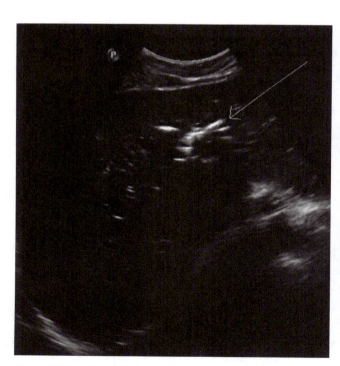

Figure 20-29 Central biliary air (*arrow*) in the liver.

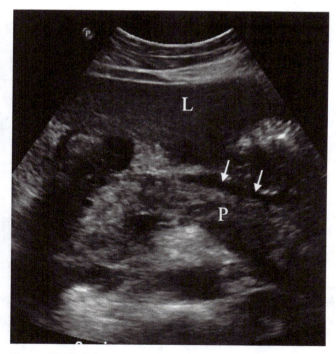

Figure 20-31 Edema (*arrows*) around pancreas (P) due to acute pancreatitis. L, liver.

CHAPTER 20 ULTRASOUND EVALUATION OF THE ABDOMEN   231

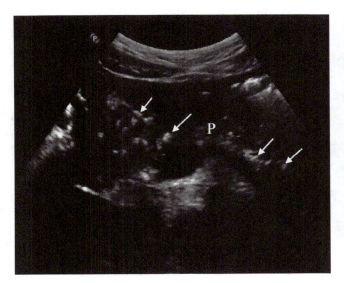

Figure 20-32 Pancreatic (P) calcifications (arrows) in chronic pancreatitis.

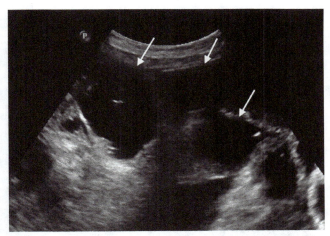

Figure 20-34 Dilated fluid-filled loops of bowel (arrows).

have both shadowing calcifications and a dilated duct due to strictures (Figure 20-32). By far, the better pancreatic imaging modality in the stable patient is CT scanning.

ULTRASOUND OF THE GASTROINTESTINAL TRACT

Sonographic imaging of gastrointestinal structures also falls into the realm of an advanced technique that is rarely helpful for the intensivist in ruling out a particular condition, although a positive finding may assist in care of the patient. The location of a nasogastric tube (by the presence of an acoustic shadow and the decompression of the stomach) may be assessed (Figure 20-33).

Pathologic intestines may be motionless or hyperactive, have thick walls >4 mm, be increased in diameter, or have anechoic fluid-filled contents (Figure 20-34). The differential diagnosis depends on ultrasound findings and clinical features and includes ileus, mechanical bowel obstruction, mesenteric ischemia, or inflammatory processes. A noncompressible thickened inflamed appendix has a target appearance in cross-section but is not usually visible in adults (Figures 20-35 and 20-36). Because of shadowing from bowel gas, intestinal pathology is better evaluated with CT (Figure 20-37). The demonstration of bowel transgressing abdominal wall can confirm hernia or dehiscence.

ABDOMINAL VASCULATURE ULTRASOUND

The aorta and IVC can be assessed in the retroperitoneum with some variability due to bowel gas. Longitudinal and transverse views are obtained. The aorta is typically round and lies just to the left of midline. Its muscular wall is echogenic and 1–2 mm thick. Pulsations are visible; the caliber does not change with respirations. The normal diameter is 2–2.5 cm. The first vessel to arise from the aorta, the celiac

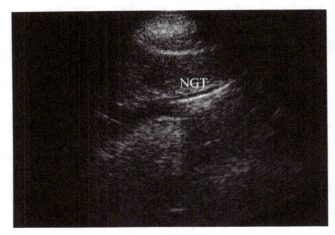

Figure 20-33 Stomach collapsed around nasogastric tube (NGT).

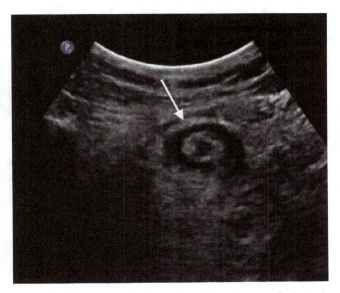

Figure 20-35 Target appearance of inflamed appendix (arrow).

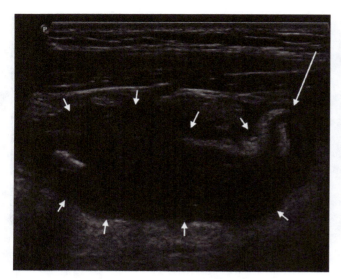

Figure 20-36 Thickened edematous blind ending (*long arrow at tip*) appendix (*short arrows*).

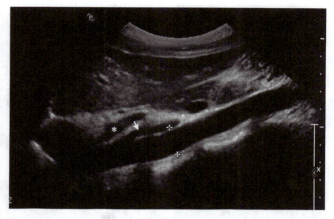

Figure 20-38 Sagittal view aorta (calipers), superior mesenteric artery (*arrow*), and celiac axis (*).

axis, arises at about the T12 level, above the renal arteries, and branches into common hepatic artery heading toward liver, splenic artery to spleen, and left gastric artery moving cephalad. The superior mesenteric artery arises next at L1 and often parallels the aorta on the longitudinal view as it passes caudad within the small bowel mesentery (Figure 20-38).

Just inferiorly, between L1 and L2 levels, the renal arteries arise and are best seen in a transverse plane. The right renal artery courses posterior to the IVC. The inferior mesenteric artery is more difficult to see because of its small size, but arises anteriorly about halfway between the renal arteries and aortic bifurcation at the L3 level. The aorta bifurcates into common iliac arteries at the L4 level at about the level of the umbilicus.

Most aortic aneurysms arise below the level of the renal arteries. They are more commonly fusiform than saccular in shape. The aorta must be measured on transverse view since many aneurysms are wider than tall. Aneurysmal dilatation of the aorta, measuring >3 cm from outer wall to outer wall, may have an anechoic lumen or an associated hypoechoic thrombus in the lumen. Rupture of an aortic aneurysm may be identified by a hyperechoic retroperitoneal hematoma with new free fluid. The treatment must not be delayed by imaging in a patient with an aneurysm in shock. Mesenteric ischemia is likely only if two of the three mesenteric vessels (celiac, superior, and inferior mesenteric arteries) are occluded. Atherosclerotic vessels will have an increased flow velocity and turbulence. These are all difficult diagnoses to make because of the interference of adjacent bowel gas.

The IVC is flatter than the aorta and to the right of midline. It demonstrates bidirectional flow, which is affected by the cardiac cycle and respiratory phase (Video 20-10). Compressibility of the IVC with inspiration in the long axis as it enters the right atrium provides a rapid assessment of a patient's

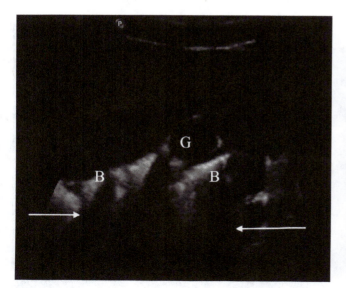

Figure 20-37 Dirty shadowing (*long arrows*) from bowel (B) gas. G, gallbladder.

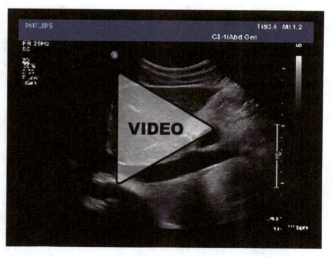

Video 20-10 Cine clip of the inferior vena cava varying in caliber with respirations. View at www.ccu2e.com

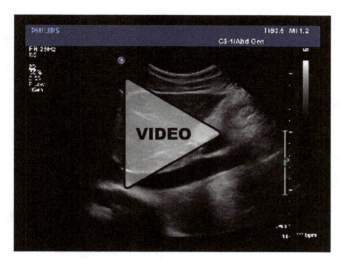

Video 20-11 Cine clip of the inferior vena cava without and with Valsalva maneuver. View at www.ccu2e.com

volume in the ICU. It will markedly decrease in caliber with Valsalva (Video 20-11). In addition to assaying this on B-mode ultrasound, this can also be measured in M-mode. The presence of positive pressure ventilation can alter the reliability of these assessments (see Chapter 10).

SUMMARY

The intensivist can obtain useful information through the use of a goal-directed abdominal ultrasound in critically ill and injured patients. The presence and nature of peritoneal fluid can be assessed as can the etiology of pain, a palpable mass, and abnormal laboratory tests, such as an elevated white cell count or bilirubin. The presence of an ileus, volume overload, and subcutaneous emphysema may render the examination difficult; however, in most cases, the point-of-care sonographer can accomplish a good screening test. As equipment continues to become more user friendly, the indications for abdominal sonography in the ICU will continue to expand.

SUGGESTED READING

Benter T, Klühs L, Teichgräber U. Sonography of the Spleen. *J Ultrasound Med*. 2011;30(9):1281–1293.

Draghi F, Rapaccini GL, Fachinetti C, et al. Ultrasound examination of the liver: normal vascular anatomy. *J Ultrasound*. 2007;10(1):5–11.

Hangiandreou NJ. AAPM/RSNA Physics Tutorial for Residents. Topics in US: B-Mode US: basic concepts and new technology. *Radiographics*. 2003;23(4):1019–1033.

Middleton WD, Kurtz AB, Hertzberg BS. Ultrasound: the Requisites. 2nd ed. St. Louis: Mosby; 2003.

Alexander NG. Trauma Ultrasonography The FAST and Beyond. Trauma.Org. Karim Brohi, Director.http://www.trauma.org/archive/radiology/FASTintro.html. Accesed January 25, 2014. <http://www.trauma.org/archive/radiology/FASTintro.html>.

O'Connor OJ, Maher MM. Imaging of Cholecystitis. *AJR*. 2011;196(4):W367–W374.

Cheng PM, Moin P, Dunn MD, Boswell WD, Duddalwar VA. What the radiologist needs to know about urolithiasis: part 1—pathogenesis, types, assessment, and variant anatomy. *AJR*. 2012;198(6):W540-W547.

Practice Guidelines. American Institute of Ultrasound in Medicine. Alentus.com. http://www.aium.org/resources/guidelines.aspx. Accessed January 25, 2014.

Rumack CM, Wilson SR, Charboneau JW, Levin D. Diagnostic Ultrasound. 4th ed. 2 vols. Philadelphia: Mosby, Elsevier; 2011.

Tchelepi H, Ralls PW, Radin R, Grant E. Sonography of Diffuse Liver Disease. *J Ultrasound Med*. 2002;21:1023–1032.

ULTRASOUND EVALUATION OF THE RENAL SYSTEM AND THE BLADDER

YEFIM R. SHEYNKIN

Scan QR code or visit www.ccu2e.com for video in this chapter

INTRODUCTION

Ultrasound is a powerful and inexpensive tool, particularly well suited for the diagnosis and monitoring of critically ill patients. While portable bedside sonography may not be the preferred tool for a detailed examination, the development of versatile portable ultrasound machines significantly improves its utility and clinical accuracy.[1]

Easy accessibility for major organs of the urinary system makes ultrasound a commonly performed test in critically ill patients. Sonography of the kidneys and bladder in critical care has multiple applications, including evaluation of patients with reduced or absent urinary output, complicated urinary tract infections (UTIs), and fever of unknown origin, renal trauma, and idiopathic hematuria. It is the most useful initial investigation in the early or late period after kidney transplantation. Sonographic study often provides the clinician with a diagnosis or guidance for rapid decision making necessary for the treatment of critically ill patients. The most important goal of ultrasound evaluation of the urinary system is to identify or rule out a problem that requires prompt, goal-directed surgical or medical intervention to improve the patient's condition. While not intended as a comprehensive formal examination, ultrasound is a convenient bedside monitoring tool for use in the intensive care unit (ICU).

In addition, many incidental abnormalities may be found during sonographic evaluation of kidneys and bladder. Whereas they may not have an impact on the immediate treatment decision, physicians should be able to recognize them and provide appropriate care if necessary.

SONOGRAPHIC ANATOMY OF URINARY TRACT

The normal adult kidney is a bean-shaped structure surrounded by a well-defined, smooth echogenic capsule representing Gerota's fascia and perinephric fat. The kidneys have a convex lateral edge and concave medial edge called the hilum. The lower pole is located more laterally and anteriorly than the upper pole. The sonographically measured normal adult kidney is between 9 and 12 cm in length and about 4–5 cm wide.

The kidney parenchyma surrounds centrally located hyperechoic fatty renal sinus, which contains renal pelvis, calyces, major branches of renal artery and vein, and lymphatic vessels. Parenchyma corresponds to the area between renal sinus and outer renal surface and has two main components: the more echogenic peripherally located cortex and centrally located hypoechoic medulla, which contains renal pyramids (Figure 21-1). The normal renal parenchyma is 1.0–1.8 cm thick. The visible distinction between the cortex and medulla is a sign of a normal kidney. While easily recognized in children and younger patients, it may not always be detectable in the elderly.

Parenchymal homogeneity is determined in comparison with that of adjacent liver and spleen. Normally, the renal cortex is hypoechoic or isoechoic to the liver (right kidney) and hypoechoic to spleen (left kidney). The collecting system of the kidney is not usually visible with ultrasound because calyces and pelvis are collapsed within renal sinus. The normal ureters measure approximately 8 mm wide and are difficult to evaluate sonographically. However, proximal or distal ends of significantly dilated ureter (hydroureter) can be seen.

The shape and appearance of the normal bladder depends on the degree of distention. When empty, the bladder lies behind the symphysis pubis. On longitudinal transabdominal view, the full bladder has a teardrop-shaped anechoic appearance, with distinct wall, while on the transverse view it appears rectangular. The thickness of the bladder wall varies with the degree of bladder filling. When mildly distended or empty, the bladder wall is thick and irregular. With full distension, the normal bladder wall is thin and smooth and does not exceed 4–5 mm in thickness (Figure 21-2).[2]

SECTION III ULTRASOUND EVALUATION OF THE NECK, TRUNK, AND EXTREMITIES

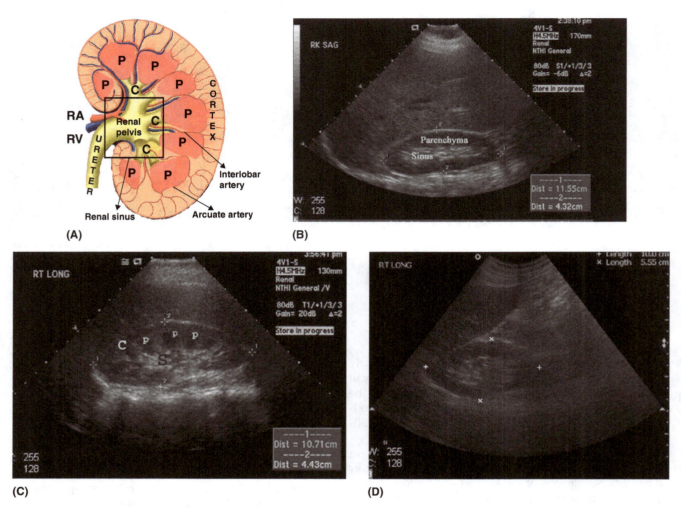

Figure 21-1 (A) Normal renal anatomy. C = calyx; P = pyramid; RA = main renal artery; RV = main renal vein. (B) Normal kidney. Longitudinal view of the kidney demonstrates peripheral hypoechoic universally thick parenchyma and central hyperechoic renal sinus. Note the echogenic white Gerota's fascia. Parenchyma is less echogenic then liver. (C) The cortical echogenicity is equal of that of the liver. Several slightly hypoechoic renal pyramids are seen. C = cortical echogenicity; L = liver. (D) Portable ultrasound of the normal right kidney. Note less contrast appearance but renal contour, parenchyma and renal sinus are clearly identified.

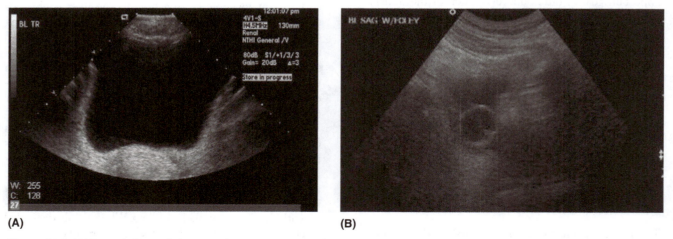

Figure 21-2 (A) Transabdominal ultrasound (transverse scan) of a normally distended bladder. (B) Foley catheter in the collapsed bladder (portable ultrasound).

IMAGING TECHNIQUE

The spectrum of urologic ultrasound includes gray-scale and Doppler evaluation of the kidneys and the bladder. In accordance with American Institute of Ultrasound in Medicine practice guideline, the examination of kidneys should include longitudinal and transverse views and assessment of the cortex and renal pelvis. Renal echogenicity may be compared with echogenicity of the adjacent liver or spleen. Kidneys and perirenal regions should be assessed for abnormalities (Table 21-1).[3]

Sonographic evaluation of a critically ill patient is typically limited by a supine position, lack of patient cooperation, presence of monitoring devices, tissue changes (e.g., bowel gas, edema, ascites), postsurgical incisions, and dressings.

TABLE 21-1
Renal Ultrasound in Critically Ill Patients

Parameter	Description
Longitudinal diameter	Easy to obtain and reproduce with less intra- and interobserve variation. Average length is between 9 and 12 cm
Parenchymal thickness	Measurements between renal surface and hyperechoic sinus, normally >1 cm
Kidney margins	Sharp and regular. V-shaped indentation may represent persistent fetal lobulation. The outline depression with rounded angles indicates inflammatory or ischemic scars
Parenchymal echogenicity	Cortex hypo/isoechogenicity compared with that of liver or spleen is usually normal, while hyperechogenicity indicates a diffuse parenchymal pathology. Medulla is slightly less echogenic than cortex
Collecting system	Visible only when dilated (hydronephrosis), mostly secondary to mechanical obstruction
Calcifications	Small hyperechogenic lesions are nonspecific and may represent small stones, vascular or intraparenchymal calcifications. Larger stones are easily diagnosed by the characteristic posterior acoustic shadowing
Renal/extrarenal masses	Solid masses are usually neoplastic and require further evaluation with CT or MRI. Simple renal cyst is anechoic thin-walled space occupying lesion with good through-transmission and no internal echoes
Resistive index	Color Doppler study of renal perfusion. Normal RI <0.70. High resistance pattern indicates decrease perfusion of various causes

CT = computerized tomography; MRI = magnetic resonance imaging; RI = resistive index.

Kidneys demonstrate a significant mobility with respiration (about 2–3 cm), which complicates the evaluation of patients on a ventilator.[4]

Commonly, a sector or curved-array transducer (3–5 MHz) is used, while higher frequency probes (5–7 MHz) with higher space resolution may be necessary to evaluate children, thin patients, and transplanted kidneys. Imaging of the urinary tract must always include evaluation of both kidneys and the bladder.

The right kidney is best examined in the supine or left lateral decubitus position through the liver, which serves as an acoustic window. The probe should be placed along the right lateral subcostal margin in the anterior axillary line, scanning through the liver to locate the right kidney. After visualization of the whole kidney, the optimal longitudinal view is obtained by slowly adjusting the probe's position up and down or side to side. The kidney is traditionally measured in the longest axis (length and width) because the longitudinal diameter has minor inter- and intraobserver variations. If needed, a transverse plane (short-axis view) can be obtained by rotating the probe 90° and evaluating upper, mid, and lower portions of the kidney separately.

The left kidney is typically less visible due to its location in a more superior position, the lack of the sonographic window generated by the liver and the overlying small bowel, and gastric gas. If possible, placing the patient in the right lateral decubitus position with the probe positioned in the posterior axillary line or left costovertebral angle may improve visualization. If bowel gas obscures the kidney (especially left) and reflects the ultrasound waves, the transducer can be positioned in the mid- or posterior axillary line.[5]

The bladder can be examined only when it is distended. Sonographic evaluation is usually performed from a transabdominal location, with the patient in a supine position. A probe is placed 1 cm above the symphysis and angled laterally, inferiorly, and superiorly. Most commonly, the transverse scan is obtained first. A normal bladder is located in the midline without deviation, and appears symmetric, smooth, and without irregularities of inner surface. On the longitudinal scan, the bladder is oriented toward the umbilicus and tapered anteriorly. Transverse and longitudinal scans provide a fairly accurate calculation of the urine volume within the bladder. If needed, postvoid residual urine volume can be automatically calculated.

Detailed bladder ultrasound may have a limited application in critically ill patients with draining indwelling Foley catheters. However, it can provide immediate bedside diagnosis of urinary retention in patients with decreased or absent urinary output.

COLOR DOPPLER ULTRASOUND

Complex Doppler studies have not been used routinely as a bedside test in critically ill patients. However, the technical improvement of portable ultrasound machines with color and power Doppler equipment enables the ability to combine gray-scale ultrasound with limited Doppler study in the critical care setting. Changes in the perfusion of renal parenchyma are commonly associated with different renal pathology. Color-flow and spectral Doppler studies are able to provide noninvasive, indirect global assessment of renal blood flow and identify the vessels at the level of the renal hilum and in the renal parenchyma. Because the spatial resolution of gray-scale sonography is much lower than frequency resolution, the Doppler study is able to detect the arteries on the basis of the flow and not the anatomic size.[2] The Doppler spectral tracing reflects a low vascular resistance and classically has a ski slope appearance. From the many different indices introduced to quantify blood flow, the most commonly used single parameter is the resistive index (RI), a ratio between end-diastolic velocity and peak systolic velocities. Restrictive index is a physiological parameter reflecting the degree of renal vascular resistance. Normal renal blood flow has a low resistance pattern, with a flow maintained throughout diastole. The normal RI values are 0.58 ± 0.10.[2] Values >0.70 are considered abnormal and may be due to lower arterial patency, although major clinical significance is observed for values >0.80. Doppler signals are commonly obtained from renal artery or interlobar arcuate arteries at the corticomedullary junction and border of medullary pyramids. However, the identification of these areas requires more training and experience in performing Doppler ultrasound. The test is routinely performed to evaluate the transplanted kidney. The RI has been proposed to assist with the differential diagnosis between obstructive and nonobstructive hydronephrosis, or diagnosis of acute obstruction when dilatation has not yet developed. A minority of patients with obstructive renal failure may not show hydronephrosis due to dehydration or decompression caused by rupture of calyceal fornix. High intrarenal pressure and changing renal hemodynamics due to the release of vasoactive substances and vasoconstriction secondary to obstruction cause an increase in intrarenal arterial resistance measured by a higher RI. While the diagnostic accuracy of RI still remains controversial due to a wide range of results, a normal RI may still be helpful in arguing against the presence of obstruction.[6-8] Color-flow Doppler ultrasound is frequently performed for the evaluation of the patency of the ureter. Jet phenomenon should be seen in the bladder when the urine bolus from the ureter is being propelled into the bladder cavity due to periodic peristalsis (1–12 jets per minute). Ureteral jets are usually identified during transverse bladder scanning as a color projecting into the bladder lumen from lateral posterior border and coursing superior and medial (Figure 21-3). While most critically ill patients have indwelling Foley catheters, bedside evaluation of ureteral jets may be limited due to the empty bladder.

CLINICAL APPLICATIONS

▶ Renal Failure

Acute and acute-on-chronic renal failure (ARF) is relatively common in critically ill patients with a reported prevalence ranging between 16% and 23%.[9] While physical examination and laboratory tests are invaluable in making a correct diagnosis, sonography rapidly provides useful information about the kidneys independent of renal function. The American College of Radiology Appropriateness Criteria suggests ultrasound as a primary imaging technique in ARF.[10]

Traditionally, renal failure is categorized as prerenal, intrinsic to the kidney, and postrenal. While prerenal kidney failure will not be associated with specific sonographic abnormalities, intrinsic and especially postrenal (obstructive) causes usually will have visible ultrasound features. Ultrasound evaluation can establish the presence of kidneys, their size, shape, and echogenicity. The absence of kidney in the normal anatomical position (pelvic kidney is usually located close to midline, just above the bladder) requires further investigation.

Renal parenchymal damage is a major cause of intrinsic renal failure. Sonographic evaluation is not helpful in providing a precise diagnosis of renal disease. However, it may provide some information regarding the nature of renal insufficiency. Normal or enlarged kidneys are likely associated with ARF. Parenchymal echogenicity is equal or greater compared to the liver. It is important to remember that liver echogenicity may also be altered in a critically ill patient. In more severe cases, the echogenicity of the renal parenchyma is equal to the renal sinus echoes.

The most common cause of ARF in critical care patients is acute tubular necrosis (ATN).[11] While sonography is not a diagnostic method used for ATN, recent research provides support for the possible use of color Doppler for the monitoring of improvement of renal hemodynamics in the critically ill patient. The recovery of renal function has been characterized by improvement in RI when there are still no significant changes in the diuresis.[2]

Chronic renal failure is associated with small (5–8 cm in length) contracted kidneys with increased echogenicity. Renal sinus echoes are still visible, but the parenchyma may show evidence of focal losses (Figure 21-4).

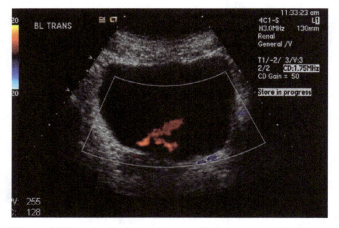

Figure 21-3 Color Doppler ultrasound of the urinary bladder shows crossing bilateral ureteral jets.

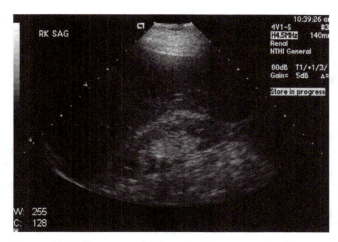

Figure 21-4 Chronic renal failure. Small contracted right kidney. Parenchymal echogenicity is equal to that of the liver and slightly less than of renal sinus.

Postrenal ARF can be efficiently corrected if promptly diagnosed. About 5% of patients with ARF suffer from obstructive uropathy (hydronephrosis). It is more common in patients with certain predisposing factors, including urolithiasis, retroperitoneal cancer, or a solitary kidney. In patients with no risk factors for urinary obstruction, only approximately 1% will have sonographically detected hydronephrosis.[9] Nevertheless, obstructive uropathy remains the most important finding that requires urgent treatment because it is likely to be reversible. Alternatively, knowing that obstruction is absent is as important a finding as treating obstruction.

Sonography can usually diagnose obstruction quickly and simply with a sensitivity of approximately 95%. The dilatation of the renal collecting system (hydronephrosis) is the most important sonographic feature of obstructive uropathy (Video 21-1). Renal pelvis and calyceal dilation

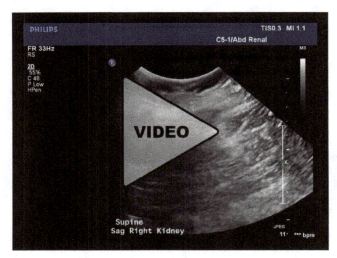

Video 21-1 Hydronephrosis due to obstructive uropathy. Note widening of the renal collecting system and loss of the parenchymal thickness. View at www.ccu2e.com

are characterized by effacement of the renal sinus fat by an anechoic-branched structure with through-transmission. Hydronephrosis is most commonly categorized as mild, moderate, or severe. The degree of renal damage can be quantified on the basis of a reduction in parenchymal thickness. Mild hydronephrosis (grade I) refers to minimal dilatation of the collecting system known as splaying. Moderate hydronephrosis (grade II) shows rounding of the calices with obliteration of the papillae. Cortical thinning is minimal in moderate hydronephrosis. Severe hydronephrosis (grade III) refers to massive dilatation of renal pelvis and calyces associated with cortical thinning (Figure 21-5).

However, the degree of dilatation does not necessarily correlate with the presence or severity of obstruction. Acute, high-grade obstruction may produce only minimal hydronephrosis on early ultrasound before significant dilatation of the collecting system develops. This problem may be common in critically ill patients with reduced renal function.

Hydronephrosis does not necessarily equate with obstruction because other factors (e.g., infection, persistent diuresis, and reflux) can cause dilatation of the pelvicocalyceal system. Doppler evaluation has been proposed for the suspected renal obstruction. Normal RIs suggest the absence of obstruction, while RIs greater than 0.70 suggest an obstructive etiology of hydronephrosis. However, this method remains controversial because of equivocal and conflicting results in detection of either acute or partial obstruction.[8]

Analysis of ureteral jets by Doppler interrogation may be another way to diagnose ureteral obstruction. The detection of intermittent flashes of Doppler color (jets) indicates patency of upper urinary tract. The absence of a unilateral jet is highly significant as an indication of obstruction. The presence or absence of ureteral jets does not correspond to the degree of hydronephrosis. The bilateral absence of jets is less specific and may indicate a lack of difference in specific gravity between urine entering the bladder and urine in the bladder. The combined Doppler study (RI and ureteral jets) improves the accuracy of renal ultrasound in the diagnosis of obstruction.[6]

Identification of the obstructing lesion remains the best way to confirm the significance of hydronephrosis. However, it is not always possible with the limited ultrasound evaluation of critically ill patient. Bilateral hydronephrosis in patients with ARF, regardless of its cause, requires emergency decompression of the kidneys to restore urinary output.

Certain sonographic findings mimicking hydronephrosis include renal cysts, an extrarenal pelvis, and polycystic renal disease (Figure 21-6). Questionable findings in patients with anuria may require an extended evaluation beyond ultrasound to confirm a diagnosis of obstruction.

Renal cysts are the most commonly found renal mass. Sonographic features of a simple cyst include a spherical appearance, an anechoic lumen without internal echoes, a well-defined back wall, clear wall demarcations, no

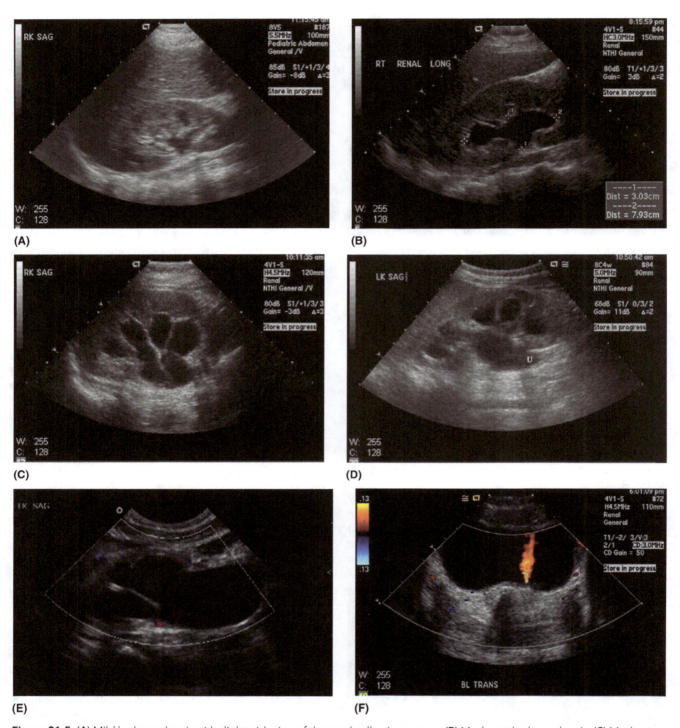

Figure 21-5 (**A**) Mild hydronephrosis with slight widening of the renal collecting system. (**B**) Moderate hydronephrosis. (**C**) Moderate hydronephrosis without loss of renal parenchymal thickness. (**D**) Hydronephrosis and proximal hydroureter (U). (**E**) Severe hydronephrosis with thinning of renal parenchyma. (**F**) Loss of the right ureteral jet in patient with right obstructive hydronephrosis.

measurable wall thickness, and an acoustic enhancement posterior to the cyst. Single or multiple cysts may be located anywhere in the kidney. A renal sinus cyst is called parapelvic and accounts for 6% of renal cysts. A parapelvic cyst does not communicate with renal pelvis and calyces. Unlike the cauliflower appearance of a dilated pelvis, a parapelvic cyst is rounder, with good through-transmission. Sonographically, the differential diagnosis between hydronephrosis and parapelvic cyst may be difficult, especially if the cysts are bilateral. Complex cysts do not meet the sonographic criteria of simple cysts. They may be septated and multilocular. While the ultrasound diagnosis of a simple cyst is

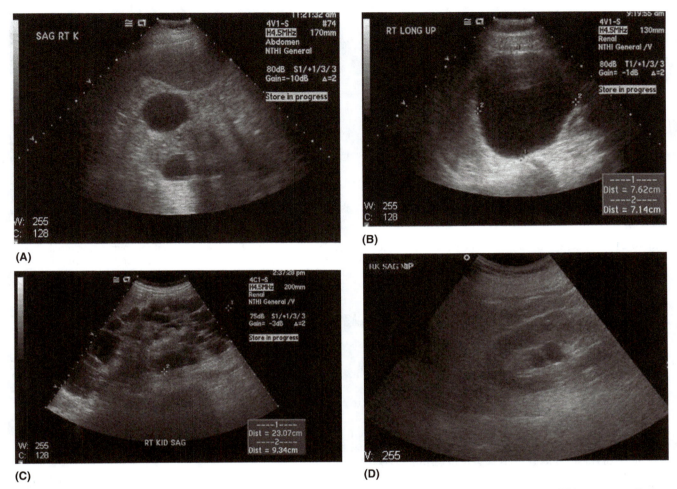

Figure 21-6 (A) Renal cyst may be single or multiple. Borders are well defined. No internal echoes are seen. (B) Large centrally located renal cyst. (C) Polycystic kidneys are usually bilateral. Normal renal parenchyma of enlarged kidney is replaced with multiple cysts of different sizes. (D) Two parapelvic cysts do not communicate with the renal collecting system (portable ultrasound).

very accurate, complex cysts may require additional imaging studies (e.g., computerized tomography [CT] or magnetic resonance imaging) to rule out malignancy.

Autosomal-dominant polycystic kidney disease is one of the etiologies of end-stage renal failure. Multiple variably sized cysts located in the cortex and medulla are characteristic for this bilateral disease. The kidneys are enlarged and the parenchyma can be identified or completely replaced by numerous cysts. The extrarenal pelvis lies largely outside the kidney rather than in its usual central location. Usually, dilatation of the calyces is not associated with nonobstructed, dilated extrarenal pelvis.

KIDNEY TRANSPLANT

Decreased renal function after transplantation is the most important indication for ultrasound evaluation. The more superficial location of the transplanted kidney requires a 5–7 MHz transducer. Longitudinal and transverse scans over the kidney provide accurate measurements of kidney size, echogenicity, shape and evidence of hydronephrosis, bladder sonogram, and the color Doppler flow studies.

The normal transplanted kidney is similar to the native kidney morphologically. It has a smooth contour and homogenous parenchyma. The urinary bladder should be visualized where possible. Normally, it must be empty because full bladder may cause hydronephrosis (Figure 21-7).[12,13]

The primary goal of ultrasound in the transplanted kidney is to differentiate between obstructive uropathy and systemic or intrinsic causes of reduced function (acute rejection [AR] or ATN) and to identify peritransplant fluid collections.

AR and ATN have no specific diagnostic sonographic features. The diagnostic value of ultrasound in ATN or AR is limited. The kidney may be enlarged, with increased cortex hyperechogenicity and occasional distortion of the renal outline. While the differential diagnosis between AR and ATN is not possible with ultrasound, obstruction

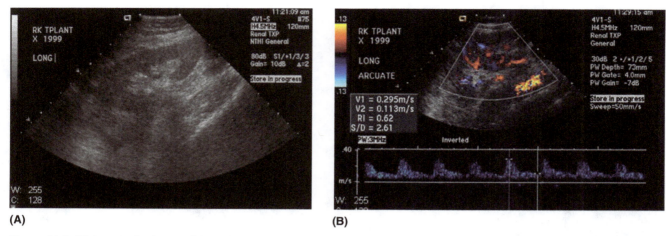

Figure 21-7 (**A**) Longitudinal view of the right transplanted kidney. The renal parenchyma is well visualized with bright renal sinus echoes centrally. (**B**) Color Doppler ultrasound image of the transplanted kidney. Spectral gate is placed over arcuate vessels. A number of indices can be measured simultaneously. Resistive index <0.7 is considered normal.

(hydronephrosis) is very distinctive and is important to rule out (Figure 21-8).

The sonography can promptly identify hydronephrosis and establish indications for surgical intervention or close follow-up. Hydronephrosis has the same appearance in the transplanted kidney as in the native kidney and may be secondary to anastomotic failure or a fluid collection due to urine leak (urinoma), lymphatic leak (seroma), or bleeding (hematoma). Peritransplant fluid collections have been reported in up to 50% of renal transplantation. The clinical relevance of these collections is largely determined by their size, location, and possible growth.[12] Peritransplant fluid collections are readily detectable by ultrasound. Regardless of their nature (urine, blood, or lymph), sonographically they may appear as well-defined anechoic areas, with or without septation, although acute hematoma may be echogenic. Internal echoes are mostly seen in hematomas where clots have become organized (Figure 21-9).

Color Doppler is used routinely to evaluate the transplanted kidney. However, RI itself is not specific for the differential diagnosis of transplant complications, although it may be helpful to confirm an obstructive hydronephrosis. The most common cause of elevated RI (over 0.70) in the absence of obstruction or infection is AR.[13] The likelihood of an AR increases as the values of RI increase.

RENAL TRAUMA

Focused assessment with sonography for trauma (FAST) has been an accurate method for detecting hemoperitoneum in unstable patients. However, ultrasound is presently not advocated as a first-line imaging modality in renal trauma because its sensitivity in diagnosing and grading renal injury remains low. Normal findings do not exclude renal injury and major injuries may not be identified.[14,15]

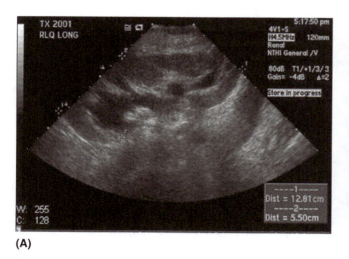
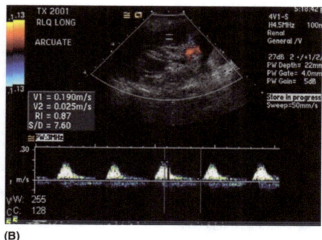

Figure 21-8 (**A**) Hydronephrosis of the transplanted kidney. (**B**) Color Doppler study shows elevated resistive index of the arcuate arteries.

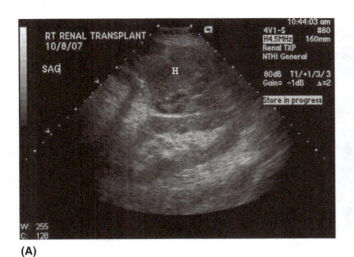 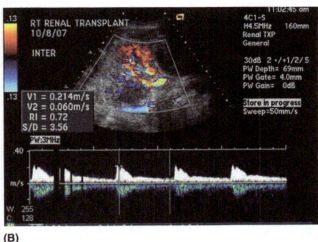

Figure 21-9 (A) Large hematoma anterior to the transplanted kidney, which does not affect kidney function. Renal parenchyma shows normal echogenicity. (B) Normal resistive index of the interlobar arteries.

While renal ultrasound may reveal subcapsular or perinephric fluid collections, it cannot provide crucial differentiation between blood, extravasated urine, and other types of free fluid. Color Doppler ultrasound can be helpful in the evaluation of renal blood flow by assessing perfusion of the whole kidney or any portion. If renal ultrasound suggests injury or if it is negative in patient with the clinical evidence of renal involvement (hematuria), a contrast CT should be provided in stable patient for further evaluation.

However, ultrasound is a very useful tool for a bedside monitoring of the resolution or expansion of hematomas in the critical care setting, as recent management of even severe isolated renal injuries is mostly conservative (Figure 21-10).

UROSEPSIS

UTI is one of the most common hospital-acquired infections and most frequent nosocomial infection in critically ill patients. Complicated UTI is not uncommon in ICU patients due to multiple predisposing factors, including compromised immune systems, associated medical problems, and indwelling urinary catheters. The spectrum of UTI extends from acute pyelonephritis with or without obstructive uropathy to renal and perirenal abscesses.

While pyelonephritis usually has no specific sonographic features; however, enlarged kidney and hyperemia of the renal parenchyma with occasional focal changes (nephronia) can be seen (Video 21-2). Ultrasound can also diagnose such abnormalities as hydro- and pyonephrosis, renal and perirenal abscesses, or emphysematous pyelonephritis.

Xanthogranulomatous pyelonephritis (XGP), a serious, chronic inflammatory disease sonographically characterized by a destructive mass in the renal parenchyma. XGP is most commonly due to *Proteus Escherichia coli* or *Pseudomonas* infection. The treatment of XGP is a nephrectomy as kidney is usually rendered nonfunctional. Most cases

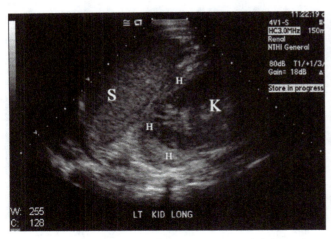 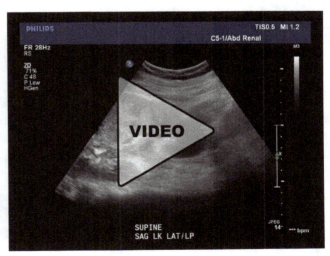

Figure 21-10 Perirenal hematoma in patient with left renal laceration. H = hematoma; K = kidney; S = spleen.

Video 21-2 Pyelonephritis with renal hyperemia. View at www.ccu2e.com

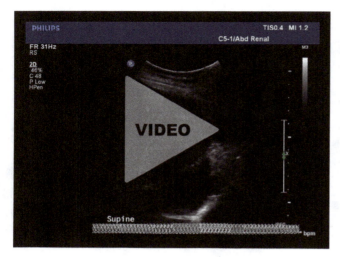

Video 21-3 Xanthogranulomatous pyelonephritis (XGP). Note destructive hypoechoic mass in the renal parenchyma. View at www.ccu2e.com

are unilateral, but bilateral disease has been reported. The overall prognosis for XGP is good, bilateral disease requires dialysis (Video 21-3).

Pyonephrosis represents pus in the obstructed and infected collecting system. It is a medical emergency requiring immediate renal decompression. Pyonephrosis must be suspected in patients with hydronephrosis, UTI, and ultrasound findings of low-level echoes with occasional layering in the dependent position of the dilated collecting system.

Renal intraparenchymal abscess appears as a complex hypoechoic mass with thick irregular walls and occasional fluid debris level. A perinephric abscess will result in a heterogeneous crescent-shaped fluid collection surrounding the kidney that may deform the renal cortex (Video 21-4). While additional tests (CT) may be necessary to differentiate between abscess and renal cancer, ultrasound can be a valuable tool to monitor the diagnosed abscess or focal pyelonephritis during medical treatment (Figure 21-11).

Emphysematous pyelonephritis is an uncommon but life-threatening diffuse infection of the renal parenchyma caused by gas-forming bacteria. Most patients are female, and 90% are diabetic. Patients are usually extremely ill, often toxic, presenting with fever, flank pain, acidosis, hyperglycemia, dehydration, and electrolyte imbalance. Ultrasound typically reveals an enlarged kidney containing high-amplitude echoes within the parenchyma/renal sinus associated with a low-level posterior acoustic shadowing. CT scan is necessary to confirm the presence of air in the renal parenchyma.

OTHER SONOGRAPHIC FINDINGS

Screening, observational, or focused ultrasound evaluation of the critically ill patient frequently reveals additional sonographic findings that have no direct impact on the patient's condition and will not change the immediate treatment. However, such incidental findings require further evaluation with additional imaging modalities to establish correct diagnosis when the patient is stable (Figure 21-12).

A solid renal mass is a heterogeneous, isoechoic, or hypoechoic lesion of variable dimensions adjacent to a normal renal parenchyma. Ultrasound is used primarily to differentiate solid masses from simple cysts. All solid renal masses in adults should be considered malignant until proven otherwise. Further evaluation with CT scan is required for appropriate diagnosis.

Nephrolithiasis is one of the most common kidney problems. Kidney stones are intensely hyperechoic linear or arching foci with posterior acoustic shadowing (Video 21-5).

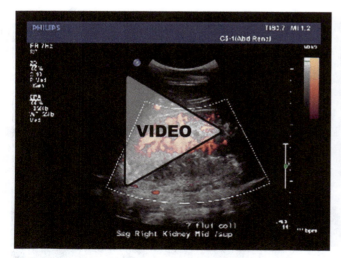

Video 21-4 Perinephric abscess. Note heterogeneous hypoechoic crescent-shaped fluid collection surrounding the kidney. View at www.ccu2e.com

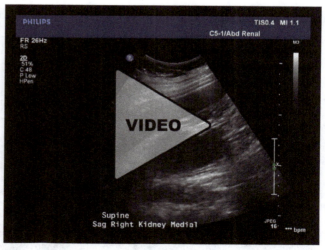

Video 21-5 Nephrolithiasis (Staghorn calculus). Note intensely hyperechoic linear and arching calculi with characteristic posterior acoustic shadowing. View at www.ccu2e.com

CHAPTER 21 ULTRASOUND EVALUATION OF THE RENAL SYSTEM AND THE BLADDER   245

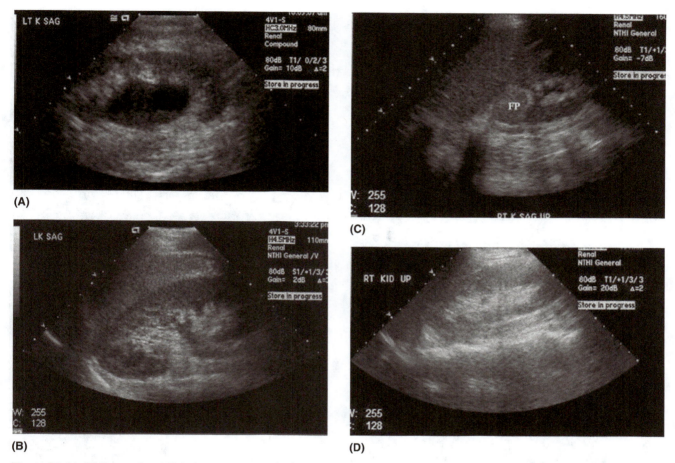

Figure 21-11 (**A**) Pyonephrosis. Moderate-to-severe hydronephrosis with fine debris in the renal collecting system. (**B**) Nonspecific finding of the enlarged kidney in patient with clinical picture of acute pyelonephritis. (**C**) Hyperechoic lesion within renal parenchyma in patient with urosepsis represents area of focal pyelonephritis (FP). (**D**) Follow-up ultrasound revealed complete disappearance of the lesion after medical treatment.

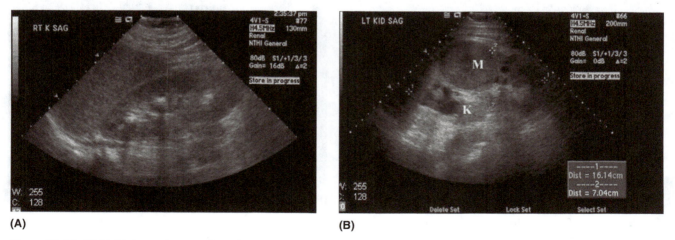

Figure 21-12 (**A**) Multiple renal stones. Nonobstructed kidney containing hyperechoic (white) calcifications with posterior acoustic shadowing. (**B**) Large solid renal mass (M) distorting renal collecting system (K).

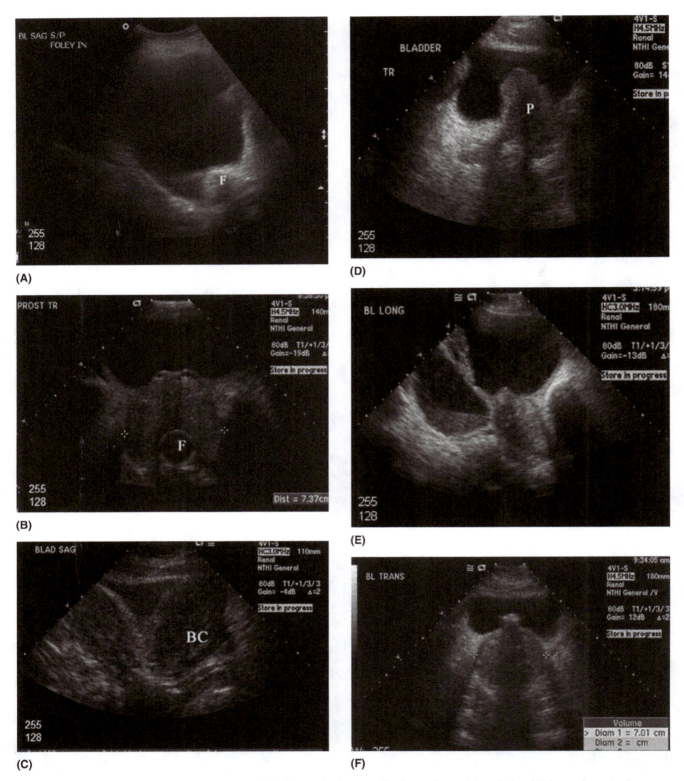

Figure 21-13 (A) Portable ultrasound. Distended bladder with obstructed Foley catheter. (B) Dislodged Foley catheter in the prostatic urethra below the bladder. (C) Large blood clot in patient with gross hematuria may simulate bladder tumor. (D) Grossly enlarged prostate protruding into the bladder lumen. (E) Large bladder diverticulum. (F) Bladder stone. BC = blood clot; F = Foley catheter.

They can be of different sizes and locations within the kidney. Obstructing stones occasionally can be seen in patients with hydronephrosis and dilated proximal or distal ureter.[16] Nonobstructing kidney stones do not require urgent treatment.

BLADDER ULTRASOUND

The sonographic evaluation of the bladder is uncommon in critically ill patients with an indwelling Foley catheter and collapsed bladder. However, it is a necessary part of renal ultrasound because urinary retention may cause hydronephrosis. Dislodged or obstructed Foley catheters are a common cause of "anuria" in critically ill patients. Bladder ultrasound allows prompt visualization of a distended bladder and can locate the balloon of the Foley catheter within or outside of a full bladder.[17] Bladder volume can be automatically calculated by measuring horizontal and vertical dimensions of the bladder on a transverse image and maximum longitudinal dimension on longitudinal image. Bladder stones appear hyperechoic with posterior acoustic shadowing. They move with changes in patient position. Blood clots may be visualized in patients with gross hematuria. The differential diagnosis must include bladder tumor, which also appears as a polypoid, hyperechoic projection from the bladder wall. Diverticula present sonographically as sonolucent masses adjacent to the bladder. Large bladder diverticula may still be visible with an empty bladder. A grossly enlarged prostate may be seen as a round or polypoid mass protrusion at the bottom of the bladder (Figure 21-13).

SUMMARY

The role of ultrasound of kidneys and bladder in critical care has been widely debated based on its usefulness and cost-effectiveness. While bedside urologic ultrasound is not a substitute for standard sonography or other important and informative imaging modalities, it certainly provides properly trained physicians with the unique ability to perform bedside ultrasound-enhanced clinical evaluations of the urinary system of critically ill patients. Whether it is a screening, observational, or emergency evaluation, this approach is helpful in expediting treatment and improving outcome.

REFERENCES

1. Kirkpatrick AW, Sustic A, Blaivas M. Introduction to the use of ultrasound in critical care medicine. *Crit Care Med*. 2007;35:S123–S307.
2. Barozzi L, Valentino M, Santoro A, Mancini E, Pavlica P. Renal ultrasound in the critically ill patient. *Crit Care Med*. 2007;35:S198–S205.
3. American Institute of Ultrasound in Medicine. AIUM Practice Guidelines for the performance of an ultrasound examination of the abdomen and/or retroperitoneum. *J Ultrasound Med*. 2008;27:319–326.
4. Heller M, Jehle D. Obstructive uropathy. In: Heller M, Jehle D, eds. *Ultrasound in Emergency Medicine*. Philadelphia, PA: WB Saunders Co; 1995:65.
5. Noble VE, Brown DFM. Renal ultrasound. *Emerg Med Clin N Am*. 2004;22:641–659.
6. Pepe P, Motta L, Pennisi M, Aragona F. Functional evaluation of the urinary tract by color Doppler ultrasonography (CDU) in 100 patients with renal colic. *Eur J Radiol*. 2005;53:131–135.
7. Gurel S, Acata D, Gurel K, et al. Correlation between renal resistive index (RI) and nonenhanced computed tomography in acute renal colic. How reliable is RI in distinguishing obstruction? *J Ultrasound Med*. 2006;25:1113–1120.
8. Cronan J. Renal failure. In: Bluth EL, Arger PH, Benson CB, Ralls PW, Siegel MJ, eds. *Ultrasound: A Practical Approach to Clinical Problems*. New York, NY: Thieme; 2000:90.
9. Keyserling HF, Fielding JR, Mittelstaedt CA. Renal sonography in the intensive care unit: when is it necessary? *J Ultrasound Med*. 2002;21:517–520.
10. American College of Radiology Appropriateness Criteria® renal failure. American College of Radiology—Medical Specialty Society. 1995. www.guideline.gov. Accessed 2005.
11. Huang SW, Lee CT, Chen CH, Chuang CH, Chen JB. Role of renal sonography in the intensive care unit. *J Clin Ultrasound*. 2005;33:72–75.
12. Park SB, Kim JK, Cho K. Complications of renal transplantation: ultrasonographic evaluation. *J Ultrasound Med*. 2007;26:615–633.
13. Baxter GM. Ultrasound of renal transplantation. *Clin Radiol*. 2001;56:802–818.
14. McGahan PJ, Richards JR, Bair AE, Rose JS. Ultrasound detection of blunt urological trauma: a 6-year study. *Injury*. 2005;36:762–770.
15. Scout LM, Sawyers SR, Bokhari J, Hamper UM. Ultrasound evaluation of the acute abdomen. *Ultrasound Clin*. 2007;2:493–523.
16. Lin EP, Bhatt S, Dogra VS, Rubens DI. Sonography of urolithiasis and hydronephrosis. *Ultrasound Clin*. 2007;2:1–16.
17. McAchran SE, Hartke DM, Nakamoto DA, Resnick MI. Ultrasound of the urinary bladder. *Ultrasound Clin*. 2007;2:17–26.

ULTRASOUND EVALUATION OF THE PELVIS

MICHAEL BLAIVAS

INTRODUCTION

Relevant pelvic pathology is periodically encountered in the intensive care unit (ICU) setting and is amenable to bedside ultrasound evaluation. The pelvic pathology of interest in point of care ultrasonography may be split into three general categories. The first is a source of blood loss and will most typically include ectopic pregnancy, hemorrhagic cyst, or bleeding mass. The second is a source of infection and is most likely to include pelvic inflammatory disease (PID), tuboovarian abscess (TOA), retained products, and endometritis. The third is a source of pain apart from the first two categories, including ovarian cysts, masses, and ovarian torsion.

ANATOMY

Sonographic pelvic anatomy can be challenging and depending on the ultrasound technique, anatomical relationships may appear confusing. The uterus, a pear-shaped muscular organ typically measuring 6–8 cm in length and 4 cm in width, is bordered anteriorly by the bladder and posteriorly by the rectum. The uterus is comprised of the fundus, body, and cervix where it narrows and protrudes into the vagina (Figure 22-1). The fallopian tubes exit the uterus on either side of the uterine fundus at the level of the cornua. The anterior cul-de-sac is a potential space between the uterus and bladder while the posterior cul-de-sac (Pouch of Douglas) is between the uterus and rectum. With the patient supine the Pouch of Douglas is the most dependent part of the pelvis and is typically the first area to collect fluid, such as blood or pus. The fallopian tubes extend laterally from the cornua in the broad ligament. An ovary attaches to the broad ligament posteriorly on each side. The iliac artery and vein run posterior and lateral to the ovaries and the two are a major landmark sonographically.

ULTRASOUND EXAMINATION: TRANSABDOMINAL

The pelvic ultrasound examination is split into two distinct types that are not mutually exclusive and one may lead to the other depending on the pathology discovered. The easiest is the transabdominal (TAS) pelvic ultrasound examination. It is typically performed utilizing a curved linear array with a typical frequency range of 5–2.5 MHz. The broad field of view afforded by this type of transducer is ideal for surveying the pelvis. In general, the TAS pelvic ultrasound examination requires a full bladder. In the case of many ICU patients, this simply means clamping the urinary catheter. An alternative is to fill the bladder with either sterile saline. The ideal volume, which allows the bladder to act as an optimum acoustic window will vary from patient to patient. Approximately 250 mm will be ample in most cases and it is possible to overfill the bladder and actually move organs of interest farther away from the transducer. Similar to the pelvic portion of the fast assessments of surgical trauma (FAST) examination, the transducer is in two standard orientations. The transverse is with the marker oriented to the patient's right hip and the longitudinal with the probe indicator pointed to the patient's head. It is critical to scan through the bladder to best image pelvic organs in the TAS approach. Pelvic organs, like most others, should be scanned in two orthogonal planes. The classic image of a distended bladder in long axis is a triangular anechoic structure. In the transverse view the bladder will typically appear rectangular in shape (Figure 22-2). The TAS examination gives limited views of the ovaries and fallopian tubes in most patients. The fallopian tubes are rarely seen on TAS unless filled with fluid. Even then it may be difficult to differentiate them from other fluid collections without using an endovaginal (EV) approach. In many cases of complicated or subtle pathologic findings, both TAS and EV scanning will be required.

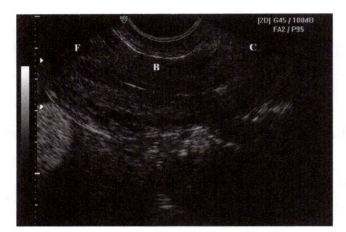

Figure 22-1 A normal uterus is seen in long axis on ultrasound. B = body of uterus; C = cervix; F = fundus of uterus.

ULTRASOUND EXAMINATION: EV

The EV ultrasound approach is generally preferred for structures within the true pelvis. The ovaries are visualized with great detail, pregnancy can be seen at a much earlier date and ectopic pregnancies can be identified with much greater accuracy than with TAS.[1] EV ultrasound is still typically described as an examination to perform after TAS. However, in clinical practice, the EV is often performed without a preceding TAS examination. The EV ultrasound examination requires an endocavity probe. These are typically microconvex and tend to range from 8 to 4 MHz, with some variation. Color or power Doppler is critical for this type of transducer in order to differentiate blood flowing in vessels from other types of fluid. The endocavity transducer is encased in a nonsterile sheath, such as a condom. Condoms with receptacle tips tend to trap air and are best avoided. The middle finger of a glove can be used as well. Hospital endocavity transducer decontamination policies and techniques should be strictly adhered to.

Prior to insertion into a sheath, the probe tip is covered with ultrasound gel. Once the sheath is slipped over the probe, the tip should be stretched tight and all air bubbles smoothed out with a finger. Additional gel is used on top of the sheath over the transducer scanning surface. Unlike the TAS approach, the EV approach requires an empty bladder. Once dressed properly, the probe is ready to insert into the vaginal vault. In modern society it is best to perform the examination in the constant presence of a chaperone, traditionally a female one. This will avoid potential questions that may be difficult to defend against if no chaperone was present. Typically, the probe is inserted too far by beginners and does not need to go beyond the anterior fornix. There are two general imaging planes in EV ultrasound. They are a coronal plane and a longitudinal plane. It may be helpful for beginners to imagine the patient standing on her head as they view the ultrasound machine screen. The anatomy will now make more sense, even though the orientation will take some time to adjust to.

With the probe indicator pointing toward the ceiling, the empty bladder, long axis of the uterus, and posterior structures are seen (Figure 22-3). A full bladder will make the examination frustrating and has to be corrected. The probe is moved from side to side to obtain images from one adnexa to the other. In addition, the transducer can be angled up and down while the indicator remains pointed toward the ceiling and introduced slightly deeper or pulled back in the vaginal vault. The fundus, cervix of the uterus, and surrounding structures can be visualized with good detail using these movements. To obtain short-axis view or coronal, the transducer is rotated toward the adnexa of interest and moved up and down or side to side (Figure 22-4). In EV scanning it is critical to image in two orthogonal planes as structures

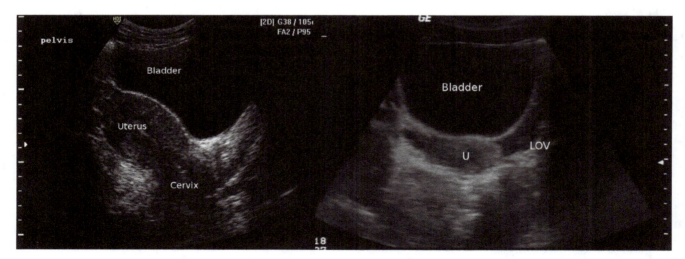

Figure 22-2 The left image shows a longitudinal cut through the bladder, uterus, and cervix. The bladder is triangular in appearance. Fluid can collect posterior to the uterus, near the cervix, or anterior to the fundus. The right image shows a transverse cut through the full bladder. The uterus (U) is shown in cross-section just below the rectangular bladder. The left ovary (LOV) is seen to the right of the uterus.

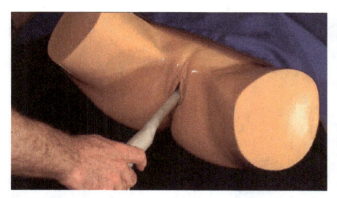

Figure 22-3 An endovaginal probe is being held in the vaginal vault of an ultrasound phantom, with the transducer indicator pointed toward the ceiling. This orientation gives a long-axis view through the uterus similar to Figure 22-1.

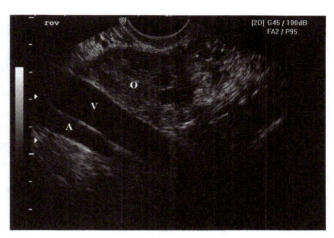

Figure 22-5 The right ovary (O) is seen adjacent to the iliac vein (V) and artery (A).

of interest are periodically seen better in one plane than another. The ovaries are located lateral to the uterus and are almost invariably anteromedial to the internal iliac artery and vein. These vascular structures are relatively easy to find on the EV examination and are an excellent landmark (Figure 22-5). The fallopian tubes can be seen leaving the cornuate portions of the uterine fundus on either side and may often be tracked nearly to each ovary, Figure 22-6. The tubes are obvious when filled with fluid, but with modern equipment they are still easily seen in most patients.

HEMORRHAGE FROM PREGNANCY

One of the best ways to rule out the presence of an ectopic pregnancy is by ruling in an intrauterine pregnancy (IUP).[2] Although ectopic pregnancies coexisting with IUPs are encountered, they were traditionally thought to be exceedingly rare in the general population, approximately 1 in 30,000.[3] However, more modern estimates demonstrate a background incidence closer to 1 in 8000.[4]

Patients undergoing any fertility treatment are at a much greater risk for heterotopic pregnancy with some studies suggesting as high as 1 in 100 for very specialized infertility practices.[5] It is important to note that as many as 70% of all ectopic pregnancies resolve spontaneously and many others can be treated medically. Thus, identifying one does not mean an impending surgical disaster if there is no evidence of rupture and if the ectopic mass is small.[6] While identifying an embryo (fetal pole), especially with a heartbeat, is the best way to diagnose an IUP, earlier embryonic structures can be used confidently to rule in an IUP. Specifically, a yolk sac is the earliest reliable embryonic structure (Figure 22-7). A gestational sac alone is insufficient to diagnoses an IUP. Having a double decidual sign increases the likelihood of an IUP to over 80%, but still does not reliably rule out an ectopic pregnancy.[7] A double decidual sign refers to the two concentric circles outlying a normal gestational sac, made up of the maternal and fetal decidua. An apparent gestational sac may, in actuality, be a pseudogestational sac, which is

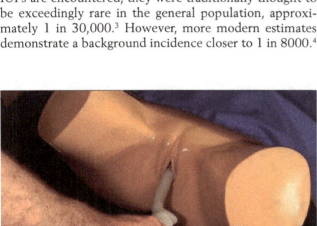

Figure 22-4 The probe inserted into the vaginal vault of the ultrasound phantom has been turned 90° counterclockwise and toward the right adnexa and is now pointed into the adnexa. Short-axis views of the uterus and both ovaries are accomplished in this orientation.

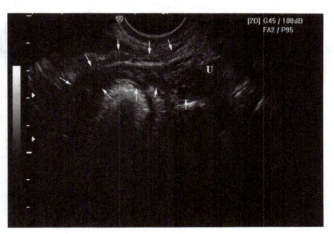

Figure 22-6 The fallopian tube (arrows) is seen leaving the uterus (U) and traveling out into the adnexa toward the ovary (not seen in this image).

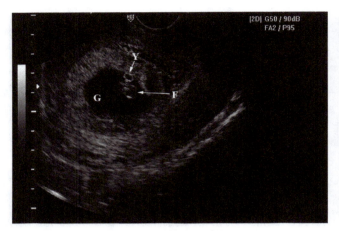

Figure 22-7 This endovaginal ultrasound of a pregnant uterus shows the gestational sac (G), yolk sac (Y), and fetal pole (F).

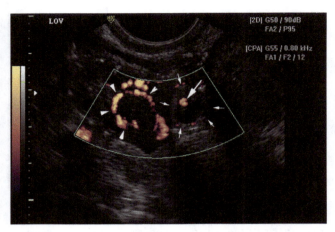

Figure 22-9 Blood flow in the heart of a live ectopic pregnancy is shown (*large arrow*). The ectopic mass (*small arrows*) sits adjacent to the left ovary, which contains a solid corpus luteum outlined with blood flow on power Doppler (*arrow heads*).

seen in a portion of ectopic pregnancies as fluid collects in the endometrial canal due to hormonal stimulation of the endometrial lining (Figure 22-8).[8] It is important to note that many radiologists will feel comfortable diagnosing an early IUP based on a double decidual sign and this is a standard in their field. Point-of-care sonologists have traditionally preferred the much higher certainty and lower risk of calling an IUP only when embryonic structures, such as a yolk sac, are documented.

TAS allows for visualization of embryonic structures as soon as 6–8 weeks with ideal ultrasound equipment, while EV approach will typically reliably show a yolk sac by 4.5 weeks gestational age. The normal location of a gestational sac is in the uterine fundus just off of the endometrial midline. The fetal pole is located next to the yolk sac, but if measured, the yolk sac should not be included in the measurement. If IUP is not confirmed on TAS, then an ectopic has not been ruled out. TAS findings suggesting ectopic pregnancy include an absence of IUP (in most cases), presence of echogenic fluid in the Pouch of Douglas, a large amount of fluid in the pelvis, or a discrete mass in the adnexa. Actual live ectopics can be seen on TAS and it may even be possible to date an embryo. This is more likely on EV however (Figure 22-9). Reported rates of live ectopic pregnancy range from 3% to 10%.[9,10] Certainty of ectopic pregnancy depends on the ultrasound findings, coupled with the clinical scenario. Obviously, having a positive pregnancy test is important for an ectopic diagnosis, but anecdotal reports of ruptured ectopic pregnancies in the setting of a negative pregnancy test do exist. Thus, never say never with ectopic pregnancy. The earliest sign of an ectopic on EV ultrasound is typically a small circular mass with central clearing, located next to the ovary. This structure is called a "tubal ring sign" and represents the fallopian tube with the ectopic pregnancy implanted in it (Figure 22-10). On the opposite

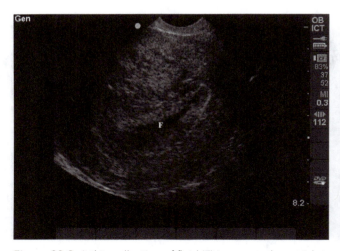

Figure 22-8 A thin collection of fluid (F) is seen endometrial canal of this patient with an ectopic pregnancy and represents a pseudogestational sac.

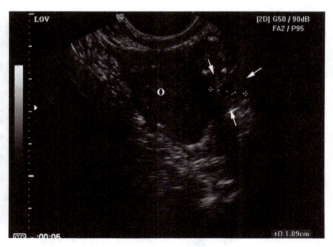

Figure 22-10 A tubal ring (*arrows*) is shown adjacent to the left ovary (O) and measures just over 1 cm across.

end of the spectrum, the tubal ring can be very subtle and may be difficult to differentiate from the corpus luteum of the ovary (which should be located on the same side as the ectopic in the majority of cases). Gently prodding the ovary with the EV probe will result in movement of the tubal ring and ovary as separate units and is a reliable sign to differentiate a corpus luteum from a tubal ring.[11] A mass next to the ovary and a large amount of echogenic fluid in the pelvis should further raise suspicion for ectopic pregnancy. Occasionally, a yolk sac or embryo may be seen in the tubal ring and this will clinch the diagnosis of ectopic pregnancy.

HEMORRHAGE IN A NONPREGNANT PATIENT

Blood loss can also occur from an ovarian cyst or mass. Hemorrhagic cysts can occasionally result in significant intraabdominal blood loss, especially when arterial bleeding is present. Typical findings include pelvic fluid and a complex ovarian cyst, which may contain evidence of thrombus in it (Figure 22-11). It may occasionally be possible to see blood flow from the offending vessel into the cyst and pelvis. Masses, especially malignant masses, may also hemorrhage, but this is less common. Fibroids can also be the source of significant hemorrhage, but typically do not bleed exclusively into the pelvis and vaginal bleeding will often be present. Fibroids take on a heterogeneous appearance and cast shadows on ultrasound examination. This shadowing can make it difficult to see other structures around the uterus (Figure 22-12). Central liquefaction may be seen in some cases as the fibroid degenerates.

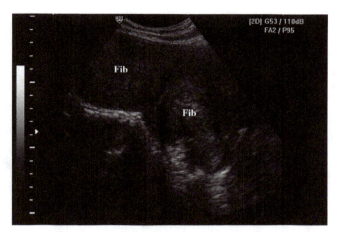

Figure 22-12 A transabdominal longitudinal image of the uterus shows two distinct masses, both fibroids (Fib). Characteristic shadows are cast by both to different degrees. The patient had pelvic pain that was worsening over several weeks.

SOURCES OF INFECTION

Sources on infection may arise from the pelvis and will most frequently include PID and may also involve abscess formation, such as TOA. If delivery complications are a possibility then retained products of conception that have become infected should also be considered as a possible source. Endometritis or infection of the endometrium can be a cause of sepsis. PID affects about 10–15% of women in the United States.[12] As many as 275,000 women are hospitalized annually for PID, with more than 100,000 surgical procedures performed.[13,14] Pus in the pelvis appears as echogenic fluid with mixed echoes. It can be confused with blood that is starting to thicken. Small amounts of fluid are first seen in the Pouch of Douglas and then extend up further along the uterus as the quantity increases. TOAs are often unilateral but occasionally appear as bilateral. Ultrasonography is most useful in differentiating TOA from other stages of PID.[15] The most common sonographic findings in PID include thickened, heterogeneous endometrium, an enlarged uterus with fluid in the endometrial cavity and fluid-filled fallopian tubes.[16,17] A tuboovarian complex (TOC) is an inflammatory pelvic mass without any pus within a cavity. A TOC consists of edematous, adherent, infected ovaries and tubes can still be visualized but cannot be separated by an EV probe. In TOA, there is a loss of the normal boundaries between the fallopian tube and ovary due to edematous inflamed tissue that is filled with pus. A variety of sonographic appearances have been described for TOA.[15] The typical sonographic appearance of a TOA is a complex adnexal mass of varying echogenicity with debris, septations, and irregular margins (Figure 22-13).[15,16,18] The other sonographic markers of TOA are pyosalpinx, and loculated or speckled, echogenic fluid in cul-de-sac (Figure 22-14).[15,16,19] Retained products after incomplete delivery of the placenta or incomplete abortion can lead

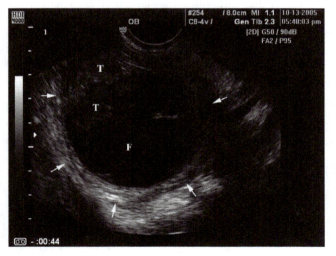

Figure 22-11 A large cyst inside of an ovary stretched around it is shown. Arrows outline the outer edge of the ovary. The cyst contains thrombus of different density (T) as well as free fluid (F) that is liquid blood.

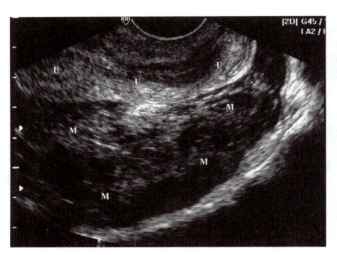

Figure 22-13 The image shows a complex mass (M) from the right adnexa extending behind the uterus (U). This patient required surgical drainage of this TOA.

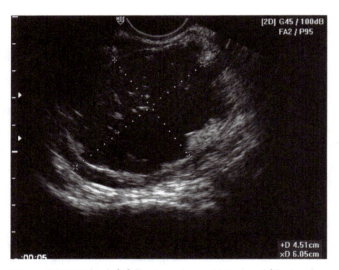

Figure 22-14 This left fallopian tube is dilated and filled with echogenic material. Measurement in the right lower corner shows its size.

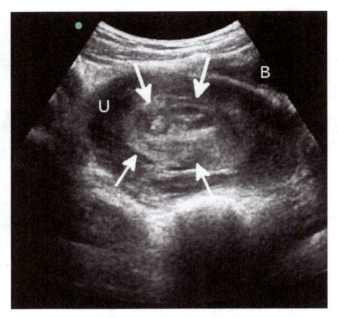

Figure 22-15 A longitudinal transabdominal image of the uterus (U) is shown. The bladder (B) is seen on the upper right of the image. Arrows outline echogenic material in the endometrial cavity.

to life-threatening infection and be a source of sepsis. A simply survey of the endometrial canal of the uterus may rule out retained products as a likely source. Figure 22-15 shows retained products in the endometrial canal after incomplete miscarriage in a patient, who presented with septic shock and pelvic pain.

Ovarian cysts or masses can cause pain by virtue of mass effect as they grow. Rupturing cysts can be the cause of surgical-type pain, which is usually self-limited. In addition, cysts or masses associated with ovaries may occasionally lead to torsion, which will result in severe pain and eventual loss of the ovary and possibly fallopian tube. Typically, a source for torsion is required and if a sizable cyst or a mass is not present on the ovary or immediately next to an ovary, torsion is unlikely. If a large cyst or a mass is present then the ovary may be at risk for torsion if clinical symptoms are present. Due to the dual arterial supply of each ovary, both ovarian and uterine arteries, it is easier to rule torsion in than out with ultrasound. If an EV examination with power Doppler shows an absence of blood flow in the ovary containing a large cyst or a mass then torsion is quite likely. However, since an EV examination showing blood flow in the ovary with a mass or cyst and a high-clinical suspicion cannot completely rule out torsion, laparoscopic evaluation may be required. Rupture of a simple cyst may cause intense pain that diminishes in intensity and should disappear completely within a day. EV examination may show a small collection of fluid in the Pouch of Douglas and occasionally immediately adjacent to the ovary in question.

SOURCES OF PAIN

Ovarian cysts, masses, and torsion are likely to be the most common sources of pelvic pain that are not associated with infection or hemorrhage. Large fibroids, especially degenerating ones, can cause severe pain and are readily detected on EV ultrasound when small, and TAS when larger. Typically, larger fibroids cause more pain than smaller ones.

REFERENCES

1. Lambert M, Villa M. Gynecologic ultrasound in emergency medicine. *Emerg Med Clin North Am.* 2004;22:683–696.
2. Kaplan BC, Dart RG, Moskos JM. Ectopic pregnancy: prospective study with improved diagnostic accuracy. *Ann Emerg Med.* 1996;28:10–17.
3. DeVoe P. Simultaneous intrauterine and extrauterine pregnancy. *Am J Obstet Gynecol.* 1948;56:1119–1126.

4. Bright DA, Gaupp FB. Heterotopic pregnancy: a reevaluation. *J Am Board Fam Pract.* 1990;3:125–128.
5. Berger MJ, Taymor ML. Simultaneous intrauterine and tubal pregnancies following ovulation induction. *Am J Obstet Gynecol.* 1972;113:812–813.
6. Elson J, Tailor A, Banerjee S, Salim R, Hillaby K, Jurkovic D. Expectant management of tubal ectopic pregnancy: prediction of successful outcome using decision tree analysis. *Ultrasound Obstet Gynecol.* 2004;23:552–556.
7. Yeh HC, Goodman JD, Carr L. Intradecidual sign: a US criterion of early intrauterine pregnancy. *Radiology.* 1986;161:463–467.
8. Dart R, Howard K. Subclassification of indeterminate pelvic ultrasonograms: stratifying the risk of ectopic pregnancy. *Acad Emerg Med.* 1998;5:313–319.
9. Nyberg DA, Hughes MP, Mack LA, Wang KY. Extrauterine findings of ectopic pregnancy of transvaginal US: importance of echogenic fluid. *Radiology.* 1991;178:823–826.
10. Adhikari S, Blaivas M, Lyon M. Diagnosis and management of ectopic pregnancy using bedside transvaginal ultrasonography in the ED: a 2-year experience. *Am J Emerg Med.* 2007;25(6):591–596.
11. Blaivas M, Lyon M. Reliability of adnexal mass mobility in distinguishing possible ectopic pregnancy from corpus luteum cysts. *J Ultrasound Med.* 2005;24:599–603.
12. Gjelland K, Ekerhovd E, Granberg S. Transvaginal ultrasound-guided aspiration for treatment of tubo-ovarian abscess: a study of 302 cases. *Am J Obstet Gynecol.* 2005;193(4):1323–1330.
13. Policy Guidelines for Prevention and Management of Pelvic Inflammatory Disease. U. S. Department of Health and Human Services, Public Health service, Centers for Disease Control, National Center for Prevention Services, From MMWR 1991; Vol. 40(RR5).
14. Pastorek JG. Pelvic inflammatory disease and tubo-ovarian abscess. *Obstet Gynecol Clin North Am.* 1989;16(2):347–361.
15. Timor-Tritsch IE, Lerner JP, Monteagudo A, Murphy KE, Heller DS. Transvaginal sonographic markers of tubal inflammatory disease. *Ultrasound Obstet Gynecol.* 1998;12:56–66.
16. Ignacio EA, Hill MC. Ultrasound of the acute female pelvis. *Ultrasound Q.* 2003;19(2):86–98.
17. Horrow MM. Ultrasound of pelvic inflammatory disease. *Ultrasound Q.* 2004;20(4):171–179.
18. Webb EM, Green GE, Scoutt LM. Adnexal mass with pelvic pain. *Radiol Clin N Am.* 2004;42(2):329–348.
19. Varras M, Polyzos D, Perouli E, Noti P, Pantazis I, Akrivis C. Tubo-ovarian abscesses: spectrum of sonographic findings with surgical and pathological correlations. *Clin Exp Obstet Gynecol.* 2003;30(2-3):117–121.

ULTRASOUND EVALUATION OF THE PERIPHERAL VASCULAR SYSTEM

JAMES E. FOSTER, II & KEVIN WISEMAN

Scan QR code or visit www.ccu2e.com for video in this chapter

INTRODUCTION

Duplex ultrasound examination of the peripheral arterial and venous systems has been refined to the point where it has become the initial modality of choice for vascular diagnosis. Technical advances have improved diagnostic accuracy such that treatment decisions previously based on angiographic studies can now be based solely on noninvasive studies. This is most evident in the noninvasive diagnosis of deep venous thrombosis (DVT),[1] and is becoming more prevalent in the management of carotid occlusive disease and atherosclerotic peripheral vascular disease.

ULTRASOUND EXAMINATION OF THE PERIPHERAL VENOUS SYSTEM

Risk factors associated with the development of DVT are common in the critical care setting. Virchow's triad of stasis, endothelial injury, and altered coagulation are readily seen in today's intensive care unit (ICU). Clinical factors such as major trauma, which include neurological injury, pelvic and long bone fractures[2,3]; prolonged immobilization due to altered mental status, paralysis, morbid obesity; multiple sites for venous access and central monitoring; and advancing age, all contribute to this increased risk.[4]

The true prevalence of acute DVT in the ICU setting is unknown. Reported incidence varies widely (4–60%) due to patient population, detection methods, and the application of surveillance programs.[5-7] Despite increased awareness and aggressive application of protocols for the prevention of DVT, postmortem studies indicate that subclinical, undetected DVT and pulmonary embolism (PE) continue to exist.[8] In addition, many ICU patients are at risk for rebleeding and are not candidates for anticoagulation.

Invasive hemodynamic monitoring or prolonged central venous access is common in the critical care environment. Catheter-associated thrombosis occurs in response to endothelial injury and the alterations in normal venous flow patterns caused by the catheter. This may be more significant in children, where small diameter veins can be functionally occluded by catheterization.[9]

Although the most common sequelae of DVT are the late problems of venous insufficiency and stasis ulceration, PE is the primary concern in the acute care setting. The present emphasis on DVT prophylaxis arises from the recognition that PE is one of the most preventable causes of death and major morbidity in hospitalized patients. Because most clinically significant PE arises from deep veins of the lower extremities, some centers have advocated routine duplex ultrasound surveillance of patients during their ICU stay (Video 23-1).

Continuous-wave Doppler ultrasound technology was introduced to clinical practice in the 1970s. Although no images were possible, these devices allowed the examiner to assess venous flow patterns by auditory waveform analysis. The combination of ultrasound imaging and Doppler spectral analysis provided the basis for current duplex ultrasound technology. By the early 1990s, the venous duplex ultrasound examination replaced contrast venography as the gold standard for the diagnosis of DVT.

Standard practice requires a trained sonographer to transport the ultrasound machine (portable but bulky) to the ICU, where a full lower extremity examination is performed and recorded on videotape or digital media. The study is reviewed by the interpreting physician who generates a report that is transcribed and returned to the patient's chart. This process, although very accurate, is time consuming and may not always serve the needs of the very dynamic and often unstable conditions in the critical care environment.

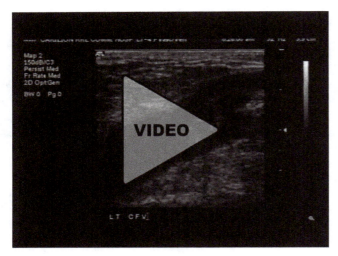

Video 23-1 Venous thromboembolism. Long-axis view of sapheno-femoral junction with thrombus extending from greater saphenous vein into common femoral vein. Note at 18 seconds of this frame the thrombus dislodges and migrates proximally (pulmonary embolism). Patient was carefully monitored for clinically significant sequelae, but none were noted. View at www.ccu2e.com

The recently developed portable, handheld, duplex scanners with multihertz transducers and color-flow Doppler capability bring the possibility of a focused venous examination to the bedside. The clinician is now able to obtain diagnostic information rapidly and interpret these results within the context of the patient's overall clinical condition. Bedside investigation can eliminate the need for patient transport to the ultrasound department or the computerized tomography (CT) scanner, often an enormous task with critically ill patients that itself has inherent risks. Where results are uncertain or equivocal, a formal diagnostic study can be obtained to assist in a definitive diagnosis. With proper training and experience, a focused venous duplex examination at the bedside can be accomplished by any clinician familiar with venous anatomy, venous flow characteristics, and the basics of duplex ultrasonography.

▶ Venous Anatomy

The venous systems of both the upper and lower extremities are divided into deep and superficial components. The deep venous system is composed of those veins draining the muscle compartments and paired with named arteries. The superficial systems drain cutaneous structures and run in the subcutaneous space. These superficial veins are not associated with adjacent arteries.

In the lower extremity, the deep venous system includes the external iliac, common femoral, superficial and deep femoral, popliteal, anterior and posterior tibial, peroneal, and soleal and gastrocnemius veins (Figure 23-1). All of the deep veins are accompanied by named arteries, except for the soleal and gastrocnemius veins. The two main veins of the superficial venous system are the greater and lesser saphenous veins. The lesser saphenous is located in the lat-

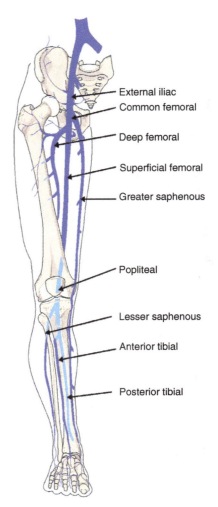

Figure 23-1 Venous anatomy of the lower extremity.

eral calf and drains into the deep system at the popliteal vein. The greater saphenous vein runs along the medial aspect of the leg from ankle to proximal thigh, where it traverses the fossa ovalis and drains into the common femoral vein. An unfortunate consequence of the traditional anatomic nomenclature is that the "superficial" femoral vein is actually a deep venous structure and is often the site of acute DVT leading to all the complications of thrombosis, including PE. Therefore, it is important to understand that thrombosis of any segment of the femoral vein (superficial, deep, or common) constitutes a DVT and should be so identified for documentation and treatment purposes.

In the upper extremity, the deep veins include the internal jugular, subclavian, axillary, brachial, radial, and ulnar veins (Figure 23-2). These veins each have a companion artery. The major components of the superficial venous system of the arm are the cephalic vein, running laterally from wrist to shoulder and draining into the subclavian vein, and the basilic vein, running medially from antecubital fossa to the axilla, where it drains into the axillary vein. When available, the superficial veins are the sites of choice for peripheral venous access.

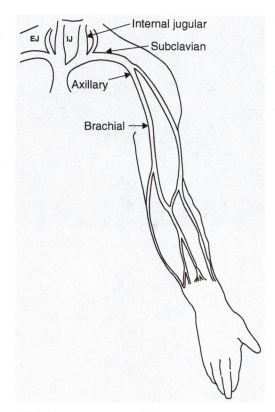

Figure 23-2 Venous anatomy of the upper extremity.

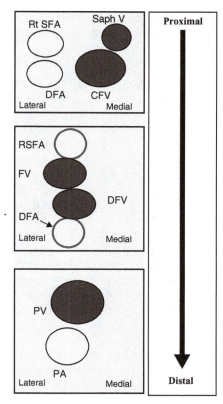

Figure 23-4 Diagrams of vessel relationships at three levels.

Sonographic imaging is performed with B-mode scanning, often using color-flow imaging to add more information. The external iliac artery and vein exit the pelvis deep to the inguinal ligament to become common femoral vessels. The common femoral vein is medial to the artery and is slightly larger in diameter. These relationships are easily identified when scanning in a transverse plane at the groin crease (Figure 23-3). The transverse plane is used to assess the veins for compressibility (see below). Moving distally along the common femoral vein, the greater saphenous can be identified as it passes from the superficial plane to drain into the femoral vein. Again, no artery accompanies the greater saphenous vein. Moving slightly more distally, common femoral vessels divide into superficial and deep femoral vessels. At this level, four vessels are seen in cross-section (Figure 23-4). From this point distally, the superficial femoral artery (SFA) and vein continue to the adductor canal, where they enter the popliteal space and are designated as popliteal vessels (Figure 23-1).

Once the distal external iliac vein is identified at the inguinal ligament, turning the transducer 90° provides a longitudinal image of the vessel. This view is best suited for a rapid survey of the veins and allows for assessment of the extent and nature of a thrombus when seen (Figure 23-5). Vein compression is not

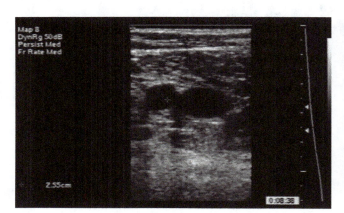

Figure 23-3 Transverse view of common femoral vessels.

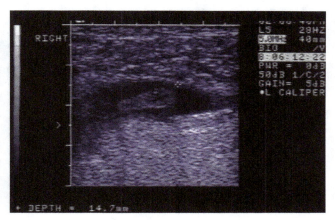

Figure 23-5 Acute deep venous thrombosis (DVT), common femoral vein (longitudinal view).

reliable while scanning in the longitudinal plane. Compressibility must be confirmed in the transverse view.

▶ Diagnostic Criteria

Diagnostic criteria for identifying DVT can be divided into vessel characteristics and flow characteristics. The primary vessel characteristic is compressibility; the ability to demonstrate wall-to-wall apposition of the vein when adequate pressure is applied using the ultrasound transducer in the transverse plane. Adequate pressure is determined by noting mild deformation of the adjacent artery (Figure 23-6). Noncompressibility indicates that intraluminal thrombus is preventing the vessel walls from collapsing. It is important to remember that fresh, immature thrombus may not be echogenic because newly formed clot has an acoustic impedance similar to blood. The second vessel characteristic is identification of intraluminal echogenic material. This can often be seen on the initial survey of the venous system and should alert the clinician to the presence of thrombus. Intraluminal echogenic material should be confirmed in both imaging planes, and when thrombus is identified, compression should be limited due to the possibility of dislodging the clot. Longitudinal imaging provides the best view for determining the extent or length of thrombus and whether it is adherent to the vessel wall or may have a free-floating tip (Figure 23-7 and Video 23-2). A third vessel characteristic that may be helpful is the assessment of valve function. Occasionally, venous valves are visible in situations where higher frequency transducers can be used (thin patients, children). Normal valves open and close in conjunction with venous flow. However, because valve cusps are often the site of thrombogenesis, an immobile valve cusp may be a clue to the presence of thrombus.

Venous blood flow characteristics are also important in assessing the presence of acute DVT. Normal venous flow patterns show a phasicity that varies with respiration. Normal inspirations decrease intrathoracic pressures and cause associated increase in venous flow. Similarly, expiration increases intrathoracic pressure and is reflected in a decrease in venous flow. A Valsalva maneuver increases intrathoracic pressure sufficiently to completely interrupt venous flow

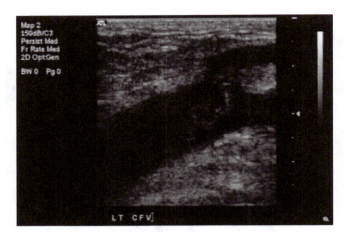

Figure 23-7 Free-floating thrombus in extending from greater saphenous vein into common femoral vein.

that is associated with an augmentation in venous flow when the Valsalva maneuver is released. These changes are easily identified by observing the Doppler waveform or by listening to flow patterns with a continuous-wave Doppler unit. Any obstructive process between the thoracic cavity and the site of insonation of the veins of the lower extremity can alter the normal phasic changes associated with respiration. Absence of phasic changes with a continuous-flow pattern or loss of augmentation with deep inspiration suggests obstruction of the venous system. Additional maneuvers to augment flow include compression of calf muscles and the distal thigh to demonstrate increased flow at the site of insonation. Loss of normal augmentation with compressions also suggests the presence of obstruction in the venous system. The assessment of both vessel characteristics and venous blood flow characteristics lead to highly accurate and reliable detection of DVT. Normal vessel and flow characteristics also provide a very high negative predictive value for DVT.

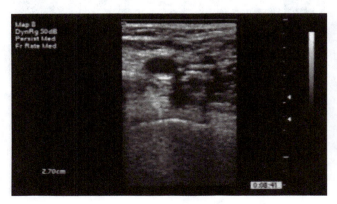

Figure 23-6 Common femoral artery and compressed common femoral vein (compare with Figure 23-3).

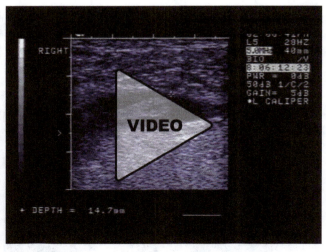

Video 23-2 Long-axis view of common femoral vein. Note echogenic intraluminal material (thrombus). It is mobile and not fully adherent to the vessel wall. Color Doppler image demonstrates restricted venous flow around the thrombus. View at www.ccu2e.com

Performing the Studies

Equipment requirements for venous duplex examinations include high-resolution gray-scale imaging, color Doppler capability, and spectral analysis directional Doppler. The transducer selection should allow for optimal imaging and Doppler analysis, and generally means using the linear-array, high-frequency (7–10 MHz) transducer for most patients. Occasionally, a low-frequency (3–5 MHz), curved-array transducer will be necessary if the patient is obese or there is considerable edema.

Patient positioning is very important, as proper positioning enhances the demonstration of abnormalities, eases the strain on the sonographer, and reduces time to complete the study. For lower extremity examinations, the patient is placed supine with the head elevated approximately 30°, if possible. The leg to be scanned is externally rotated with the knee flexed (Figure 23-8). For upper extremity studies, the patient is also placed supine, with the head turned away from the side being scanned. The chin should be raised (neck extended) slightly, if possible (Figure 23-9).

The first component of the lower extremity protocol involves transverse compressions in gray-scale imaging mode. Beginning at the femoral crease, with the transducer in a transverse (cross-section) orientation, identify the common femoral vein. There should be one artery and the saphenofemoral junction should be visible. Using gentle-to-moderate probe pressure applied toward the femur, observe the femoral vein compression with wall-to-wall contact. Identification of intraluminal echogenic material mandates gentle pressure only. Visualization of a mobile thrombus within the vein precludes further compression to avoid dislodging an embolus. If compressions are easy and complete, the probe can be moved a few centimeters distally, and the division of the common femoral vein into the deep and superficial femoral veins can be observed. Repeat the compression maneu-

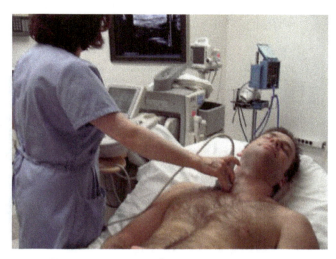

Figure 23-9 Patient position for upper extremity venous examination.

ver every 5 cm, proceeding distally along the superficial femoral vein. At the distal thigh, the vein traverses the adductor canal and enters the popliteal space. At this point, position the transducer in the popliteal space, identify the popliteal artery and vein, and compress the vein to assure wall-to-wall contact.

The second phase of the lower extremity venous examination evaluates flow characteristics using color Doppler imaging and Doppler spectral analysis. The transducer is returned to the groin and the common femoral vein is again identified in the transverse view. The transducer is then rotated 90° to obtain a longitudinal (sagittal) image of the vein (Figure 23-10). Observe the Doppler signal for flow that is spontaneous and phasic with respiration. A Valsalva maneuver will halt flow at end-inspiration and will demonstrate augmented flow when respiration resumes. Flow can also be augmented by squeezing the calf muscles. This should produce a spike in the spectral signal. These observations are made in the superficial femoral and popliteal veins to complete the study (Videos 23-3 and 23-4).

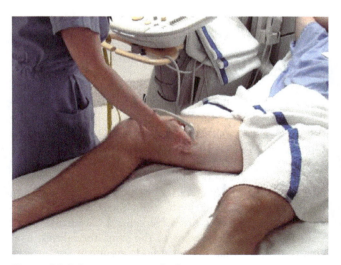

Figure 23-8 Patient position for lower extremity venous examination.

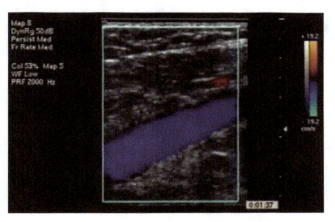

Figure 23-10 Normal color-flow image of common femoral vein. *Note:* direction of flow is away from transducer.

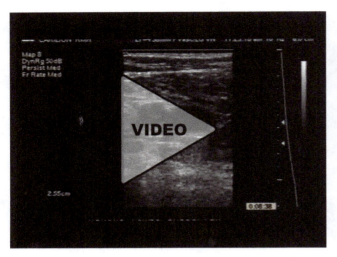

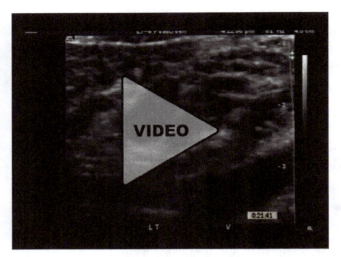

Video 23-3 Normal Venous Study (Two-Dimensional and Pulsed Doppler).

Time frames:

0:00–0:05 seconds: Compression of common femoral vein in short axis (transverse) plane.
0:06–0:14 seconds: Normal respiratory phasicity in long-axis (longitudinal) view.
0:15–0:18 seconds: Valsalva maneuver resulting in the cessation of venous flow.
0:19–0:27 seconds: Release phase of the Valsalva maneuver resulting in flow augmentation, followed by the return of normal respiratory phases (compare frame 0:06).
0:27–0:30 seconds: Augmentation of venous flow resulting from compression of the calf and the thigh (respectively).
0:31 seconds: End of the video femoral vein compression in short-axis (transverse) view. View at www.ccu2e.com

Video 23-5 Subclavian vein thrombosis associated with central venous catheter.

Time frames:

0:00–0:10 seconds: Note mobile echogenic material in left subclavian vein.
0:11–0:28 seconds: Intraluminal central venous catheter (hyperechoic), with thrombus adherent to the outer surface.

Note: Mobile echoes at the catheter tip are due to the eddy current from the hypotonic fluid infusion into the bloodstream and can be easily differentiated from the thrombus by the interruption of the intravenous infusion. View at www.ccu2e.com

A similar protocol is used to evaluate the upper extremities. Transverse compressions of the internal jugular, axillary, and brachial veins should be demonstrated. The subclavian vein cannot be compressed because of the clavicle. Therefore, color Doppler and spectral analysis are used to obtain signals from the subclavian vein and its confluence with the internal jugular vein. Flow in the subclavian and internal jugular should be spontaneous and somewhat pulsatile. These indirect findings confirm the patency of the brachiocephalic veins and the superior vena cava, which cannot be routinely imaged directly on the Duplex examination (Video 23-5).

INTERPRETATION OF RESULTS

Table 23-1 shows the sensitivity, specificity, positive and negative predictive values for the vessel, and flow characteristics assessed in the venous study.[10] It is readily seen that a combination of noncompressible veins with intraluminal echogenic material and abnormal flow characteristics is diagnostic for DVT. The absence of these abnormal findings correlates with no venous pathology.

The venous duplex study is straightforward and easily accomplished at the bedside. But besides the information on venous pathology, a variety of additional information can be obtained while performing these studies. Associated arterial disease is often recognized because adjacent arteries are easily viewed with the same modalities. Atherosclerosis, arterial injury, pseudoaneurysm, or arterial embolization may be evident and are described more fully below. Flow abnormalities may be a clue to increased

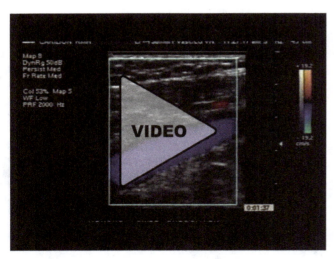

Video 23-4 Normal Venous Study (Color Doppler).

Time frames:

0:00–0:07 seconds: Normal venous flow with respiratory variations (phasicity).
0:08–0:11 seconds: Valsalva maneuver resulting in the cessation of venous flow.
0:12–0:20 seconds: Augmentation of venous flow resulting from compression of the calf and the thigh (respectively).
0:20 seconds: End of the video aliasing due to too low filter gate setting (for the venous examination). View at www.ccu2e.com

TABLE 23-1
Diagnostic Value of Venous Duplex Parameters for Diagnosis of Acute DVT

Criteria	Sensitivity	Specificity	PPV	NPV
Thrombus seen	50	92	95	37
Incompressible	79	67	88	50
No spontaneous flow	76	100	100	57
Absent phasic flow	92	92	97	79

DVT, deep venous thrombosis; NPV, negative predictive value; PPV, positive predictive value.

central venous pressures or valvular heart abnormalities. Mass effects with extrinsic compression may show altered flow patterns, with no evidence of intraluminal pathology. Central venous catheters are easily recognized and may demonstrate catheter-associated thrombus. The internal jugular exam may suggest associated thyroid abnormalities.

The availability of high-quality portable bedside duplex scanners has advanced the ability to accurately diagnose acute DVT within the capability of every physician dealing with critically ill patients. The education and skills required to become comfortable with the techniques are basically extensions of the physical examination skills. And it is almost axiomatic that the individual, who is best able to interpret the findings, is the one with daily responsibility for the care of the patient and who can correlate the results within that individual patient's clinical context.

ULTRASOUND EXAMINATION OF THE PERIPHERAL ARTERIAL SYSTEM

The most common application of ultrasound in the evaluation of the arterial system is to assess the presence and degree of atherosclerotic peripheral vascular disease. Atherosclerotic plaque and calcification of arterial walls are easily demonstrated by gray-scale imaging. Duplex imaging and Doppler waveform analysis provide reliable information related to flow characteristics and arterial stenosis.

Perhaps the most common ultrasound-based assessment is the ankle–brachial ratio, which utilizes continuous-wave Doppler instruments to identify arterial flow, while blood pressures are obtained to calculate the index. Although the baseline assessment of peripheral vascular disease is valuable, in the ICU setting screening ultrasound examinations are most often directed to determining the presence or absence of flow and indications of arterial injury, such as arterial dissection, pseudoaneurysm, or arteriovenous (AV) fistula. Diagnosis of these problems is based on the accurate assessment of flow characteristics and requires a basic understanding of arterial anatomy, hemodynamics, and the fundamentals of pulsed Doppler ultrasound to optimize results. Because bedside arterial examinations may be technically challenging, suspected abnormalities are best con-

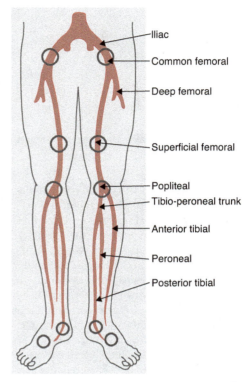

Figure 23-11 Arterial anatomy of the lower extremity.

firmed by formal complete sonographic examination or by angiographic modalities.

Arterial anatomy of the upper extremity is consistent and generally accessible to ultrasound examination. Examination of the great vessels is best performed with a transesophageal approach (see Chapter 8). Peripheral vessels amenable to ultrasound evaluation include the carotid and vertebral arteries supplying the head, face and brain, and the subclavian, axillary, brachial, radial, and ulnar arteries in the upper extremities. The arterial supply of the lower extremities consists of the external iliac vessels, the common, deep, and SFA in the thigh, the popliteal artery and its branches—the anterior and posterior tibial arteries along with the peroneal artery (Figure 23-11).

The common carotid arteries are readily identified in the cervical region, lateral to the trachea and deep to the internal jugular veins. The right common carotid arises from the innominate artery. The left common carotid arises directly from the aortic arch. At the level of the larynx, the common carotid bifurcates into the internal and external carotid vessels. The external is more medial, has multiple branches, and supplies the face and scalp. The internal carotid is lateral, has no branches in the neck, and supplies the brain.

Normal peripheral arterial hemodynamics are characterized by laminar flow in a high-resistance system that generates a characteristic triphasic waveform (Figure 23-12). The initial forward flow is generated by ventricular systole (phase 1). The second phase is a short period of reversed flow that occurs as the aortic valve closes. Phase 3 reflects

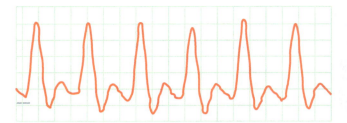

Figure 23-12 Normal triphasic waveform of a peripheral artery.

forward flow generated by the elastic recoil of normal arterial walls. The normal triphasic waveform is easily recognized by Doppler spectral analysis or color-flow imaging (Videos 23-6 and 23-7). In addition, the characteristic auditory signal is easily recognized when using continuous-wave Doppler instruments without imaging capability. Arterial flow in low-resistance systems, such as the internal carotid and vertebral arteries, show characteristic changes in the waveform due to the requirement for continuous forward flow to high-demand organs, such as the brain. Low-resistance waveforms show forward flow during systole and maintain forward flow through the entire cardiac cycle with no phase 2 flow reversal. These characteristics are helpful in distinguishing internal carotid artery (ICA; low-resistance) from the external carotid artery (high-resistance).

Various disease processes produce changes in the flow patterns that form the basis for duplex evaluation and diagnosis. Medial calcinosis of peripheral arteries seen in diabetes leads to decreased vascular elasticity and a loss of phase 3 of the normal arterial waveform. Atherosclerosis can cause similar changes in its early stages. As plaque deposition increases, normal laminar flow becomes more turbulent, leading to spectral broadening seen on ultrasound examination. As stenosis progresses, flow velocities and turbulence increase. Turbulent flow is associated

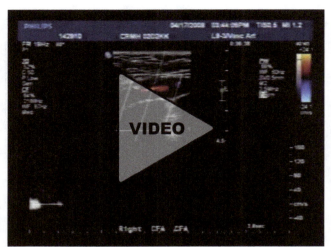

Video 23-7 Abnormal arterial Doppler signal (monophonic). View at www.ccu2e.com

with spectral broadening and generates audible bruits. The ultrasound manifestation of the high-grade stenosis is a Doppler artifact known as "aliasing." Aliasing occurs when the flow velocity exceeds the ability of the pulsed Doppler signal to accurately describe the flow rate (see Chapter 2; Video 23-8). The duplex instrument falsely generates an opposite image or color map of the arterial flow. Aliasing is beneficial in quickly directing the sonographer to a point of maximum stenosis. When aliasing is identified, the sonographer should change instrument settings to eliminate the artifact. Only after appropriate adjustments can accurate flow information be obtained. Critical degrees of arterial stenosis eventually lead to low flow states and occlusion, often as result of thrombosis. Arterial occlusion is characterized by the absence of a Doppler signal or color-flow signal in the vessel distal to the point of obstruction. Duplex findings consistent with

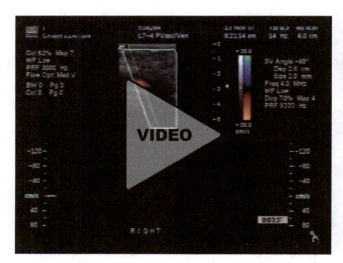

Video 23-6 Normal (high resistance) pattern of arterial flow. Note triphasic arterial Doppler waveform. View at www.ccu2e.com

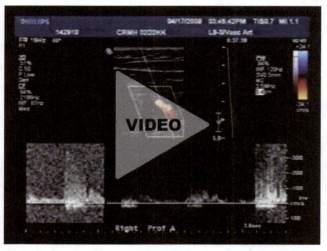

Video 23-8 High grade stenosis of the artery. Note elevated Doppler flow velocities, marked spectral broadening and signal aliasing of the pulsed Doppler. View at www.ccu2e.com

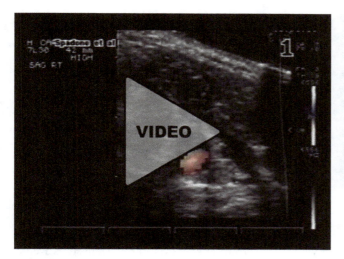

Video 23-9 Carotid artery dissection.
Time frames:
0:00–0:10 seconds: Short-axis view demonstrating the false lumen above the true lumen. Note flow is present in both.
0:25–0:41 seconds: Long-axis view of the dissection flap (intraluminal septum).
0:42–1:00 seconds: Color flow image of the dissection (dual flow channels). View at www.ccu2e.com

arterial occlusion should be confirmed by some angiographic technique, as a "string sign" with extremely low flow can be missed by ultrasound. In addition, embolic events can lead to acute arterial occlusion that can be recognized by duplex examination. Emboli to the carotid arteries can be a cause of stroke, and in the extremities lead to acute arterial insufficiency. These events require a search for the source including mural thrombi from the heart, large vessel aneurysms, and possible paradoxical emboli originating in the venous system and traversing an intracardiac shunt.[11] All of these etiologies can be evaluated using various sonographic techniques.

Arterial injuries also have characteristic ultrasound findings. Aortic dissection is the most common and may be best evaluated by transesophageal echocardiography (see Chapter 8). The increase in cervical trauma related to shoulder belt injuries from motor vehicle collisions has also raised the awareness of carotid artery dissection. These

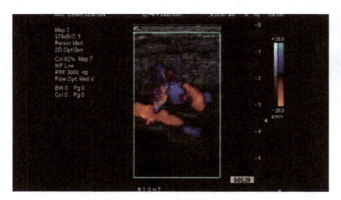

Figure 23-13 Common femoral artery pseudoaneurysm.

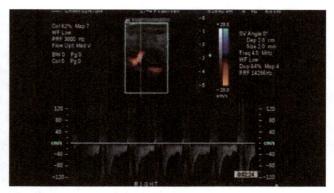

Figure 23-14 High-velocity, turbulent flow seen in tract of pseudoaneurysm.

injuries are characterized by altered flow in the affected artery. Gray-scale imaging sometimes demonstrates an intra-arterial echogenic line that represents the separated intima. Doppler or color-flow analysis may show different flow patterns on either side of the septum[12,13] (Video 23-9). Additional imaging with magnetic resonance angiography or CT angiography may be warranted to confirm the ultrasound findings.[14]

Advances in percutaneous intravascular procedures from coronary angiography to intravascular stent placement have led to an increased incidence of arterial injuries and pseudoaneurysm formation. Iatrogenic femoral artery pseudoaneurysm is reported to occur in up to 6% of diagnostic and therapeutic catheterizations.[15] These pseudoaneurysms can be recognized as extravascular fluid collections that communicate with the arterial system by a narrow tract. Duplex examination demonstrates high-flow velocity with marked turbulence in the tract and a swirling, turbulent flow pattern within the pseudoaneurysm itself (Figures 23-13 and 23-14, and Video 23-10).

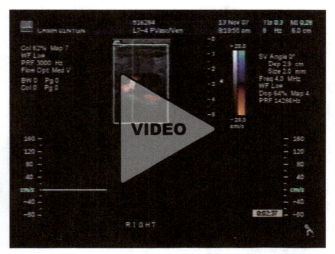

Video 23-10 Right common femoral artery pseudoaneurysm.
Time frames:
0:00–0:16 seconds: High-velocity bidirectional Doppler flow signal in the neck of the pseudoaneurysm.
0:17 seconds: End of the video low-velocity "drumbeat" signal in the pseudoaneurysm sac. View at www.ccu2e.com

Current treatment options include ultrasound-guided thrombin injection.[16] Care must be taken to avoid delivery of thrombin to the native artery. Repeat injections can be performed for persistent or recurrent pseudoaneurysms. AV fistula can result from blunt or penetrating trauma or attempts at vascular access for a variety of purposes. AV fistula at the peripheral level changes a high-resistance system to a low-resistance system. As such, the resulting changes in sonographic flow patterns are predictable. Marked turbulence is identified at the site of the abnormal communication. The presence of aliasing artifact is helpful in identifying the site. The arterial waveform takes on the low-resistance characteristic of higher-end diastolic flow. The flow pattern in the adjacent involved vein will be "arterialized," reflecting the pulsatile waveform of the high-pressure artery.

▶ Performing the Studies

Carotid duplex examination

Equipment: Ultrasound system with high-resolution gray-scale imaging, color Doppler capability, and spectral analysis directional Doppler for velocity measurements.

Transducer: Linear-array, high-frequency transducer (7–10 MHz), with the occasional use of curved-array transducer (3–5 MHz) for deep vessels.

The patient is placed supine, with the head elevated slightly without a pillow and turned away from the side of the examination; the chin should be raised slightly. This approach helps to extend the neck. The patient's head position can and should be altered during the examination to obtain the best image (Figure 23-15). Examination Protocol:

Step 1: Gray-Scale
Examine the carotid arteries in at least two long-axis views and one transverse view. Identify the bifurcation of the common carotid into internal and external carotid arteries. Document the extent and severity of plaque formation (location, characteristics, luminal reduction).

Step 2: Color Doppler
Examine the carotid arteries in a transverse plane with color Doppler to demonstrate the patency of the vessels and to determine the flow disturbances caused by plaque formation or other abnormalities.

Step 3: Spectral Analysis
Obtain a velocity spectrum from the following locations:
Subclavian artery (high-resistance waveform);
Proximal and distal common carotid artery (CCA);
Proximal external carotid artery (high-resistance waveform); and
Proximal ICA (low-resistance waveform).
Vertebral artery: the vertebral is found by rotating the transducer laterally and identifying the vessel between the transverse processes of the cervical vertebrae.

Note: All velocity recordings should be made with an angle of insonation of 60° or less, parallel to the vessel wall, and in the center of the vessel where flow is highest. Obtain a velocity spectrum at the level of any stenosis as well as immediately distal to the lesion to assess flow disturbance. The aliasing artifact can be very helpful at this time in identifying the areas of maximum flow velocity/stenosis.

Arterial duplex examination of the lower extremities

Equipment: Ultrasound system with high-resolution, gray-scale imaging, color Doppler capability, and spectral analysis directional Doppler for velocity measurements.

Transducer: Linear-array, high-frequency transducer (7–10 MHz), with the occasional use of a curved-array transducer (3–5 MHz) for deep vessels.

Patient Positioning: Supine, with head slightly elevated. Examined leg is flexed at the knee and externally rotated.
Examination Protocol:

Step 1: Gray-Scale
Beginning in the groin with a transverse probe position, identify the common femoral artery (CFA). Rotate to a longitudinal probe position in line with the CFA. Follow the CFA distally to identify the bifurcation into profunda and superficial femoral arteries (SFA). Continue to follow the SFA to the distal thigh. Change probe position to the popliteal fossa. Begin again in the transverse probe position to identify the popliteal artery. Rotate to a longitudinal probe position in line with the popliteal artery. All arteries should be examined in gray-scale first to look for acute emboli, plaque formation, or other abnormalities.

Step 2: Color Doppler and Spectral analysis
Repeat step 1 following the CFA, SFA, and popliteal arteries, using color-flow and spectral Doppler modes. Signals should be obtained in the CFA, SFA (proximal, mid, and distal segments), and the popliteal artery.

Note: All velocity recordings should be made with an angle of insonation of 60° or less, parallel to the vessel wall, and in the center of the vessel, where flow is highest. Obtain a velocity spectrum at the level of any stenosis as well as immediately distal to the lesion to assess flow disturbance. The aliasing artifact can be very helpful at this time in identifying the areas of maximum-flow velocity/stenosis.

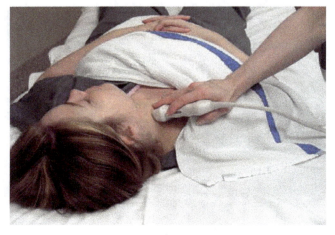

Figure 23-15 Patient position for carotid arterial examination.

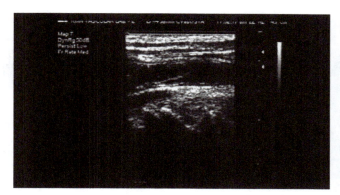

Figure 23-16 Intra-arterial (carotid) embolus. Longitudinal view.

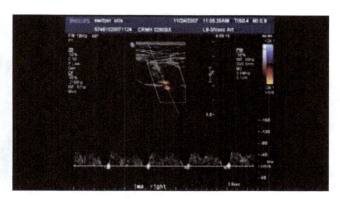

Figure 23-18 Double systole waveform of a patient on intra-aortic balloon assistance.

Examination of the upper extremities follows a similar pattern to that described above for the lower extremities.

▶ Interpreting the Findings

The diagnosis of arterial stenosis depends on elevated flow velocities when seen in the appropriate clinical setting. In high-resistance vessels, a doubling of the flow velocity at a site of stenosis when compared with the arterial flow velocity immediately prior to the suspicious area suggests a hemodynamically significant stenosis when accompanied by characteristics of Doppler spectral broadening and turbulent flow.[17] Such findings may warrant a formal arterial duplex exam for confirmation.

Diagnosis of hemodynamically significant stenosis in the ICA is somewhat more refined. Peak systolic velocity >145 cm/s is associated with stenosis >50%. An associated end-diastolic velocity >140 cm/s identifies the critical stenosis in the range of 80–99%. An additional criterion is the ratio of peak ICA velocity divided by the peak velocity in the CCA; the ICA/CCA ratio. A ratio >3.7 helps confirm the critical stenosis. The ICA/CCA ratio can also be helpful when flow in the carotids is restricted, as in the case of associated aortic stenosis or conditions of decreased cardiac output.[10]

Vascular occlusion is identified by complete absence of color-flow or Doppler signal in the examined artery.

Intraluminal emboli may be seen on gray-scale imaging (Figures 23-16 and 23-17). Patent collateral vessels may be identified; however, these are not often seen in the acute setting. Suspected ICA occlusion should be confirmed by another angiographic modality prior to deciding the patient is not a candidate for endarterectomy.

ADDITIONAL INFORMATION

Duplex arterial exams can yield associated information that can be helpful in recognizing pathologic conditions. Generally, reduced arterial flow may be an indication of left ventricular failure (Figure 23-18 and Video 23-11). Valvular heart disease can be suspected from alterations in the arterial waveforms. Ventricular and valve function can then be evaluated with transthoracic echocardiography. Associated venous disease can be recognized, along with nonvascular problems, such as cysts and tumors.

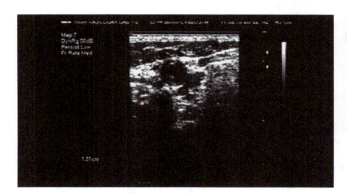

Figure 23-17 Intra-arterial (carotid) embolus. Transverse view.

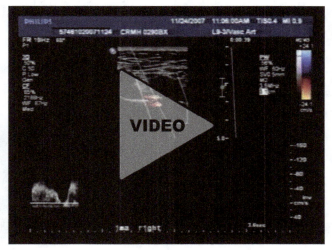

Video 23-11 Intra-aortic balloon pump. Internal mammary arterial Doppler flow signal with intra-aortic balloon pump in place to assist with the management of cardiogenic shock with 1:2 ratio. Note diastolic flow augmentation in alternative beats indication proper balloon timing and function. View at www.ccu2e.com

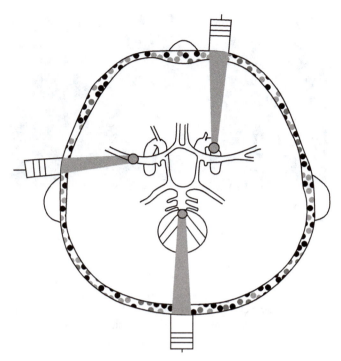

Figure 23-19 Transcranial Doppler: acoustic windows.

TRANSCRANIAL DOPPLER (TCD)

The application of TCD ultrasound technology to the evaluation of the cerebral circulation was introduced by Aaslid et al. in 1982.[18] The initial technique involved a handheld, low-frequency pulsed-wave transducer and relied on waveform analysis and depth of insonation to identify cerebral vessels. With current duplex technology, color-flow imaging serves as an adjunct to vessel location, identification, and flow assessment. Areas of clinical application include assessment of arterial stenosis and occlusion, identification of vascular anomalies, assessment of blood flow in the posterior cerebral circulation, intraoperative monitoring during carotid endarterectomy, assessment of vasospasm in relation to subarachnoid hemorrhage (SAH) and in sickle cell anemia, autoregulation of cerebral blood flow, and as an adjunct in assessment of brain death.[10] Compared with other duplex vascular examinations, TCD is more technically demanding due to limited acoustic access to the cerebral circulation and requirements to alter power levels and Doppler parameters to insure an optimal study with reliable and reproducible results.

Study protocols are generally standardized. A 2 MHz pulsed-wave signal is used for insonation. Access to the cranial vessels is obtained via any of three common acoustic windows: transtemporal, transforaminal, and transorbital (Figure 23-19). The transtemporal window allows evaluation of the middle cerebral, anterior cerebral, and posterior cerebral arteries (Figure 23-20). Ipsilateral and contralateral vessels may be insonated from the same window. It should be noted that 8–12% of patients may have inadequate acoustic windows.[19] The transforaminal window allows access to the vertebral and basal arteries via the foramen magnum. The transorbital window is used to insonate the ophthalmic artery and the carotid siphon. Care must be exercised to reduce power settings to prevent adverse bioeffects to the eye. Several parameters are combined to confirm the vessel being insonated. These include depth of the sample volume in relation to the acoustic window being utilized; orientation of the transducer; direction of blood flow in relation to the transducer; and relationship of the examined artery to the junction of middle cerebral and internal carotid arteries. Duplex machines add the benefit of color imaging, which can assist in vessel identification and demonstration of the circle of Willis (Figure 23-21). Flow velocities are calculated as time-average means and normal values vary by vessel. Tables of norms are published,[20] and it is suggested that each vascular laboratory validate its own results in comparison with these norms (Table 23-2). Perhaps the most significant application in the ICU setting is monitoring middle cerebral artery (MCA) vasospasm following SAH. In a recent review, Springborg et al. reported a high sensitivity and specificity for serial TCD studies when compared to arteriography.[21] Sharp

TABLE 23-2
Transcranial Doppler Parameters

Artery	Depth (mm)	Mean Velocity	Direction	Peak Systolic	End Diastolic	Children Mean Level
MCA	45–65	32–82	Toward	63–110	23–52	<170
ACA	62–75	18–82	Away	53–93	20–45	<150
ICA siphon	60–64	20–77	Bidirectional	–	–	<130
OA	50–62	20 ± 6	Toward	38 ± 11	11 ± 4	–
PCA	60–68	16–58	Bidirectional	–	–	<100
Basilar	80–100	12–66	Away	32–64	12–32	<100
Vertebral	60–80	12–66	Away	32–64	12–32	<80
MCA > ACA > ICA > PCA ≥ Basilar > Vertebral						

ACA, anterior cerebral artery; ICA, internal carotid artery; MCA, middle cerebral artery; OA, ophthalmic artery; PCA, posterior cerebral artery.
Source: Modified from Aaslid R, et al: Noninvasive transcranial Doppler ultrasound recording of flow velocity in the casal cerebral arteries. J Neurosurg. 1982;57:769–774.

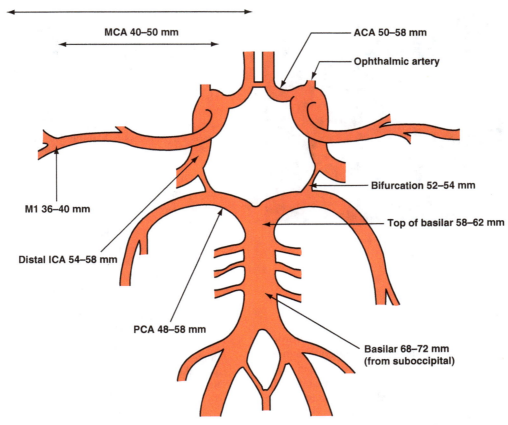

Figure 23-20 Diagram of circle of Willis with depths of insonation from ipsilateral transtemporal window.

increases in MCA flow velocities when compared with baseline values predicted the development of MCA vasospasm. The role of TCD in the diagnosis of brain death remains ill defined. Several patterns of altered waveforms have been described, but the most accurate has not been determined (Figures 23-22 and 23-23). Sensitivity >90% and specificity of 100% have been reported.[22] However, limitations to the diagnostic value of TCD still present problems. Premorbid TCD studies must be available to confirm that an absent signal is not due to the absence of a suitable acoustic window. Isolated anterior or posterior circulation blood flow may be demonstrated despite clinical evidence of brain death. Although TCD may be useful in patients known to have received sedative drugs, its current role in the diagnosis of brain death remains adjunctive.

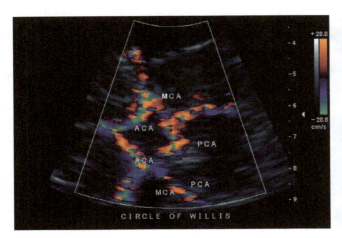

Figure 23-21 Transcranial color image of the circle of Willis. ACA, anterior cerebral artery; MCA, middle cerebral artery; PCA, posterior cerebral artery.

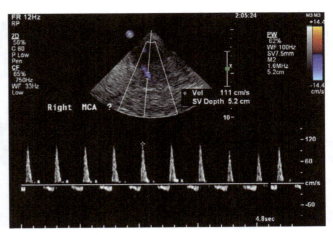

Figure 23-22 Abnormal middle cerebral artery (MCA) waveform seen in brain death. Note the high-resistance pattern with end-diastolic flow reversal.

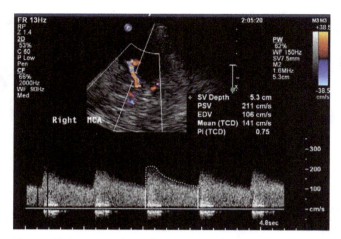

Figure 23-23 Normal middle cerebral artery (MCA) waveform. This is a low-resistance pattern with flow throughout the cardiac cycle.

CONCLUSION

The availability of high-quality, portable bedside duplex scanners has brought the ability to accurately diagnose acute DVT within the capability of every physician dealing with critically ill patients. The education and skills required to become comfortable with the techniques are basically extensions of the physical examination skills. And it is almost axiomatic that the individual who is best able to interpret the findings is the one who has daily responsibility for the care of the patient and who can correlate the results within the clinical context for that individual patient. A working knowledge of arterial anatomy and a basic understanding of arterial hemodynamics provide the bedside sonographer a solid foundation on which to perform and interpret the arterial duplex examination. Current portable duplex equipment provides high-quality information and puts this modality in the armamentarium of every clinician willing to gain the necessary experience with this modality.

REFERENCES

1. Blaivas M. Ultrasound in the detection of venous thromboembolism. *Crit Care Med.* 2007;35(Suppl 5):S224–S234.
2. Knudson MM, Collins JA, Goodman SB, et al. Thromboembolism following multiple trauma. *J Trauma.* 1992;32:2–11.
3. Kudsk KA, Fabian TC, Baum S, et al. Silent deep vein thrombosis in immobilized multiple trauma patients. *Am J Surg.* 1989;158:515–519.
4. Cook D, Attia J, Weaver B, et al. Venous thromboembolic disease: an observational study in medical-surgical intensive care unit patients. *J Crit Care.* 2000;15:127–132.
5. Burns GA, Cohn SM, Frumento BJ, et al. Prospective ultrasound evaluation of venous thrombosis in high-risk trauma patients. *J Trauma.* 1993;35:405–408.
6. Harris LM, Curl GR, Booth FV, et al. Screening for asymptomatic deep vein thrombosis in surgical intensive care patients. *J. Vasc Surg.* 1997;26:764–769.
7. Marik PE, Andrews L, Maini B. The incidence of deep venous thrombosis in ICU patients. *Chest.* 1997;111:661–664.
8. Stein PD, Henry JW. Prevalence of acute pulmonary embolism among patients in a general hospital and at autopsy. *Chest.* 1995;108:978–981.
9. Massicotte MP, Dix D, Monagle P, et al. Central venous catheter related thrombosis in children: analysis of the Canadian Registry of Venous Thromboembolic Complications. *J Pediatr.* 1998;133:770–776.
10. Strandness DE. Ultrasonic duplex scanning. In: Ascher E, ed. *Haimovici's Vascular Surgery.* Malden, MA: Blackwell Science, Blackwell Publishing Co; 2004:7–34.
11. Beaulieu Y, Marik PE. Bedside ultrasonography in the ICU: part 2. *Chest.* 2005;128:1766–1781.
12. Panetta TF, Sales CM, Marin ML, et al. Natural history, duplex characteristics, and histopathologic correlation of arterial injuries in a canine model. *J Vasc Surg.* 1992;16:867–874.
13. Tola M, Yurdakul M, Cumhur T. B-flow imaging in low cervical internal carotid artery dissection. *J Ultrasound Med.* 2005;24:1497–1502.
14. Davison BD, Polak JF. Arterial injuries: a sonographic approach. *Radiol Clin North Am.* 2004;42:383–396.
15. Imsand D, Hayoz D. Current treatment options of femoral pseudoaneurysms. *Vasa.* 2007;36:91–95.
16. Hanson JM, Atri M, Power N. Ultrasound-guided thrombin injection of iatrogenic pseudoaneurysm: Doppler features and technical tips. *Br J Radiol.* 2008;81:154–163.
17. Kohler TR, Nance DR, Cramer MM, Vandenburghe N, Strandness DE Jr. Duplex scanning for diagnosis of aortoiliac and femoropopliteal disease: a prospective study. *Circulation.* 1987;76:1074–1080.
18. Aaslid R, Markwalder TM, Nornes H. Noninvasive transcranial Doppler ultrasound recording of flow velocity in the casal cerebral arteries. *J Neurosurg.* 1982;57:769–774.
19. Otis SM, Ringelstein FB. Transcranial Doppler sonography. In: Zweibel WJ, ed. *Introduction to Vascular Ultrasonography.* Philadelphia: WB Saunders; 1992:145–171.
20. White H, Venkatesh B. Applications of transcranial Doppler in the ICU: a review. *Intensive Care Med.* 2006;32:981–994.
21. Springborg JB, Frederikson HJ, Eskesen V, et al. Trends in monitoring patients with aneurysmal subarachnoid haemorrhage. *Br J Anaesthesia.* 2005;94(3):259–270.
22. Ducrocq X, Braun M, Debouverie M, et al. Brain death and transcranial Doppler: experience in 10 cases of brain dead patients. *J Neurol Sci.* 160:41–46.

SECTION IV

Ultrasound Guidance for Procedures

24

ULTRASOUND-GUIDED TRANSTHORACIC PROCEDURES

PETER DOELKEN & PAUL H. MAYO

Scan QR code or visit www.ccu2e.com for video in this chapter

INTRODUCTION

Ultrasonographic guidance of thoracic drainage and biopsy procedures is an attractive alternative to computerized tomography (CT) or fluoroscopic guidance. While CT scanning is the standard for overall imaging of the chest in all cases of malignancy and many nonmalignant conditions, ultrasound may be used for procedure guidance. Ultrasound guidance eliminates further radiation exposure and is often less time consuming and more comfortable for the patient. The intensivist–sonographer, who engages in thoracic interventions, must possess the cognitive and manual skills required for pleural and lung sonography; and, in the case of anterior mediastinal biopsy, must be familiar with the ultrasound anatomy of the mediastinal organs. The ability to visualize inserted hardware and to recognize and interpret reverberation artifact associated with hardware is required for all but thoracentesis and some simple biopsy procedures.

HARDWARE

Convex-array or sector-scanning probes with frequencies between 2 and 5 MHz (typically 3.5 MHz) are most suitable for thoracic sonography and are also the most versatile for thoracic procedure guidance.[1] Higher frequency transducers do have better near-field resolution at the expense of penetration depth. We do not recommend probes with a biopsy channel for thoracic interventions due to the common problem of ribcage interference with imaging. Instead, an approach combining imaging with traditional bony landmark detection, that is, finding the upper rib margin with a finder needle prior to insertion of other hardware, is generally preferred. As in general thoracic sonography, the mark on the probe is oriented cephalad and the corresponding mark on the screen is placed at the upper left of the image. Thus, the orientation of standard views, which is imaging in the longitudinal axis, is cephalad left and caudal right on the screen. However, during procedure planning and visualization of hardware, nonstandard imaging planes are routinely used.

POSITIONING FOR PROCEDURES

Proper patient positioning is essential in interventional chest sonography. Free-flowing pleural effusions follow the gravitational gradient and collect in the most dependent part of the thoracic cavity. In the patient sitting upright, an effusion will collect in the inferior and posterior chest and is most easily accessed from a position behind the patient. The approach to positioning the critically ill patient varies with the size of the effusion, presence of obesity, number and type of support devices, and physiologic compromise, such as hemodynamic instability. Large effusions may be accessed with the patient in the supine position, which presents few problems during access. However, lateral access may be impossible in the very obese even with very large effusions. Adduction of the ipsilateral arm across the chest greatly improves lateral access and should uniformly be attempted. Posterior access may be facilitated by having the patient held in a sitting position but also by placing the patient at the very edge of the bed or even in the full lateral decubitus position. These positions require assistants to assure safety and prevent inadvertent movement of the patient. Occasionally, simply elevating the head of the bed allows lateral access even in cases where this was not possible in the fully supine position. Careful monitoring of endotracheal tubes and vascular access devices is required at all times during patient positioning.

Patient positioning for biopsy of lung or pleural lesions depends on the location of the lesion. The ability of the patient to comfortably maintain position for the duration of the procedure is essential for successful performance of the procedure and for maintaining sterility throughout. The overall guiding principle for positioning for sonographically guided procedures is the individualized approach that fully exploits the flexibility of sonographic imaging.[2]

THORACENTESIS

By adding sonographic guidance, the success rate of the thoracentesis procedure increases and the complication rate decreases likely by eliminating inadvertent attempts to drain fluid when no fluid is present. Proficiency in diagnostic sonography of pleural effusion is therefore a prerequisite for the successful use of sonographically guided thoracentesis (see Chapter 18). The issues pertaining to sonographic guidance in particular, such as patient positioning and access site selection, are described here. The more common complications of thoracentesis include pneumothorax, pain, shortness of breath, cough, and vasovagal reactions. Other complications that have been described are re-expansion pulmonary edema, inadvertent liver or splenic injury, hemothorax, infection, subcutaneous emphysema, air embolism, and chest wall or subcutaneous hematoma. Of all the complications, sonographic guidance appears to result in lower rates of traumatic pneumothorax; with rates between 5–18% for clinically guided versus 1–5% for sonographically guided thoracentesis. Obviously, the likely reduction of traumatic pneumothorax is especially important in the mechanically ventilated patient, who is at much higher risk for tension pneumothorax than the spontaneously breathing patient.

In patients not receiving mechanical ventilation, the risk of pneumothorax associated with thoracentesis performed by a radiologist has been reported to be 2.7%[3]; in a surgical intensive care unit setting, the complication rate was found to be 2.4%.[4] Ultrasound guidance for therapeutic thoracentesis appears to almost eliminate needle trauma as the immediate cause of postprocedure pneumothorax in spontaneously breathing patients. Pneumothorax in this setting has been reported to be associated with unexpandable lung and not laceration of the visceral pleura in almost all cases.[5] The incidence of pneumothorax in mechanically ventilated patients has been reported by radiologists to be higher than in spontaneously breathing patients, with an overall rate of only 2%,[6] but with a rate of 7% in intubated patients. However, Godwin and Sahn reported a similar risk of pneumothorax in patients receiving mechanical ventilation when compared with spontaneously breathing patients.[7] Other studies have reported low pneumothorax rates in the mechanically ventilated patient.[8-11] Although no direct comparison between thoracentesis with versus without ultrasound guidance has been performed, Diacon et al. found that the use of ultrasonography for site location for thoracentesis was more accurate than standard physical examination.[12]

In addition to the apparent safety of sonographically guided thoracentesis in regard to pneumothorax, physician-performed bedside ultrasound guidance may obviate the need to transport the critically ill to interventional radiology, thus eliminating the indirect risks related to the transport of the critically ill.

Because the pulmonary and critical care physician is already familiar with the basic procedure, thoracentesis is ideally suited for the initial adoption of sonographic guidance for thoracic interventions. While diagnostic sonography of pleural effusion is concerned with the detection and characterization of pleural fluid and the size of the effusion, sonographic guidance has the selection of a suitable access site and avoidance of organ puncture as the primary goals.

For ultrasound-guided thoracentesis to be performed safely and successfully, particular attention must be directed toward patient and operator positioning relative to the ultrasound machine to allow unencumbered use of the device without compromising sterility. The procedure field needs to be free of monitoring and support devices. Determination of a suitable access site requires the demonstration of pleural fluid immediately adjacent to the parietal pleura and sufficient distance from organs throughout the respiratory cycle. The diaphragm, liver, or spleen should be identified unequivocally. This is necessary so as not to confuse the curvilinear line of Morrison's pouch (hepatorenal recess), located between the liver and kidney, with the diaphragm (Figure 24-1 and Video 24-1). On the left, a curvilinear line may also be seen between spleen and kidney, and this line may also be mistaken for the diaphragm by the inexperienced sonographer. Misidentification of these lines can result in inadvertent hepatic or splenic injury. After marking

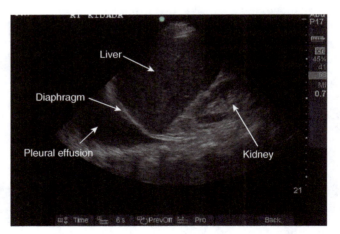

Figure 24-1 This image shows a pleural effusion above the diaphragm, the liver, the hepatorenal recess, and the kidney. The inexperienced scanner may identify the recess as the diaphragm and the liver as an echodense pleural effusion with inadvertent subdiaphragmatic device insertion. It is required to positively identify the kidney, the liver (or spleen), and the diaphragm when accessing a pleural effusion. The 3.5 MHz transducer is in longitudinal orientation and placed perpendicular to the chest wall to scan through the 9th intercostal space in the right mid-axillary line.

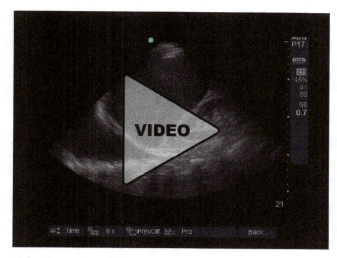

Video 24-1 This video shows a pleural effusion above the diaphragm, the liver, the hepatorenal recess, and the kidney. The inexperienced scanner may identify the recess as the diaphragm and the liver as an echodense pleural effusion with inadvertent subdiaphragmatic device insertion. It is required to positively identify the kidney, the liver (or spleen), and the diaphragm when accessing a pleural effusion. The 3.5 MHz transducer is in longitudinal orientation and placed perpendicular to the chest wall to scan through the 9th intercostal space in the right mid-axillary line. View at www.ccu2e.com

the access site, position of the mark should once again be sonographically verified. Sonography allows the measurement of the distances between the parietal pleura and the various underlying organs. Provided that the patient does not change position between the ultrasound examination and needle insertion and does not cough during the procedure, these distance measurements are reliable and are not subject to compression artifact as are measurements of chest wall thickness.[2,13-15] As the depth of the parietal pleural surface is indicated by pleural fluid return when the needle is advanced under aspiration, the measured distances between parietal pleural surface and underlying organs are measures of how much further and at which angle the needle may be safely advanced. An important caveat is related to possible occlusion of the needle lumen by clot or the solid contents of a complex effusion. This pitfall may be avoided by remembering that fluid return is expected approximately within 5 mm after passing the upper margin of the inferior rib. The needle lumen may also be cleared by injecting small amounts of local anesthetic if occlusion is suspected.

We do not routinely use real-time visualization of the thoracentesis needle during insertion. Real-time visualization adds complexity due to the need for a sterile sleeve, and may interfere with maintaining the proper needle insertion angle.[16]

After achieving proper local anesthesia and pleural fluid return, the needle is withdrawn and a small incision is made to allow insertion of the thoracentesis catheter if large volume thoracentesis is performed. Care must be taken that no air is inadvertently introduced during catheter inser-

tion and connection to the drainage system.[17] In case only a diagnostic sample is required, we withdraw the needle into the rib interspace until fluid return stops. We then exchange the syringe containing the local anesthetic with a clean syringe and reinsert the needle to the same depth at which pleural fluid was obtained before and begin aspiration of the sample. Anterior lung sliding may be documented prior to the procedure, and its continued presence after the procedure will reliably exclude an immediate postprocedure pneumothorax.

ULTRASOUND-GUIDED TUBE THORACOSTOMY

Indications for sonographically guided tube thoracostomy include complicated parapneumonic effusion, empyema, malignant pleural effusion, and pneumothorax. The type and size of the chest tube is dictated by the underlying condition. Large bore tubes are typically inserted for acute hemothorax or for pneumothorax and bronchopleural fistula in the mechanically ventilated patient; whereas small-bore pigtail catheters are the most versatile of chest tubes and are suitable for most other conditions. For chronic outpatient management of malignant pleural effusion, tunneled catheters may be used. Regardless of the type of tube used, the principles of ultrasound guidance are similar to those of simple ultrasound-guided thoracentesis. We routinely image a guide wire in real time, if applicable, to ascertain proper placement prior to use of dilators or catheter insertion (Figure 24-2 and Video 24-2). In order to image hardware, the transducer is rotated along its long axis to bring the wire or catheter into the sonographic image plane. The tip of a typical J-type guide wire can easily be seen with ultrasonography.

As the drainage devices remain in place, consideration has to be given to patient comfort whenever feasible and

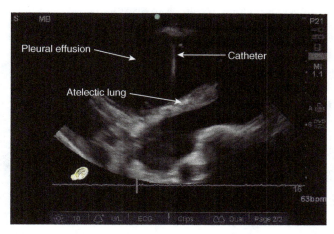

Figure 24-2 This image shows and large pleural effusion, atelectic lung, and a drainage catheter situated in the fluid. The 3.5 MHz transducer is in longitudinal orientation and placed perpendicular to the chest wall to scan through the 6th intercostal space in the right mid-axillary line.

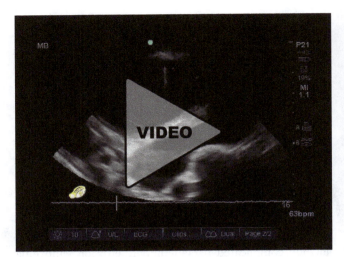

Video 24-2 This image shows a large pleural effusion, atelectatic lung, and a drainage catheter situated in the fluid. The 3.5 MHz transducer is in longitudinal orientation and placed perpendicular to the chest wall to scan through the 6th intercostal space in the right mid-axillary line. View at www.ccu2e.com

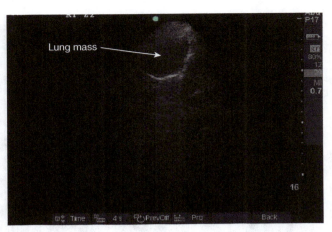

Figure 24-3 This image shows a lung mass adjacent to the chest wall that is suitable for ultrasound-guided aspiration or biopsy. The 3.5 MHz transducer is in longitudinal orientation and placed perpendicular to the chest wall to scan through the 6th intercostal space in the right posterior axillary line.

the device preferably should be inserted more laterally than during typical thoracentesis. However, this is not always possible and occasionally a pigtail catheter must be inserted posteriorly.

The use of sonography in catheter placement for pneumothorax is limited, as the distance between parietal and visceral pleura cannot be visualized in the presence of intrapleural air. However, sonography is useful in order to exclude underlying organs touching the parietal pleura immediately at the intended insertion site. We recommend CT guidance for pneumothorax in a complex pleural space due to adhesions from previous pleural injury or disease.

TRANSTHORACIC BIOPSY PROCEDURES

Ultrasound-guided needle biopsy is suitable for peripheral lung lesions, anterior mediastinal masses, and lesions of the pleura itself. However, any lesion must abut an accessible area of the parietal pleura and must be readily visualized by sonography (Figure 24-3 and Video 24-3). Critical to the success of the biopsy is operator proficiency in chest ultrasonography and the ability to correlate CT images with ultrasound findings. CT imaging is essential for procedure planning in order to characterize the lesion and document the extent and local topography, such as proximity of the heart or other structures (Figure 24-4 and Video 24-4). However, sonographic guidance is preferred to CT guidance of device insertion due to lack of radiation exposure and better patient comfort. Accessibility of the lesion with ultrasound guidance is determined by imaging of the lesion and confirmation of a clear needle path without intervening air, bone, organs, or vasculature. The angle of needle entry and penetration depth is then determined. Determination of penetration depth is susceptible to skin compression artifact, and this requires employment of strategies similar to the ones described above (see discussion on thoracentesis).

Although the needle may be tracked in real time after insertion by keeping the scanning plane parallel to the needle path, this is difficult due to the anatomy of the chest wall especially during biopsy of a superficial lesion. Needle guides may help keep the needle in the scanning plane, thereby simplifying real-time visualization. However, this benefit is outweighed by limitations imposed on needle angulation due to the more cumbersome device.[13–15,18] We do not routinely use real-time visualization during biopsy of superficial lesions of the lung or pleura.

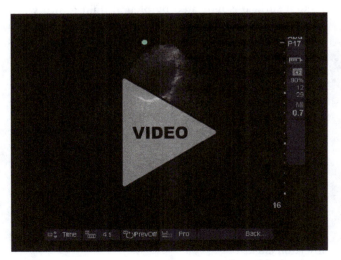

Video 24-3 This image shows a lung mass adjacent to the chest wall that is suitable for ultrasound guided aspiration or biopsy. The 3.5 MHz transducer is in longitudinal orientation and placed perpendicular to the chest wall to scan through the 6th intercostal space in the right posterior axillary line. View at www.ccu2e.com

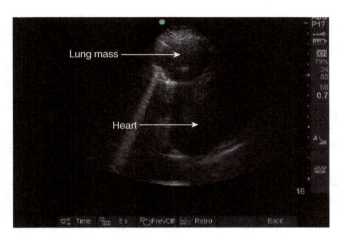

Figure 24-4 This image shows a lingular lung mass adjacent to the chest wall and heart that is suitable for ultrasound-guided aspiration or biopsy. Determination of safe needle trajectory must take into account adjacent anatomic structures, as indicated in this image. The 3.5 MHz transducer is in an oblique orientation and placed perpendicular to the chest wall to scan through the 5th intercostal space in the left anterior axillary line.

Eighteen or 20 gauge needles are appropriate for fine needle aspiration. After local anesthesia, and once the lesion is entered, suction is applied and the needle is moved in a to-and-fro motion in a fanlike pattern. Suction is then released and the needle withdrawn. It is important to release suction before the needle is withdrawn to avoid contamination of the specimen and to avoid aspiration of the specimen into the syringe used to apply suction. Specimens are immediately transferred to microscopy slides and

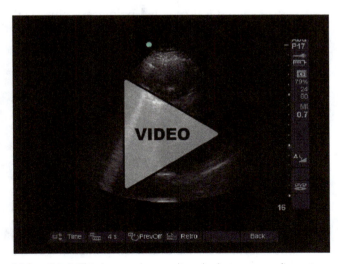

Video 24-4 This image shows a lingular lung mass adjacent to the chest wall and heart that is suitable for ultrasound-guided aspiration or biopsy. Determination of safe needle trajectory must take into account adjacent anatomic structures, as indicated in this image. The 3.5 MHz transducer is in an oblique orientation and placed perpendicular to the chest wall to scan through the 5th intercostal space in the left anterior axillary line. View at www.ccu2e.com

air-dried or fixed in alcohol. Media for flow cytometry or cellblock preparations should also be readily available.

Core biopsies of pleural or lung lesions require the use of cutting needle devices. The standard coaxial cutting needle technique is suitable for the purpose, and kits are commercially available. The kits contain an introducer with stylet and a spring-loaded cutting needle. Cutting needles are available with and without adjustable throw. We use needle sizes 16–20 G and reserve the largest size for pleural biopsy.

After site verification by ultrasound, the introducer assembly is advanced into the intercostal space. The patient is asked to hold their breath while the introducer assembly is introduced into the target lesion. Resistance may be encountered upon entering the lesion. Once the desired position is attained, the introducer assembly is locked in place. Whenever the stylet or biopsy needle is removed from the introducer lumen, the patient is asked to hold their breath to prevent inadvertent air entry. With the introducer assembly in place, the stylet is removed, the charged cutting needle advanced and locked, and immediately discharged. The cutting side of the needle is always oriented caudally to help avoid injury to the intercostal vasculature. Core biopsies allow histologic diagnosis. Onsite cytopathologic examination to determine specimen adequacy is possible by rolling the tissue cylinder on a microscopic slide prior to transfer into fixative.[19–21]

There are few absolute contraindications to biopsy. These include an uncooperative patient, a patient who cannot be maintained in position for the duration of the procedure, and intractable coughing. Mechanical ventilation and severe pulmonary hypertension are relative contraindications. The feasibility of biopsy has to be considered on a case-by-case basis. Other relative contraindications are coagulopathies, thrombocytopenia (platelet count <50K), and uremic platelet dysfunction. Some of these abnormalities can be corrected prior to the procedure.

The risks of biopsy of lung lesions are similar to the risks of fiberoptic transbronchial biopsy. The most common complication is pneumothorax, with an occurrence rate of about 3%, and is typically associated with pleuritic chest pain. Unfortunately, when pneumothorax does occur, the ultrasound image is lost, and the procedure has to be aborted. This need to stop mid-procedure is a disadvantage of using ultrasonography when compared with CT guidance.[22,23] Obviously, underlying lung disease or having only a single lung increases the risk of complications of pneumothorax. In this case, a pneumothorax often requires immediate treatment.[24–28]

Hemoptysis occurs in up to 10% of cases after core biopsy but is typically self-limited. Massive hemoptysis may occur and result in a poor outcome. The management of massive hemoptysis is no different from the management of hemoptysis from transbronchial biopsy: tamponade with the bronchoscope, endobronchial balloon occlusion, and selective intubation of the contralateral side.[28] Coughing may cause tearing of the pleura and air embolism, which can also occur without coughing. The risk of air embolism may be lower with ultrasound-guided than with CT-guided biopsy due to the generally peripheral location of lesions accessible to ultrasound guidance. Occluding the introducer cannula between passes of the needle may prevent this complication. If air embolism is suspected, the patient should be placed in the left lateral decubitus position and given 100% oxygen. Hyperbaric oxygen treatment is an option to be considered. Other risks include inadvertent puncture of other vital organs, which should be an extremely rare occurrence with an experienced operator.[29]

BIOPSY OF LUNG LESIONS

A requirement for ultrasound guidance for lung biopsy is the ability to visualize the target. Any intervening aerated lung will make sonographic visualization impossible and initial determination of suitability for sonographic guidance may be made by careful examination of the chest CT. One of the advantages of sonographic guidance when compared with CT guidance is the superior ability of sonography in distinguishing solid from liquid in a partially necrotic lesion. Using ultrasound, the biopsy needle may be confidently directed toward solid areas.[30] Cavitary lesions containing air need to be considered individually. Chronic cavitating or bronchiectatic lesions are commonly highly vascularized and have a higher risk of bleeding. It has been shown recently that important staging information in primary lung cancer can be derived by the determination of presence or absence of movement of lung lesions relative to the parietal pleura. With higher frequency transducers, interruption of the pleural reflection and invasion of the ribs or chest wall may be demonstrated. Any of these findings indicates chest wall invasion and may affect staging of nonsmall cell lung cancer.[31]

PLEURAL BIOPSY

Indications for sonographically guided pleural biopsy include suspected pleural malignancy, especially when pleural fluid cytology is negative; suspected malignant mesothelioma; and suspected tuberculous pleural effusion. Ultrasonography may detect abnormal areas of the pleura that may be targeted for biopsy. The yield is improved with this approach when compared with random pleural sampling.[19,32] For the diagnosis of malignant pleural mesothelioma, a tissue sample demonstrating invasiveness is often required and ultrasound-guided biopsy should be considered as the initial diagnostic procedure. We include part of the chest wall in the biopsy. Demonstration of invasiveness requires inclusion of chest wall tissue with the biopsy core. This may be achieved by partial withdrawal of the introducer assembly into the rib interspace prior to discharge of the cutting apparatus. The cutting aspect of the needle is oriented caudally, away from the neurovascular bundle. A sensitivity of 77% and a specificity of 88% may be attained with sonographically guided core biopsy in cases of malignant pleural mesothelioma.[33]

ANTERIOR MEDIASTINAL BIOPSY

Anterior mediastinal masses may be accessible to sonographically guided biopsy provided that aerated lung is displaced sufficiently to open a sonographic window through the anterior rib cage. It is essential that the needle path is well clear of the mammary vessels as well as the aorta, pulmonary artery, and the heart. The procedure is performed in the supine position after careful review of the chest CT. Generally, core biopsy is necessary for the diagnosis of anterior mediastinal masses, unless metastatic carcinoma is suspected, in which case fine needle aspiration may be sufficient.[34–37]

SUMMARY

The use of ultrasound for guidance in procedures involving the pleural space has become routine and has an excellent safety record. Once understanding of the pleural anatomy as seen on ultrasonography is learned, the techniques for intervention can be easily mastered by the physician–operator. Ultrasound guidance is in many cases preferable to CT guidance, as transport of the critically ill patient is avoided. Sonography does not subject the patient to the radiation effects of CT and comes at a lower cost. The operator must be familiar with all the possible complications of these procedures and their treatment. The need to understand pleural ultrasonography, especially its role in interventions, will continue to grow and become important part of the critical care and pulmonary physician's armamentarium.

PERICARDIOCENTESIS

Ultrasonography allows safe performance of pericardiocentesis. Seward et al. described 1127 serial pericardiocenteses with a very low complication rate.[16] Ultrasound-guided pericardiocentesis should completely replace fluoroscopic guidance. Fluoroscopic guidance requires subcostal needle insertion during which the position of the liver is unknown; and the relationship of the needle to the myocardium is uncertain, as fluoroscopy is a two-dimensional (2D) technique. Ultrasound-guided pericardiocentesis is so clearly superior to fluoroscopic guidance, that the critical care ultrasonographer should develop proficiency in the procedure to improve patient safety.

▶ Overview of Procedure

Ultrasonographic guidance of pericardiocentesis has features in common with thoracentesis and paracentesis. The operator identifies the fluid collection, and then chooses a safe site, angle, and depth for needle insertion. While the principles are the same, pericardiocentesis is different because of its intrinsic hazard. Laceration of the myocardium or of a coronary artery is a catastrophic complication of pericardiocentesis. The operator needs to be highly skilled at image acquisition and interpretation as well completely proficient with the manual skills related to hardware insertion. Pericardiocentesis is not a procedure for the entry-level ultrasonographer. The teacher attending is advised to supervise the fellow very closely during the procedure.

▶ Equipment Requirements

An ultrasound machine equipped with a cardiac transducer is required. Doppler capability is not required for ultrasound guidance of pericardiocentesis. Regarding equipment for the procedure itself, there are kits that are marketed specifically for pericardiocentesis. Another approach is to use a generic wire insertion approach. Central venous insertion kits can be used for pericardiocentesis, as can widely available cavity drainage systems. Manufacturers also market as stand-alone items, wire/catheter combinations. These are supplemented with appropriate equipment of the operator's choice. Whatever equipment is chosen, the clinician should choose the shortest possible needle length for the initial pericardial penetration. Some kits provide a 20-cm needle. These are difficult to manipulate, and therefore dangerous to use. Some clinicians prefer to insert an angiocath into the space, followed by the wire. Others prefer to use a wire-through-needle approach. Either way, a general principle always holds. The needle is inserted to the most minimal depth possible to obtain free flow of fluid, and for the shortest possible time. Once the wire is in place and the needle removed, the risk of myocardial of coronary artery or myocardial laceration is no longer present. Whatever hardware is used for the procedure, the operator must be completely proficient in all aspects of wire placement, dilatation over the wire, and insertion of a catheter over the wire. This chapter will not discuss the technical aspects of hardware use, but will concentrate on the use of ultrasonography to guide the procedure.

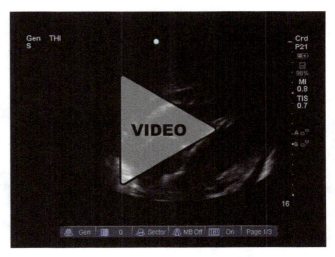

Video 24-5 This image shows a pericardial effusion from a subcostal window with the liver interposed between the heart and the abdominal wall. This would contraindicate needle insertion at this site. The 3.5 MHz transducer is in a subxiphoid position to obtain a long-axis subcostal view of the heart. View at www.ccu2e.com

▶ Site Selection and Preparation

With fluoroscopic guidance, the operator is limited to the subcostal approach with liver and other vital organs in close but uncertain proximity to the needle path (Figure 24-5 and Video 24-5). Using ultrasonography, the best site is determined by where the most fluid is found. This may be subcostal or at any point on the anterior or lateral chest. Frequently, the best site is identified on the lateral chest using the apical four-chamber view (Figure 24-6 and Video 24-6). If the effusion is very large, a parasternal view

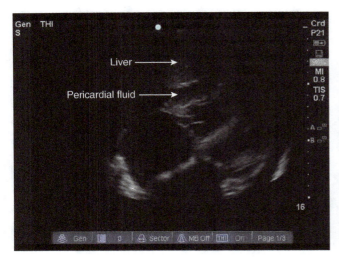

Figure 24-5 This image shows a pericardial effusion from a subcostal window with the liver interposed between the heart and the abdominal wall. This would contraindicate needle insertion at this site. The 3.5 MHz transducer is in a subxiphoid position to obtain a long-axis subcostal view of the heart.

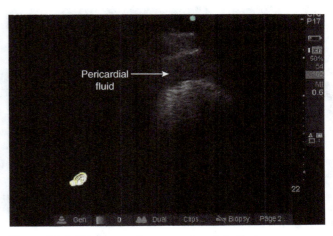

Figure 24-6 This image shows a pericardial effusion from an apical window with sufficient fluid to permit safe pericardiocentesis. The 3.5 MHz transducer is in an apical position to obtain an apical four chamber view of the heart.

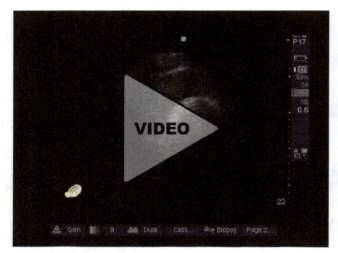

Video 24-6 This image shows a pericardial effusion from an apical window with sufficient fluid to permit safe pericardiocentesis. The 3.5 MHz transducer is in an apical position to obtain an apical four chamber view of the heart. View at www.ccu2e.com

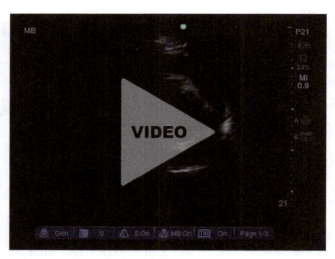

Video 24-7 This image shows a pericardial effusion from parasternal sort-axis window with sufficient fluid to permit safe pericardiocentesis. The 3.5 MHz transducer is in a parasternal position to obtain a parasternal short-axis view of the heart. View at www.ccu2e.com

may offer a good approach (Figure 24-7 and Video 24-7). Frequently, the effusion will be predominately posterior in location. This being the case, changing the patient's body position may distribute the fluid into a more favorable position. For example, the semisupine position may improve the subcostal view, while a left lateral decubitus position may move the fluid for improved apical view.

The heart is a highly mobile organ. It changes in size throughout the contractile cycle, it is subjected to respiratory effects that are accentuated if the patient has respiratory distress, and cardiac "swinging" is a common phenomenon in severe tamponade. The apparent thickness of the pericardial effusion may rapidly change to major extent during cardiac movement (Figure 24-8 and Video 24-8). The distance between the site of needle penetration

into the pericardium and the heart itself is a major determinant of safety (Figure 24-9 and 24-10 and Video 24-9 and 24-10). There is no absolute rule for how much fluid must be present to allow safe needle entry. A reasonable approach is to require at least 1 cm of fluid depth between the heart and the proposed needle entry point into the pericardial space, while taking into account the change in this distance that occurs during cardiac and respiratory cycle movement (Figure 24-11 and Video 24-11).

An important element in safe site selection is the avoidance of injury to adjacent structures. The lung is of concern. Fortunately, aerated or consolidated lung is easy to identify and therefore to avoid (see Chapter 19). The same holds for the liver, which may be readily identified and

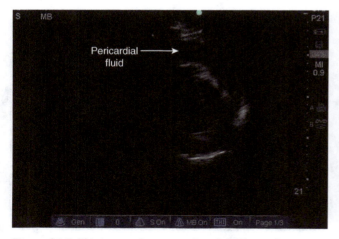

Figure 24-7 This image shows a pericardial effusion from a parasternal short-axis window with sufficient fluid to permit safe pericardiocentesis. The 3.5 MHz transducer is in a parasternal position to obtain a parasternal short-axis view of the heart.

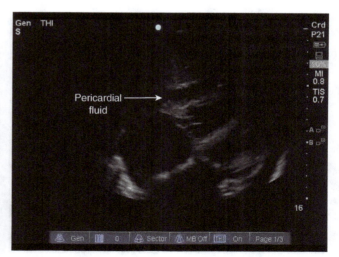

Figure 24-8 This image shows a pericardial effusion from a subcostal window with insufficient fluid depth for safe pericardiocentesis. This would contraindicate needle insertion at this site. The 3.5 MHz transducer is in a subxiphoid position to obtain a long-axis subcostal view of the heart.

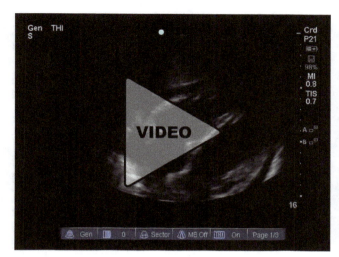

Video 24-8 This image shows a pericardial effusion from a subcostal window with insufficient fluid depth for safe pericardiocentesis. This would contraindicate needle insertion at this site. The 3.5 MHz transducer is in a subxiphoid position to obtain a long-axis subcostal view of the heart. View at www.ccu2e.com

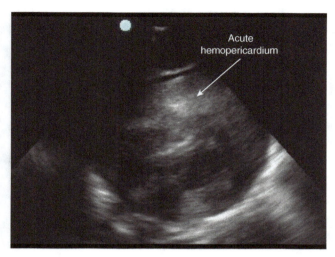

Figure 24-10 This image shows an acute hemopericardium that resulted from an attempt to perform pericardiocentesis from the subcostal position as indicated in Figure 24-8 and Video 24-8. This image emphasizes the need to have an adequate depth of fluid to permit safe needle insertion into the pericardial fluid. The 3.5 MHz transducer is in a subxiphoid position to obtain a long-axis subcostal view of the heart.

therefore avoided when using the subcostal approach. If using a parasternal approach, the internal mammary artery is an issue. Color Doppler of the proposed needle track is mandatory when using the parasternal approach in order to avoid the internal mammary vessels. Pleural effusion may be identified in association with the pericardial effusion, and may be large enough to interfere with pericardial access. In this case, the best approach is to drain the pleural effusion first, followed by rescanning to determine best approach to the pericardial effusion.

The depth of needle penetration is a critical element to safe pericardiocentesis. The ultrasound machine allows accurate measurement of the distance required for needle penetration. However, skin compression artifact is a concern. The transducer is pressed into the patient's skin with some degree of force in order to obtain good image quality. In the edematous or obese individual, this compression artifact may be several centimeters in depth. This results in a significant underestimation of the distance required to access the pericardium during the actual procedure. The last factor in determining safe needle trajectory for pericardiocentesis is to ascertain the best angle of approach. This is determined by the angle at which the transducer is held to obtain the best site of access.

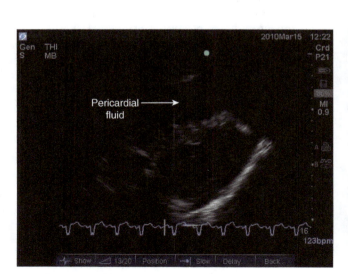

Figure 24-9 This image shows a pericardial effusion from a subcostal window with adequate fluid depth for safe pericardiocentesis. The 3.5 MHz transducer is in a subxiphoid position to obtain a long-axis subcostal view of the heart.

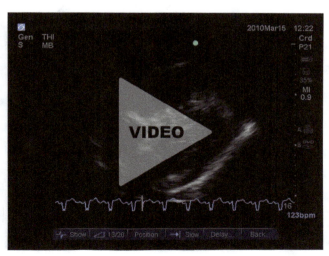

Video 24-9 This image shows a pericardial effusion from a subcostal window with adequate fluid depth for safe pericardiocentesis. The 3.5 MHz transducer is in a subxiphoid position to obtain a long-axis subcostal view of the heart. View at www.ccu2e.com

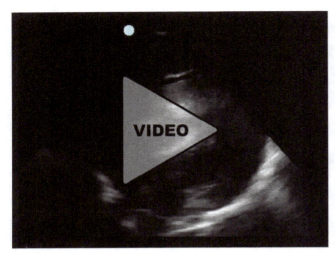

Video 24-10 This image shows an acute hemopericardium that resulted from an attempt to perform pericardiocentesis from the subcostal position as indicated in Figure 24-8 and Video 24-8. This image emphasizes the need to have an adequate depth of fluid to permit safe needle insertion into the pericardial fluid. The 3.5 MHz transducer is in a subxiphoid position to obtain a long-axis subcostal view of the heart. View at www.ccu2e.com

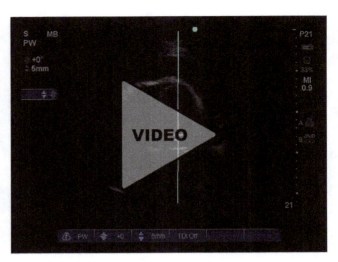

Video 24-11 This image shows a pericardial effusion from an apical window with sufficient fluid to permit safe pericardiocentesis. The 3.5 MHz transducer is in an apical position to obtain an apical four chamber view of the heart. View at www.ccu2e.com

▶ Site Preparation

It is advisable to scan the patient before sterile skin preparation. The best site and angle of needle insertion is determined and the site is marked. The skin may be marked with ink. Alternatively, it may be indented with a needle cap. Depth measurement includes an estimate of skin compression artifact. The depth of needle penetration is measured from a frozen image on the ultrasound screen using the calipers function. The skin is then prepared for sterile procedure. The patient should be covered with a full body drape, and the team use sterile coverings (mask, gown, eye protection, and caps). The transducer should be covered with a sterile sleeve and be part of the sterile field setup.

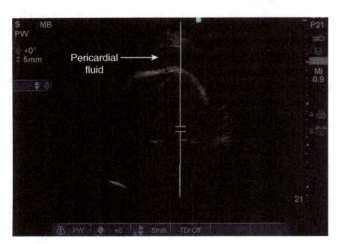

Figure 24-11 This image shows a pericardial effusion from an apical window with sufficient fluid to permit safe pericardiocentesis. The 3.5 MHz transducer is in an apical position to obtain an apical four chamber view of the heart.

Before the final confirmatory scan, all aspects of the equipment setup should be completed, such as needle–syringe assembly, lidocaine, wire layout, and tubing connections. This minimizes the time between the final scan and needle insertion. Following full equipment set-up, the operator once again confirms the site and depth of needle penetration using the transducer with sterile probe cover, and notes the angle of the transducer. This angle will be carefully duplicated by the angle of the needle–syringe assembly during device insertion. The operator proceeds with needle–wire insertion, followed by catheter insertion. Confirmation of wire or catheter insertion may be accomplished by direct visualization using 2D ultrasonography. If there is question of position, several cubic centimeters of agitated saline may be injected through the catheter to document catheter position movement (Figure 24-12 and Video 24-12). Malignant pericardial effusions are frequently hemorrhagic. The team may be apprehensive about this result, so documentation of pericardial placement with bubble study is a reassuring result.

Similar to thoracentesis and paracentesis, pericardiocentesis does not require real-time guidance with ultrasonography. The largest published study on the subject did not use real-time guidance.[16] However, it is important to have the transducer with sterile cover in place for immediate use throughout the procedure, in case there is need to rescan and document successful device insertion.

▶ Pitfalls: Common and Uncommon

Skin compression artifact is a common problem (see above). It causes an underestimation of the depth for needle insertion. During needle insertion, the operator is appropriately concerned, if there is no fluid obtained at the depth measured from the ultrasound machine screen. After all,

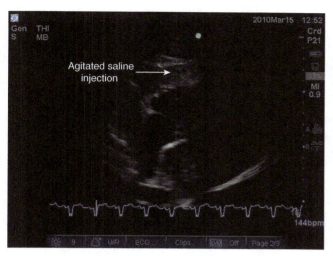

Figure 24-12 This image shows agitated saline injection into a pericardial catheter following successful pericardiocentesis. This confirms appropriate device position. The 3.5 MHz transducer is in a subxiphoid position to obtain a long-axis subcostal view of the heart.

coronary or ventricular laceration may result in lethal outcome to the patient. The solution to this problem is to rescan the patient, confirm angle of insertion, and estimate compression artifact more accurately. Another cause for difficulty is movement of the mark that designates the appropriate site for needle insertion. Skin is movable, so that the injudicious force application by the operator's hand may shift the skin mark. The needle should be inserted at the mark without any tension applied to the area that might shift mark position. Similarly, a "dry tap" might result from inaccurate duplication of the angle at which the transducer was held or inaccurate skin mark. The solution remains to rescan the patient to recheck angle and site. Generally, it is easier to duplicate a perpendicular transducer angle than one that is acutely angled. This favors an anterior or lateral chest wall approach (if fluid is accessible), as the transducer is often perpendicular to the chest wall when scanning in these areas. This is not the case in the subcostal approach.

An unusual cause of a "dry tap" is a blocked needle, resulting in overly deep needle insertion. Clotted blood or skin plug may be the culprit. Overly vigorous probing of the anterior costal cartilage (if using a parasternal approach) may also block the needle with cartilage so that the operator inserts too deeply with potential complication to the patient.

A large anterior pericardial fat pad may be mistaken for a pericardial effusion by the inexperienced ultrasonographer, with potentially catastrophic consequences to the patient. Pericardial fat has some element of echogenicity and moves in synchrony with cardiac contraction. In addition, it is very uncommon for a consequential pericardial effusion to occur anterior to the heart without a significant posterior pericardial effusion also being present.

An uncommon pitfall of pericardiocentesis occurs when the anesthesia needle penetrates the pericardium after having traversed the pleural space. The pericardial effusion may then drain into the pleural space through the defect in the pericardium made by the anesthesia needle. This may occur if there is a delay before definitive pericardial device insertion. The operator is unpleasantly surprised by the lack of pericardial effusion and the presence of a new pleural effusion. To avoid this situation, device insertion should promptly follow infiltration of the local anesthesia.

▶ **Summary**

Ultrasonography permits safe pericardiocentesis. Ultrasonography allows the intensivist to select a safe site, angle, and depth for needle and device insertion. Meticulous attention to image acquisition and interpretation allows the operator to avoid the serious complication of myocardial or coronary artery laceration. The critical care ultrasonographer is strongly encouraged to develop proficiency in ultrasound guidance of pericardiocentesis, as it is superior to subcostal fluoroscopic guidance.

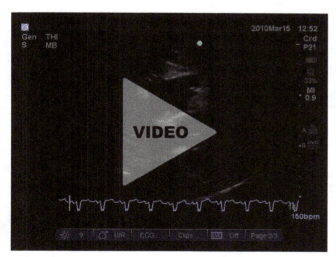

Video 24-12 This image shows agitated saline injection into a pericardial catheter following successful pericardiocentesis. This confirms appropriate device position. The 3.5 MHz transducer is in a subxiphoid position to obtain a long-axis subcostal view of the heart. View at www.ccu2e.com

REFERENCES

1. Reuses J. Interventional chest sonography. In: Mathis G, Lassa KD, eds. *Atlas of Chest Sonography.* Berlin, Germany: Springer-Verlag; 2003:147–162.
2. Lichtenstein DA. Interventional ultrasound. In: Lichtenstein DA, ed. *General Ultrasound in the Critically Ill.* Berlin, Germany: Springer-Verlag; 2005:170–174.
3. Jones PW, Moyers JP, Rogers JT, Rodriguez RM, Lee YC, Light RW. Ultrasound-guided thoracentesis: is it a safer method? *Chest.* 2003;123:418–423.
4. Petersen S, Freitag M, Albert W, Tempel S, Ludwig K. Ultrasound-guided thoracentesis in surgical intensive care patients. *Intensive Care Med.* 1999;25:1029.

5. Heidecker J, Huggins JT, Sahn SA, Doelken P. Pathophysiology of pneumothorax following ultrasound-guided thoracentesis. *Chest*. 2006;130:1173–1184.
6. Gervais DA, Petersein A, Lee MJ, Hahn PF, Saini S, Mueller PR. US-guided thoracentesis: requirement for postprocedure chest radiography in patients who receive mechanical ventilation versus patients who breathe spontaneously. *Radiology*. 1997;204:503–506.
7. Godwin JE, Sahn SA. Thoracentesis: a safe procedure in mechanically ventilated patients. *Ann Intern Med*. 1990;113:800–802.
8. Lichtenstein D, Hulot JS, Rabiller A, Tostivint I, Meziere G. Feasibility and safety of ultrasound-aided thoracentesis in mechanically ventilated patients. *Intensive Care Med*. 1999;25:955–958.
9. Mayo PH, Goltz HR, Tafreshi M, Doelken P. Safety of ultrasound-guided thoracentesis in patients receiving mechanical ventilation. *Chest*. 2004;125:1059–1062.
10. McCartney JP, Adams JW 2nd, Hazard PB. Safety of thoracentesis in mechanically ventilated patients. *Chest*. 1993;103:1920–1921.
11. Gordon CE, Feller-Kopman D, Balk EM, Smetana GW. Pneumothorax following thoracentesis: a systematic review and meta-analysis. *Arch Intern Med*. 2010;170(4):332–339.
12. Diacon AH, Brutsche MH, Soler M. Accuracy of pleural puncture sites: a prospective comparison of clinical examination with ultrasound. *Chest*. 2003;123:436–441.
13. Beckh S, Bolcskei PL, Lessnau KD. Real-time chest ultrasonography: a comprehensive review for the pulmonologist. *Chest*. 2002;122:1759–1773.
14. Dubs-Kunz B. Sonography of the chest wall. *Eur J Ultrasound*. 1996;3:103–111.
15. Reuss J. Sonographic imaging of the pleura: nearly 30 years experience. *Eur J Ultrasound*. 1996;3:125–139.
16. Tsang TS, Enriquez-Sarano M, Freeman WK, et al. Consecutive 1127 therapeutic echocardiographically guided pericardiocenteses: clinical profile, practice patterns, and outcomes spanning 21 years. *Mayo Clin Proc*. 2002;77:429–436.
17. Doelken P, Sahn SA. Thoracentesis. In: Ayres SM, ed. *Textbook of Critical Care*. Philadelphia, PA: Elsevier Saunders; 2005:1845–1848.
18. Matalon TA, Silver B. US guidance of interventional procedures. *Radiology*. 1990;174:43–47.
19. Chang DB, Yang PC, Luh KT, Kuo SH, Yu CJ. Ultrasound-guided pleural biopsy with Tru-Cut needle. *Chest*. 1991;100:1328–1333.
20. McLoud TC. Should cutting needles replace needle aspiration of lung lesions? *Radiology*. 1998;207:569–570.
21. Yang PC, Lee YC, Yu CJ, et al. Ultrasonographically guided biopsy of thoracic tumors. A comparison of large-bore cutting biopsy with fine-needle aspiration. *Cancer*. 1992;69:2553–2560.
22. Brown KT, Brody LA, Getrajdman GI, Napp TE. Outpatient treatment of iatrogenic pneumothorax after needle biopsy. *Radiology*. 1997;205:249–252.
23. Yankelevitz DF, Davis SD, Henschke CI. Aspiration of a large pneumothorax resulting from transthoracic needle biopsy. *Radiology*. 1996;200:695–697.
24. Charboneau JW, Reading CC, Welch TJ. CT and sonographically guided needle biopsy: current techniques and new innovations. *AJR Am J Roentgenol*. 1990;154:1–10.
25. Heilo A. US-guided transthoracic biopsy. *Eur J Ultrasound*. 1996;3:141–151.
26. Klein JS. Interventional techniques in the thorax. *Clin Chest Med*. 1999;20:805–826, ix.
27. Moore EH. Technical aspects of needle aspiration lung biopsy: a personal perspective. *Radiology*. 1998;208:303–318.
28. Weisbrod GL. Transthoracic percutaneous lung biopsy. *Radiol Clin North Am*. 1990;28:647–655.
29. Moore EH, Shepard JA, McLoud TC, Templeton PA, Kosiuk JP. Positional precautions in needle aspiration lung biopsy. *Radiology*. 1990;175:733–735.
30. Pan JF, Yang PC, Chang DB, Lee YC, Kuo SH, Luh KT. Needle aspiration biopsy of malignant lung masses with necrotic centers. Improved sensitivity with ultrasonic guidance. *Chest*. 1993;103:1452–1456.
31. Bandi V, Lunn W, Ernst A, Eberhardt R, Hoffmann H, Herth FJ. Ultrasound vs. CT in detecting chest wall invasion by tumor: a prospective study. *Chest*. 2008;133:881–886.
32. Diacon AH, Theron J, Schubert P, et al. Ultrasound-assisted transthoracic biopsy: fine-needle aspiration or cutting-needle biopsy? *Eur Respir J*. 2007;29:357–362.
33. Heilo A, Stenwig AE, Solheim OP. Malignant pleural mesothelioma: US-guided histologic core-needle biopsy. *Radiology*. 1999;211:657–659.
34. Pedersen OM, Aasen TB, Gulsvik A. Fine needle aspiration biopsy of mediastinal and peripheral pulmonary masses guided by real-time sonography. *Chest*. 1986;89:504–508.
35. Saito T, Kobayashi H, Sugama Y, Tamaki S, Kawai T, Kitamura S. Ultrasonically guided needle biopsy in the diagnosis of mediastinal masses. *Am Rev Respir Dis*. 1988;138:679–684.
36. Wernecke K, Vassallo P, Peters PE, von Bassewitz DB. Mediastinal tumors: biopsy under US guidance. *Radiology*. 1989;172:473–476.
37. Yu CJ, Yang PC, Chang DB, et al. Evaluation of ultrasonically guided biopsies of mediastinal masses. *Chest*. 1991;100:399–405.

ULTRASOUND GUIDANCE FOR ABDOMINAL AND SOFT TISSUE PROCEDURES

Scan QR code or visit www.ccu2e.com for video in this chapter

SAMEH AZIZ, WILLIAM J. BRUNELLI, JR., & JAMES S. CAIN

INTRODUCTION

Ultrasound technology is readily available and can provide guidance for invasive abdominal procedures in multiple planes without ionizing radiation. Further, real-time guidance of the needle tip position allows the operator to avoid inadvertent puncture of vital structures during the performance of invasive and soft tissue procedures of the abdominal cavity. Recently, this technology has a demonstrated benefit in abdominal procedures, such as paracentesis, liver and kidney biopsy, percutaneous gallbladder drainage, and abscess drainage.

Transducer selection for abdominal procedures most commonly includes a curved or phased array. A curved array allows the user to visualize a larger field, but the actual transducer size is larger than a phased array. Curved array is the transducer of choice for most abdominal procedures since a larger field can be visualized during the exam. A sector array is smaller and is most commonly used for abscesses that are close to the diaphragm and allows for an intercostal approach.

PARACENTESIS

Ultrasound use in paracentesis improves both the ease and efficiency of the procedure and reduces unnecessary abdominal punctures in patients with scant fluid. It is particularly helpful in obese patients to assess the depth to the peritoneum and in patients with loculated effusions to define the largest locule for drainage. Ultrasound use can identify intra-abdominal pathology that may increase the risk of bowel perforation during the procedure.[1]

▶ Indications

Diagnostic paracentesis is indicated as a part of the initial evaluation of patients with new onset ascites and in patients with a known history of ascites secondary to liver cirrhosis, who develop clinical deterioration, including the signs and symptoms of fever, abdominal pain, rapid worsening of renal function, worsened hepatic encephalopathy, leukocytosis, acidosis, gastrointestinal bleeding or sepsis, and to rule out underlying spontaneous bacterial peritonitis (SBP).[2] Paracentesis can also be used for the evaluation of intra-abdominal fluid in trauma patients. Therapeutic paracentesis is performed in patients with tense or diuretic-resistant ascites to alleviate difficulty with breathing or abdominal pain.

▶ Contraindications

Paracentesis is contraindicated in patients with disseminated intravascular coagulation, a platelet count $<50 \times 10^9$ per liter, an international normalized ratio (INR) >2, and a local skin infection, visible scar, hematoma, or cutaneous vein at the site of needle entry.[3] Patients with underlying renal insufficiency who have an increased tendency for bleeding should be carefully evaluated prior to the procedure.

▶ Equipment and Procedure Tray

A 3.5–5 MHz broadband curved array is preferred for the evaluation of ascites and for assistance with ultrasound-guided paracentesis.[1,4] Prepackaged paracentesis procedure kits are commercially available and contain all necessary equipment, including an aspiration catheter, catheter bag, blood collection tubing, 19-gauge introducer needle with 5-French catheter, lidocaine for skin anesthesia, skin preparation solution, and dressing pack with sterile draping (Figure 25-1). For real-time ultrasound-guided procedures, a sterile sleeve is used to cover the ultrasound probe.

▶ Site

The optimal site for paracentesis is where the depth of ascitic fluid is maximal and the abdominal wall is the thinnest.[5] It is common practice to perform a paracentesis in the left

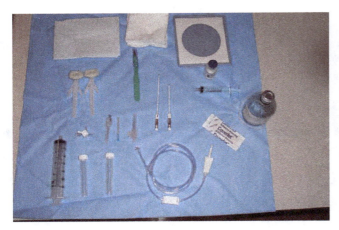

Figure 25-1 Paracentesis tray showing equipment including 5-French catheter.

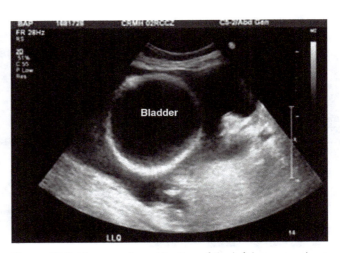

Figure 25-3 Ultrasound examination of the left lower quadrant in a patient with ascites demonstrates a collection of ascites adjacent to a full urinary bladder. A full bladder poses an increased risk of bladder perforation; therefore, the patient should be asked to empty bladder prior to the procedure.

lower quadrant (LLQ). Paracentesis in the right lower quadrant is generally avoided because of an increased risk of bowel perforation in patients with a distended cecum. The best location for paracentesis is 5 cm superior and medial to the anterior superior iliac spine. One prospective study of 52 patients with ascites secondary to cirrhotic liver disease demonstrated that the LLQ was the optimal location for paracentesis because it was easier and safer than an infraumbilical, midline approach because of a lower incidence of "dry tap" and bleeding.[5] Preprocedure scanning with ultrasound is recommended to avoid complicating factors like cutaneous veins, the inferior epigastric artery, and areas with previous scars and operations (Figure 25-2).

▶ **Procedure Description**

After obtaining informed consent, the patient is asked to empty the bladder prior to the procedure to decrease the risk of urinary bladder perforation (Figure 25-3). The patient is positioned supine. Prior to starting the procedure, the four abdominal quadrants are scanned to evaluate the extent of the ascites. The liver and spleen should also be evaluated. Scanning the entire abdomen allows the identification of complicating factors for intra-abdominal paracentesis, like intraperitoneal septation (Figure 25-4). Noncomplicated ascites usually has a characteristic anechoic contrast on ultrasound (Figure 25-5). An abnormal density, loculation, or septation may be identified on ultrasound and presents visually as an echogenic mass.[6]

After screening the abdominal cavity with ultrasound, the optimal site is identified, cleaned, and draped. The ultrasound probe is covered with a sterile sheath and the abdomen is rescanned to confirm the site of needle entry. Using a 25–30 gauge needle, the skin is infiltrated with local anesthetic using 1% or 2% lidocaine. A combination of lidocaine and sodium bicarbonate may be used to reduce the burning associated with the local injection of lidocaine. Next, a 22-gauge 1.5 cm needle can be used to

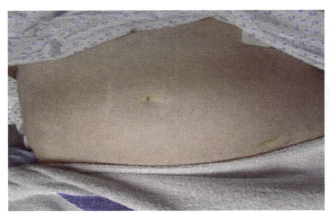

Figure 25-2 The abdomen of a patient with malignant ascites is shown. This patient had a history of a previous cholecystectomy, with a paraumbilical scar. Paracentesis was performed in the left lower quadrant, as demonstrated by the Band-Aid, to avoid possible adhesions in the right lower quadrant.

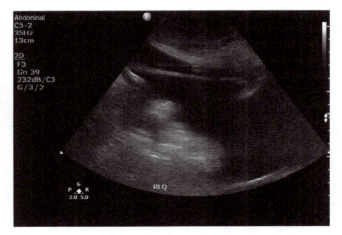

Figure 25-4 Right lower quadrant ultrasound examination for the evaluation of ascites demonstrates the presence of peritoneal fluid with intra-abdominal separation representing complicated intra-abdominal ascites.

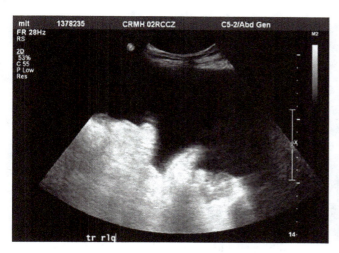

Figure 25-5 Ultrasound evaluation of the right lower quadrant demonstrated clear anechoic peritoneal fluid.

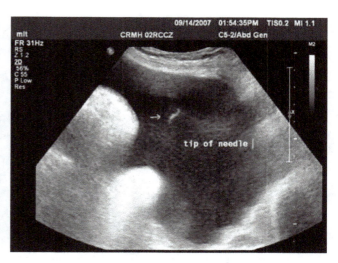

Figure 25-7 Ultrasound examination of the abdomen during real-time paracentesis demonstrates the position of the needle tip.

infiltrate the local anesthetic to the subcutaneous tissues and anterior abdominal wall. A 19-gauge needle with an echogenic tip is then introduced into the peritoneal cavity. To avoid precipitating a peritoneal fluid leak, a "Z-line technique," which introduces the needle at an angle and avoids creating a direct tract, is recommended. A 5-French catheter can be used for drainage of the peritoneal fluid.

A free-hand technique, in which paracentesis is guided by real-time ultrasound, is recommended to avoid direct injury to the bowel for a small pocket of peritoneal fluid (Figure 25-6). In this approach, the needle is introduced into the peritoneal cavity and fluid collected under direct vision (Figure 25-7). A sample of fluid is submitted to the clinical laboratory for appropriate diagnostic studies.

For a therapeutic tap of a large volume of ascites, a catheter-over-the-needle assembly can be used. In this approach, a needle is introduced into the peritoneal cavity, and once the needle passes through the ascitic collection, a catheter is introduced over the needle. Follow-up imaging with ultrasound can document the proper and safe position of the tip of the catheter. Then, drainage tubing connected to a vacuum device can be attached to the catheter. On occasion, the bowel will obstruct the catheter; when this occurs, the drainage tubing can be clamped with hemostats and the tubing separated from the catheter. This allows the suction to be temporarily removed from the catheter. The catheter can then be pulled back a few millimeters until ascites again begins to escape from the catheter. The drainage tubing is reattached and the hemostats removed to continue draining the ascites (Video 25-1).

▶ Fluid Analysis

A number of diagnostic tests can be performed on the ascitic fluid to assist with clinical interpretation.[7-9] These include:

- *Gram stain and culture:* A gram stain and culture is recommended to rule out infection of the peritoneal fluid and may identify secondary peritonitis.
- *Cell count and differential:* This test allows for the diagnosis of inflammation or SBP. The sensitivity and specificity

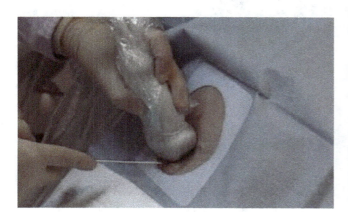

Figure 25-6 A demonstration of the "freehand technique" during ultrasound-guided paracentesis.

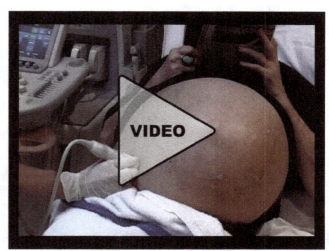

Video 25-1 Ultrasound guided paracentesis. View at www.ccu2e.com

depends on the polymorphonuclear (PMN) count. A PMN count >500 cells/mm³ has a sensitivity of 70–100% and a specificity of 86–100%.
- *Glucose:* Ascitic fluid glucose is low in secondary peritonitis.
- *Albumin:* Albumin levels allow for a determination of the etiology of the ascitic fluid. The serum-ascites albumin gradient (SAAG) is the absolute difference between the serum albumin and the ascitic albumin level. A SAAG >1.1 g/dL identifies ascites due to portal hypertension. A SAAG <1.1 g/dL indicates an exudative ascites that can be due to infection or malignancy.[10]
- *Total protein:* An ascitic fluid protein level >2.5 g/dL supports a diagnosis of an exudative peritoneal effusion, while a protein level <2.5 g/dL supports a diagnosis of a transudative effusion. The differential diagnosis associated with a transudate includes cirrhosis, congestive heart failure, portal vein thrombosis, and myxedema, and that associated with an exudative effusion includes peritoneal carcinomatosis, tuberculosis, infection, connective tissue disease, bowel obstruction, and infarction.
- *Amylase:* A high amylase level in ascitic fluid >1000 indicates leakage of pancreatic enzymes into the peritoneal cavity.
- *Triglycerides:* Chylous ascites with triglycerides level >200 mg/dL is highly suggestive for intra-abdominal malignancy or infection (filariasis, tuberculosis).
- *Bilirubin:* High ascites bilirubin >6 mg/dL indicates choleperitoneum (bile in the peritoneal cavity).
- *Cytology:* Malignant cells may be present in the peritoneal fluid and indicate carcinomatosis.[7-9]

▶ Complications

The incidence of bleeding from diagnostic paracentesis is estimated at approximately 0.2%. This was found to increase cost-related procedure by about $19,066 and increase length of hospital stay.[11] Hemorrhage related to large volume therapeutic abdominal paracentesis >4 L is estimated at approximately 2%.[12] An inferior epigastric artery pseudoaneurysm has been reported in two cases after large volume paracentesis. These were treated by percutaneous embolization.[13,13a] This complication can be avoided by scanning of the abdomen with ultrasound to define the optimal entry site that is lateral to the rectus abdominis muscles and avoids large intra-abdominal veins. It was found that ultrasound had decrease the risk of bleeding after paracentesis by 19%.[11]

Other complications may include intestinal or urinary bladder perforation, secondary peritonitis, and reaccumulation of peritoneal fluid. Large volume paracentesis, >10 L, is usually avoided because it may lead to a reduction in central venous pressure and associated hypotension. In addition, activation of the rennin-angiotensin-aldosterone system occurs, which is extremely sensitive in patients with liver cirrhosis. This phenomenon is worse in patients who have liver cirrhosis with ascites but without peripheral edema, and may precipitate hyponatremia, renal insufficiency, and hepatorenal syndrome if the patient does not receive simultaneous intravenous albumin.[13,13a,14] This is due to the absence of edema, which can functionally re-equilibrate with plasma.

ABSCESS DRAINAGE

Drainage of an intra-abdominal abscess by using puncture and aspiration was described in the 1930s.[15]

▶ Role of Ultrasound Guidance

Real-time sonography has the advantages of being portable, readily available at the bedside, and a success rate of approximately 90% for intra-abdominal abscesses.

Ultrasound is able to differentiate between a solid mass and cyst in approximately 95% of cases.[16] Using a gray scale, the cyst will appear bright white, while the adjacent organs appear gray. This is referred to as the "light bulb" sign.[17] Ultrasound provides real-time imaging during catheter placement. Color-Doppler flow can be used to identify crossing blood vessels, which allow proper planning of an optimum approach.[18] When compared with computerized tomography (CT), ultrasound is more accurate in localizing and guiding the drainage of small, deep abscesses[19] (Figure 25-8).

▶ Indications

The drainage of abnormal fluid collections is recommended for fluid that is suspicious for infection. Percutaneous fluid drainage is a safe and expeditious option for critically ill patients, who are too unstable for an operative intervention or need a temporizing measure to improve their condition and reduce morbidity. Percutaneous drainage provides a rapid, inexpensive, and immediate treatment in elderly, unstable patients. While this procedure is usually performed in the radiology department with the

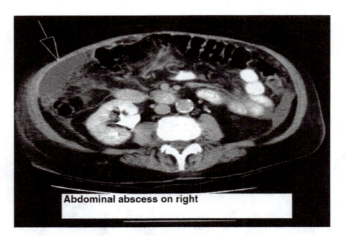

Figure 25-8 Computerized tomography (CT) scan of the abdomen demonstrating an intra-abdominal abscess.

assistance of CT or fluoroscopy, the role of bedside ultrasound is important for those patients, who are too sick for transportation to the radiology suite and whose transportation conveys additional risks for potential complications.

▶ Contraindications

Percutaneous abscess drainage is contraindicated if the catheter path is through a vital organ (lack of safe route). If possible, consider correction of coagulopathy prior to the procedure.[1,17] Ultrasound may be limited in differentiating between an abscess and other abdominal fluid collections, such as blood. Bowel gas may reduce image quality. Surgical dressing or drains may limit ultrasound evaluation.

▶ Site

The site of the abscess must be evaluated by ultrasound prior to the procedure by using a 5–7 MHz transducer; for very superficial abscesses a 10 MHz transducer may provide better resolution.[16] One needs to evaluate a safe path for catheter placement, the size of the abscess, the content of the abscess (light bulb sign), and the proximity to the skin surface.[17] The key to a successful procedure is a careful, well-planned needle path and an appropriate angle of entry prior to starting.

▶ Equipment

The catheter chosen for the procedure depends on the indication, with smaller catheters (6–8 French) used for aspiration of fluid collections, while larger caliber catheters (10–14 French) may be needed for more viscous fluid collections.

▶ Procedure Description

The procedure site is sterilized and draped. Lidocaine 1–2% is used to anesthetize the skin. A sterile sheath is used to cover the ultrasound probe. The catheter is introduced into the abscess under direct ultrasound visualization.

Different techniques are available for abscess drainage. The trocar technique is the preferred method for a large abscess with thick fluid; however, this method is associated with more severe complications due the large size of the introducer needle. In the Seldinger technique, a needle, guide wire, and dilators are sequentially introduced prior to the introduction of the catheter.

For a superficial abscess, a 22-gauge needle can be used; for deeper collections, a larger bore needle is recommended. For deeper abscesses using a Seldinger technique, the skin is prepped and draped and the ultrasound probe is covered with a sterile sleeve. The probe is held in parallel with the needle tract and the skin is anesthetized. The 18-gauge introducer needle is advanced along the parallel ultrasound plane (beam), carefully observing and avoiding surrounding anatomical structures. After placing the needle tip into the collection, a syringe is attached to the needle and a sample of aspirate is removed for cultures. The syringe is removed and a 0.035 guide wire is placed through the needle lumen

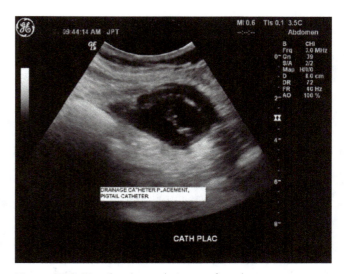

Figure 25-9 Pigtail catheter drainage of an abscess.

into the collection. Direct visualization of the wire can be achieved by carefully tugging on the wire while observing for movement within the collection. The tract is dilated to the desired size of the catheter, most commonly a 10-French, 30 cm, multipurpose "pigtail" catheter. Starting with a 6-French dilator, sequential dilation can occur with 8- and 10-French dilators. The drainage catheter is advanced over the wire and into the abscess (Figure 25-9). The metal stiffener (inner portion of the catheter mechanism) should only be advanced a few millimeters passing through the border of the collection; the catheter is slightly longer than the stiffener. After passing through the wall of the collection, hold the stiffener while advancing the catheter over the stiffener into the collection. Remove the stiffener from the catheter, remove the wire, and pull the string, which causes the distal end of the catheter to coil (pigtail). The catheter is secured using either suture or an adhesive device. The catheter is attached to the drainage bag and a dressing placed over the catheter entry site. If it is difficult to visualize catheter placement, push a combination of 3 cc of sterile saline with 1 cc of air through the catheter. Perform this technique while scanning; you should see air bubbles floating within the collection.

Aggressive manipulation of the catheter after placement is discouraged to prevent bacteremia.[20] The abscess contents should be aspirated as completely as possible, followed by gentle irrigation with sterile saline. Once the catheter is in place, it should be secured and allowed to drain to gravity. Irrigation of the catheter with normal saline is recommended every 4 hours until the drainage fluid clears. A precise recording of daily output of the drainage is important.

Once the patient becomes more stable and the condition improves, a follow-up imaging study, such as a CT, is recommend to evaluate the position of the catheter, the extent of the abscess, and identification of nondraining areas. After completion of antibiotics, a trial of catheter lock for 24 hours is recommended prior to removal of the catheter.

▶ Complications

Risks range from minor bleeding in 9.8% of the cases to serious complications, such as perforation and bacteremia, in 5% of the cases. Uncooperative patients increase the risk of complications.[20]

LIVER BIOPSY

Percutaneous liver biopsy was first described at the end of the 19th century. A second liver biopsy was described by Menghini in the 1950s, and ultrasound guidance for percutaneous biopsy was introduced in the late 1970s.[21] Ultrasound can provide a real-time evaluation of the liver, the lesion, and needle placement. The addition of color Doppler improves the ability to visualize and avoid blood vessels that may be in the track of the needle.[22] While diagnostic yield may not be improved with ultrasound-guided liver biopsy, it often results in fewer attempts, fewer complications, less pain, and shorter procedure times.[23]

▶ Indications

The most common indications for liver biopsy are:
- Diagnosis and staging of hepatitis B or C
- Chronic alcoholism
- Diagnosis of Wilson's disease
- α-1 antitrypsin deficiency
- Hemochromatosis
- A liver mass
- A focal liver lesion
- Elevated liver enzymes after liver transplantation
- Unexplained abnormal liver biological tests[2]

▶ Contraindications

Liver biopsy is considered a safe procedure when performed by skilled practitioners. The reported incidence of bleeding ranges from 0.06% to 1.7%, with an associated mortality rate between 0.009% and 0.33%.[23] Most of the bleeding complications are caused by a penetrating injury to a branch of the hepatic artery, portal vein, or puncture of the gallbladder. There is controversy about the need to withhold aspirin or nonsteroidal anti-inflammatory drugs prior to the procedure due to their potential affect on platelets. Relative contraindications to liver biopsy include ascites, empyema, or infection below the right diaphragm. Absolute contraindications include coagulopathy, an INR >1.4, a platelet count <60,000/mm^3, a prolonged bleeding time, a liver mass with suspicion of a hemangioma, or an uncooperative patient.

▶ Role of Ultrasound Guidance in Liver Biopsy

Ultrasound-guided biopsy of the liver can be performed either by the free-hand technique, in which the operator holds the probe in one hand and the biopsy needle in the other, or by using a biopsy adaptor, which is a tool that attaches to the ultrasound probe and guides the needle to the target area.

For the diagnostic accuracy of fibrotic liver disease, a biopsy sample of >25 mm is needed. After evaluation of the liver lesion with B-mode, gray-scale sonography, a color Doppler sonogram is used for evaluation to view the anatomic course of blood vessels and biliary ducts and to provide a precise evaluation of vasculature of the liver mass. Highly vascular liver lesions, like hemangiomas, may be echo-poor and show heterogeneity.[24]

Ultrasound-guided liver biopsy improves specimen adequacy regardless of operator experience.[25] By providing guidance for needle angulation, ultrasound helps to guide the operator with positioning the needle.[26] This is particularly helpful because selective clinical criteria like obesity, difficult liver percussion, or chest deformity alone are often insensitive selection criteria for determining which patients may need an ultrasound-guided biopsy.[27-29] In children, ultrasound-guided percutaneous liver biopsy has been more accurate, has had a higher success rate and fewer complications likely due to a reduced number of passes, and has allowed the needle to be directed away from large intrahepatic vessels, gallbladder, lungs, and kidneys.[29,30] Ultrasound also allows the operator to detect significant postprocedure complications, such as hepatic hematomas, following percutaneous liver biopsy.

Tense ascites often prevents adequate tissue sampling because the liver may "bounce" away during the procedure. In addition, bleeding may be difficult to control. Ultrasound guidance positively influences these outcomes by directly visualizing the liver; avoiding intervening structures within the procedure track, such as the lung, gallbladder, a large central vessel, or colonic loop; and reducing the incidence of bleeding. In one study, ultrasound guidance led to a change in procedure site in 15.1% of patients.[31]

▶ Equipment and Needles

There are three types of needles that can be used in liver biopsy: (1) suction needles (like Menghini needle), (2) cutting needles (like Tru-cut needles), and (3) spring-loaded cutting needles.

Fine needle aspiration biopsy is preferred for focal liver lesions because it has a high sensitivity and specificity for the detection of malignancy. A Tru-cut needle has a high diagnostic yield in patients with liver cirrhosis because of the ability to cut through the liver, which results in better preservation of tissue architecture.[32,33] However, there is a higher risk of bleeding with Tru-cut needles.

▶ Procedure Description

Ultrasound-guided percutaneous liver biopsy is usually performed with the patient in the supine position, with the right arm raised above the head. The patient is asked to take a deep breath and hold it. Percussion is performed between the anterior and mid-axillary lines during deep inspiration

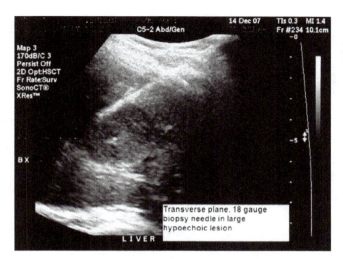

Figure 25-10 Liver biopsy of hypoechoic liver lesion.

beginning under the right breast and progressing in a caudal direction to the point of first maximal dullness; a site for biopsy is marked on the skin in the interspace below the percussion line, usually at the mid-axillary line. The liver biopsy is performed in expiratory apnea. A transthoracic approach is preferred. First, a longer needle (22-gauge) is used to administer local anesthetic along the needle track, a small skin incision is then performed to alleviate skin resistance. After identifying the safe needle tract to the lesion that avoids the bowel, major vessels, diaphragm, and gallbladder, the needle is introduced adjacent to the transducer into the peritoneal cavity and into the biopsy site while maintaining visualization of the needle in the middle of the ultrasound field using a slow, rocking motion of the transducer. A steering attachment can be applied to the transducer to help guide the needle into the exact location. Alternatively, the coaxial technique allows the lesion to be visualized and focused in the center of the field and the needle is introduced along the longitudinal axis of the transducer as a straight arrow entering the biopsy site (Figure 25-10). Postprocedure ultrasound evaluation is recommended to rule out acute hematoma formation. After the procedure, the patient is positioned on the right side for at least 2 hours, with frequent monitoring of vital signs. Prophylactic antibiotics are recommended for patients with underlying heart disease who are at risk for endocarditis.

▶ Complications

Pain, ranging from moderate to severe in intensity, is the most frequent complication of percutaneous liver biopsy occurring in approximately 30% of cases, and is responsible for approximately 4% of postprocedure hospital admissions.[34-36] The most common source of postprocedure pain is related to injury to the lung, irritation to the pleural, and subcapsular bleeding.

The mortality related to percutaneous liver biopsy is 0.01–0.1%, and is mainly related to bleeding or biliary peritonitis due to puncture of the gallbladder. The risk of major bleeding secondary to injury to intra- or extrahepatic vasculature is 0.12–0.34%. Intrahepatic bleeding is associated with pain due to stretching of the capsule. Severe intrahepatic bleeding requires evaluation with angiography and potentially embolization of the bleeding artery. Resection of a portion of the liver may be needed if bleeding is uncontrollable. One reported case of a delayed hemorrhage after percutaneous liver biopsy occurred 17 days postprocedure and was related to a pseudoaneurysm of a branch of the right hepatic artery and associated with an arterioportal venous fistula.[35]

GALLBLADDER DRAINAGE

▶ Indications

Acute cholecystitis is one of the main indications for drainage of the gallbladder and achieves similar clinical outcomes to percutaneous cholecystostomy.[37] Percutaneous cholecystostomy is recommended in critically ill patients when surgical intervention is considered risky. Percutaneous cholecystostomy can provide easy access for cholangiography prior to surgery, allowing for identification of the anatomy of the biliary duct and the pathogenesis of the underlying disease.[38] The failure to drain the gallbladder may lead to empyema, perforation, abscess, peritonitis, and sepsis. There is a high positive predictive value to diagnosing cholecystitis when ultrasound evaluation shows gallstones, gallbladder wall thickening, and a positive Murphy's sign.

Acute acalculous cholecystitis (AAC) is a serious disease with high mortality and morbidity in contrast to calculous cholecystitis. Percutaneous cholecystostomy is the best therapy for critically ill patient with AAC.[39] Surgical consultation for patients that undergo percutaneous cholecystostomy but do not improve within 24 hours is important to ensure that early surgical intervention can be provided if needed.[40]

▶ Contraindications

The contraindications for the procedure include coagulopathy, INR above 1.2, platelets <80.000/mm^3, prolonged bleeding time, liver masses with suspension of hemangioma, and an uncooperative patient.[41]

▶ Equipment and Procedure Tray

A 0.035 guide wire, such as a 3 mm J-type, 18-gauge needle with echogenic tip (7, 10, or 15 cm), 6- and 8-French dilators, 8-French multipurpose catheter, 3.5 or 5.0 MHz transducer with curved array.

▶ Procedure Description

The procedure is usually performed with the patient in the supine position, with right arm raised above the head. The fundus of the gallbladder is the preferred entry point to be used for the needle and the catheter. The gallbladder may be drained through a transhepatic or direct transperitoneal approach. The transhepatic approach is preferred because of the lower risk of bowel perforation, peritonitis, and loss of access after decompression of the gallbladder. In patients with acute cholecystitis, the distended gallbladder usually extends below the liver margin and is easier to access for direct puncture.[40]

The entry point for the needle is marked, the skin is cleaned, and appropriate drapes are placed. The skin is anesthetized and a 3-mm incision is made with a #11 blade. Placing the transducer parallel to the needle tract, the needle is traversed through the tissues and into the gallbladder, assuring that the gallbladder is entered through the fundus. About 5 mL of bile is removed to partially decompress the gallbladder and the fluid is sent for gram stain and cultures. Placement of a drainage catheter can be performed using a trocar device or for placement of pigtail-shaped drainage using the Seldinger technique.

In the Seldinger technique, a guide wire is placed through the needle into the gallbladder, with real-time observation of the ultrasound monitor. The needle is removed, and the tract is dilated sequentially using first a 6-French and then an 8-French dilator. If there is resistance when advancing the dilator, smaller dilators can be used and sequential one-size increments can be attempted. The catheter and stiffener are then advanced over the wire, into the lumen of the gallbladder. Direct visualization is necessary to ensure that the catheter has advanced past the gallbladder wall. While holding the stiffener, advance the catheter into the gallbladder. It is essential to advance the catheter far enough so that the drainage ports are inside the gallbladder. After placing the catheter, the stiffener and wire are removed and the distal end of the catheter is coiled by pulling the string. The catheter is then secured and attached to a drainage bag. A final scan should be performed and an image recorded. If catheter placement is not achieved, a contrast study may be performed. Up to 90% of patients with cholecystitis show an improvement in symptoms after drainage.[40]

▶ Complications

The most common complications of the procedure are bleeding, bile leakage, and catheter dislodgment. Failure to develop a mature track may occur in critically ill patients with underlying medical problems that intervene with the healing process. Other complications, such as bowel perforation and vasovagal reactions, have been reported.[41]

RENAL BIOPSY IN THE INTENSIVE CARE UNIT (ICU)

▶ Indications

The renal biopsy is used to diagnose and guide the treatment of kidney disease. In the ICU setting, renal biopsy should be performed rarely to determine the cause of renal dysfunction in situations where the added information will guide therapy. The cause of acute renal failure in ventilated patients can be determined without biopsy in most cases.[42]

The most likely ICU scenarios calling for a kidney biopsy are the pulmonary renal syndromes (PRS) due to Goodpasture syndrome, the antineutrophil cytoplasmic antibody vasculidites, or rapidly progressive glomerulonephritis (RPGN).[43,44] The combination of respiratory failure with acute renal failure can rapidly lead to death, while the diagnostic differential of the condition leads to therapeutic dilemmas (antibiotics vs. immunosuppression). Biopsy can provide the correct information for treating the condition. Histologic confirmation of diagnosis should be obtained, if possible, prior to initiating therapy.[42]

Biopsy should be performed when:

1. The diagnosis cannot be obtained by other tests
2. The disease appears to be renal and diagnosable (this presumes a high likelihood of renal disease and pathology support to rapidly process and interpret the biopsy)
3. The patient will benefit from the information obtained
   - The interpretation will be timely
   - There are therapeutic choices that depend on the result
   - The patient agrees to the potential treatment change
4. There are no contraindications to biopsy[45,46]

Nephrotic syndrome

The nephrotic syndrome, edema with heavy proteinuria, and low serum albumin could potentially require renal biopsy in the ICU. Usually, however, the nephrosis of diabetes, membranous, IgA, human immunodeficiency virus (HIV)-associated nephropathy, heroin-associated nephropathy, or focal and segmental glomerulosclerosis can await stabilization and biopsy can be done in the routine manner.

Acute nephritic syndrome

RPGN requires renal biopsy to diagnose and guide therapy. The diseases involved are often aggressive and fatal. The primary diagnoses to be considered are systemic lupus erythematosus (SLE) and the vasculidites (Wegener's granulomatosis and their variants). In the ICU setting, these syndromes may be confused with severe pneumonia.[43,44] Immunosuppressive treatment is indicated for SLE and Wegener's granulomatosis (with or without plasmapheresis). It is contraindicated for an infectious process.

Acute renal failure

A renal biopsy for the diagnosis of the commonly diagnosed acute renal failure, the result of low blood flow, or pressure in the setting of infections, nephrotoxins, or shock does not usually require renal biopsy. The occasional patient with unexpected failure to recover can usually be stabilized and biopsied in a controlled setting.[45]

Chronic renal failure

Several chronic renal diseases have the potential to complicate acute critical care, and renal biopsy may be considered to guide therapy. Diabetic nephropathy is the most common cause of chronic kidney disease in the United States (US). Additional renal insults can result in additional loss of renal function. The resulting "acute on chronic" renal failure can cloud the diagnosis and treatment of critical illness, especially when the diagnosis of RPGN must be excluded. Renal biopsy is rarely required.

Allograft dysfunction

Biopsy of a dysfunctional renal allograft in the ICU is easier than the biopsy of native kidneys. The allograft is closer to the surface and is relatively immobile. Acute rejection must be ruled out, while other causes of acute renal failure, such as acute tubular necrosis, cyclosporine toxicity, and recurrent primary glomerulonephritis, are considered. Ultrasound guidance is helpful in determining the depth to the organ and the method for avoiding other structures.

▶ Risks

The primary risk from the standard percutaneous renal biopsy is bleeding. Gross hematuria is present in low percentages of patients.[46] Properly performed renal biopsies can result in hematuria, both gross and microscopic. The uncomplicated renal biopsy in the past was admitted for at least 24 hours of observation, but recent advances in biopsy preparation and technique have allowed this to become an outpatient procedure in most cases. Some recommend a 24-hour period of observation due to the late appearance of some complications.[46] These improvements apply to the ICU setting as well, allowing much more flexibility and safety in the procedure. The advent of ultrasonography allows bedside real-time guidance in the ICU, as opposed to the former practice of finding the general location and depth of the kidney for the US-guided operator, and the use of intravenous pyelogram-guided or open renal biopsy in the past.

In addition, the use of the "free-hand" biopsy gun allows more flexibility in patient position, as experienced user of the ultrasound machine can guide the needle safely to the target organ. These guns have also smaller needles, which results in less bleeding while still obtaining adequate specimens for diagnosis. Voss et al. reported no reduction in bleeding compared with a Vim Silverman needle, apparently with excellent results, but did report shorter hospital stays.

The use of a trocar to relocate the kidney for second and third biopsy has reduced the time and number of passes required to perform the procedure. This should facilitate biopsy of ventilated patients.

In some institutions, the use of transvenous renal biopsy has been advocated in the patient with bleeding problems. These improvements allow more aggressive diagnostic approaches to be taken without compromising patient safety.[47]

Other risks to consider in addition to bleeding include pain, infection, transfusion, loss of renal function, loss of limb or organ function, and loss of life. In the ICU setting, with PRS as a diagnosis, these are manageable with relatively less significant issues.

▶ Contraindications

In the past, several renal conditions have been considered too risky to biopsy due to the danger in outcome, but the low rate of complication for renal biopsy in general coupled with recent technical advances have allowed most of these conditions to be biopsied. The physician is responsible for weighing the risks and benefits and determining the best course of action.[42,45,47,48]

Solitary and horseshoe kidney

The risk for a solitary or horseshoe kidney is that controlling bleeding could require a nephrectomy. Newer, intra-arterial techniques to occlude bleeding arteries and avoid loss of organ can be used in most cases.[46]

Urinary tract infection (UTI)

The presence of a UTI is a relative contraindication to renal biopsy due to the risk of bacterial spread outside of the urinary tract. The use of antibiotics may allow a biopsy of the patient with a UTI. In general, the biopsy of anyone with pyelonephritis is contraindicated.[45,46]

Renal tumor

The risk of spreading malignant cells to extrarenal sites must be considered. The usual practice is to perform a nephrectomy for suspected malignancy if the patient's renal function is adequate and age and condition do not preclude it. Urologic consultation is often helpful in these circumstances. In the setting of a PRS, pulmonary metastasis may be the cause of the problem.[46]

Bleeding disorders

Correction of a bleeding disorder from a factor deficiency, anticoagulation, or platelet deficiency or dysfunction before the biopsy will allow the procedure to proceed safely. Uremic platelet dysfunction can be controlled with estrogen therapy or transfusion,[49] thrombocytopenia with transfusion. An open biopsy would have been the primary recommendation in the recent past, but the advent of transjugular biopsies[47] and biopsy guns[9,10] has made these the preferred approaches.

Anemia

Anemia, especially a hematocrit <30%, is associated with prolonged postbiopsy bleeding. Transfusion and erythropoietin therapy will often correct the problem. The correction of ongoing losses and evaluation for the cause of the anemia are advised.

Hypertension

Correction of uncontrolled hypertension is advised prior to renal biopsy due to an increased risk of hemorrhage. Donadio and Buxo report a higher incidence of postbiopsy bleeding in hypertensive patients.[50]

Patient unable to cooperate with procedure

The noncompliant patient is a contraindication to the procedure; the patient is asked to hold breath briefly to stop the movement of the kidney, which occurs normally with respiration. The patient must be awake and cooperative. Light sedation to relieve anxiety is administered; general anesthesia is not routinely used.

The intubated patient can be fully anesthetized. Assistance to provide an expiratory hold to complete the biopsy will be needed. In both of these settings, the option of transjugular biopsy or open biopsy should be chosen if that is in the best interest of the patient.

The original position for performing a renal biopsy was sitting up on the edge of the bed, and the right kidney was usually biopsied. The usual procedure now is to have the patient prone, and the left organ is usually the target of choice. There is no contraindication to creative positioning of the patient to allow for mechanical ventilation. No other requirements are necessary, as long as the procedure is performed by the experienced sonographer using real-time guidance and reasonable caution.

▶ Procedure Description

Prebiopsy preparation

Review of the history and physical, removal, or correction of anticoagulation, control of blood pressure, review for and correction of UTI. A renal ultrasound, if not previously done, may be performed at the time of the procedure. Review for obstruction, mass, polycystic kidney disease, or nephrolithiasis. Gross hematuria, if present, should be explained and other causes that may mimic PRS ruled out. Rule out pregnancy with a b human chorionic gonadotropin. Proper permission must be obtained. Appropriate laboratory testing must be performed, including a prothrombin time, a partial thromboplastin time, a basic metabolic panel, and complete blood count; type and screen two units of packed red blood cells. Anemia should be corrected as needed prior to the procedure. Sedation may be given 30 minutes prior to the procedure.

The procedure

The patient is placed face down; this may be difficult for a ventilated patient, and pulmonary or anesthesia support may be needed to ensure the patient's safety. The kidney is localized, and the presence of two kidneys free of obstruction, mass, or tumor is documented. With ultrasound guidance, the skin over the lower pole of the kidney is marked at end-inspiration. The skin is prepped in a sterile manner and lidocaine injected superficially. A nick in the skin with a small blade is made to pass the needle through. Bleeding is controlled with direct pressure.[46]

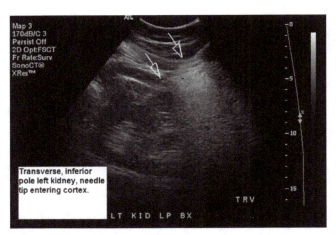

Figure 25-11 Renal biopsy showing the position of the needle tip entering the cortex.

A small-gauge spinal needle is introduced to the surface of the kidney and the location is verified either by direct visualization or using ultrasound (Figures 25-11 and 25-12). The needle will move in a vigorous arc cephalad to caudad with respiration when it is in the renal parenchyma. The operator's hands should not impede movement of the needle. When renal tissue has been reached, the surface of the kidney is anesthetized with 1% lidocaine. The depth of the needle needs to be marked closely and lidocaine injected as the spinal needle is withdrawn. The patient needs to be told to stop breathing when the operator has contact with the needle and the operator needs to be mindful of the patient's respiratory status because discomfort and incomplete exhalation may occur during a biopsy pass. The danger here is that a firmly held needle could tear the renal tissue when the kidney moves with respiration. The spinal needle is withdrawn and a biopsy needle inserted to the same depth. Once again, the location of the needle at the surface of the

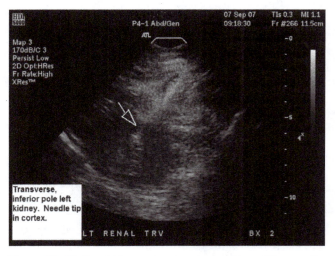

Figure 25-12 Renal biopsy showing the position of the needle tip in the cortex.

organ is verified by movement with respiration or by real-time ultrasound (Figures 25-11 and 25-12). Respirations are held and the biopsy device, Tru-cut needle or biopsy gun, is activated. The needle is withdrawn and the patient instructed to breathe. The patient should be asked how he or she is doing, which allows the operator to assess pain and also verifies responsiveness. The tissue is removed from the needle and the presence of glomeruli verified by direct inspection. A magnifying lens or dissecting microscope is helpful here. This procedure is repeated until adequate tissue for diagnosis is obtained. The tissue is submitted to nephropathology for light microscopy, immunofluorescent microscopy, and electron microscopy. The light microscopy specimen is placed in formaldehyde, the electron microscopy specimen is submitted in glutaraldehyde, and the immunofluorescence is submitted on ice for immediate frozen sections or is placed in Michel's fixative.[46]

Postbiopsy care

After the biopsy, vital signs should be closely monitored for hypotension, tachycardia, and signs of internal bleeding. Urinalysis to detect hematuria and serial hematocrit determinations is performed. Most complications are evident within 8 hours. A total of one third of complications occur after the first 8 hours, so patients must continue to be watched closely.[51] Most light microscopy and immunofluorescence can be processed and interpreted within 24 hours. Direct and clear communication with the pathologist will be helpful.

▶ Soft Tissue Ultrasound (Skin and Subcutaneous Structures)

Soft tissue ultrasound has been recently utilized for successful diagnosis of the depth of skin and soft tissue infections (Cellulitis vs. Fasciitis vs. Myositis/myonecrosis). Detection of the air in the soft tissues may be used for the early detection of the necrotizing fasciitis and used for the timing of fasciotomy. Ultrasound guidance can greatly assist with the percutaneous drainage of the soft tissue abscesses for diagnosis or where surgery may not be tolerated.

SUMMARY

Overall, there are a number of benefits to the use of ultrasound for abdominal and soft tissue procedures that make it an ideal technique for the critically ill patient. The technique improves the safety and efficiency of bedside procedures and prevents the difficult and often dangerous transportation of the critically ill patient to the radiology suite. In trained and experienced hands, it is a powerful diagnostic tool.

REFERENCES

1. Shameem RN, Dewbre H, Miller AH. Ultrasound-assisted paracentesis performed by emergency physicians vs. the traditional technique: a prospective randomized study. *Am J Emerg Med.* 2005;23:363–367.
2. Thomsen TW, Shaffer RW, White B, et al. Paracentesis. *N Eng J Med.* 2006;355:e21.
3. Mc Vay PA, Toy PT. Lack of increased bleeding after paracentesis and thoracentesis in patients with mild coagulation abnormalities. *Transfusion.* 1991;31:164–171.
4. Nicolaou S, Talsky A, Khashoggi K, et al. Ultrasound-guided interventional radiology in critical care. *Crit Care Med.* 2007;35(Suppl 5):S186–S197.
5. Sakai H, Sheer TA, Mendler MH, et al. Choosing the location for non-image guided abdominal paracentesis. *Liver Intern.* 2005;25:984–986.
6. Blavias M. Emergency diagnostic paracentesis to determine intraperiotneal fluid identity discovered on bedside ultrasound of unstable patients. *J Emerg Med.* 2005;29: 461–465.
7. McGibbon A, Chen GI, Peltekian KM, et al. An evidence-based manual for abdominal paracentesis. *Dig Dis Sci.* 2007;52:3307–3325.
8. Mittal R, Dangoor A. Paracentesis in the management of ascites. *Br J Hosp Med.* 2007;68(9):M162–M165.
9. Lipsky MS, Sternbach MR. Evaluation and initial management of patients with ascites. *Am Fam Phys.* 1996;15:1327–1333.
10. Wong CL, Holroyd-Leduc J, Thorpe KE, Straus SE. Does this patient have bacterial peritonitis or portal hypertension? How do I perform a paracentesis and analyze the results? *JAMA.* 2008;299(10):1166–1178.
11. Mercaldi CJ, Lanes SF. Ultrasound guidance decreases complications and improves the cost of care among patients undergoing thoracentesis and paracentesis. *Chest.* 2013;143(2):532–538.
12. Webster ST, Brown KL, Lucey MR, et al. Hemorrhagic complications of large volume abdominal paracentesis. *Am J Gastroenterol.* 1996;91:366–368.
13. Lam EY, Mclafferty RB, Taylor LM, et al. Inferior epigastric artery pesudoaneurysm a complication of paracentesis. *J Vasc Sur.* 1998;28:566–569.
13a. Schouten J, Michielsen PP. Treatment of cirrhotic ascites. *Acta Gastroenterol Belg.* 2007;70(2):217–222.
14. Zakim B. *Hepatology.* 4th ed. Philadelphia: Saunders; 2003.
15. Rumack CM, Wilson SR, Charboneau JW. *Diagnostic Ultrasound.* 4th ed. Philadelphia: Elsevier Science; 2004.
16. Tibbles CD, Porcaro W. Procedural applications of ultrasound. *Emerg Med Clin N Am.* 2004;22:797–815.
17. Conard MR, Sanders RC, James E. The sonolucent "Light Bulb" sign of fluid collections. *J Clin Ultrasound.* 1976;4:409–415.
18. Nicolaou S, Talsky A, Khashoggi K, Venu V. Ultrasound-guided interventional radiology in critical care. *Crit Care Med.* 2007;35(Suppl. 5):S186–S197.
19. McGahan JP. Aspiration and drainage procedures in the intensive care unit: percutaneous sonographic guidance. *Radiology.* 1985;154:531–532.
20. Irwin RS, Rippe JM, Curley FJ, Heard SO. *Procedures and Techniques in Intensive Care Medicine.* 3rd ed. Philadelphia: Lippincott Williams & Wilkins; 2003.
21. Bravo AA, Sheth SG, Chopra S. Liver biopsy. *N Engl J Med.* 2001;344:495–500.
22. Polakow J, Ladny JR, Dzieciol J, et al. Ultrasound guided percutaneous fine-needle biopsy of the liver: efficacy of color Doppler sonography. *Hepatogastroenterology.* 1998; 45:1829–1830.

23. Farrell RJ, Smiddy PF, Pilkington RM, et al. Guided versus blind liver biopsy for chronic hepatitis C: clinical benefits and cost. *J Hepatol.* 1999;30:580–587.
24. Duysburgh I, Michilesen P, Fierens H, et al. Fine needle trucut biopsy of focal liver lesions. *Dig Dis Sci.* 1997;42:2077–2081.
25. Shiffman AK. Percutaneous liver biopsy in clinical practice. *Liver Int.* 2007;27:1166–1173.
26. Caturelli E, Giacobbe A, Facciorusso D, et al. Percutaneous biopsy in diffuse liver disease: increasing diagnostic yield and decreasing complications rate by routine ultrasound assessment of puncture site. *Am J Gastroenterol.* 1996;91:1318–1320.
27. Terjung B, Lemnitzer I, Ludwig F, et al. Bleeding complications after percutaneous liver biopsy. *Digestion.* 2003;67:138–145.
28. Ahmed M, Riley T. Can one predict when ultrasound will be useful with percutaneous liver biopsy? *Am J Gastroenterol.* 2001;96:547–549.
29. Nobili V, Comparcola D, Sartorelli MR, et al. Blind and ultrasound-guided percutaneous liver biopsy in children. *Pediatr Radiol.* 2003;33:772–775.
30. Michielsen PP, Duysburgh IK, Francque SM, et al. Ultrasonically guided fine needle puncture of focal liver lesions: review and personal experience. *Acta Gastro-Enterologica Belgica.* 1998;61:158–163.
31. Chevallier P, Ruitort F, Denys A, et al. Influence of operator experience on performance of ultrasound-guided percutaneous liver biopsy. *Eur Radiol.* 2004;14:2086–2901.
32. Colombo M, Del Ninno E, De Franchis R, et al. Ultrasound-assisted percutaneous liver biopsy: superiority of the Tru-Cut over the Menghini needle for diagnosis of cirrhosis. *Gastroenterology.* 1988;95:487–489.
33. Lindor KD, Bru C, Jorgensen RA, et al. The role of ultrasonography and automatic-needle biopsy in outpatient percutaneous liver biopsy. *Hepatology.* 1996;23:1079–1083.
34. Riley T. How often does ultrasound making change the liver biopsy site? *Am J Gastroenterol.* 1999;94:3320–3322.
35. Sherlock S. Aspiration liver biopsy. *Lancet.* 1945;29:397–401.
36. Kowdley KV, Aggarwal AM, Sachs PB. Delayed hemorrhage after percutaneous liver biopsy. *J Clin Gastroenterol.* 1994;19:50–53.
37. Chopra S, Dodd GD III, Mumbower AL, et al. Treatment of acute cholecystitis in non-critically ill patient at his surgical risk: comparison of clinical outcomes after gallbladder aspiration and after percutaneous cholecystostomy. *AJR.* 2001;176:1025–1031.
38. Ralls PW, Colletti PM, Lapin SA, et al. Real-time sonography in suspected acute cholecystitis, prospective evaluation of primary and secondary signs. *Radiology.* 1985;155:767–771.
39. Wong S-R, Lee K, Kuo K-K, et al. Ultrasound-guided percutaneous transhepatic drainage of gallbladder followed by cholecystectomy for acute cholecystitis. 10 years' experience. *Kaohsiung J Med Sci.* 1998;14:19–24.
40. Hultman CS, Herbst CA. The efficacy of percutaneous cholecystostomy in critically ill patients. *Am Surg.* 1996;62(4):263–269.
41. Kadir S. *Teaching Atlas of Interventional Radiology, Non-Vascular Interventional Procedures.* New York, NY: Thieme Medical Publishers; 2005.
42. Conlon PJ, Kovalik E, Schwab SJ. Percutaneous renal biopsy of ventilated intensive care unit patients. *Clin Nephrol.* 1995;43:309–311.
43. Falk RJ. ANCA-associated renal disease. *Kidney Int.* 1990;38:998–1010.
44. Urizar RE, Mcgoldrick D, Cerda J. Pulmonary renal syndrome its clinicopathologic approach in 1991. *NYS Med J Med.* 1991;91:212–221.
45. Parrish AE. Complications of percutaneous renal biopsy. *Clin Nephrol.* 1992;38:135–141.
46. Radford MG, Donadio JV, Holley KE, Bjornsson J, Grande JP. Renal biopsy in clinical practice. *Mayo Clin Proc.* 1994;69:983–984.
47. Rychlik I, Petrtýl J, Tesar V, Stejskalová A, Zabka J, Br ha R. Transjugular renal biopsy. Our experience with 67 cases. *Kidney Blood Press Res.* 2001;24:207–212.
48. Voss DM, Lynn KL. Percutaneous renal biopsy: an audit of a 2 year experience with the Biopty gun. *New Zealand Med J.* 1995;25(108):8–10.
49. Sloand JA, Schiff MJ. Beneficial effect of low dose transdermal estrogen on bleeding time and clinical bleeding in uremia. *Am J Kidney Dis.* 1995;26:22–26.
50. Diaz-Buxo JA, Donadio JV. Complications of percutaneous renal biopsy: an analysis of 1000 consecutive biopsies. *Clin Nephrol.* 1975;4:223–227.
51. Whittier WL, Korbe SM. Renal biopsy update. *Curr Opinion Nephrol Hypertens.* 2003;13:661–665.

26

PERIPHERAL AND CENTRAL NEURAXIAL BLOCKS IN CRITICAL CARE MEDICINE

SANTHANAM SURESH

INTRODUCTION

The role of neuraxial blocks and peripheral nerve blocks in the critical care setting has vastly improved due to the use of ultrasonography. Despite the available technology, the use of these techniques in critical care remains rare. This chapter will provide examples of current and potential uses for the use of central and peripheral nerve blocks using ultrasound in a critical care setting.

EQUIPMENT

Although the physics and the use of equipment have been described previously (Chapter 2), specific discussion of the use of particular transducers for certain procedures is important. The use of a linear probe can help to localize nerve using ultrasonography. Sterile precautions should always be exercised prior to the performance of these blocks. Although the use of a sterile sheath can be very helpful, in an acute setting, a sterile Tegaderm can be used to cover the probe and effectively place nerve blocks in an intensive care unit (ICU). Nerves can appear anechoic, hypoechoic, or hyperechoic, depending on the particular plexus. Unlike vascular structures, they are not always hypoechoic and, therefore, color is unable to delineate them. A portable ultrasonography machine that can be brought to the patient's bedside to scan the patient and place the blocks is most useful in the ICU. Although sedation may be required in some instances, especially if infants and children are involved, most blocks can be performed with the superficial subcutaneous injection of local anesthetic. The advantage of ultrasonography is the ability to have a single pass directly to the proximity of the nerve structure and provide the block without the need for nerve stimulation. Nerve blocks are performed for a variety of reasons in the ICU, including diagnostic reasons, pain control, and managing vascular insufficiency (Table 26-1).

LOCAL ANESTHETIC SOLUTION

Any long-acting local anesthetic solution, mostly amides, are used for pain control using a regional anesthetic technique.[1] Although the commonly used, long-acting, local anesthetic bupivacaine is a dextroenantiomer and may have greater cardiovascular toxicity compared with the levoenantiomer, it is still routinely used in most clinical practices.[2,3] The dose of local anesthetic solution has to be contained within the toxic dosage allowable. A dose of <4 mg/kg will ensure a reasonable degree of safety, although careful aspiration should be carried out prior to injection. Ultrasonography has advanced our ability to identify vascular structures prior to injection. Newer levoenantiomers, ropivacaine, and levobupivacaine, although safe, cannot be considered completely immune to the cardiovascular and neurotoxicity of local anesthetic solutions. A detailed description of local anesthetics and their toxicity can be found in many standard pharmacology and anesthesia textbooks. A rule of thumb is that toxicity varies for different blocks decreasing in the progression from intercostal block, caudal blocks, epidural blocks, to peripheral nerve blocks. Local anesthetic toxicity includes seizures and cardiovascular collapse. A newer modality of treating the toxicity with intravenous intralipid is gaining popularity.[4] In the ICU, it may be reasonable to have the availability for lipid rescue in the event there is accidental injection of local anesthetic solution into the intravascular compartment.

CENTRAL NEURAXIAL BLOCKS

Central neuraxial blocks are performed for diagnosis or for pain control. A common central neuraxial procedure in the ICU is a diagnostic lumbar puncture. Although this can be performed with ease in most patients, the depth of the epidural space and the dura from the skin may be

TABLE 26-1
Ultrasonography in Critical Care
Diagnostic
Lumbar puncture
Pain control
Epidural analgesia
Upper extremity blocks
Lower extremity blocks
Truncal blocks
Vascular insufficiency
Epidural analgesia
Upper extremity blocks
Lower extremity blocks

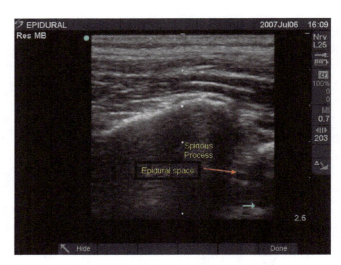

Figure 26-1 Ultrasound image of the epidural space.

difficult to ascertain both in younger populations, such as in infants and children,[5] and in the obese older patient, particularly in the obstetrical suite. The use of ultrasound may be a helpful diagnostic tool to determine the exact depth of the epidural space and the dura in children and adults.[6,7] Although the curvilinear probe may be helpful in the older adult, a transverse probe capable of scanning deeper (7 MHz) may be helpful in children and infants. The epidural and dural area can be scanned for depth using a transverse axial approach and in a sagittal longitudinal plane. A cadaver-based teaching model for ultrasonography has recently been described for learning ultrasound imaging for central neuraxial sonoanatomy.[8] It is important to understand that the transverse axial plane can be used to discern the sonoanatomy of the vertebral column, while the longitudinal sagittal plane can be used for recognizing the spinous, articular, and transverse processes. Real-time use of the sonoanatomy for placement of epidural catheters can be applied in children, where there is less calcification and an improved ability to visualize structures.[7] The use of epidural analgesia for pain control has traditionally been reserved for patients in the postoperative period. The use of this technique for pain control in the ICU has been reported anecdotally for vascular insufficiency by providing a sympathetic blockade.[9] Epidural analgesia can be provided for pain control following vascular crisis in sickle cell disease in an intensive care setting.[10]

The technique for epidural analgesia is presented in Figure 26-1.

▶ Axial Plane

1. Place the ultrasound probe between the spinous process.
2. Determine the location of the spinous and transverse processes.
3. Gently slide the probe cephalad or caudad until the dura and the epidural space can be located.
4. Use the depth indicator to measure the exact distance of the epidural space from the skin.
5. Mark the ends of the probe bilaterally and in the midline.
6. A line intersecting these two lines will provide a point of entry of the needle.
7. The exact distance for the needle to enter into the epidural space to the predetermined area allows the operator to advance the needle to the specified depth.
8. If real-time ultrasonography is used, it is imperative to use loss of resistance with saline or local anesthetic solution for determining the depth of the space.

UPPER EXTREMITY BLOCKS

The brachial plexus supplies the pain fibers to the upper extremity. It is derived from the cervical roots C5, C6, C7, C8, and T1. It is important to understand the multiple approaches to the brachial plexus for a variety of surgical procedures, depending on the area that is being operated on (Table 26-2). This technique can also be used for pain relief in critically ill trauma victims in the ICU.[11] This block has the advantage of increasing blood supply, thereby potentially improving perfusion to the compromised upper extremity.[12] The approach to the brachial plexus is at the interscalene (roots), supraclavicular (trunks), infraclavicular (divisions and cords), and axillary (branches) levels of the brachial plexus in the arm (Tables 26-2 and 26-3).[13,14] If an indwelling catheter is placed for trauma

TABLE 26-2
Brachial Plexus Block
Interscalene block: For shoulder pain
Supraclavicular block: For pain relief from fractures, vascular insufficiency
Infraclavicular: For longer duration of pain relief with catheter
Axillary: Single shot for immediate pain relief and vascular insufficiency

Dose: Adults = 15 mL, 0.2% ropivacaine or 0.25% bupivacaine; Children = 0.2 mL/kg, 0.2% ropivacaine or 0.25% bupivacaine.

TABLE 26-3
Approaches and Probes for Brachial Plexus Blocks

Axillary block	Linear probe	In-plane approach
Infraclavicular	Linear probe	In-plane approach
Supraclavicular	Linear probe	In-plane or out of plane
Interscalene	Linear probe	In-plane

or vascular insufficiency, we prefer using the infraclavicular approach.[15,16] The supraclavicular approach is an easier approach, especially if there is significant trauma in the upper extremity, because this can reduce arm movement during performance of the block. The ultrasound technique for each one of these approaches is well described. Often, operator preference determines the approach used. We tend to use the supraclavicular approach for most fractures. For larger limb salvage procedures that require multiple days of intense pain control, an indwelling infraclavicular approach is preferred. The volume of local anesthetic solution varies, depending on the access. For most pain control, however, a volume of 15 mL of local anesthetic solution (0.2% ropivacaine or 0.25% bupivacaine) can provide adequate analgesia. In children, a dose of 0.2 mL/kg of local anesthetic solution is used.

▶ Supraclavicular Approach

Ultrasound-guided approach to the supraclavicular plexus is an easy and rapidly achieved block in the ICU. The ultrasound probe is placed above the clavicle, and the nerves are seen surrounding the subclavian artery. We prefer using an in-plane approach to the nerves. Local anesthetic solution is deposited and the spread of local anesthetic is seen in real time as the injection proceeds. A "donut sign" of the nerves surrounded by the local anesthetic solution denotes correct placement of the local anesthetic solution (Figure 26-2).

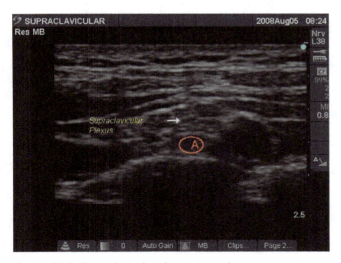

Figure 26-2 Supraclavicular plexus. Note the arrow pointing to the plexus surrounding the subclavian artery.

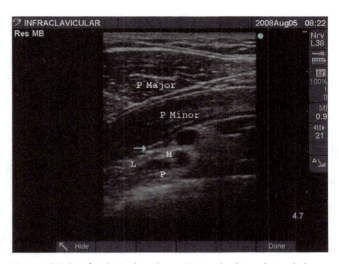

Figure 26-3 Infraclavicular plexus. Note the lateral, medial, and posterior cords surrounding the subclavian artery.

▶ Infraclavicular Approach

The infraclavicular approach is preferred for placement of a catheter for pain control.[17] A linear ultrasound probe is placed below the clavicle and medial to the acromial process. The cords are seen surrounding the subclavian artery; the medial, lateral, and posterior cords can be easily identified (Figure 26-3). The pectoralis major and minor have to be traversed prior to access to the cords. If a catheter is placed in the area for continuous infusion of local anesthetic, it can be introduced using an 18-G Touhy needle with the tip of the catheter close to the posterior cord. If a continuous infusion is sought postoperatively, an infusion rate of 3 mL/h is usually adequate for providing pain relief and also a sympathetic blockade for vascular insufficiency.

▶ Axillary Block

The axillary approach to the brachial plexus is easy and can be performed in most ICU patients with ease using a linear probe or a hockey stick probe in younger children and infants. The probe is placed with the orientation of the median, radial, and ulnar nerves in close proximity to the axillary artery (Figure 26-4). The plexus is very superficial even in obese individuals. If there is any doubt about the position of the nerves, color Doppler is used to check the position of the vessels. A total volume of about 15 mL of local anesthetic solution is injected into the area providing adequate relief of pain. The efficacy of the block is increased if the local anesthetic solution is seen surrounding the nerves completely.

▶ Complications from Brachial Plexus Blocks

Intravascular injection is an inherent problem due to the close proximity of the great vessels. Injection into the vertebral artery and the intrathecal space can be a complicating factor while performing the supraclavicular approach.

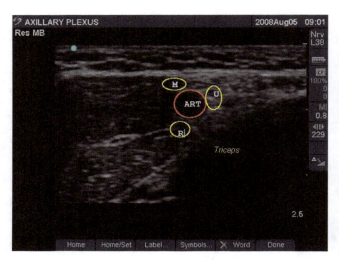

Figure 26-4 Axillary plexus ultrasound image.

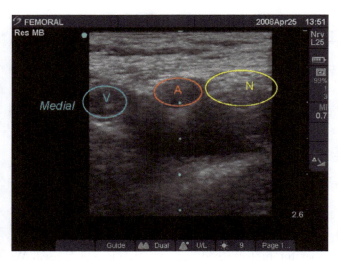

Figure 26-5 Ultrasound image of femoral nerve. Note the vein, artery, and nerve located in a single plane.

LOWER EXTREMITY BLOCKS

The lumbar (L2, L3, L4) and sacral roots (S1, S2, S3) supply the sensory and motor supply to the lower extremity. Although it is of academic importance to understand the regional anesthetic techniques for lower extremity in the ICU, it is important to understand its utility for major trauma, particularly femur fractures, and for patients with vascular insufficiency.[18]

▶ Femoral Nerve Block (Table 26-4)

The femoral nerve is located lateral to the femoral artery as it leaves the femoral triangle. The nerve supplies the anterior portion of the thigh and the femur and is blocked for managing pain. A nerve stimulator can be used to localize the nerve, eliciting a "patellar snap" denoting a quadriceps muscle contraction. Ultrasonography can be used for performing this block.

Technique

A linear ultrasound probe is placed below the ilioinguinal ligament along the crease. The femoral artery is identified. The femoral nerve is located lateral to the femoral artery. It can be visualized as a hyperechoic structure (Figure 26-5). With slight angling of the probe, the fascicles of the nerve can be seen under ultrasound imaging.[19] A needle is then placed using an in-plane technique to block the femoral nerve. Adequate blockade is noted when the nerve is encircled with local anesthetic solution (donut sign). A volume of 15 mL of 0.2% ropivacaine or 0.25% bupivacaine can provide adequate blockade of the femoral nerve. In children and infants, a dose of 0.2 mL/kg is used to provide blockade of the femoral nerve. A catheter can be left in place for managing severe pain due to trauma in adults and children. This may facilitate a reduction in the use of opioids and associated adverse effects including somnolence, nausea, and vomiting.

Complications

Intravascular placement of needle and catheter, injury to femoral nerve due to intravascular injection.

▶ Sciatic Nerve Block

The sciatic nerve is derived from the lower lumbar and the upper sacral roots. It supplies the sensory and motor block to the leg and foot. Sciatic nerve blockade is easy to perform under ultrasound guidance, although the need for sciatic nerve block in the ICU is less than the femoral nerve. In our institution, we have used ultrasound-guided sciatic nerve blocks for a child with severe acute respiratory distress syndrome and hemodynamic instability who required a fasciotomy for compartment syndrome. The block can be performed at the popliteal fossa or at the subgluteal area.

Technique

Popliteal Fossa Block. The patient is kept prone or supine depending on his or her hemodynamic stability. A linear ultrasound probe is placed in the popliteal fossa. The popliteal artery is identified. The common peroneal and the tibial nerves are identified. The ultrasound probe is moved cephalad until the coalition of the two peripheral branches is seen. A needle is inserted using the in-plane approach. A total of 15–20 mL of local anesthetic solution is deposited around the nerve to completely encircle the nerve (donut sign; Figure 26-6).

TABLE 26-4
Femoral Nerve Block
Indications: Femur fracture, vascular insufficiency Technique: In-plane approach, linear probe Landmarks: Vein, artery, and nerve from medial to lateral orientation, color used to identify vascular structures Complication: Intraneural injection, intravascular injection

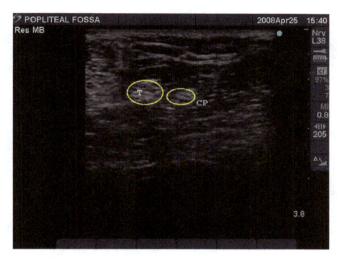

Figure 26-6 Ultrasound image of the popliteal fossa. Note the common peroneal (CP) and tibial nerve (T) in the popliteal fossa distal to their bifurcation.

Subgluteal Approach. The subgluteal approach to the sciatic nerve is another approach to the nerve as it exits the pelvis. This is another easy approach using ultrasonography and can be utilized for leaving an indwelling catheter for pain control after major trauma. The ultrasound probe is placed along the gluteal crease and the biceps femoris and the semitendinosus are identified. The sciatic nerve is seen as a hyperechoic shadow at this level. Using an in-plane approach we block the sciatic nerve at this site (Figure 26-7). Usually, a volume of 15–20 mL of local anesthetic solution is needed to block the nerve effectively (Figure 26-7).

TRUNCAL BLOCKS

Truncal blocks can be of value inpatients, who may have significant pain secondary to rib fractures. In fact, we note that the use of these blocks may enhance the ability of these patients to take deep breaths and may reduce the incidence of atelectasis due to decreased efforts at breathing.

▶ Intercostal Block

Anatomy

The intercostal nerves are derived from thoracic nerves T1–T12. As the nerves emerge from their respective intervertebral foramina, they divide into four branches:

1. The first branch is the paired gray and white anterior ramii communicans, which pass anteriorly to the sympathetic ganglion.
2. The second branch is the posterior cutaneous branch, which supplies the skin and muscle in the paravertebral region.
3. The third branch is the lateral cutaneous branch, which then branches to an anterior and posterior branch to supply the midline portion of the chest and abdomen.
4. The ventral ramus, which is the intercostal nerve.

The intercostal nerves carry both sensory and motor fibers and pierce the posterior intercostal membrane distal to the intervertebral foramen to enter the subcostal grove and continue to run parallel to the rib. Its course within the thorax is between the parietal pleura and innermost intercostals muscle and the external and internal intercostals muscles.

Indications

Intercostal nerve blocks (ICBs) can be used for chest trauma associated with rib fractures,[18] thoracotomy,[20] and upper abdominal surgery, including cholecystectomy and appendectomy, and for pain control following breast surgery. The 10th intercostal nerve (umbilical nerve) can also be blocked for umbilical hernia repair.[21] ICBs with the use of neurolytics can be used to manage chronic pain conditions, such as postmastectomy pain, herpetic neuralgia, and post-thoracotomy pain syndromes.[22]

Technique

Ultrasound guidance has significantly improved the performance of this block. Although not described in detail in the literature, there is growing interest in using ultrasound guidance to perform this block. We prefer using a mid-axillary approach to the intercostal nerve. A linear ultrasound probe is placed alongside the mid-axillary line overriding two ribs. The pleura can be seen moving with every breath. The innermost intercostal muscle is identified. Using an off-plane approach, a 27-gauge needle is introduced into the innermost intercostal muscle; local anesthetic solution is injected after careful aspiration to rule out intravascular placement (Figure 26-8).

Complications

The major complication is pneumothorax, the rate of which is below 1%.[23] Tension pneumothorax is rare, and

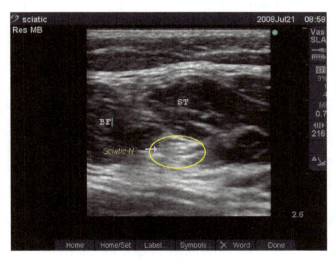

Figure 26-7 Subgluteal approach to sciatic nerve. Note the biceps femoris and the semitendinosus. Arrow points to the sciatic nerve.

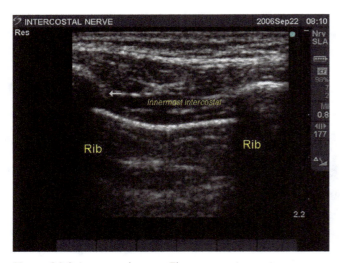

Figure 26-8 Intercostal space. The arrow points to innermost intercostal muscle, where the neurovascular bundle is seen.

the need for chest tube placement is dictated by presence of respiratory or cardiovascular compromise. Absorption of the local anesthetic from the intercostal space is rapid and has a higher incidence of toxicity when compared with other nerve blocks.[24] Peak plasma concentrations develop rapidly and toxicity is a concern, especially with multiple or continuous intercostal injections. Peak arterial plasma concentration develops rapidly and toxicity is always a concern with multiple or continuous intercostal injections.[24] The use of more dilute local anesthetic concentrations, smaller volumes, and incremental injection with frequent aspiration may reduce the probability of excess vascular absorption. The peritoneum and abdominal viscera are at risk of penetration when the lower intercostal nerves are blocked. A high subarachnoid blockade is possible when a posterior approach to the intercostal space is utilized.

CONCLUSION

The use of ultrasonography to provide analgesia may provide a safe and standardized method for critically ill patients. The techniques are still early in their development, but demonstrate promise in clinical care to relieve pain outcomes of ICU patients. Prospective randomized, controlled trials can help to determine the efficacy of these nerve blocks in critically ill patients to the current approaches to pain control in the ICU.

REFERENCES

1. Mather LE, McCall P, McNicol PL. Bupivacaine enantiomer pharmacokinetics after intercostal neural blockade in liver transplantation patients. *Anesth Analg.* 1995;80:328–335.
2. Foster RH, Markham A. Levobupivacaine: a review of its pharmacology and use as a local anaesthetic. *Drugs.* 2000;59:551–579.
3. McClellan KJ, Faulds D. Ropivacaine: an update of its use in regional anaesthesia. *Drugs.* 2000;60:1065–1093.
4. Weinberg G. Lipid rescue resuscitation from local anaesthetic cardiac toxicity. *Toxicol Rev.* 2006;25:139–145.
5. Suresh S, Wheeler M. Practical pediatric regional anesthesia. *Anesthesiol Clin North Am.* 2002;20:83–113.
6. Arzola C, Davies S, Rofael A, Carvalho JC. Ultrasound using the transverse approach to the lumbar spine provides reliable landmarks for labor epidurals. *Anesth Analg.* 2007;104:1188–1192.
7. Willschke H, Bosenberg A, Marhofer P, et al. Epidural catheter placement in neonates: sonoanatomy and feasibility of ultrasonographic guidance in term and preterm neonates. *Reg Anesth Pain Med.* 2007;32:34–40.
8. Tsui B, Dillane D, Pillay J, Walji A. Ultrasound imaging in cadavers: training in imaging for regional blockade at the trunk. *Can J Anaesth.* 2008;55:105–111.
9. Chiafery MC, Stephany RA, Holliday KJ. Epidural sympathetic blockade to relieve vascular insufficiency in an infant with purpura fulminans. *Crit Care Nurse.* 1993;13:71–76.
10. Yaster M, Tobin JR, Billett C, et al. Epidural analgesia in the management of severe vaso-occlusive sickle cell crisis. *Pediatrics.* 1994;93:310–315.
11. Clark F, Gilbert HC. Regional analgesia in the intensive care unit. Principles and practice. *Crit Care Clin.* 2001;17:943–966.
12. Szili-Torok T, Paprika D, Peto Z, et al. Effect of axillary brachial plexus blockade on baroreflex-induced skin vasomotor responses: assessing the effectiveness of sympathetic blockade. *Acta Anaesthesiol Scand.* 2002;46:815–820.
13. Brull R, Perlas A, Chan VW. Ultrasound-guided peripheral nerve blockade. *Curr Pain Headache Rep.* 2007;11:25–32.
14. Perlas A, Chan VW, Simons M. Brachial plexus examination and localization using ultrasound and electrical stimulation: a volunteer study. *Anesthesiology.* 2003;99:429–435.
15. Sandhu NS, Manne JS, Medabalmi PK, Capan LM. Sonographically guided infraclavicular brachial plexus block in adults: a retrospective analysis of 1146 cases. *J Ultrasound Med.* 2006;25:1555–1561.
16. Ilfeld BM, Morey TE, Enneking FK. Continuous infraclavicular brachial plexus block for postoperative pain control at home: a randomized, double-blinded, placebo-controlled study. *Anesthesiology.* 2002;96:1297–1304.
17. Sandhu NS, Capan LM. Ultrasound-guided infraclavicular brachial plexus block. *Br J Anaesth.* 2002;89:254–259.
18. Burton AW, Eappen S. Regional anesthesia techniques for pain control in the intensive care unit. *Crit Care Clin.* 1999;15:77–88, vi.
19. Oberndorfer U, Marhofer P, Bosenberg A, et al. Ultrasonographic guidance for sciatic and femoral nerve blocks in children. *Br J Anaesth.* 2007;98:797–801.
20. Cook TM, Riley RH. Analgesia following thoracotomy: a survey of Australian practice. *Anaesth Intensive Care.* 1997;25:520–524.
21. de Jose Maria B, Gotzens V, Mabrok M. Ultrasound-guided umbilical nerve block in children: a brief description of a new approach. *Paediatr Anaesth.* 2007;17:44–50.
22. Doi K, Nikai T, Sakura S, Saito Y. Intercostal nerve block with 5% tetracaine for chronic pain syndromes. *J Clin Anesth.* 2002;14:39–41.
23. Moore DC, Bridenbaugh PO. Pneumothorax: its incidence following intercostal nerve block. *JAMA.* 1960;174:842.
24. Behnke H, Worthmann F, Cornelissen J, et al. Plasma concentration of ropivacaine after intercostal blocks for video-assisted thoracic surgery. *Br J Anaesth.* 2002;89:251–253.

ULTRASOUND GUIDANCE FOR VASCULAR ACCESS

CHRISTIAN H. BUTCHER

Scan QR code or visit www.ccu2e.com for video in this chapter

INTRODUCTION

Vascular access procedures, such as central venous and arterial catheterization, are commonly performed in the critical care setting. An estimated 5 million central venous catheters (CVCs) are placed annually in the United States[1] in a variety of settings, including critical care units, emergency departments, operating rooms, and in outpatient venues. The usual indications for CVC placement are to assist in hemodynamic monitoring; as a route for the administration of vasoactive medications, total parenteral nutrition, or other vascular irritants; and as a route for drawing blood. In addition, the Surviving Sepsis guidelines advocate measuring mixed venous oxygen saturation in the management of septic shock, which could ultimately lead to increased utilization of oximetric CVCs.

Arterial catheters are an important tool in the management of many intensive care unit (ICU) conditions, including shock, severe hypertension, and other circumstances, in which blood pressure monitoring is important. For a number of reasons, it seems that the role for arterial catheterization in the ICU may also increase. First, with the introduction of "minimally invasive" techniques now available to help estimate cardiac output, arterial catheter placement is becoming increasingly important for the management of selected patients with heart failure. Second, arterial catheterization can be used to assess the response to therapy in patients with pulmonary hypertension. Finally, there has been a significant amount of attention focused recently on respiratory variation of the peak arterial pressure as a means to predict fluid responsiveness in shock states.[2]

Peripherally inserted CVCs (PICCs) and peripherally inserted catheters sited in a midline position (midlines) have gained increased popularity as an alternative to CVCs in the care of selected patients because of their ease of insertion, longevity, and low rate of early complications.

They have become an important component of the central venous access armamentarium. Peripheral intravenous (IV) catheters, long overlooked by the medical ultrasound community, can be placed with very high success rates even in very difficult to cannulate patients when performed under ultrasound guidance.

Vascular access is associated with a relatively low rate of serious complications.[1] However, an improved understanding of complications and why they occur may help the provider to reduce their risk. Complications associated with vascular access procedures are well described,[1] and can be categorized as patient or operator dependent (Table 27-1). Patient-dependent factors include body habitus, coagulopathy, and anatomic variation. Operator-dependent factors include the operator's level of experience, time allotted to perform the procedure, and human factors, like fatigue and lack of ultrasound guidance.[3-5] The most common complications of CVC placement include accidental arterial puncture, failed placement, malposition of the catheter tip, hematoma, pneumothorax, and hemothorax, the frequency of which vary depending on the site of catheter insertion (Table 27-2). Arterial catheter placement can be complicated by venous puncture, multiple arterial punctures, significant hematoma, and failed placement. PICCs and midline placement are also associated with hematomas and arterial insertions. A common complication of PICC line placement is malposition of the catheter tip into the ipsilateral internal jugular (IJ) vein, or coiling in the subclavian vein or a thoracic branch, such as the thoracodorsal vein (Figure 27-1).

Complications from these procedures are associated with excess direct costs derived from prolonged hospital and ICU lengths of stay (LOS) and additional procedures, such as chest tube insertion or hematoma evacuation, to treat the complications. For example, a single episode of iatrogenic pneumothorax has an attributable LOS of

TABLE 27-1
Patient and Operator-Associated Risk Factors for Central Line Complications

Patient-dependent	Operator-dependent
Body habitus	Experience
Coagulopathy	Time allotted for procedure
Vascular anatomic variation	Fatigue
Prior surgery with distortion of anatomy	Lack of ultrasound use

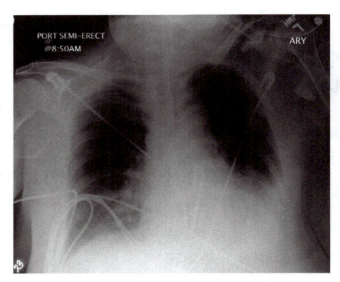

Figure 27-1 Peripherally inserted central venous catheter (PICC) tip malposition. The catheter tip is visualized in the ipsilateral internal jugular vein.

3–4 days.[6] Indirect costs, such as additional provider time and patient suffering, are also important considerations.

ULTRASOUND USE FOR VASCULAR ACCESS

There are several studies that assess the impact of ultrasonography in improving the success of vascular access procedures. In 1984, Legler et al. published a brief report describing the use of Doppler ultrasonography to locate the IJ vein for cannulation.[7] Since then, three meta-analyses investigating the use of ultrasound for CVC placement or dialysis catheter placement,[8–10] several review articles, standardized procedure guidelines,[11,12] large case series,[13,14] and the SOAP-3 trial[15] have been published. The body of evidence from these and other studies demonstrates that the use of two-dimensional (2D) ultrasound during central venous access is associated with fewer complications, fewer attempts before successful cannulation, shorter procedure times, and fewer failed procedures when compared with a landmark-based approach. As a result, the Agency for Healthcare Research and Quality and the British National Institute of Clinical Excellence have issued statements advocating the use of ultrasound guidance in central venous access procedures.[16,17] In addition, International Evidenced-based Recommendations on Ultrasound Guided Vascular Access have also been published.[18]

Despite these evidence-based guidelines, some providers continue to resist and use ultrasound only in potentially "difficult to cannulate" patients, such as the morbidly obese, or in cases of failed cannulation.[19] Unfortunately, it is difficult to predict which patients will be difficult to cannulate, and the recognition of a failed attempt, as may arise from an occluded vessel, can only be viewed retrospectively after the failure has occurred and the patient has been adversely affected.[20] Some complications from CVC are considered preventable medical errors, which refers to either mistakes or poor outcomes that could potentially have been prevented or hospital-acquired conditions, which is a medical problem not present on admission.[21] Although barriers to widespread adoption exist, such as a lack of training programs,[22] ultrasound is a noninvasive tool that can help prevent complications and assists the operator in achieving optimal care for patients with less discomfort and fewer risks. Therefore, developing a strategy to overcome these barriers, both at the local and national level, is a worthwhile goal. It should be noted that even modest training programs have shown the potential to increase success rates and decrease complications.[23,24] Therefore, the consideration of ultrasound to improve safety in all central venous access procedures is recommended.

REVIEW OF ULTRASOUND

▶ Transducer Selection

As described before (see Chapter 2), transducers come in a variety of frequencies, each with different properties and clinical applications. Two important concepts are important for ultrasonography in central venous access and need to be reviewed here. First, the relationship between ultrasound frequency and the depth of tissue penetration is an inverse relationship. This implies that low-frequency ultrasound (1–3 MHz) penetrates more deeply than high-frequency ultrasound (7–10 MHz). Second, the relationship between frequency and image detail, or resolution, is *proportional*. This means that low-frequency ultrasound has poorer resolution than high-frequency ultrasound. Therefore, high-frequency ultrasound provides a very detailed image of superficial structures, to a depth of approximately

TABLE 27-2
The Most Common Complications of Central Venous Catheterization by Site of Insertion

	Internal Jugular	Subclavian	Femoral
Pneumothorax	0–1%	2–3%	N/A
Hemothorax	0	<1%	N/A
Arterial puncture	5–10%	3–5%	5–15%
Failed attempt	15–20%	5–15%	15–40%

5 cm, but cannot penetrate into deeper tissues. Alternatively, lower frequency ultrasound is capable of reaching into deeper structures, but provides a less detailed image. These relationships form the basis for transducer selection. For percutaneous vascular access, which is a procedure that is superficial, higher frequency transducers are ideal.

▶ Modes

A-mode ultrasound has very few clinical applications and is not discussed further here. B-mode ultrasound creates recognizable 2D images. B-mode is the most common mode currently employed in diagnostic medical ultrasound. M-mode ultrasound uses information obtained with B-mode to create an image that demonstrates the movement of structures over time (Figure 27-2). The most common application of M-mode is to assess valve leaflet movement and wall motion in cardiac ultrasound.

Doppler mode also has several forms. The simplest produces no image; there is only an audible signal that varies in intensity with the velocity of the structure being studied (e.g., blood; Figure 27-3). Recently available ultrasound equipment uses Doppler in combination with B-mode to both create an image and give information about velocity (Figure 27-4). Color Doppler takes velocity information obtained by the Doppler shift and applies color to it. The Doppler is then superimposed on the B-mode image (Figure 27-5). Color Doppler is very commonly used in vascular applications, such as vascular access. The strength of the Doppler signal is related to the velocity of the target tissue (e.g., blood) and the angle of incidence. The best estimate of velocity occurs at an angle approaching zero (Figure 27-6). However, if the same vessel is imaged at 90°, there is no perceived motion of blood either toward or away from the transducer, and the Doppler signal fades. When the angle of incidence changes from one "side" of the 90° mark to the other "side," the color of the blood within the target vessel changes (from red to blue). This is very important and a potential source of error when a beginner is becoming familiar with orientation and selecting a vessel for cannulation.

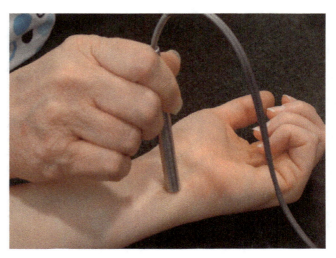

Figure 27-3 Continuous-wave Doppler "wand" seen during evaluation of the ulnar artery.

▶ Techniques of Ultrasound Guidance

Ultrasound is not a substitute for a thorough knowledge of the landmark-based technique for central venous cannulation. Frequently, the beginner may focus on the image on the screen and be inattentive to anatomic landmarks and the position of the needle (Figure 27-7).

Ultrasound-guided procedures can be categorized as static or dynamic. Static guidance refers to the use of ultrasound

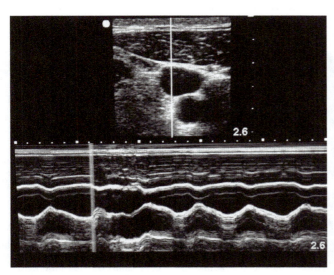

Figure 27-2 2D image through the internal jugular (IJ) vein transversely, with the common carotid artery inferior and to the right (top). M-mode image through the IJ (see vertical line in 2D image) showing changes in vessel diameter with respiration (bottom). IJ = internal jugular.

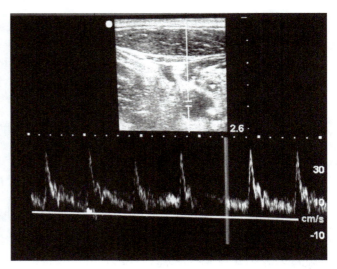

Figure 27-4 Doppler mode showing target of sample in the common carotid artery. Bottom image shows typical arterial waveform.

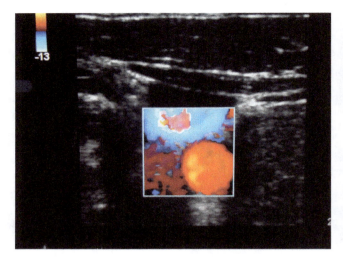

Figure 27-5 Transverse view through right internal jugular vein and common carotid artery, showing color Doppler. Vein is superior to the artery, and is depicted as blue.

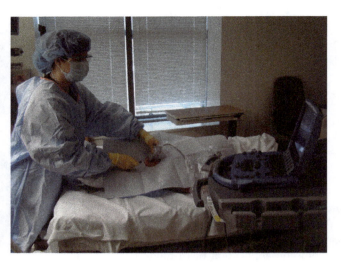

Figure 27-7 A combination of landmark-based and ultrasound-based techniques is optimal. Paying particular attention to the ultrasound screen, and ignoring the patient, can be disastrous.

to localize and mark a site on the skin to facilitate a subsequent percutaneous procedure, much like a traditional landmark-based approach. B-mode or Doppler ultrasound is used to locate the IJ vein, assess its patency, and mark a suitable site on the skin for cannulation. The cannulation itself is not performed with ultrasound. Dynamic guidance refers to performing the procedure in "real time," with ultrasound imaging viewing the needle puncturing the vessel wall. For vascular access, static guidance appears to be inferior to dynamic, but still better than the landmark-based technique alone.[12] This is due to the time interval between marking with static guidance and the puncture, during which patients may move, or marks removed during skin preparation, both of which can lead to complications. Table 27-3 provides a comparison between static and dynamic guidance techniques. Dynamic guidance is more technically demanding because it requires significant eye–hand coordination. Another distinction is that cannulation can be performed either free hand or with needle guides. Recent data suggest that needle guides may help keep the needle tip in view which, theoretically, could lead to a reduced risk of mechanical complications.[25]

▶ **Planes and Views**

For our purposes, there are two planes to be considered: transverse and longitudinal, which refer to the orientation of the ultrasound transducer and the image to the vessel axis. A transverse view is a cross-section and provides the operator with information about structures that lay adjacent to the vessel of interest. For example, a cross-sectional view of the IJ vein will enable visualization of the adjacent common carotid artery and, perhaps, the vagus nerve, thyroid gland, and trachea (Figure 27-8).

A longitudinal view will depict structures anterior and posterior to the vessel of interest and may allow for visualization of the entire needle during cannulation, but does

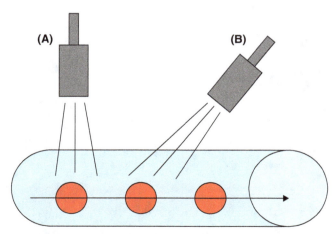

Figure 27-6 Relationship between angle of incidence of the ultrasound beam and the strength of the Doppler signal. As the angle approaches zero, the signal strength is maximized; as the angle approaches 90°, the strength is reduced.

TABLE 27-3	
Differences Between Static and Dynamic Guidance Techniques for Central Line Placement	
Dynamic Guidance	**Static Guidance**
Ultrasonic localization and image-guided cannulation	Ultrasonic localization and marking of landmarks only
More precise and "real-time"	Cannulation is not image guided
More difficult to maintain sterility	Time delay between marking and cannulation
Requires significant hand–eye coordination	Less difficult to maintain sterility
	Less technically demanding

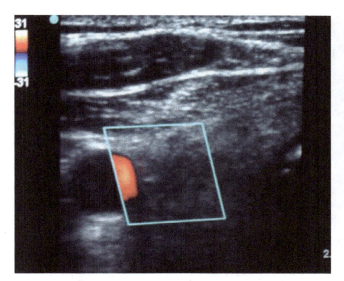

Figure 27-8 Transverse (short-axis) view at the level of the internal jugular vein (to the left of the carotid artery and not shown). The right carotid artery and right thyroid lobe can be seen. The lateral wall of the trachea can be seen to the far right of the picture.

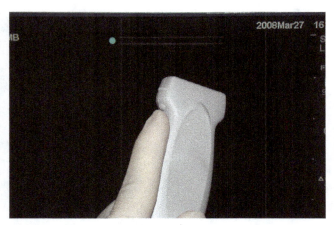

Figure 27-10 To gain orientation, the "notch" on the transducer (just distal to fingertip) should be matched to the "dot" on the screen (blue circle, upper left side).

not allow simultaneous visualization of structures lateral to the vessel (Figure 27-9). All commonly utilized central venous and peripheral arterial sites can be visualized in either orientation.

▶ **Methods of Orientation**

Orientation is probably the most important step to a successful procedure. Most transducers have an identifiable mark, known as a "notch," on one side. This corresponds to a mark displayed on one side of the image, and allows right–left, or lateral, orientation (Figure 27-10). In rare instances, where the orientation is uncertain, a finger can be rubbed on one side of the transducer surface to produce an image and confirm the orientation (Figure 27-11).

Problems with orientation can largely be prevented by ensuring proper patient, transducer, and ultrasound console positioning adjacent to each other. The operator, transducer, and console should be arranged in a straight line (Figure 27-12). In this way, the vessel to be cannulated and the image screen will be in the direct line of sight of the operator. When accessing the IJ vein, the console should be on the *same* side as the vessel to be cannulated, usually at the level of the patient's, to ensure that transducer orientation—the right side of the transducer, the right side of the patient, and the right side of the image—are all aligned. When cannulating the subclavian or axillary vein, the console should be on the *opposite* side of the patient,

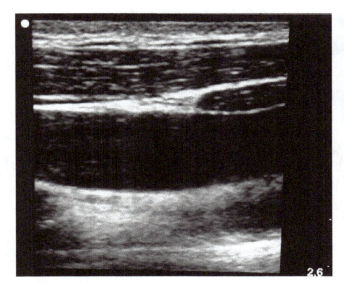

Figure 27-9 Longitudinal view through the internal jugular vein. Information regarding the location of surrounding structures is limited when compared with the transverse view.

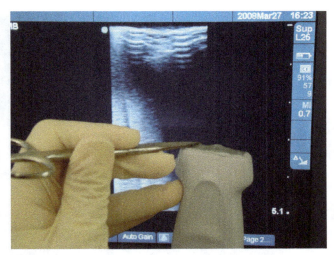

Figure 27-11 During a procedure, the probe surface can be rubbed with a finger or instrument to determine orientation; in this case, the scissors are placed on the left side of the probe and are seen on the screen as an artifact on the left side. This can also be easily accomplished while the probe is on the patient.

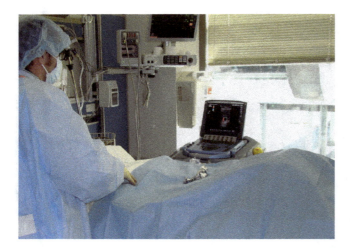

Figure 27-12 To optimize comfort, the patient, the target vessel/probe, and the screen should be in the line of vision of the operator; this minimizes operator movement during the procedure.

directly across from the operator, again, in the direct line of vision of the operator. In this example, the right side of the transducer corresponds to the inferior aspect of the patient, but everything else is the same.

Once the proper orientation is assured, the area of interest is scanned and the operator needs to be able to differentiate an artery from vein, which can be done in several ways. The first and easiest method is to assess vessel compressibility by applying downward pressure with the transducer while visualizing the vessel on the monitor. Veins will typically compress at a lower applied pressure than arteries, unless a clot is present (Figure 27-13). The second technique is to assess for the influence of respiratory variation on vessel diameter. Veins usually have easily identifiable respiratory variation as compared with arteries. The third technique is to apply standard Doppler or color Doppler to the vessel and listen to the audible signal or observe the character of the color "pulsation," both of which give an estimation of blood velocity inside the target vessel. Remember, as previously discussed, the color (red vs. blue) of the blood in the vessel is dependent on transducer position. It is useful to compare color Doppler signals of all vessels in the area of interest, paying close attention to the angle of incidence; with a little practice, arterial flow is easily differentiated from venous flow. Large, rapid fluctuations in intrathoracic pressure can create very high venous blood flow velocities that can mimic arterial flow, which may require the use of the other two methods of respiratory variation and compressibility to help differentiate the vessel type.

Occasionally, the vein cannot be visualized. The most common reason for this is hypovolemia with associated venous collapse; this can be remedied by placing the patient in the Trendelenburg position or applying a Valsalva maneuver or fluid administration. Other less common causes are agenesis, chronic occlusion or scarring of the vessel, and clot that is completely occluding the lumen. Clot may be difficult to distinguish from the surrounding tissue, and may appear similar to that of an absent vessel. In this case, a thorough examination of the proximal and distal parts of the vessel should be performed and a formal venous Doppler should be performed to evaluate for deep venous thrombosis prior to any attempted central venous cannulation. If access is critical and vessel presence or patency cannot be assured, a different vessel should be cannulated.

HOW TO PERFORM ULTRASOUND-GUIDED CANNULATION

▶ IJ Vein

The first step in successfully cannulating the IJ vein is proper positioning of the patient. The head should be rotated slightly contralaterally, with the neck extended. Severe rotation of the neck and head should be avoided because this may lead to significant distortion of the anatomy, and may increase the amount of overlap of the carotid artery and jugular vein. The bed should be placed in Trendelenburg position and the ultrasound machine should be placed by the ipsilateral side of the bed, at about the level of the patients' waist.

An initial examination of the landmarks, without ultrasound, should be performed, followed by selection of an insertion site. The site should then be confirmed with ultrasound. There are two reasons for this. Not only does it provide the operator with immediate feedback regarding landmark-based positions, but it also facilitates teaching both the landmark-based approach and ultrasound-guided approach. During this process, proper orientation, both transverse and longitudinal, should be ensured. The target vessel and surrounding structures should be identified and the patency of the vessel should be confirmed.

The patient's skin can now be prepped in the usual manner, and full barrier precautions should be used to maintain sterility and reduce the incidence of catheter-related

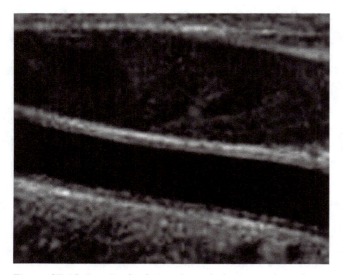

Figure 27-13 Longitudinal view through the internal jugular vein (top) and carotid artery (bottom) showing thrombus in the internal jugular vein.

infections.[26] Ultrasound use introduces another piece of equipment onto the sterile field, making the maintenance of sterility more difficult. While learning, special attention should be paid to this issue in order to develop good habits: a recent study by Latif et al. showed that simulation-based training in aseptic technique is helpful in that regard.[27] A sterile ultrasound sheath should be placed on the sterile field for when an assistant hands you the ultrasound transducer.

After the patient is prepped and draped, the catheter is set up as per normal routine. All ports should be flushed with bacteriostatic saline to remove air and to test for occlusion caused by manufacturing defects. The components needed for catheter insertion, including needles, wire, dilator, scalpel, and catheter, should be arranged in an orderly fashion and placed within easy reach. The assistant holds the transducer, with ultrasound gel applied (can be nonsterile gel), in a position such that the operator can both acquire the transducer and place it in the sterile sheath in one motion (Figure 27-14). Note that instead of utilizing an assistant, the transducer can be "picked up" by the operator, whose hand is inside the sterile sheath. The sheath is then extended to cover the transducer cord, and sterile rubber bands are applied to secure the sheath in place.

A second ultrasound examination should be performed to ensure that the original insertion site is still viable. Remember that proper orientation every time the probe is applied to the patient is essential for assuring an appropriate procedure.

When cannulating the vessel, use the same insertion site and needle trajectory that you would if you were using the landmark-based approach (lateral, medial, etc.). If using the transverse plane for ultrasound guidance, be sure to center the vessel lumen on the screen; remember that if the

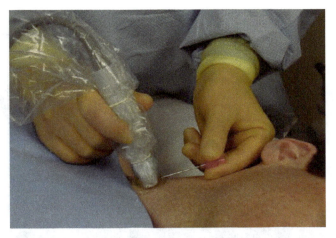

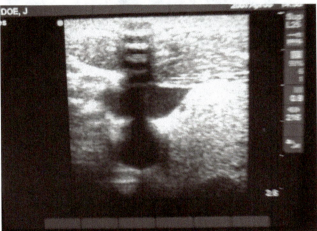

Figure 27-15 Technique of performing a "mock poke"; the needle is placed on the skin surface, and then imaged with ultrasound (top). The needle will cast an acoustic shadow on underlying structures. If the needle directly overlies the vein, the acoustic shadow will bisect the vein (bottom).

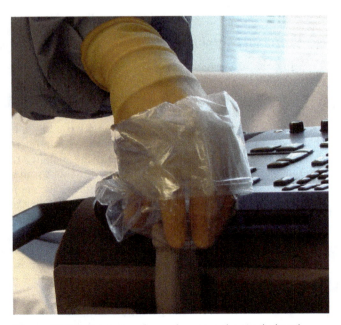

Figure 27-14 Retrieving the probe using the single-hand technique to maintain sterility. Once covered, the probe is placed on the sterile field.

vessel is centered on the screen, it is directly underneath the middle of the transducer head. Sometimes, it is useful to perform a "mock poke" to confirm your proposed insertion site relative to the underlying vessel (Figure 27-15). This is done by laying the needle on the skin surface, then placing the transducer over it. The acoustic shadow produced by the needle should be visualized directly over, or superimposed on, the target vessel (Figure 27-15). The skin puncture should be approximately 1 cm proximal to the transducer, which in most cases will result in visualization of the needle tip entering the vessel without having to move the probe much. If the needle tip cannot be visualized indenting either the subcutaneous tissue overlying the vessel or the vessel itself, move the probe along the axis of the vessel while slightly "agitating" the needle; this will accentuate the image of the needle and tip. The point of the "V" caused by indenting the subcutaneous tissue above the vein with the needle tip should be directly over the vessel (Figure 27-16). Be sure to visualize the tip of the

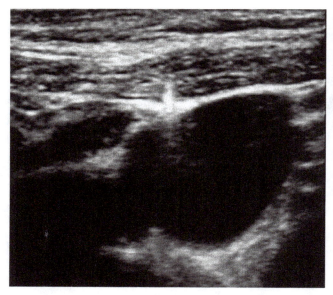

Figure 27-16 Transverse view of the internal jugular vein during cannulation. The needle tip (bright white) is seen penetrating the internal jugular vein at about 11 o'clock. Note that the probe is typically placed approximately 1–2 cm distal to the needlestick to ensure that the tip will remain in the ultrasound view. The probe can be moved proximally or distally to keep the needle tip in view.

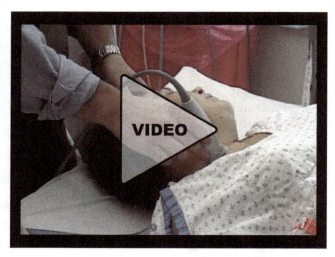

Video 27-1 Ultrasound guidance for jugular vein placement: Time frames
0:0–0:06 seconds: Prescreening of the target vessel transducer position
0:07–0:23 seconds: Identifying jugular vein by compressibility
0:24–0:43 seconds: Identifying jugular vein by colored Doppler
0:43–end of the video: Direct ultrasound-guided vessel cannulation in the short-axis view (note needle coming into the vessel from above). View at www.ccu2e.com

needle at all times; it is very easy to misinterpret the shaft of the needle as the tip; be sure to move the probe axially along the vessel frequently to maintain imaging of the tip. If done properly, the needle tip should be seen entering the lumen at about the same time as the flash of blood is obtained in the syringe. Recent data indicate that longitudinal guidance, or so-called "in-plane" technique, may reduce both inadvertent arterial puncture and puncture of the posterior wall of the vein.[28] This is achieved by keeping the needle tip in view at all times with this technique. A hybrid approach (medial-oblique) has also been described.[29]

Once the vessel has been successfully cannulated, the transducer can be set aside and the procedure can proceed normally with wire placement. Intravascular position of the wire can be confirmed with ultrasound, which can be saved for documentation in the medical record. Advance the wire slowly; there should be little to no resistance. Based on practical experience, the distance from the insertion site to the distal superior vena cava (SVC) in the average person is no more than 17–18 cm, so the wire should not be advanced farther than this. Once the wire is in place, the needle is removed, and a "stab" incision is made through the dermis at the point where the wire enters the skin. The tract is then dilated. Care should be taken not to insert the dilator too far, as this can potentially cause vessel perforation. After removal of the dilator, the catheter is then advanced to the desired distance, which is usually no more than 17–18 cm. Once the line is in place, flushed, secured, and dressed, a quick ultrasound examination of the anterior chest wall can be performed to evaluate for a pneumothorax (see Chapters 18 and 19).[30]

The use of ultrasound should be documented in the medical record. Typically, a statement regarding the use of ultrasound to assess the location and patency of the vessel and an image of the wire or catheter in the vessel lumen is sufficient for documentation and often provide sufficient documentation for reimbursement. In addition, a statement about the presence or absence of sliding pleura should be included (Video 27-1).

▶ **Subclavian Vein**

Typically, the subclavian vein is more difficult to visualize ultrasonographically than the IJ, axillary, or femoral veins. This is due to its position under the clavicle, which requires significant angulation and manipulation of the transducer to acquire a useful image (Figure 27-17). Two additional challenges are the difficulty of visualizing the vein in obese patients using an infraclavicular view and the inability to externally compress the vein, making it difficult to adequately assess the vein for clot. However, studies have demonstrated the usefulness of ultrasound in cannulating the subclavian vein in terms of reducing mechanical complications, increasing success, and decreasing procedure times.[31]

In our experience, it is usually easier to visualize the subclavian with a longitudinal, supraclavicular view because an adequate transverse view is often technically challenging, especially in obese patients. However, other operators prefer an infraclavicular transducer position. If a transverse view is desirable, using a small footprint curvilinear probe allows better angulation under the clavicle and improves imaging of the entire vein. Figure 27-17 shows the typical

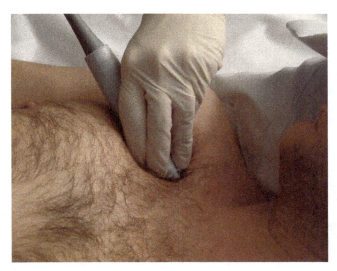

Figure 27-17 Probe position required to image the subclavian vein longitudinally. Note the cephalad angulation that is necessary to obtain a good view, which can become cumbersome during image-guided cannulation.

transducer placement for imaging the subclavian vein and Figure 27-18 provides the ultrasound image. Note that the patient is relatively thin, so an infraclavicular window is used. Except for the relative difficulty in cannulating the subclavian under dynamic guidance and the longer "learning curve" associated with it, the procedure itself is largely the same as that outlined above under "IJ Vein" cannulation, except for the use of the longitudinal view as described.

▶ **Axillary Vein**

Using the axillary vein for central venous access has many unique advantages over other sites.[32-36] Although not well studied, because the insertion site is on the anterior chest, axillary catheterization likely shares a lower incidence of catheter-related infections than the subclavian approach. Unlike the subclavian vein, using the axillary vein may be associated with fewer complications, such as pneumothorax, hemothorax, and chylothorax. The axillary vein is usually easier to compress than the subclavian vein and allows for an easier recognition of clots. There is, however, the additional potential complication of causing a brachial plexus injury, particularly if a far lateral approach is used.[34] One distinct disadvantage of the axillary approach is the unique dependence on ultrasound to ensure localization and subsequent cannulation; landmark techniques are not as effective as with the other common sites used to access the central venous system. Figure 27-19 shows proper transducer placement for viewing the axillary vein transversely. As with IJ and subclavian access approaches, a quick postprocedure scan of the chest should be performed to ensure sliding pleura, which essentially eliminates the possibility of pneumothorax.[30]

▶ **Femoral Vein**

Femoral cannulation remains a popular approach due to its relatively low incidence of life-threatening complications. Aside from the well-described risk of infection, there are several clinically important complications that may occur, which may lead to significant morbidity. Accidental (or intentional) femoral arterial cannulation, especially in coagulopathic patients, may cause life-threatening retroperitoneal hemorrhage and hematoma. Inadvertent

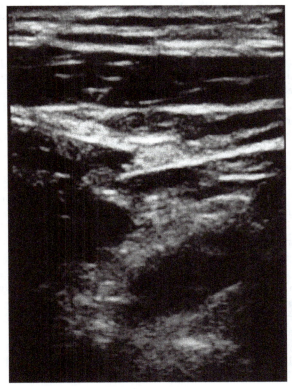

Figure 27-18 Longitudinal view of the subclavian vein (dark, round structure just left of center) and subclavian artery (bottom toward the right).

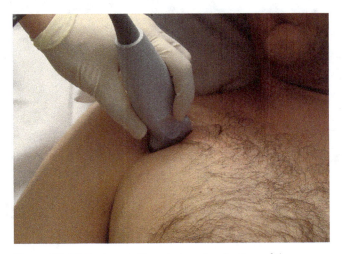

Figure 27-19 Probe position during visualization of the axillary vein.

stimulation of the femoral nerve with the cannulation needle can cause intense pain. A puncture site that is too proximal can also result in inadvertent puncture of intraperitoneal structures. Ultrasound can help avoid some of these important complications.

As with IJ, subclavian, and axillary cannulation, the first step in successful femoral access is achieving proper orientation. The ultrasound machine should be placed on the contralateral side of the patient, directly across from the operator. The entire area should be scanned, with identification of all vascular structures, including the femoral artery, common femoral vein, and saphenous or profunda femoris vessels, if possible. Once the vein is identified, it should be evaluated for the presence of clot. In addition, a longitudinal view of the vein should be obtained as it dives under the inguinal ligament, and the ligament itself should be marked on the skin (Figure 27-20). This ensures that an intraperitoneal puncture will not occur.

Regardless of the site chosen for cannulation, ultrasound guidance has other advantages over landmark-based technique. These include assessment for complications, such as pneumothorax and/or hemothorax, or even catheter tip malposition. Zanobetti et al. in 2013 showed that ultrasound has a 94% sensitivity and 89% specificity in detecting mechanical complications when compared to chest radiography, and in much less time (5 minutes vs. 65 minutes).[37]

ARTERIAL CATHETER PLACEMENT WITH ULTRASOUND GUIDANCE

The principles and techniques of ultrasound guidance for CVC insertion can be easily adapted to the placement of arterial cannulae. From an ultrasound guidance perspective, the procedures are very similar. There are, however, some factors associated with arterial catheter placement that deserve special consideration.

The most commonly cannulated arteries include the radial, axillary, and femoral approaches. The radial approach significantly exceeds the others in terms of popularity. The reasons for this are easy accessibility of the wrist, the presence of a dual circulation of the hand (in most patients), and the fact that the wrist is a relatively clean site. It is important to understand, however, that radial artery catheterization is not risk-free.

In 1929, Dr. Edgar van Nuys Allen described a maneuver in which the dual palmar circulation could be tested by obstructing both radial and ulnar arterial flow, then releasing either ulnar or radial to see if palmar circulation was restored. The test was repeated to assess flow in the other of the two arteries. The importance of this test is to ascertain the duality of the circulation, so that if one of the arteries was obstructed (from thrombus or spasm after puncture), the palmar circulation would not be compromised. Although there is some debate as to the value of Allen's test in predicting who is at risk of hand ischemia, the test continues to be performed on a routine basis, especially in the setting of radial artery harvesting for coronary bypass grafting. Ultrasound use may improve the accuracy of Allen's test, first reported in 1973.[38] This test requires ultrasonic localization of the palmar arteries with Doppler, followed by occlusion of the radial artery; if flow is maintained, there is adequate dual circulation, suggesting that radial artery cannulation or harvesting is safe (Figure 27-21).

Unsuccessful attempts at radial artery catheterization can be associated with hematoma formation. While this is usually insignificant and without clinical consequence, hematomas can seriously impair further attempts at cannulation by obscuring the arterial pulsation during palpation. As a result, procedure times are prolonged, pain is increased, and procedures fail. Using either static guidance to mark a suitable site for cannulation or cannulation under dynamic guidance reduces the number of unsuccessful attempts (Figure 27-22),[39–41] and may increase the first pass success rate as much as 71%.[42] If a hematoma occurs while using ultrasound, arterial flow is still readily apparent with application of Doppler or color Doppler to the 2D image, enabling subsequent attempts.

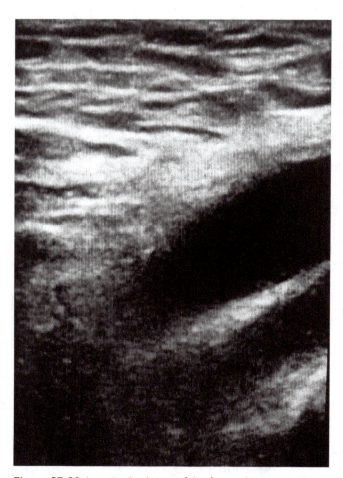

Figure 27-20 Longitudinal view of the femoral vein as it dives posteriorly under the inguinal ligament. The artery is superior to the vein in this example. The inguinal ligament is seen as a bright area to the left.

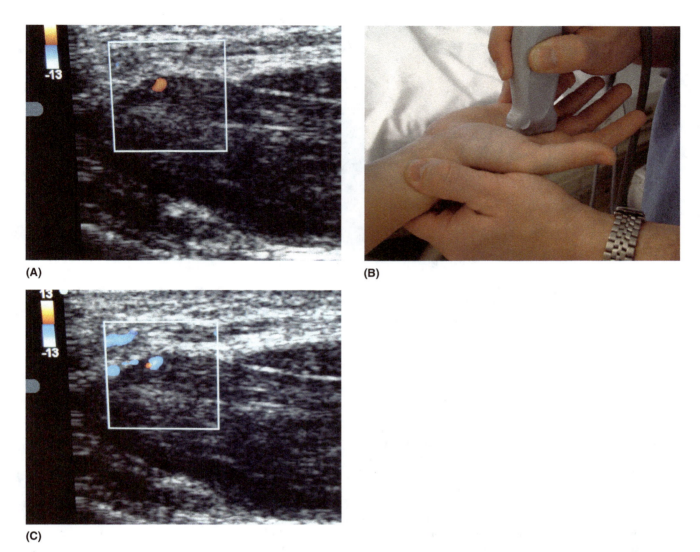

Figure 27-21 (**A**) Color Doppler image of the palmar arch. (**B**) Occlusion of the radial artery while imaging the palmar arch. (**C**) Reversal of flow in the palmar arch after occlusion, which indicates flow is maintained by the ulnar artery.

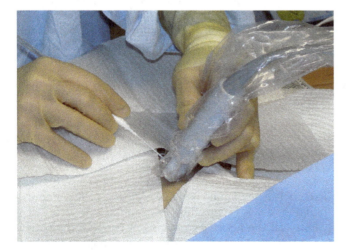

Figure 27-22 Cannulation of the radial artery under dynamic guidance.

Interestingly, Yokoyama et al. demonstrated anatomic variations using ultrasound in 11 of 115 (2.6%) patients scheduled to undergo percutaneous coronary intervention via a radial artery approach. Of these, only three were inaccessible for cannulation. These findings confirm that although anatomic variations exist, ultrasound guidance can identify many of these in anticipation of the procedure.[43]

PICC LINES/MIDLINES

PICC lines have gained significant popularity in recent years, presumably because of a low incidence of complications from insertion, improved patient comfort as compared with standard CVCs, safety and ease of care in the outpatient setting, and a relatively low incidence of catheter-related infections.[44,45] First described as an alternative to CVCs placed in the IJ, subclavian, or femoral veins, PICCs

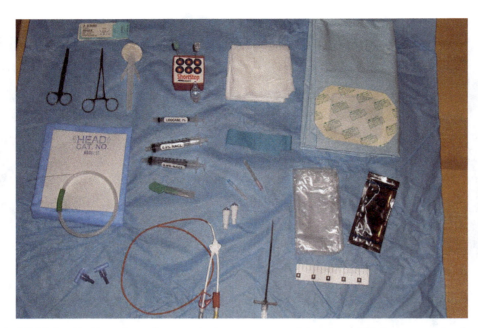

Figure 27-23 Typical PICC line kit. Note the catheter at the bottom center of the photo. This is an example of a guide wire–based introducer system (peel-away introducer is to the bottom right). PICC indicates peripherally inserted central venous catheter.

are placed in peripheral veins of the upper extremities and "threaded" into the central venous system (Figure 27-23).

There are fair amount of data on long-term complications of these catheters. The most common complications include thrombosis, catheter-related infection, catheter tip malposition or migration, vessel or heart chamber perforation, deep venous thrombosis, and malfunction.[44–46] Factors associated with a higher risk of thrombosis include larger catheter size, cephalic vein placement, "peripheral" placement (outside of the vena cava), duration of catheterization, and presence of underlying solid-tumor malignancy or hypercoagulation disorders. Note that the best catheter tip position is the distal third of the SVC at the SVC–right atrial junction. This position causes the catheter tip to "float" within the lumen, which is associated with a lower incidence of thrombus formation.[46] Also, the SVC has a higher flow rate compared with the axillary, subclavian, or brachiocephalic veins, which has implications for thrombus formation and damage to the vessel from infusion of caustic substances.[46]

The risk of catheter-related infection with PICCs is substantially lower than that with CVCs, but is still a significant problem.[41] Factors associated with higher infection rates are use of any skin prep other than 2% chlorhexidine, lack of full barrier precautions (cap, mask, gown, gloves, and large drape), and use of catheters with more than a single lumen (the more lumens, the higher the risk). Antimicrobial PICC lines may reduce this risk, but the evidence at this point is inconclusive.

There are several PICC line kits on the market. It is important to review the needs of your particular patient when selecting a catheter. A "power PICC," which is capable of handling high-pressure infusions, such as may be used with IV contrast agents, may be indicated. PICCs also come with one, two, or three lumens, which should be selected depending on the patient's needs.

There are two basic methods of PICC placement. First, the Seldinger technique, where the vessel is cannulated with a needle, a wire is threaded through the needle followed by needle withdrawal, and a dilator/tear-away introducer is then inserted. The dilator is removed from the introducer, and the PICC is inserted to the appropriate position, followed by removal of the introducer. The second method requires cannulation with a device similar to an angiocath, where the vessel is cannulated by a needle/catheter combination, and then the catheter is advanced over the needle into the vessel. The PICC is advanced through this catheter, which is then "torn away." This method tends to be more cumbersome.

An institutional algorithm that governs IV access taking into consideration indications, patient factors, and alternatives when deciding on the type of vascular access device may avoid excessive and inappropriate PICC line use. One approach is shown in Figure 27-24.

For PICC line insertion, 2D and color Doppler ultrasound is used to "map" the extremity of interest. All superficial vascular structures of the distal brachium are identified, paying particular attention to differentiating artery from vein, and assessing vein size. Figure 27-25 shows the typical venous anatomy of the upper extremity. After mapping is complete, a candidate vein is selected for insertion and marked. Patency should be assessed, by ensuring compressibility, as well as venous flow.

Once all the necessary equipment is ready, the patient is positioned and sterilely prepped and draped. The ideal position for successful catheter insertion is depicted in Figure 27-26. The right arm is preferable due to the higher

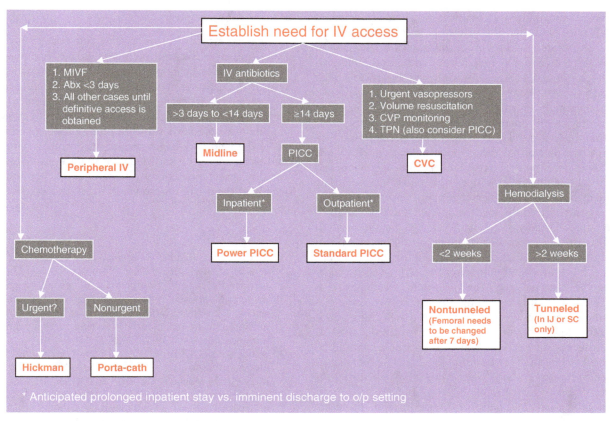

Figure 27-24 An example of an IV access algorithm. IV, intravenous.

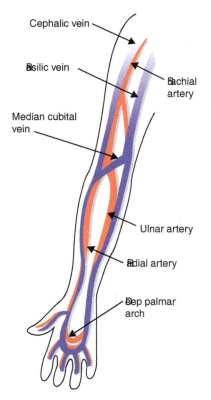

Figure 27-25 Typical venous anatomy of the upper extremity.

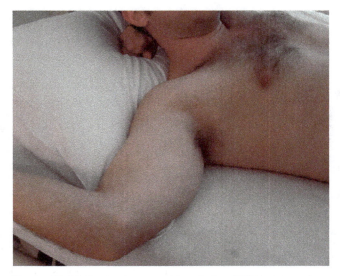

Figure 27-26 Optimal arm position during PICC line insertion. Shoulder abducted and externally rotated, arm flexed 90°. This maneuver exposes the basilic vein.

incidence of catheter tip malposition when inserted in the left arm. Note that the extremity is abducted, slightly externally rotated, and secured; this allows easy access to the basilic vein, and may help reduce catheter tip malposition by forming a straight line from the insertion site to central venous system. If the arm is left at the patient's side, the catheter tip must negotiate a turn when entering the subclavian; this increases the risk of the catheter either entering the ipsilateral IJ vein or coiling in the subclavian. There are no data on the risk of air embolization with PICC or midline placement; the risk is likely to be negligible and roughly the same as that with peripheral IV insertion. The Trendelenburg position, therefore, is not necessary.

Next, the desired PICC kit is opened and the line itself is prepared. Usually, these catheters have a long metallic obturator that provides stiffness during insertion; this should be partially withdrawn to allow for catheter trimming. The desired catheter length is estimated by measuring the distance from the proposed insertion site to the glenohumeral joint, adding the distance from the glenohumeral joint to the sternal notch, then adding about 6 cm to allow for proper positioning in the distal SVC. Once this distance is determined, the catheter should be trimmed to length. *The obturator should not be cut because this will produce a sharp point capable of puncturing the vessel.*

Rescan the area and confirm the position of the target vein. Cannulate the vessel under dynamic guidance as described above in the CVC section. When access to the vein is obtained, remove any dilators that may be present with the introducer, and advance the catheter slowly to the hub. Quickly advancing the catheter increases the risk of catheter tip malposition. By slowing the rate of advancement, the catheter becomes more "flow directed" and follows the flow into the correct position. Remember that the catheter was trimmed to an appropriate length already, so advancing the hub will ensure correct tip position. When the catheter is fully advanced, remove the inner stylette or obturator, attach a syringe, and aspirate blood to confirm an intravascular position. Ultrasound can also be used to evaluate for catheter tip malposition by scanning the ipsilateral IJ vein and contralateral subclavian, if possible. The line can then be secured by a suture or one of several commercially available adhesive devices and dressed appropriately. Of course, a portable chest radiograph should be obtained to confirm correct placement.

▶ Peripheral IV Access

One of the most common reasons cited for placing PICC and midline devices is difficulty obtaining adequate peripheral access. This can, in part, be avoided by providing nursing and support personnel with ultrasound guidance principles for peripheral IV access. Multiple studies have shown this strategy to be effective in increasing successful peripheral cannulation, decreasing PICC and central line utilization, or both.[47,48]

SUMMARY

Vascular access can be made safer and easier with ultrasound guidance. The basic technique is the same regardless of the procedure being performed. Once the technique of dynamic guidance is mastered, it can be applied to almost any procedure. Recently published (and developing) practice guidelines provide additional information.[49] Ultrasound should not be used as a substitute for a proper understanding of the landmark-based technique. Rather, it should be used to augment the knowledge of the venous system and vascular access procedures. Remember to appropriately document the use of ultrasound in the medical record.

REFERENCES

1. McGee DC, Gould MK. Preventing complications of central venous catheterization. *N Engl J Med*. 2003;348:1123–1133.
2. Brennan JM, Blair JE, Hampole C, Goonewardena S. Radial artery pulse pressure variation correlates with brachial artery peak velocity variation in ventilated subjects when measured by internal medicine residents using hand-carried ultrasound devices. *Chest*. 2007;131:1301–1307.
3. Polderman KH, Girbes AJ. Central venous catheter use. Part 1: mechanical complications. *Intensive Care Med*. 2002;28:1–17.
4. Merrer J, De Jonghe B, Golliot F, et al. Complications of femoral and subclavian venous catheterization in critically ill patients: a randomized controlled trial. *JAMA*. 2001;286:700–707.
5. Mansfield PF, Hohn DC, Fornage BD. Complications and failures of subclavian vein catheterization. *New Engl J Med*. 1994;331:1735–1738.
6. Light RW. *Pleural Diseases*. 5th ed. Philadelphia, PA: Lippincott Williams & Wilkins; 2007.
7. Legler D, Nugent M. Doppler localization of the internal jugular vein facilitates central venous cannulation. *Anesthesiology*. 1984;60:481–482.
8. Randolph AG, Cook DJ, Gonzales CA, et al. Ultrasound guidance for placement of central venous catheters: a meta-analysis of the literature. *Crit Care Med*. 1996;24:2053–2058.
9. Hind D, Calvert N, McWilliams SR, et al. Ultrasonic locating devices for central venous cannulation: meta-analysis. *BMJ*. 2003;327:361.
10. Rabindranath KS, Kumar E, Shail R, Vaux E. Use of real-time ultrasound guidance for the placement of hemodialysis catheters: a systematic review and meta-analysis of randomized controlled trials. *Am J Kidney Dis*. 2011;58:964–970.
11. Feller-Kopman D. Ultrasound-guided internal jugular access. *Chest*. 2007;132:302–309.
12. Maecken T, Grau T. Ultrasound imaging in vascular access. *Crit Care Med*. 2007;35:S178–S185.
13. Cavanna L, Civardi G, Vallisa D, et al. Ultrasound-guided central venous catheterization in cancer patients improves the success rate of cannulation and reduces mechanical complications: a prospective observational study of 1,978 consecutive catheterizations. *World J Surg Oncol*. 2010;8:91.
14. Peris A, Zagli G, Bonizzoli M, et al. Implantation of 3951 long-term central venous catheters: performances, risk analysis, and patient comfort after ultrasound-guidance introduction. *Anesth Analg*. 2010;111:1194–1201.

15. Milling TJ Jr, Rose J, Briggs WM, et al. Randomized, controlled clinical trial of point-of-care limited ultrasonography assistance of central venous cannulation: the third sonography outcomes assessment program (SOAP-3) trial. *Crit Care Med.* 2005;33:1764–1769.
16. NICE Guidelines. http://www.nice.org.uk/nicemedia/pdf/Ultrasound_49_GUIDANCE.pdf. Accessed March 3, 2009.
17. Rothschild J. AHRQ evidence based practice. http://www.ahrq.gov/clinic/ptsafety/pdf/chap21.pdf. Accessed March 3, 2013.
18. Lamperti M, Bodenham AR, Pittiruti M, et al. International evidence-based recommendations on ultrasound-guided vascular access. *Intensive Care Med.* 2012;38(7):1105–1117.
19. Muhm M. Ultrasound guided central venous access (letter). *BMJ.* 2002;325:1374–1375.
20. Forauer A, Glockner J. Importance of US findings in access planning during jugular vein hemodialysis catheter placements. *J Vasc Interv Radiol.* 2000;11:233–238.
21. http://www.cms.hhs.gov/HospitalAcqCond/Downloads/HAC-POA-Listening12-17-2007.pdf. Accessed: March 19, 2013.
22. Matera JT, Egerton-Warburton D, Meek R. Ultrasound guidance for central venous catheter placement in Australasian emergency departments: potential barriers to more widespread use. *Emerg Med Australas.* 2010;22(6):514–523.
23. Dodge KL, Lynch CA, Moore CL, et al. Use of ultrasound guidance improves central venous catheter insertion success rates among junior residents. *J Ultrasound Med.* 2012;31(10):1519–1526.
24. Sekiguchi H, Tokita JE, Minami T, et al. A prerotational, simulation-based workshop improves safety of central venous catheter insertion: results of a successful internal medicine house staff training program. *Chest.* 2011;140(3):652–658.
25. Ball RD, Scouras NE, Orebaugh S, et al. Randomized, prospective, observational simulation study comparing residents' needle-guided vs. free-hand ultrasound techniques for central venous catheter access. *Br J Anaesth.* 2012;108(1):72–79.
26. Mermel LA. Prevention of intravascular catheter-related infections. *Ann Intern Med.* 2000;132:391–402.
27. Latif RK, Bautista AF, Memon SB, et al. Teaching aseptic technique for central venous access under ultrasound guidance: a randomized trial comparing didactic training alone to didactic plus simulation-based training. *Anesth Analg.* 2012;114(3):626–633.
28. Stone MB, Moon C, Sutijono D, Blaivas M. Needle tip visualization during ultrasound-guided vascular access: short axis vs. long axis approach. *Am J Emerg Med.* 2010;28(3):343–347.
29. Dilisio R, Mittnacht AJ. The "medial-oblique approach to ultrasound-guided central venous cannulation-maximize the view, minimize the risk. *J Cardiothorac Vasc Anesth.* 2012;26(6):982–984.
30. Mayo PH, Doelken P. Pleural ultrasonography. *Clin Chest Med.* 2006;27:215–227.
31. Fragou M, Gravvanis A, Dimitriou V, et al. Real-time ultrasound-guided subclavian vein cannulation versus the landmark method in critical care patients: a prospective randomized study. *Crit Care Med.* 2011;39(7):1607–1612.
32. Sandhu NS. Transpectoral ultrasound-guided catheterization of the axillary vein: an alternative to standard catheterization of the subclavian vein. *Anesth Analg.* 2004;99:183–187.
33. Mackey SP, Sinha S, Pusey J. Ultrasound imaging of the axillary vein-anatomical basis for central access (Letter). *Br J Anaesth.* 2003;93:598–599.
34. Galloway S, Bodenham A. Ultrasound imaging of the axillary vein-anatomical basis for central venous access. *Br J Anaesth.* 2003;90:589–595.
35. Sharma S, Bodenham AR, Mallick A. Ultrasound-guided infraclavicular axillary vein cannulation for central venous access. *Br J Anaesth.* 2004;93:188–192.
36. Uhlenkott MC, Sathishkumar S, Murray WB, et al. Real-time multimodal axillary vein imaging enhances the safety and efficacy of axillary vein catheterization in neurosurgical intensive care patients. *J Neurosurg Anesthesiol.* 2013;25(1):62–65.
37. Zanobetti M, Coppa A, Bulletti F, et al. Verification of correct central venous catheter placement in the emergency department: comparison between ultrasonography and chest radiography. *Intern Emerg Med.* 2013;8(2):173–180.
38. Mozersky DJ, Buckley CJ, Hagood CO Jr, et al. Ultrasonic evaluation of the palmar circulation. A useful adjunct to radial artery cannulation. *Am J Surg.* 1973;126:810–812.
39. Maher JJ, Dougherty JM. Radial artery cannulation guided by Doppler ultrasound. *Am J Emerg Med.* 1989;7:260–262.
40. Levin PD, Sheinin O, Gozal Y. Use of ultrasound guidance in the insertion of radial artery catheters. *Crit Care Med.* 2003;31:481–484.
41. Shiver S, Blaivas M, Lyon M. A prospective comparison of ultrasound-guided and blindly placed radial artery catheters. *Acad Emerg Med.* 2006;13:1275–1279.
42. Shiloh AL, Savel RH, Paulin LM, Eisen LA. Ultrasound-guided catheterization of the radial artery: a systematic review and meta-analysis of randomized controlled trials. *Chest.* 2011;139(3):524–529.
43. Yokoyama N, Takeshita S, Ochiai M, Koyama Y. Anatomic variations of the radial artery in patients undergoing transradial coronary intervention. *Catheter Cardiovasc Interv.* 2000;49:357–362.
44. Schmid MW. Risks and complications of peripherally and centrally inserted intravenous catheters. *Crit Care Nurs Clin North Am.* 2000;12:165–174.
45. Maki DG, Kluger DM, Crnich CJ. The risk of bloodstream infection in adults with different intravascular access devices: a systematic review of 200 published prospective studies. *Mayo Clin Proc.* 2006;81:1159–1171.
46. National Association of Vascular Access Networks (NAVAN). Tip location of peripherally inserted central catheters. NAVAN position statement. *JVAD.* 1998;3:9–10.
47. Shokoohi H, Boniface K, McCarthy M, et al. Ultrasound-guided peripheral intravenous access program is associated with a marked reduction in central venous catheter use in noncritically ill emergency department patients. *Ann Emerg Med.* 2013;61(2):198–203.
48. Au AK, Rotte MJ, Grzybowski RJ, et al. Decrease in central venous catheter placement due to use of ultrasound guidance for peripheral intravenous catheters. *Am J Emerg Med.* 2012;30(9):1950–1954.
49. Troianos CA, Hartman GS, Glas KE, et al. Guidelines for performing ultrasound guided vascular cannulation: recommendations of the American Society of Echocardiography and the Society of Cardiovascular Anesthesiologists. *J Am Soc Echocardiography.* 2011;24:1291–1318.

28

OCULAR ULTRASOUND

DAVID EVANS

Scan QR code or visit www.ccu2e.com for video in this chapter

INTRODUCTION

Nearly 3% off all visits to emergency departments in the United States involve ocular complaints. Bedside ultrasound has become an indispensable tool for both traumatic and nontraumatic eye complaints. While ocular ultrasonography is not a new concept, its application in the critical care setting is new. Traditional fundoscopic-based eye exams are not only difficult to perform in the acute care setting; they are notoriously unreliable in the setting of trauma. The physical exam of the eye requires controlled conditions and appropriate equipment not often found in the ICU. Intensivists can use familiar ultrasound-based principles to develop a limited ocular exam capable of ascertaining a rage of pathological conditions not previously detectable on a physical exam. The eye itself is a fluid-filled structure ideal for sonographic imaging. The use of ultrasound allows the provider to perform a detailed exam of the ocular structures without the patient opening his or her eyes. This limited sonographic exam allows the practitioner to evaluate ocular movement, the anterior chamber, the posterior chamber, and the retrobulbar space, including the optic sheath to assess intracranial pressure.

SONOGRAPHIC ANATOMY OF THE EYE

The eye and the surrounding orbit offer perhaps one of the most acoustically friendly areas of the body. The surrounding bony orbit should be intensely hyperechoic with a posterior shadow. The anterior cortex of the orbital bones should be smooth with a sharp edge and display no irregularity, which could be a sign of pathology. The globe itself should be round, completely anechoic with the exception of the anterior structures, and posterior acoustic enhancement should be apparent (Figure 28-1). The anechoic fluid-filled anterior chamber is easily identified along with the thin hyperechoic cornea, which lies just superior to this space. Inferior to the anterior chamber lies the hyperechoic iris. Just posterior to the iris the elliptical shape of the lens is noted. Behind the lens lies the large echo-lucent posterior chamber. The posterior portion of the eye is hyperechoic and is made up of several layers, including the retina, choroid plexus, and sclera as the outermost layer. The optic nerve and sheath travel posterior to the globe as is seen as a long straight anechoic nerve bounded by hyperechoic sheath (Figure 28-2).

IMAGING TECHNIQUE

The eye is a delicate structure and requires the examiner to pay explicit attention to technique. The patient should be placed in the supine to semirecumbent position. If the patient is noted to have obvious globe rupture the exam should not be preformed at the bedside. A high-frequency (7.5–15 MHz) linear transducer should be used for the exam. Most ultrasound machines currently have an "ophthalmological" setting, though other presets, such as small parts, musculoskeletal, or superficial, can be used if output power is reduced (please consult with the specific ultrasound system manufacturer to assure safety compliance). The patient should be advised to keep his or her eyes shut during the exam. Alternatively, a clear bio-occlusive IV dressing can be placed over the affected eye if the patient has difficulty keeping his or her eyes closed during the exam (Figure 28-3). A copious amount of ultrasound gel should be applied to the preorbital space (Figure 28-4). The high-frequency linear array transducer should be placed in the sagittal plane with the transducer marker toward the patient's head (Figure 28-5). Care should be taken to not place pressure on the ocular structures but rather using the mound of gel as a standoff pad between the transducer and the patient's eye. The examiner's hand can rest on the bridge

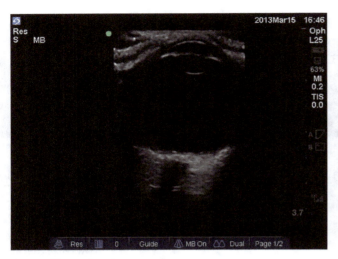

Figure 28-1 Normal eye.

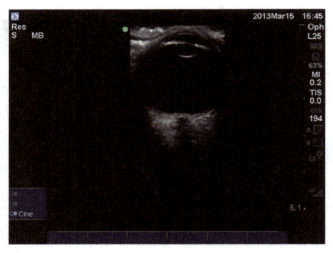

Figure 28-2 Normal eye with optic sheath.

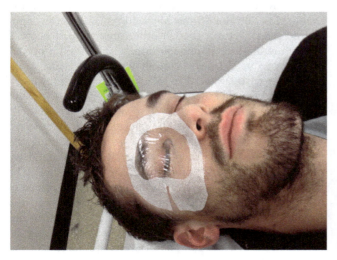

Figure 28-3 Bio-occlusive dressing for ocular ultrasound.

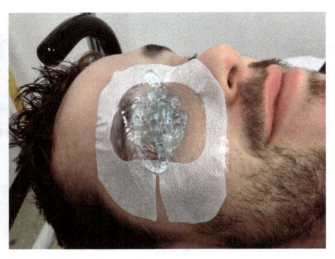

Figure 28-4 Copious gel for ocular ultrasound exam.

of the nose or the eyebrow to steady the image and limit arm fatigue. The transducer should then be swept medially and laterally to identify any pathology. After a full evaluation in the sagittal plane, the transducer should be rotated to the left 90° to the transverse plane. The transducer should be swept from cranial to caudal to identify any pathology. In addition to this sweeping motion, it is sometimes helpful to have the patient shift his or her gaze from side to side or up to down (Video 28-1). These so-called kinetic eye movements can sometimes help elucidate underlying pathology, like posterior vitreous hemorrhage or retinal detachment. It will be important during the exam to be able to increase the gain multiple times throughout the ultrasound.

CLINICAL APPLICATIONS

▶ Ocular Trauma

Trauma to the orbit or surrounding structures is often difficult to evaluate for a nonophthalmological specialist.

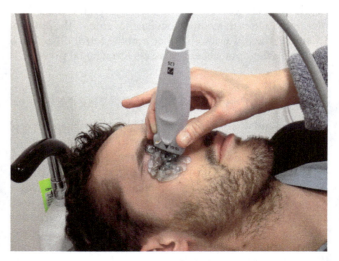

Figure 28-5 Transducer in sagittal plain.

CHAPTER 28 OCULAR ULTRASOUND 321

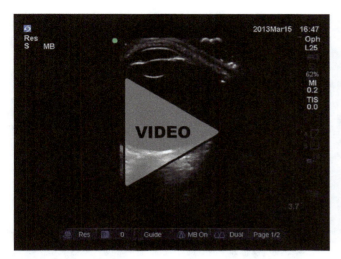

Video 28-1 Normal kinetic eye movements. View at www.ccu2e.com

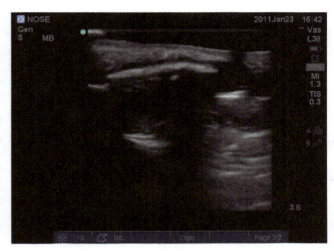

Figure 28-6 Nasal bone fracture.

With concomitant head injury and concern over intracranial pressure, prying the patients swollen eyelids open to perform a limited physical exam is typically dissuaded. It is therefore not surprising that in the setting of multisystem trauma the vast amount of ocular injuries go unrecognized for this reason. Ocular ultrasound allows the provider to perform a rapid examination of the surrounding orbit, the globe, the internal structures, and the retrobulbar space for pathological conditions that would require urgent ophthalmological consultation.

▶ Periorbital Trauma

The role of computerized tomography (CT) in the diagnosis of periorbital injuries is well established; however, bedside ultrasound offers real advantages for the diagnosis of orbital pathology. Ultrasound is performed in real time and is highly specific, noninvasive, inexpensive, portable, safe, and does not expose the patient to radiation. The use of CT is often limited by coexistent injuries, patient positioning, and CT availability; all which may prevent or delay the diagnosis of significant orbital wall defects.

Therefore, the periorbital structures should be imaged first during the examination of any trauma patient, who sustained significant periorbital injuries. Fractures will appear as an abrupt disruption of the bright hyperechoic cortex (Figure 28-6). If any displacement has occurred the most anterior fracture segment will cast a posterior shadow.

▶ Vitreous Hemorrhage

Vitreous hemorrhage commonly occurs with ocular trauma and nontraumatic conditions, such as diabetic retinopathy and central vein occlusion. The patient will typically describe floaters and reduced visual acuity following the trauma. On sonographic examination there will be areas of "spider webs" in the posterior chamber (Figure 28-7). It is important during this exam to increase the gain systematically in order to reliably identify any hemorrhage.

During kinetic movements, the organized portion of the hemorrhage will appear to tumble around in the posterior chamber in what is described as a "washing machine" type of movement (Video 28-2).

▶ Globe Rupture

Performing an ultrasound of obvious globe rupture is typically discouraged. If globe rupture is possible, care should be taken during the exam to not place any pressure on the globe itself. Sonographically the globe will appear to have lost its round shape due to decreased amount of vitreous, which can lead to bulking of the sclera. Typically, in globe rupture there will be a component of vitreous hemorrhage that can be appreciated (Figure 28-8).

▶ Lens Dislocation

Traumatic vision loss occurring after a direct blow can be a symptom of lens dislocation. The patient will complain of blurry vision and the patent will typically exhibit

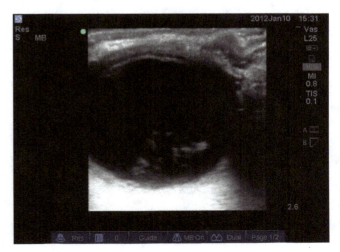

Figure 28-7 Posterior vitreous hemorrhage.

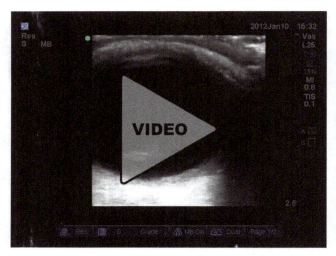

Video 28-2 Posterior vitreous hemorrhage. View at www.ccu2e.com

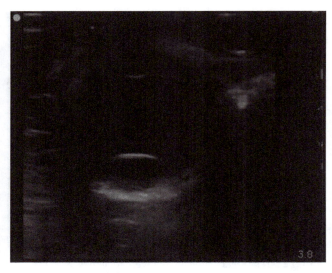

Figure 28-9 Lens dislocation.

a pupillary defect. Lens dislocation is easily identified on bedside ultrasound by directly visualizing the displacement of the lens from its normal location. Lens dislocation can by partial or complete. If the lens is completely dislocated it will be found in the posterior chamber and will move independently during kinetic movements (Figure 28-9).

▶ **Foreign Body**

Ocular foreign bodies can be precisely located using bedside ultrasound. Foreign bodies will appear as hyperechoic entities within the posterior chamber, regardless of the object's composition (Figures 28-10A and B). If the foreign body is very stiff, like metal, a reverberation artifact may be seen posterior to the object. The additional application of color Doppler to this area of reverberation will cause a rapidly changing red–blue "twinkle" effect, useful in identifying the foreign body. If the foreign body is located in the posterior fat behind the globe it can be hard to identify due to the fact it my blend in with the hyperechoic nature of the fat (Video 28-3).

ACUTE VISION LOSS

Acute visual disturbance is a common condition encountered in the acute care setting. Patients routinely complain of flashes of light, blurry vision, or even complete blindness. Acute visual loss can occur for a multitude of reasons either related to traumatic or nontraumatic conditions. Atraumatic visual loss tends to be multifactorial and as such harder to diagnosis. For the intensivist it is important to identify true ophthalmic emergencies that need urgent consultation with ophthalmic specialist.

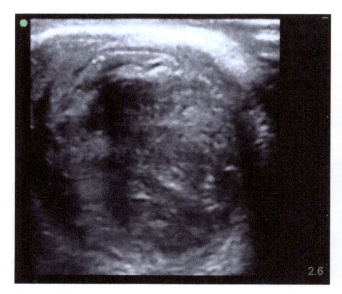

Figure 28-8 Globe rupture.

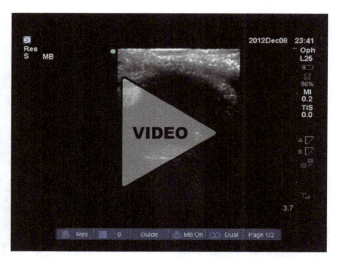

Video 28-3 Ocular foreign body. View at www.ccu2e.com

CHAPTER 28 OCULAR ULTRASOUND 323

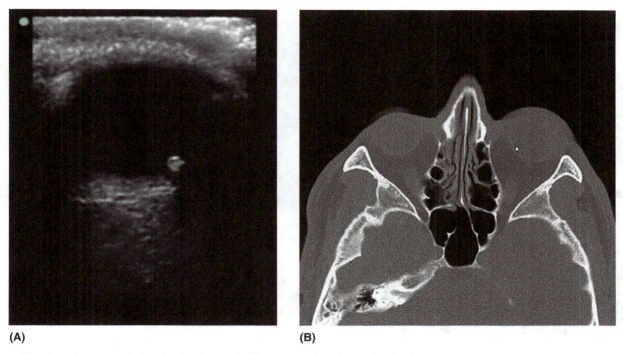

Figure 28-10 (A) Ultrasound of ocular foreign body. (B) CT scan of ocular foreign body.

▶ Retinal Detachment

Retinal detachment typically presents with flashes of light and decreased visual acuity. It occurs when the sensory layer of the retina separates from the pigment layer. Retinal detachments are classified as rhegmatogenous, tractional, or exudative. Rhegmatogenous detachment is typically seen in vitreous detachment; tractional detachment is commonly seen in diabetic retinopathy and aging, but can occur in other conditions, like sickle cell disease; finally, exudative detachment can be caused by inflammatory, infectious, vascular, degenerative, malignant, or genetically determined pathological conditions. It is vital for the intensivist to properly identify retinal detachment. Untreated retinal detachment can progress to full and permanent visual loss. Bedside ultrasound helps the examiner quickly identify retinal detachment and distinguish it from other causes of acute visual disturbance. Retinal detachment will appear as a hyperechoic line in the posterior chamber (Figure 28-11). During kinetic movements the hyperechoic membrane will have a tethered appearance. When the detachment is complete it will have a V shape as the retina will maintain a connection to the optic nerve head (Figure 28-12). During the examination the gain should be slowly increased to properly identify retinal detachment.

▶ Central Retinal Artery/Vein Occlusion

Acute, sudden, painless visual loss is associated with central retinal artery or vein occlusion. This condition can be assessed with bedside ultrasound via the use of Doppler. Once the optic nerve is identified color Doppler should be placed on the posterior portion of the globe at the attachment of the optic nerve. Pulsatile arterial flow and continuous venous flow should be identified (Video 28-4). In the hands of a skilled sonographer, spectral Doppler can be used to observe the flow patterns of both the artery and the vein (Figure 28-13). The absence of either arterial or

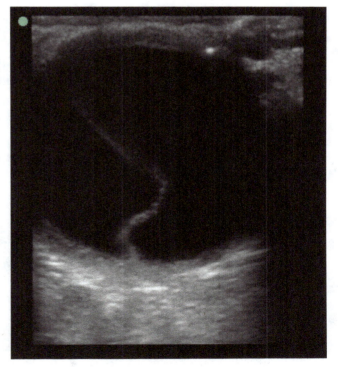

Figure 28-11 Retinal detachment, partial.

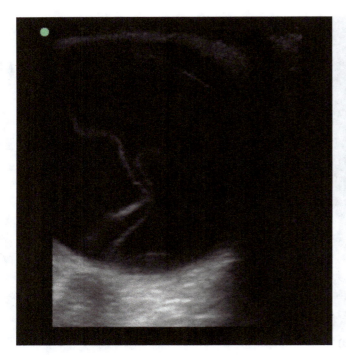

Figure 28-12 Retinal detachment, complete.

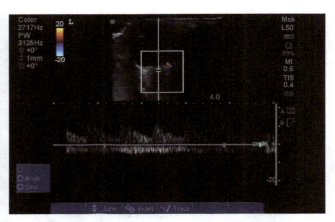

Figure 28-13 Spectral Doppler of normal central retinal arterial flow.

venous flow strongly suggests there is a vascular cause for the patient's loss of vision.

ASSESSING INTRACRANIAL PRESSURE

It is important for the intensivist to be able to assess intracranial pressure rapidly and reliably at the bedside. While many modalities exist for screening patients for increased intracranial pressure none of them are as easy, rapid, reproducible, or as safe as bedside ultrasound. CT is expensive, exposes the patient to radiation, requires patients to be transported to radiology, and is impractical to repeat multiple times over. Lumbar puncture is dangerous to perform in the setting of increased intracranial pressure. Fundoscopy is often difficult to perform on a patient with increased intracranial pressure and altered mental status. Ultrasound examination for increased intracranial pressure relies on a standard measurement of the optic sheath. During episodes of increased intracranial pressure fluid is pushed from the subarachnoid space into the optic sheath causing swelling and enlargement of the optic sheath.

Using linear array transducer, the optic nerve and sheath is identified under B-mode ultrasound. Care must be taken to ensure the best B-mode image possible is obtained. Once the optic nerve is identified, the image is frozen and a measurement is made from the posterior optic disk to 3 mm into the optic nerve. At this point the optic sheath is measured from outer to outer and should not exceed 5mm (Figure 28-14). Both optic sheaths should be measured for confirmatory purposes. If there is a question as to whether optic sheath enlargement exists, the patient should be asked to shift his or her gaze lateral 30° which should reduce the optic sheath diameter by 10% if the enlargement is truly due to fluid shift. This measurement will continue to increase in size as

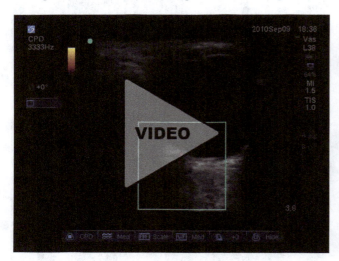

Video 28-4 Power Doppler of normal central retinal artery flow. View at www.ccu2e.com

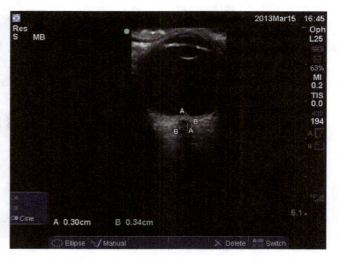

Figure 28-14 Normal optic sheath measurement.

the patient's intracranial pressure rises to a measurement around 7.5 mm at its max. Conversely, as the patient's intracranial pressure is corrected the optic sheath will decrease in size giving the intensivist a noninvasive monitoring system for intracranial pressure. During episodes of severe elevations in intracranial pressure, an echolucent "crescent sign" may develop in the optic nerve.

SUMMARY

Ophthalmic emergencies are often overlooked due to the fact that most intensivists lack the tools necessary to properly examine the eye in the ICU setting and most patients are unable to participate in the ophthalmic examination. Furthermore, it has been shown that during episodes of extremis, such as multisystem trauma, ocular emergencies are often overlooked. Ocular ultrasound is a powerful tool in the hands of an intensivist, it enables the provider to rapidly and reliably assess the patient for ophthalmic emergencies and increased intracranial pressure at the bedside and in real time.

SUGGESTED READING

Blavis M, Theodoro D, Sierzenski PR. A study of bedside ocular ultrasonography in the emergency department. *Acad Emerg Med.* 2002;9(8):791–799.

Byrne SF, Green RL. *Ultrasound of the Eye and Orbit.* 2nd ed. St. Louis, MO: Mosby Year Book; 2002.

Coleman DJ, Silverman RH, Lizzi FL, Rondeau MJ. *Ultrasonography of the Eye and Orbit.* 2nd ed. New York, NY: Lippincott Williams & Wilkins; 2006.

Geeraets T, Launey Y, Martin L, et al. Ultrasonography of the optic nerve sheath may be useful for detecting raised intracranial pressure after severe brain injury. *Intensive Care Med.* 2007;33(10):1704–1711.

Guthoff RF, Berger RW, Winkler P, Helmke K, Chumbley LC. Doppler ultrasonography of the ophthalmic and central retinal vessels. *Arch Ophthalmol.* 1991;109(4):532–536.

Shinar Z, Chan L, Orlinsky M. Use of ocular ultrasound for the evaluation of retinal detachment. *J Emerg Med.* 2011;40(1):53–57.

Yoonessi R, Hussain A, Jang TB. Bedside ocular ultrasound for the detection of retinal detachment in the emergency department. *Acad Emerg Med.* 2010;17(9):913–917.

Appendix A

GLOSSARY

Absorption
Conversion of ultrasound energy into heat.

Active element
Integral part of all ultrasound transducers. Also called a crystal, it is made of piezoelectric material (lead zirconate titanate or PZT) that converts electrical energy into ultrasound and vice versa.

Acoustic variables
Parameters that define a sound wave, such as pressure and density, that changes rhythmically.

AIUM
American Institute of Ultrasound in Medicine.

AIUM 100 mm test object
Standard phantom used for quality assurance.

Akinetic
Organ or its part that should be moving, but is not.

Aliasing
Sampling error characteristic of the inability of pulsed-wave Doppler to accurately measure high-flow velocities.

Ambiguity (range)
Characteristic of continuous-wave Doppler describing its inability to define the position of the sample. Caused by an overlap between transmitting and receiving beams.

A-mode ultrasound
Antiquated mode of ultrasound used to depict the position of a reflector as well as the strength of the returning echo by its amplitude. Seldom used in modern practice.

Amplification (receiver gain)
Increases signal strength in the receiver of the ultrasound system and therefore overall brightness of the image.

Amplitude
The difference between the average value of the acoustic variable and its maximum value through the duration of the sound wave; the "loudness" of the ultrasound.

Analog image
Image on the screen of the cathode-ray tube (TV screen) prior to any computer processing.

Anechoic
Area producing no-echo reflections and appearing black on the ultrasound image.

Archiving
Storage of images.

Array transducer
Transducer with multiple active elements, arranged in a certain order.

Artifact
Image errors or any image that differ from true anatomy of the reflector. Can be caused by malfunction of the ultrasound system, physical limitations of ultrasound, or operator error.

As low as reasonably achievable (ALARA)
AIUM principle, limiting possible bioeffects of acoustic radiation.

APPENDIX A GLOSSARY

Attenuation
Reduction of amplitude of an ultrasound wave, as it propagates through the medium.

Attenuation coefficient
Attenuation in negative decibels per one centimeter (cm) travel. In soft tissues, **0.5 dB/cm/MHz**.

Augmentation
Increase in venous flow with distal compression; a sign of venous patency.

Axial resolution
The minimal distance between two objects positioned along a line parallel to the ultrasound beam where both can be distinguished as separate objects. Defines longitudinal or depth resolution or the distance between two reflectors, measured in millimeters (mm), at which the reflectors are still imaged as separate. It is measured as a half of the ultrasound pulse length, with typical values in diagnostic ultrasound of **0.05–0.5 mm**.

Backing material
Backing also known as damping material consists of the layer of epoxy resin impregnated with tungsten and placed behind the active element of the ultrasound transducer. It improves axial resolution by decreasing pulse duration (after-ringing), much like a hand placed on a guitar string.

Banding
Hyperechoic artifact within the focal zone. Appears as a bright, horizontal stripe.

Beam (ultrasound beam)
Bundle of acoustic radiation transmitted by the transducer, caused by wavelet interactions, and shaped like an hourglass.

Bernoulli equation (simplified)
Converts maximal flow velocity into a pressure gradient used to assess the severity of either valvular or vascular stenosis. Pressure gradient (mm Hg) = $4 \times [(\text{Max flow velocity (m/sec)})]^2$.

Bioeffects
All patient-related effects of acoustic radiation.

Bistable image
Black-and-white image characterized by excessively high contrast and a narrow dynamic range (see **Dynamic range**).

B-mode ultrasound
Imaging mode where echoes are represented by dots with the brightness corresponding to the strength of the signal. Though two-dimensional ultrasound is often called B-mode, this use of the terminology is technically incorrect.

Case
The outer shell of the transducer that prevents electrical injury to the patient and the operator.

Cavitation
Biological effect of the ultrasound on the tissues, caused by expansion and bursting of air bubbles in tissue.

Color Doppler
Pulsed Doppler technique that converts flow velocity information into color. Color Doppler measures the "mean" velocity of the moving reflector.

Color map
Depicts the direction and velocity (sometimes also the variance) of the flow with relationship to the transducer. It is presented as a colored stripe in the corner of the image. The upper color represents maximal flow velocity toward the transducer; the lower color represents maximal flow velocity away from the transducer.

Compensation [also known as TGC or DGC (time or distance gain compensation]
Image processing technique that is used to selectively amplify distant (deeper), and therefore weaker, echoes, making all similar reflectors look the same irrespective of the depth.

Compression
Image processing technique that diminishes the difference between the strongest and the weakest echo signal (the brightest and the darkest parts of the image) by reducing the dynamic range.

Constructive interference
Summation of two in phase sound waves to form a wave with greater amplitude.

Continuous-wave Doppler (CW)
Nonimaging ultrasound modality measuring flow velocity by Doppler shift. One active element continuously emits and the other receives ultrasound signals. CW measures maximal (peak) flow velocity, but cannot measure velocity at a selected point of flow due to signal overlap (range ambiguity).

Convex (curved)-array transducer
Transducer with active elements arranged in an arc and activated in the same manner, as in a linear-array transducer. Curved-array transducers tend to be lower-frequency abdominal transducers characterized by a large image both in the near and far field with a blunted or trapezoid sector image.

Crosstalk
Doppler mirror-image artifact.

Crystal
Active element of the ultrasound transducer.

Curie point (temperature)
The temperature (360°C) at which the active element irreversibly loses its piezoelectric properties. As a result, the transducer should never be exposed to heat sterilization.

Decibel dB (0.1 Bell)
Unit of amplitude or intensity. In audible sound, it is perceived as loudness. The decibel scale is logarithmic and relative such that a 3 dB difference indicates a 2-fold change in the intensity or loudness of a sound, while a 10 dB difference indicates a 10-fold change in the intensity or loudness of a sound.

Demodulation
Image processing technique that makes echo signals suitable for screen display.

Destructive interference
Summation of two counterphase sound waves to form a wave with lesser amplitude.

Diffraction
The ability of sound to spread in more or less concentric circles in all directions. Higher-frequency sounds (ultrasound) diverge less than lower-frequency sounds. Diffraction allows a listener to hear sound around corners.

Digital converter
Converts images into digital format for archiving and display.

Display (screen, glass)
That part of the ultrasound system where the image is observed.

Divergence
Spreading out of the ultrasound beam beyond the focal point. Higher-frequency transducers produce less divergence.

Doppler effect
Change in frequency of the emitted or reflected sound produced by the moving object. If the object is moving toward the receiver, the frequency increases (positive Doppler shift); if it is moving away, the frequency decreases (negative Doppler shift).

Doppler packets (ensembles)
Series of multiple pulses in color Doppler.

Doppler transducer
Utilizes Doppler effect (frequency difference between emitted and reflected ultrasound) to measure the velocity of the moving reflector.

Dosimetry
Study of the biological effects of acoustic radiation.

Duplex imaging
Modality providing an anatomical image and Doppler flow information simultaneously.

Duty factor (DF)
Percentage of time when the transducer emits sound (usually **0.1–1%** in imaging and pulsed Doppler transducers). If DF is 0%, the system is off; if it is 100%, continuous-wave Doppler is on.

dV/dP
Compliance.

Dynamic frequency tuning
An imaging technique utilizing higher-frequency signals to visualize superficial structures and lower-frequency signals to image deeper structures.

Dynamic range
The ratio of the strongest to the weakest signal in the ultrasound system (image gray scale). The narrower the dynamic range, the higher the image contrast.

Dyskinetic
Organ or its part moving in the direction opposite to what is expected (e.g., aneurysmal dilatation during systole).

Echo
Any reflected sound.

Echocardiography (Echo)
Ultrasound study of the heart, so named by cardiologists to differentiate the cardiac examination from other applications of ultrasonography.

Echoencephalography
Archaic A-mode technique used to detect the position of midline brain structures in head trauma.

Energy (acoustic)
Amount of energy delivered by the sound beam into the tissue; proportional to the bioeffects of the ultrasound radiation.

Enhancement
Low-attenuation artifact resulting in a hyperechoic (bright) image distal to a hypoechoic structure.

Five-chamber view
Apical echocardiographic view that visualizes both atria, ventricles, and the aorta. Useful for measurement of stroke volume and aortic flow velocity.

Focus or focal zone
Narrowest area (waist) of the hourglass-shaped ultrasound beam. Technically, the focus is a single point in the middle of the focal zone. The narrower the focus, the better the lateral resolution of the image.

Focusing
Techniques diminishing the size of the focus [acoustic lenses in single-crystal transducers (fixed focus) or electronic focusing on phased-array probes (adjustable focus)]. Focusing improves lateral resolution.

Footprint (acoustic footprint)
Area of the direct contact between the transducer and the surface of the skin. Curved-array probes, used in the abdominal ultrasound, have the largest footprint.

Fourier transform
Form of spectral analysis of Doppler signal.

Frame
One complete sweep of the mechanical or the phased-array two-dimensional transducer. The frame is a basic element of the movie of the mobile reflector.

Frame rate
Number of frames produced by the ultrasound system per unit of time. Measured in Hz, it should not be confused with the frequency of the ultrasound wave. The higher the frame rate, the more fluid the motion and the more "real time" the two-dimensional image. Higher frame rates result in better temporal resolution.

Fraunhofer or far zone
The area of the ultrasound beam distal to the focus where there is beam divergence.

Frequency
The number of sound oscillations (periods) occurring per unit of time (1 sec). It is measured in Hertz (one period per second). This parameter is reciprocal to period (frequency × period = 1). Any sound with frequency of >20,000 Hz is an ultrasound; diagnostic ultrasound frequency is between 2,000,000 and 20,000,000 Hz (2–20 MHz). Sound with frequency <20 Hz is an infrasound. Neither ultrasound nor infrasound is audible.

Fresnel or near zone
The area of the beam between the transducer and the focus (where the beam is converging).

Gain (receiver gain)
A knob controlling amplification. Higher gain increases screen brightness (see **Amplification**).

Ghosting
Doppler artifact caused by registering the movements of adjacent structures rather than the flow of blood.

Harmonic imaging (tissue harmonics, THI)
Technique utilizing echoes with frequencies that are multiples of that of the emitted signal for image formation. The frequency of the emitted sound is known as fundamental (Ff); therefore, harmonic frequency will be the fundamental frequency × 2, × 4, etc. (i.e., if Ff = 2 MHz, then with THI the image will be formed from the echoes with the frequency of 4 MHz). THI signals are generated in the tissues, eliminating some artifacts and very often (but not always) improving overall quality of the image.

Heterogeneous
Displaying multiple echo characteristics throughout the image or area of an image.

Homogeneous
Displaying the same echo characteristics throughout the image or area of an image.

Huygens' principle
Explains the formation of the hourglass shape of the ultrasound beam by the algebraic sum of the constructive and destructive interference of the individual wavelets within the beam.

Hyperechoic
Containing more echoes than usual or expected resulting in a brighter image.

Hyperkinetic
Moving more than expected.

Hypoechoic
Containing fewer echoes than usual or expected resulting in a darker image.

Hypokinetic
Moving less than expected.

Impedance
Calculated by multiplying density and propagation speed, and measured in rayls. Impedance describes the sound-transmitting and sound-reflecting properties of the medium. The boundary between two mediums with different impedance will produce reflection, but the boundary between two mediums with identical impedance will produce no reflection. The greater the difference in impedance, the greater the reflective property of the boundary. Impedances of 1,200,000–1,800,000 rayls are usual at human tissue boundaries.

Intensity
Power over area (measured in watts/cm^2). Power correlates with bioeffects. Multiple ways of measuring intensity exist, but spatial peak-temporal average (SPTA) best predicts thermal energy transfer, and therefore thermal bioeffects.

Jellyfish sign
Chest ultrasound term that describes compressed lung visualized floating in pleural fluid, undulating with the respiratory cycle.

Jet
High-velocity Doppler flow signal (high pitch and amplitude) due to valvular or vascular (arterial) stenosis.

Knobology
Knowledge of the particular controls of the ultrasound. Controls differ greatly from one ultrasound system to another, and require specific training that is unique to each device.

Laminar (parabolic) flow
Bullet-shaped, orderly flow of blood through a vessel, where the blood at the center of the vessel moves faster than that at the periphery, but the movement is in parallel lines. Associated with a spectral Doppler envelope with a thin outer line that delineates a clear space or spectral window. Distinguished from disturbed or turbulent flow associated with an obstructive lesion.

Lateral resolution (angular or transverse resolution)
The minimal distance between two objects positioned along a line perpendicular to the ultrasound beam where both can be distinguished as separate objects.

Line density
The number of ultrasound beams (lines) per unit of surface forming two-dimensional images. Increased line density improves spatial but reduces temporal resolution.

Linear array
Common transducer design that uses a series of piezoelectric elements arrayed in a straight line. Neighboring elements are excited simultaneously, resulting in individual scan lines parallel to one another. Often used in vascular transducers, linear arrays are usually high-frequency probes designed to visualize relatively shallow structures. They are characterized by a square image.

Lobes (side and grating)
Artifacts caused by the echoes of ultrasound beams transmitted in a secondary direction (other than that of the main axis).

Long-axis plane
In echocardiography, the ultrasound plane parallel to the long axis of the left ventricle (LV). This is defined by a line that goes through the LV apex and the center of the base of the LV intersecting with the center of the aortic valve (AoV). In vascular and general ultrasound, the plane that parallels the longest dimension of the anatomical structure.

Lung flapping
Chest ultrasound term that describes compressed lung visualized floating in pleural fluid, undulating with the respiratory cycle.

McConnell sign
Diffuse hypokinesis of the right ventricular (RV) free wall sparing the apex. It is an echocardiographic finding suggestive of pulmonary embolism.

Mirror-image artifact
In two-dimensional imaging, where an object adjacent to a curved-tissue plane is duplicated on the other side of the curved surface in mirror orientation, most commonly seen adjacent to the diaphragm or other highly reflective boundary (mirror). In Doppler imaging, a symmetric spectral image on the opposite side of the baseline from the true signal (crosstalk).

M-mode
An early application of diagnostic ultrasound utilizes a single line of ultrasound interrogation with the signal-plotting reflector position against the time. Useful for high temporal resolution of rapidly moving cardiac structures (i.e., valves).

Moderator band
A normal right ventricular (RV) structure housing the right bundle that can be confused with a mural RV thrombus.

Nyquist frequency limit
Pulsed-wave Doppler frequency at which aliasing occurs. Nyquist frequency limit (kHz) = PRF/2.

Oscillation
A rhythmic change in a parameter that may produce a wave.

PACS
Picture Archiving and Communication System, digital archiving.

Period
Time needed to complete one wave cycle. This parameter is reciprocal to frequency (frequency × period = 1). A typical value in diagnostic ultrasound is 1–5 × 10^{-7} sec.

Phased-array transducers
Transducer design where the image sector is triangular and both focusing and steering are achieved electronically. Relatively high-frequency phased-array transducers offer good real-time images of moving structures. This transducer type has a small acoustic footprint, so it is useful for imaging through the intercostal spaces as in echocardiography.

Pixel
The smallest distinct element of the digital picture or movie. Increased pixel density of the image improves image quality (spatial resolution).

Power Doppler
Color Doppler modality detecting presence of flow regardless of direction or velocity (used to detect presence or absence of flow in ischemic organs). The only color Doppler modality not susceptible to aliasing.

Processing (signal processing)
Conversion of the ultrasound signal into the image.

Pulse repetition frequency (PRF)
The number of pulses emitted by imaging or pulsed-wave (PW) transducer per unit of time (usually 1 sec); measured in Hz. Not to be confused with the frequency of the ultrasound waves.

Pulsed-wave Doppler (PW)
Single crystal Doppler modality offering range resolution but subject to aliasing.

Range equation
Distance to the boundary (mm) = time of flight (μsec) × 0.77 (mm/μsec); used by the ultrasound system to position the object on the screen (13 μsec flight = 1 cm depth).

Range resolution
Ability to identify the location of the pulsed-wave Doppler sample.

Rayleigh scattering
Equal reflection in all directions occurring when the reflector is significantly smaller than the wavelength of the ultrasound.

Reflection
Return of ultrasound beam (energy) from the reflective boundary to the source in a form of an echo.

Refraction
Change in the direction of the ultrasound beam when it encounters a boundary with different propagation speed at an angle. Governed by Snell's law.

Refraction artifact
Side-by-side copy of the anatomical structure.

Regional wall motion abnormalities (RWMA)
Echocardiographic term indicating segmental ventricular wall contractile dysfunction; often associated with coronary artery disease.

Reverberation artifact
Multiple, equally spaced hyperechoic horizontal lines ("Venetian Blinds") perpendicular to the direction of the ultrasound beam. Caused by the presence of two strong adjacent reflectors (i.e., parietal and visceral pleura).

Ring-down (comet-tail) artifact
Solid hyperechoic vertical line (form of reverberations).

Ringing
Internal vibrations in the active element that continue after the echo signal has been received. Ringing deteriorates the image quality. Ringing is reduced by backing of "damping" material in the transducer.

Sagittal view
Long axis.

SAM
Systolic Anterior Motion of the mitral leaflet (sign of hypertrophic cardiomyopathy).

Scattering
Reflection of sound in all directions.

Sector
Imaging area in two-dimensional studies. Limiting sector size improves temporal resolution.

Segmental Doppler, Doppler segmental pressures (DSP) analysis
Flow velocity detection in specific places usually utilized in arterial studies to detect the location of a stenotic area.

Snell's law: Governs refraction (see Refraction). Sine (transmission angle): Sine (incident angle)
Propagation speed A and propagation speed B, where A and B are two layers at the boundary.

Spatial resolution
Ability to show image in more detail (see **Pixel**).

Spectral waveform analysis
Graphic display of flow velocity against time.

Speed of sound
Propagation speed (in soft tissue = 1540 m/sec).

Shadowing
Hypoechoic vertical linear artifact caused by the ultrasound beam encountering a high-attenuation reflector (i.e., gallstone).

Short-axis plane
Plane perpendicular to the long axis also referred to as the transverse or cross-section plane. In echocardiography and vascular ultrasound, the imaged organ appears round.

Transcranial Doppler (TCD)
Doppler study designed to detect the flow velocity of intracranial arteries (can be used to diagnose vasospasm after intracranial trauma or to document brain death).

Transmission
Onward propagation of the unreflected portion of the ultrasound beam at the reflective boundary.

Transverse view
Short-axis plane.

Turbulent flow
Chaotic disorganized flow pattern indicative of vascular stenosis or valvular heart disease. In color Doppler echocardiography, turbulent flow is also called **mosaic** flow pattern.

Two-dimensional imaging (2D)
Two-dimensional images offering gray scale "slices" of anatomic structures in the plane of the steered or serially activated ultrasound beam. Sometimes called B-mode imaging, which is technically incorrect.

Two-dimensional phased-array transducers
Are used to form three-dimensional real-time (four-dimensional) images.

Velocity
Directional speed.

Vortex shed
Area distal to the jet where laminar flow becomes disturbed.

VTI
Velocity Time Integral. Used in calculation of the stroke volume and CO.

Wave
Rhythmical transmission of energy (measured as an oscillating parameter) through the medium.

Wavelength
Length of the single cycle within the wave, measured in the units of distance (mm). Wavelength (mm) = 1.54 (mm)/frequency (MHz) in human tissues (0.1 – 1 mm is typical).

Window (acoustic window)
The part of the body surface through which the ultrasound image is obtained.

Z transform
Algorithm for spectral analysis.

Zone
Ultrasound image for fixed-focus transducers (**near** = from the transducer to the focus, **far** = beneath or deeper then the focus). For multifocus transducers, the zone division is not as well defined. In most portable ICU systems, there are two separate knobs that control near-field and far-field gain. These gain areas correspond to the near and far zones.

Zoom
The ability to enlarge the image of the structure for close-up view. Preprocessing zoom increases the number of pixels per cm^2 and does not deteriorate the spatial resolution; postprocessing zoom increases the size of the individual pixels and worsens the resolution.

Appendix B

DRAFT ULTRASOUND REPORTS BY BODY REGION

The technical and interpretive skills of the physician–sonographer will be judged by peers, including radiologists and cardiologists, and potentially in a court of law if misinterpretations occur and adverse events result. The ultrasound report is an important tool for assuring that physicians document their findings on the data gathered, the interpretation of those data, their decision about what, if anything to do with the acquired information, and the actions, if any, that were taken for the patient's benefit.

Reports should be constructed in such a manner as to provide the necessary information to those interested in understanding the procedure within the context of the patient's condition. The report serves not only for documentation, but as a communication tool from one provider or group of providers to another.

This appendix includes several report templates that can be useful in assuring that the reports of intensive care unit (ICU) ultrasound procedures for different body regions contain the relevant information. Ultimately, each physician–sonographer will find his or her own method of relating findings in the chart to the patient's family and to other medical professionals; however, the following examples provide a reasonable starting point.

I. Ultrasound of the neck or larynx
   A. General information
      i. State the indication for the examination (e.g., neck mapping prior to percutaneous tracheostomy or evaluation of endotracheal tube (ETT) placement)
      ii. Provide patient identifying information (name, age, and medical record number)
      iii. Time the beginning and the end of the examination
   B. Specific information
      i. Report your findings
      ii. Begin with an overall assessment of the technical quality of the study. For example, were all views obtained? Can all the appropriate structures be visualized? Is the study adequate to answer the clinical question?
      iii. The physician should pay particular attention to the stated reason for the examination. The examination details should be described including the anatomic or physiologic findings. For example, the neck was mapped prior to percutaneous tracheostomy. There was a bridging anterior jugular vein at the level of the second tracheal cartilage, and a midline inferior thyroid artery, visualized in transverse and longitudinal views, with two-dimensional and color Doppler. A suitable window for the puncture was located in between the second and third tracheal ring, and the site was marked on the skin
      iv. For neck mapping prior to tracheostomy, make note of the tracheal anatomy itself, such as the number of tracheal rings visible superior to the sternal notch, the width of the trachea at the proposed insertion site, which may impact the size of the inserted tube, and the angle that the trachea makes with the skin surface (e.g., parallel vs. "diving")
      v. Examine the entire trachea for overlying vascular structures, paying particular attention to any aberrant thyroid vessels or bridging jugular vessels. Note the depth of the trachea from the skin
      vi. For ETT placement, assure that the tip is in the trachea and not the esophagus. If the tip is seen, note its distance from the cricoid cartilage and the sternal notch. Perform a bilateral pleural examination to evaluate for sliding pleura
      vii. If anything else is seen during the examination, note it. For example, "the neck was examined

for ETT placement. The visualized portions of the thyroid gland, carotid arteries, and jugular veins were unremarkable. There were no clots present in the jugular veins"
    viii. Summarize the findings in a report and place the report on the chart

II. **Ultrasound examination of the chest**
  A. General information
    i. State the indication for the examination (e.g., to determine the presence, size, and characteristics of a pneumothorax or pleural effusion)
    ii. Provide patient identifying information (name, age, and medical record number)
    iii. Time the beginning and the end of the examination
  B. Specific information
    i. Report your findings
    ii. Begin with an overall assessment of the technical quality of the study. For example, were all views obtained? Can all the appropriate structures be visualized? Is the study adequate to answer the clinical question?)
    iii. The examination details should be described next, including the anatomic or physiologic findings. The physician should pay particular attention to the stated reason for the examination. For example, "The patient underwent ultrasonography of the chest. Interrogation along the midclavicular and anterior axillary lines in a supine position along X to X intercostal spaces demonstrated presence (absence) of the lung sliding consistent with absence (presence) of pneumothorax." The operator should state when the sliding was noted (lung point). There was an anechoic (state ultrasound description) area consistent with the presence of pleural fluid (define anatomical borders of fluid collection, i.e., diaphragm, atelectatic lung, chest wall)
    iv. State the condition of the lung parenchyma (i.e., local or global increased echogenicity consistent with consolidation, alveolar filling)
    v. Describe other important findings (e.g., lymph nodes, vascular abnormalities)
    vi. Summarize you findings in final report
    vii. Define the plan (e.g., proceed with thoracentesis or chest tube placement)

III. **Focused transthoracic echocardiography report**
  A. General information
    i. State the indication for the examination (e.g., volume status assessment, differential diagnosis of shock)
    ii. Provide patient identifying information (name, age, and medical record number)
    iii. Time the beginning and the end of the examination
    iv. Type of examination: two-dimensional, Doppler, color flow, M-mode
  B. Specific information
    i. Report your findings
    ii. Begin with an overall assessment of the technical quality of the study. For example, were all views obtained? Can all the appropriate structures be visualized? Is the study adequate to answer the clinical question?
    iii. The examination details should be described next including the anatomic or physiologic findings. The physician should pay particular attention to the stated reason for the examination describing the findings in a systematic fashion. For example, the patient underwent a two-dimensional, Doppler, and M-mode examination (state only the examinations actually performed and recorded). The technical quality of the study was (e.g., optimal, suboptimal, technically limited, uninterpretable)
    iv. If M-mode was used to measure chamber dimensions and wall thicknesses, present the numbers and state any abnormalities ("the left atrium was enlarged to 5 centimeters")
    v. Proceed with the description of the two-dimensional examination. A two-dimensional study was performed in parasternal, apical, subcostal, and suprasternal views [assess technical quality of each view and state which views could be analyzed and interpreted (e.g., "only the subcostal views could be analyzed due to technical limitations"] (Figure B-1)
    vi. Begin with the left ventricle (LV): State if regional wall motion abnormalities (RWMA) were encountered and in which segments; correlate the abnormalities to the coronary artery anatomy and distribution/territory of blood flow (Figure B-2). For example: "RWMAs consistent with segmental disease were present, involving the mid and apical segments of the anterior free wall of the LV and adjacent apical segments of intraventricular septum." Describe the overall LV function and, if necessary, link it to the previous paragraph ("stated RWMA resulted in a reduction of overall left ventricular performance"). Absence of RWMA may be an important negative ("there were no RWMAs, but overall LV function was decreased"). Define left ventricular ejection fraction (LVEF) and clearly state how the number was estimated (shortening fraction, biplane Simpson). Link it to the prior paragraph ("Left ventricular function was reduced with estimated LVEF of 45%")
    vii. Characterize hydration status by describing LV diastolic dimensions and, if possible, LV compliance. For example, "LV diastolic diameter

APPENDIX B   DRAFT ULTRASOUND REPORTS BY BODY REGION   337

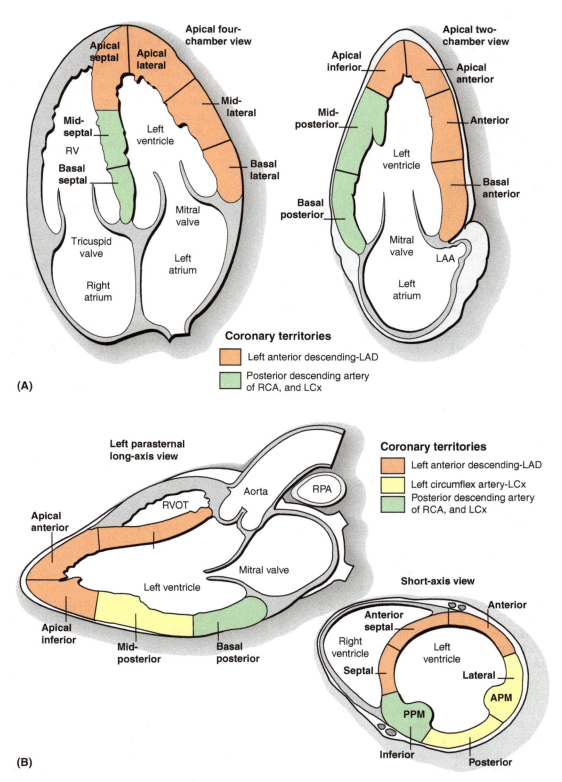

Figure B-1 Standard transthoracic echocardiographic views and regional wall motion abnormalities chart. Reproduced with permission from Yale University Echocardiography laboratory educational website http://www.med.yale.edu/intmed/cardio/echo atlas/contents/index.html.

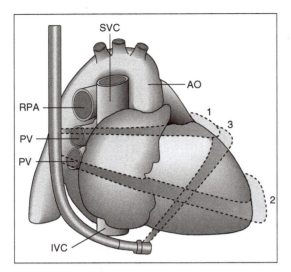

Figure B-2 Standard transesophageal echocardiographic views.

is normal (decreased, increased), and diastolic dysfunction with decreased diastolic compliance was noted"

viii. Describe the visual condition of the mitral and aortic valves, including the number of aortic cusps. The mitral valve apparatus appears normal (calcified) with good (decreased) leaflet separation. If prolapsed, identify which leaflet and give possible explanations. Are abnormal echo densities present or absent? Remember that the presence of any vegetation is a pathologic diagnosis

ix. Describe the right ventricle (RV) in the same systematic manner. Address RV function and condition of the ventricular septum with regard to RV pressure (flatten, paradoxical septal motion). If secondary RV failure is likely, a follow-up venous study to define the possible source of pulmonary embolism may be necessary

x. Characterize the condition of great vessels including the inferior and superior vena cava and aorta

xi. Pericardium: Is a pericardial effusion present? Assure that you define the reasons why it is pericardial and not pleural. Are there findings of pericardial tamponade (e.g., diastolic collapse of RV)? If a pleural effusion is present, some consideration should be given to proceeding with chest ultrasound and thoracentesis

xii. Use Doppler studies to corroborate the findings and link them to previous findings. For example, a Doppler study demonstrated moderate mitral regurgitation consistent with previously described abnormal appearance of mitral valve. You may allow a hypothetical diagnosis here. (The presence of mitral regurgitation and an abnormal echo density on the flow side of the posterior leaflet of the mitral valve makes the diagnosis of mitral valve endocarditis likely.)

xiii. Summarize you findings in a final report. Start by answering the initial reason for the examination in the most direct manner (e.g., decreased RV and LV diastolic dimensions with good preservation of systolic function consistent with hypovolemic shock or RV dilatation, increase in RV systolic pressure with decrease of RV systolic function in all but apical segments, makes the diagnosis of pulmonary embolism a likely explanation for the patient's hypotension)

xiv. Define the future plan. Remember that you are not attempting to perform a definitive diagnostic study but rather incorporating the examination into an overall care plan [e.g., will reassess cardiac function and hydration status after an attempt at fluid resuscitation using 30 cc/kg isotonic fluids or will proceed with anticoagulation and computerized tomography (CT) angiogram of the chest]. May have to link to a procedure or other bedside examination as stated previously (e.g., will use ultrasonic guidance for pericardiocentesis or, because sepsis with an abdominal source is highly suspected, will follow with bedside examination of the abdomen

IV. Transesophageal echocardiography (TEE) report
   A. General information
      i. State the indication for the examination (e.g., volume status assessment, differential diagnosis of shock)
      ii. Provide patient identifying information (name, age, and medical record number)
      iii. Time the beginning and the end of the examination
      iv. Personnel: Physician performing study
      v. Medication used to facilitate the procedure (sedatives, analgesics)
      vi. Equipment and modalities used including which TEE probe and system, two-dimensional imaging, color flow, spectral Doppler
      vii. Complications: Clearly state if none were encountered
   B. Specific information
      i. Report your findings:
      ii. Begin with an overall assessment of the technical quality of the study. For example, were all views obtained (esophageal, transgastric)? Can all the appropriate structures be visualized (great vessels, cardiac chambers, valves)? Is the study adequate to answer the clinical question?
      iii. The examination details should be described next, including the anatomic or physiologic findings. The physician should pay particular

attention to the stated reason for the examination, describing the findings in a systematic fashion. For example, the patient underwent a two-dimensional, Doppler, and M-mode examination (state only the examinations actually performed and recorded). The technical quality of the study was (e.g., optimal, suboptimal, technically limited, uninterpretable)

    iv. Procedural information should begin with the LV and comment on:
        a) Size: (normal, reduced, mildly dilated, moderately dilated, severely dilated)
        b) Global systolic function: (normal, hyperdynamic, mildly reduced moderately reduced, severely reduced)
        c) RWMA: (present or absent, and characterize)
    v. Doppler findings may be included here including:
        a) Color-flow Doppler: Valvular regurgitation may be qualitatively described as well as semiquantitated based upon visualization (absent/none, mild regurgitation, moderate regurgitation, severe regurgitation)
        b) Spectral Doppler: Report pertinent findings of a focused examination (e.g., pulmonary vein flow)
    vi. Summarize the pertinent findings and specifically state how the findings relate to the primary indication for the study. Include a statement about chamber sizes, the LV, and the presence or absence of significant valvular disease. Other categories, such as great vessels and pericardium, may be included if positive findings are noted

V. Ultrasound examination of the abdomen and retroperitoneal space
  A. General information
    i. State the indication for the examination (e.g., differential diagnosis of pain, including location or abnormal laboratory values or other test results)
    ii. Provide patient identifying information (name, age, and medical record number)
    iii. Time the beginning and the end of the examination
    iv. Personnel: Physician performing study
    v. Medication used to facilitate the procedure (sedatives, analgesics)
    vi. Equipment used: Scan performed using ultrasound instrument and a () MHz curved transducer
  B. Specific information
    i. Report your findings
    ii. Begin with an overall assessment of the technical quality of the study. For example, were all views obtained? Can all the appropriate structures be visualized? Is the study adequate to answer the clinical question?
    iii. The examination details should be described next, including the anatomic or physiologic findings. Table B-1 provides an opportunity to present the findings in a tabular rather than

TABLE B-1

An Example of a Templated Report for Detailing an Abdominal and Pelvic Ultrasound in the Intensive Care Unit

Structure	Normal	Abnormal	Not Seen	Comments
Liver				
Gallbladder				☐ Stones, ☐ sludge, ☐ wall thickness___mm ☐ CBD dilated___mm, Other:
Spleen				
Left kidney				
Left adrenal				
Left ovary				
Bladder				
Pelvic region				
Right kidney				
Right adrenal				
Right ovary				
IVC/aorta				
Pancreas				
Duodenum				
Ascites	☐ Absent	☐ Present		
Pericardium				
Left costophrenic angle				
Right costophrenic angle				
Other				

CBD, common bile ducts; IVC, inferior vena cava.

descriptive form. This approach adds the value of assuring that all elements of the examination are addressed in the template and that appropriate descriptors are used between different physicians in a given department. The physician should pay particular attention to the stated reason for the examination describing the findings in a systematic fashion. The technical quality of the study was (e.g., optimal, suboptimal, technically limited, uninterpretable)

    iv. Summarize you findings in a final report and suggest repeat examinations if necessary

VI. Venous duplex examination of the extremities

A. General information
  i. State the indication for the examination (e.g., assess for presence of deep venous thrombosis in a patient with significant oxygen requirement and possible pulmonary embolism)
  ii. Provide patient identifying information (name, age, and medical record number)
  iii. Time the beginning and the end of the examination
  iv. Personnel: Physician performing study
  v. Equipment used: Scan performed using ultrasound instrument and a () MHz curved transducer

B. Specific information
  i. Report your findings
  ii. Begin with an overall assessment of the technical quality of the study. For example, were all views obtained? Can all the appropriate structures be visualized? Is the study adequate to answer the clinical question?
  iii. The examination details should be described next, including the anatomic or physiologic findings
  iv. Venous duplex examination of the venous system of the (right, left, both) lower (upper) extremity (extremities) was/were performed using the duplex ultrasound instrument and a () MHz (linear/curved) phased-array transducer
  v. Gray-scale imaging demonstrated (good) incomplete compressibility of the (name the abnormal vessels) veins. Intraluminal echogenic material was seen in the (location) veins. The proximal tip of the intraluminal material was (mobile/stable)
  vi. Doppler waveform analysis demonstrated (did not demonstrate) loss of phasicity with respiration/no flow signal) suggesting outflow obstruction
  vii. Color-flow imaging demonstrated (did not demonstrate) abnormal/absent flow
  viii. Summarize your findings in final report and suggest repeat examinations if necessary (e.g., duplex ultrasound findings consistent with deep venous thrombosis involving (name the veins) of the (right/left/both) lower extremity (extremities) or no evidence of deep venous thrombosis)

VII. Procedures

A. Vascular access procedures
  i. General information
    a) State the indication for the examination (e.g., ultrasound-guided vascular access for shock)
    b) Provide patient identifying information (name, age, and medical record number)
    c) Time the beginning and the end of the examination
    d) Personnel: Physician performing study
    e) Equipment used: Scan performed using ultrasound instrument and a () MHz curved transducer
    f) Complications: Clearly state if none were encountered
  ii. Specific information
    a) Preprocedure ultrasound assessment: Patients (state vein location, e.g., internal jugular, common femoral, deep veins of upper extremities) were assessed with ultrasound for patency and position, and marked
    b) If static guidance was used, that is all that should be reported, and representative image should be retained for the chart
    c) If dynamic guidance was used, the following report may be helpful: The patient was placed in (state position), prepped in the usual manner, and placed under sterile drapes. An ultrasound probe was placed into the sterile sheath and sterile ultrasound gel was applied to the site of the procedure. (Name vein) was adequately (or not) visualized. Under direct ultrasound visualization, the needle was positioned into the vein, good blood return assured. A J-wire easily passed, with the position of the wire in the vein, was (was not) confirmed ultrasonographically. Proceed with the remaining description of the modified Seldinger technique
    d) Remember that this may link with an ultrasound of the chest if axillary, subclavian, or internal jugular veins were cannulated to rule out procedure-related complications (i.e., pneumothorax), particularly if immediate use of the line is highly desirable

B. Thoracentesis, paracentesis, pericardiocentesis
  i. General information
    a) State the indication for the examination (e.g., suspected empyema or spontaneous peritonitis)
    b) Provide patient identifying information (name, age, and medical record number)

c) Time the beginning and the end of the examination
d) Personnel: Physician performing study
e) Equipment used: Scan performed using ultrasound instrument and a () MHz curved transducer
f) Complications: Clearly state if none were encountered

ii. Specific information
a) Preprocedure ultrasound assessment: Patient was placed in (state position). A collection of pleural (peritoneal) fluid was visualized via ultrasound (state anatomical boundaries and ultrasound characteristics of the fluid and its estimated volume) and marked. For pericardiocentesis, state which echo view was used
b) If static guidance was used, that is all that should be reported, and representative image should be retained for the chart
c) If dynamic guidance was used, the following report may be helpful: The patient was placed in (state position), prepped in the usual manner, and placed under sterile drapes. An ultrasound probe was placed into the sterile sheath and sterile ultrasound gel was applied to the site of the procedure. A fluid collection was adequately (or not) visualized. Under direct ultrasound visualization, the needle was positioned into the collection and good fluid return assured. Proceed with describing procedure. If a pigtail catheter or other device is retained, remember to state if its position was confirmed by the ultrasound

INDEX

Note: Page numbers followed by *f* and *t* indicates figures and tables, respectively.

A
Abdominal procedures
  fluid analysis, 287–288
  invasive, guidance for, 285
  transducer selection for, 285
Abdominal ultrasound, 50, 50*f*
  AIUM indications for, 220
  anatomic correlation, 220
  biliary ultrasound, 228–231
  gastrointestinal tract ultrasound, 231
  image orientation, 220
  liver ultrasound, 224–226
  overview, 219
  pneumoperitoneum identification, 222
  of retroperitoneum, 231
  splenic ultrasound, 227–228
Abdominal vasculature ultrasound, 231–233
Abscess drainage
  catheter for, 289
  complications associated with, 290
  indications and contraindications for, 288–289
  pigtail catheter drainage of, 289
  site of, 289
  ultrasound guidance role in, 288
Absolute hypovolemia, 105
Acoustic artifacts, 33
Acoustic enhancement, 35*f*
Acoustic shadowing, 35*f*
Acute acalculous cholecystitis (AAC), 291
Acute cor pulmonale (ACP)
  apical four-chamber view, 106*f*
  causes of, 116, 116*t*
  clinical scenarios leading to
    acute RV failure of sepsis, 123–124
    ARDS, 123
    massive PE, 122–123
    recruitment maneuvers, 123
    RV infarction, 124
  definition of, 115
  parasternal short-axis view, 106*f*
  and pulmonary hypertension, 121–122
  volume resuscitation in, 105
  vs. chronic right heart failure, 121
Acute dyspnea, GDE for, 60
Acute myocardial infarction (AMI)
  cardiogenic shock in, 139–140, 140*f*
  echocardiography for
    technical and administrative issues in, 135, 137
  left bundle branch block, 138
  left ventricular thrombi, 141–142, 142*f*
  and murmur, 138–139
  myocardial rupture following, 138–139
  non–ST-segment elevation MIs, 140
  pacemaker therapy for, 137–138
  postmyocardial infarction pericarditis, 140
  symptoms of, 135, 137
  true posterior MIs, 140–141
Acute nephritic syndrome, 292
Acute renal failure
  cause of, 238
  respiratory failure with, 292
Acute respiratory distress syndrome (ARDS), 105, 123
Acute respiratory failure, lung ultrasonography in, 214
Acute RV failure of sepsis, 123–124
Acute vision loss, 322–323
Acute visual disturbance, 322
Adult respiratory distress syndrome (ARDS), 209
Advanced CCE
  examination
    apical five-chamber view, 72–73, 73*f*
    apical four-chamber view, 72
    apical three-chamber view, 73, 74, 74*f*
    apical two-chamber view, 73, 73*f*
    IVC longitudinal view, 74
    parasternal long-axis view, 71
    parasternal short-axis view, 71–72, 72*f*
    right ventricular inflow and outflow long-axis views, 71, 71*f*
    subcostal four-chamber view, 74, 74*f*
    subcostal short-axis view, 74, 74*f*
    suprasternal and supraclavicular views, 75, 75*f*
  proficiency in, 65, 163
Aliasing, 18–19
  methods of controlling, 19–20, 20*f*
  Nyquist limit and, 19*f*
A lines, lung ultrasonography, 211
Allograft dysfunction, 293
American College of Chest Physicians (ACCP), 38
American College of Graduate Medical Education (ACGME), 39
A-mode ultrasound, 305
Anatomic correlation, in abdominal ultrasound, 220
Anemia, 293
Annular phased arrays, 27
Anterior mediastinal biopsy, 278
Aortic duplication, 36*f*
Aortic injury, 177–178
Aortic regurgitation (AR), evaluation of, 166–167, 167*f*
Aortic stenosis (AS)
  causes of, 165
  methods for identifying, 165–166, 165*f*
Arrhythmogenic right ventricular dysplasia (ARVD), 158–159
Arterial catheters
  for managing ICU conditions, 303
  placement factors associated with, 312
  radial approach, 312–313
Arterial injuries, 265
Arterial occlusion, 264–265
Arterial stenosis
  carotid duplex examination of
    critical degrees of, 264
    equipments for, 266
    examination protocol, 266
  diagnosis of, 267
Artifacts
  acoustic, 33
  causes of, 33
  terminology, 33*t*
  ultrasound, 33–36, 34*t*
Artifacts and image alterations, 31
Ascites evaluation, 286
Athlete's heart, 156
Autosomal-dominant polycystic kidney disease, 241
Axial resolution, 16
Axillary plexus ultrasound image, 300
Axillary vein
  for central venous access, 311
  ultrasound-guided cannulation of, 312

B
Basic CCE
  examination
    apical four-chamber view, 69, 69*f*
    IVC longitudinal view, 70–71, 70*f*
    parasternal long-axis view, 67–68, 67*f*
    parasternal short-axis midventricular view, 68–69, 68*f*
    subcostal four-chamber view, 69–70, 70*f*
  proficiency in, 65, 163

INDEX

Bedside critical care ultrasonography in PICU
  airway ultrasound, 50
  benefits of CVLs, 44
  FAST examination, 50, 50f
  focused echocardiography, 45–47
  indications for, 44t
  novel uses of, 51–52
  procedural ultrasound, 51
  thoracic ultrasound
    for lung consolidation, 49–50
    for neonatal RDS, 50
    for pleural effusion, 47–48, 47f
    for pneumothorax assessment, 48–49
  vascular access, 43–45, 44f, 45f
  value of, 3
Bedside echocardiography, 45–46, 127, 137, 140–141, 164
Biliary ultrasound, 228–231
Biopsy of lung
  contraindications to, 277
  patient positioning for, 273
  ultrasound guidance for, 278
Biplane Simpson's method of left ventricular assessment, 92–94, 94f
  CO calculations, 92
  endocardial border, 94f
  end systolic and end diastolic Frames, 93t
  TTE calculations, 92
Bladder
  bladder volume, 247
  color Doppler, 237–238
  diverticuli, 247
  Foley catheter localization, 246, 247
  shape and appearance of, 235–236
  transabdominal, 236–237
  ultrasound of, 247
Bleeding disorders, 293
B lines, lung ultrasonography, 211–212
Blunt cardiac injury
  sequela after, 175–176
  traumatic injuries, 175
B-mode ultrasound, 305
Brachial plexus block
  approaches and probes for, 298–299
  from cervical roots, 298
  complications from, 299
  pain control
    axillary approach for, 299
    infraclavicular approach for, 299
    supraclavicular approach for, 299

C

Cardiac arrest and TEE, 78
Cardiac function assessment, 46
Cardiac output calculation, with pulsed-wave Doppler, 94–95
Cardiac tamponade
  clinical and laboratory investigation of, 128–129
  definition of, 127
  echocardiography in
    pericardial effusions, 129, 130f, 131f
    pleural effusions, 129
    two-dimensional, 131–132, 131f, 132f
  epidemiology and etiology of, 128
  pathophysiology of, 127–128
  pulsed-wave Doppler imaging, 132–133, 132f, 133f
  treatment of, 133, 133f
Cardiac trauma
  diagnostic approach to, 180, 180f
  transthoracic echocardiogram of, 175
    aortic injury, 177–178
    electrical and heat stroke-related cardiac injury, 179–180
    penetrating cardiac injury, 176–177
    pericardial effusion, 178–179, 178f
    septal and valvular injury, 176
Cardiogenic shock and AMI, 139–140, 140f
Cardiomyopathy (CMP)
  definition of, 143
  dilated (See Dilated cardiomyopathies)
  endocardial fibroelastosis, 159
  hypertrophic (See Hypertrophic CMP)
  left ventricular noncompaction, 159–160, 159f
  restrictive (See Restrictive CMP)
  transient LV apical ballooning syndrome, 160–161, 161f
  WHO classification of, 143, 144t
Carotid duplex examination, 266
Catheter
  arterial, 303, 312–313
  long-term complications of, 314
  for pain control, 303–301
  for paracentesis, 287
  placement for abscess drainage, 289
  in prostatic urethra, 246
  safe path for, 289
  sonography use for, 276
  tip malposition, 315–316
  for trauma/vascular insufficiency, 298–299
Catheter-associated thrombosis, 257, 268
Cavitation, 22
Central neuraxial blocks, 297–298
Central venous cannulation
  ultrasound-guided procedures for, 305–306
Central venous catheterization
  complications, 304
  insertion, ultrasound guidance for, 312
  placement, complications of, 303
Central venous line (CVL) placement, 44, 44f
Cervical lymph node, 31
Chest x-rays (CXR), 129
Chronic renal failure (CRF), 238–239, 293
Circle of Willis, schematics, 269
Cleaning transabdominal transducers, 220
Coaxial cutting needle technique, 277
Color-flow Doppler, 20–21, 21f
  of palmar arch, 313
  technical issues related to, 66
  of urinary bladder, 238
  in vascular applications, 305
Common carotid arteries
  carotid duplex examination of
    equipments for, 266
    examination protocol, 266
  in cervical region, 263
Competence
  CCUS elements required for, 38
  cognitive elements required for, 37
  definition of, 38
  with "on the job" training, 37
Continuous wave (CW) Doppler, 18, 18f
  technical issues related to, 66
Continuous-wave doppler transducer, components of, 24, 24f
Convex sequential-array probes
  for thoracic sonography, 273
Critical care echocardiography (CCE), 65
  advanced (See Advanced CCE)
  basic (See Basic CCE)
  Doppler measurement, 66
Critical care TEE
  endotracheally intubated, 78
  equipments, 79
  examination, 79–80, 80f
  indications for, 78
  in large ICUs, 77
  patient selection and preparation for, 78
  probe cleaning, 86
  probe insertion, 79
  training in, 77, 78
  transducer movement, 79
  value of, 77
  view orientation, 79
  views
    fractional area change, 84, 84f
    midesophageal ascending aorta short-axis view, 85–86, 86f
    midesophageal AV long-axis view, 81, 81f
    midesophageal AV short-axis view, 80, 80f
    midesophageal bicaval view, 81, 81f
    midesophageal four-chamber view, 82, 82f
    midesophageal long-axis view, 82–83, 83f
    MV inflow, 83
    SVC M mode view, 81f, 82
    TDI, 83
    transgastric long-axis view, 84, 85f
    transgastric midpapillary short-axis view, 83, 84f
  vs. standard cardiology TEE, 77

Critical care ultrasonography (CCUS)
  epidural analgesia, 298
  lower extremity blocks, 300–301
  skills required for, 37
  training in
    challenge to attending level intensivist, 37
    competence (*See* Competence)
    international patterns of, 39–41
    recommendations for, 38–39, 39t, 40t
  truncal blocks, 301–302
  upper extremity blocks, 298–299
Critical care ultrasound
  advantages of, 4
  bedside chest ultrasound, 4
  challenges of, 5–6
  factors influencing, 6
  hand-carried ultrasound devices, 4
  impact on
    cost reduction, 7
    patient experience, 6–7
    population health, 7
  neonates and children, 5
  provider training and education, 6
  pulmonary ultrasonography, 4
  role of "FADE," 4, 5
  role of "FAST," 5
  and triple aim, 6, 6f
CVP, 106–107

D
Deep venous thrombosis (DVT)
  diagnosis of, 257
  diagnostic criteria for, 260
  equipment requirements for, 261–262
  flow characteristics, 261–262
  patient positioning, 261
  risk factors associated with development of, 257
  sequelae of, 257
  transverse compressions, 261–262
Depth-gain compensation (DGC), 29
Dilated cardiomyopathies
  classification of, 143
  echocardiographic diagnosis of, 143–144
    aortic root motion, 146f, 147
    aortic valve opening and closing, 146f, 147
    diasystolic function assessment, 149–152, 150f, 151f, 152f
    Doppler assessment, 148
    e-point septal separation, 146f, 147
    LV dilatation, 144–145, 145f
    LV thrombus, 148, 148f
    LV wall motion and thickening, 145–147, 146f
    mitral regurgitation, 147, 147f
    M-mode features, 146f, 147
    myocardial performance index (MPI), 152
    right heart-related findings, 148, 149f
    systolic and diastolic performance, 148
    systolic function assessment, 149
    two-dimensional imaging, 152–153
  etiologies of, 143
Doppler modalities
  continuous-wave Doppler, 18, 18f
  pulsed-wave Doppler, 18, 18f
Doppler phenomenon, 17, 17f
Doppler shift and transducer frequency, 19
Doppler training, 163
Doppler ultrasound
  bullet-like pattern, 19–20, 20f
  hypertrophic CMP, 154–155, 155f
  mitral stenosis (MS), 168–169, 169f
  restrictive CMP, 158, 158f
  technical issues related to, 66
Duplex scanners, 258, 263
Dynamic echocardiographic parameter estimation
  mechanically ventilated patient, 109–111
    induced preload changes, 111
    IVC and SVC diameter changes, 109–110
    respiratory changes of LV SV, 109
  spontaneously breathing patients, 112–114
    respiratory cyclic variations of pulse pressure, 112
    response to PLR, 112–113
    SV, 114

E
Echo, 9
Echocardiographic image of phased-array probe, 26f
Ectopic pregnancy
  blood flow in heart of, 252
  fluid in endometrial canal, 252
  with IUPs, 251–253
  TAS and EV ultrasound of, 252–253
Electrical and heat stroke-related cardiac injury, 179–180
Emphysematous pyelonephritis, 244
Endocardial fibroelastosis, 159
Endotracheal intubation, 187–191
Endotracheal tube, 52f
Endotracheal tube malposition, 188
Endotracheal tube (ETT) position, 187–191
  algorithm for determining satisfactory, 191
  pleural ultrasound, 190–191
  translaryngeal 2D ultrasound for visualization of, 189
Endovaginal (EV) ultrasound approach, 250–251
Epidural analgesia for pain control, 298
Euvolemia, 105
Extremity blocks, for pain control
  lower, 300–301
  upper, 298–299
Eye, 319, 320f
  imaging technique, 319–320, 320f
  optic sheath, 320f

F
"FADE" (Fast Assessment Diagnostic Echocardiography), 4, 5
Femoral artery
  and compressed common femoral vein, 260
  pseudoaneurysm, 265
Femoral nerve blockage, 300–301
Femoral vein
  acute deep venous thrombosis, 259
  and artery, relationship between, 259
  color-flow image of, 261
  and common femoral artery, 260
  free-floating thrombus in, 260
  longitudinal view of, 312
  ultrasound-guided cannulation of, 311–312
Femoral vessels
  superficial and deep, 259
  transverse view of, 259
Fluid analysis, 287–288
Fluid challenge *vs.* volume responsiveness, 105–106
Fluid resuscitation
  benefits and pitfalls of, 105
  pressure parameters, 106–107
Focused abdominal sonography in trauma (FAST), 242
  for hemoperitoneum detection, 242
  pneumoperitoneum identification, 222
Focused assessment with sonography for trauma (FAST), 5, 50, 50f
Focused echocardiography, pediatric cardiac ICU, 45–47
Focused transthoracic echocardiography report, 336–338
Foley catheter
  in collapsed bladder, 236
  critically ill patients with draining indwelling, 237
  distended bladder with obstructed, 246–247
  localization, 246, 247
Fractional area change, 97–98, 98f
Fractional shortening and M-mode derived modality, 96–97, 97f
Frank–Starling curve, 106f
Free-floating thrombus, in femoral vein, 260

G
Gallbladder
  drainage of complications associated with, 292
  indications and contraindications for, 291
  procedure, 291–292
Gastrointestinal tract ultrasound, 231

Goal-directed echocardiography (GDE), 57
  for acute dyspnea and hypotension, 60
  clinical applications of, 58–61
  competence in
    skills in clinical syndrome recognition, 59
    skills in image interpretation, 58
  definition of, 57
  for hypotension and urosepsis, 58
  for hypotension related to urosepsis, 61
  for hypotension with left ventricular dysfunction, 61
  limitations of, 61–62
  for pneumonia with septic shock, 62
  for progressive hypotension, 60
  for severe hypotension and respiratory distress, 60
  for severe hypotension and respiratory failure, 59
  with TEE, 57, 58
  training in, 58
  with TTE, 57, 58
Globe rupture, 321
Guitar string vibration, 9, 10f

H
Healthcare delivery, essential areas of, 3
Healthcare improvement, paradigm shift for, 3
Heart
  M-mode examination of, 25f
  standard tomographic views of, 66
Hemodynamic failure assessment and TEE, 78
Hemoptysis, 277
Hemorrhage
  in nonpregnant patient, 253
  from pregnancy, 251–253
Hemorrhagic cysts, 253
High-frequency ultrasound
  for percutaneous vascular access, 305
High-grade stenosis, ultrasound manifestation of, 264
Horseshoe kidney, risk for, 293
Hydronephrosis
  categorization of, 239
  kidney, 238, 239, 241
  mild/moderate, 240
  in patients with ARF, 239
Hyperechoic (white) calcifications, in kidney, 245
Hypertrophic CMP
  apical, 155
  and athlete's heart, 156
  clinical features of, 153
  Doppler assessment of, 154–155, 155f
  of elderly, 155
  M-mode and two-dimensional assessment of, 153–154, 153f
  secondary, 155–156
Hypoechoic liver lesion, 291

Hypotension
  GDE for, 60
  with left ventricular dysfunction, GDE for, 61
  related to urosepsis, GDE for, 61
  and urosepsis, GDE for, 58
Hypovolemia
  absolute/relative, 105
  fluid resuscitation for, 105

I
Image formation, 14
Imaging transducer, components of, 24f
Imaging transducers, 23
Infective endocarditis, evaluation of, 171–173, 172f
Inferior vena cava (IVC) diameter assessment, 47, 47f
Infraclavicular plexus, 299
Institute for Healthcare Improvement's (IHI)
  domains of quality improvement, 3, 4f
  "Triple Aim Initiative"
    goal of, 3
    key elements of quality in, 5f
    schematic of, 4f
Institute of Medicine, domain definitions of, 4t
Intensive care ultrasound. See Critical care ultrasound
Intercostal nerve blocks (ICBs), 301
Intercostal nerves, branches of, 301
Internal jugular (IJ) vein
  accessed with an introducer needle, 44f
  2D image through, 305
  with intraluminal guidewire, 45f
  longitudinal view through, 308
  transverse view through right, 306
  ultrasound-guided cannulation of, 308–310
Interventional chest sonography
  patient positioning for, 273
Intraarterial (carotid) embolus, 267
Intracranial pressure, 324-325, 325f
Intrauterine pregnancy (IUP), 251–253
Invasive hemodynamic monitoring, 257
Ionizing radiation exposure, pediatric patients, 7
IV access algorithm, 315

K
Kidney
  anatomy of, 235–236
  Color Doppler, 242
  hydronephrosis, 238, 239, 241
  hyperechoic (white) calcifications, 245
  longitudinal diameter and transverse plane, 237
  peritransplant fluid collections, 242
  renal failure, 238–241
  renal obstruction, 239
  transplanted, ultrasound evaluation of AR and ATN, 241–242

  ultrasound examination of conditions affecting, 237
  ureteral obstruction, 239

L
Iatrogenic femoral artery pseudoaneurysm, 265
Left atrial dilatation, 148
Left atrial pressure (LAP) estimation
  ASE algorithm for, 100f
  2D echocardiography, 99
Left bundle branch block (LBBB), 138
Left bundle branch block and AMI, 138
Left internal jugular vein with juxtaposed carotid artery, 44f
Left ventricle, segments of, 90–91, 91f, 136f
Left ventricular diasystolic function assessment
  ASE algorithm, 102f
  lung ultrasonography, 101
  LV filling pressures, 99, 101
  measurement techniques, 99–101, 100f
  problems with, 101–102
Left ventricular (LV) dysfunctions, 89
Left ventricular end-diastolic area (LVEDA), 107, 107f
Left ventricular end-systolic area (LVESA), 107, 107f
Left ventricular enlargement, 46
Left ventricular (LV) functions, 89
Left ventricular hypertrophy (LVH), 156t
Left ventricular noncompaction, 159–160, 159f
Left ventricular outflow tract (LVOT), 95, 95f
Left ventricular systolic function
  estimates of, 90
  and LVEF assessment, 90
  qualitative assessment of
    with echocardiography, 92–96
    with standard 17-segment model, 90–92
  semiquantitative methods of assessing
    3D image, 98–99, 99f
    fractional area change, 97–98, 98f
    fractional shortening and M-mode derived modality, 96–97, 97f
Left ventricular thrombi and AMI, 141–142, 142f
Lens dislocation, 321, 322f
Linear array transducer, 324
Linear sequential arrays, 26f
Linear sequential array transducer, vascular image of, 26f
Liver biopsy
  complication of, 291
  contraindications for, 290
  of hypoechoic liver lesion, 291
  indications for, 290
  mortality related to, 291
  needles used in, 290

percutaneous, 290
specimen adequacy, 290
transthoracic approach, 291
ultrasound-guided free-hand technique for, 290
Liver ultrasound, 224–226
Local anesthetic bupivacaine, 297
Local anesthetic solution, 297
Loculated effusions, pleural ultrasound, 202
Lower extremity
  arterial anatomy of, 263
  arterial duplex examination of, 266–267
  blockage of
    femoral nerve, 300
    sciatic nerve, 300–301
  venous examination, 261
  venous systems of, 258
Lower extremity blocks, for pain control, 300–301
Low-frequency ultrasound, 304
Lung consolidation
  with air-filled bronchi, 49f
  thoracic ultrasound for, 49–50
Lung lesions
  risks of biopsy of
    hemoptysis, 277
    pneumothorax, 277
  ultrasound guidance for biopsy of, 278
Lung sliding, 208–210
Lung ultrasonography
  advanced applications of, 215
  basic principles of, 207
  B lines, 211–212
  clinical applications of, 214–215
  consolidated lung, 212–213
  key findings of, 208–214
  limitations of, 215–216
  A lines, 211
  lung point, 210–211
  lung sliding, 208–210
  machine requirements, 207–208
  performance of, 208
  pleural effusion, 213
  sonographic signs on, 47t

M

Mechanically ventilated patients
  dynamic echocardiographic parameter estimation, 109–111
    induced preload changes, 111
    IVC and SVC diameter changes, 109–110
    respiratory changes of LV SV, 109
    traumatic pneumothorax in, 274
  vs. spontaneously breathing patient, 108–109
Mechanical scanning and phased-array probes, 25f
Medical errors, 3
Middle cerebral artery (MCA)
  waveforms, 269

Mitral regurgitation (MR), 169–171, 170f
Mitral stenosis (MS)
  Doppler measurements of, 168–169, 169f
  hemodynamic consequences of, 168
Mitral valve inflow tracing, 101f
Multidimensional transducers, 27
Murmur and AMI, 138–139
Myocardial rupture and AMI, 138–139

N

Nasogastric tube (NGT), 231
Neonatal respiratory distress syndrome, lung ultrasound for, 50
Neonates and children, critical care ultrasound for, 5
Nephrotic syndrome, 192
Nonimaging continuous-wave (CW) Doppler transducers, 23
Non–ST-segment elevation MIs, 140
Nyquist limit and aliasing, 19, 19f, 19f

O

Ocular ultrasound, 319–325
  bio-occlusive dressing for, 320f
  clinical applications, 320–321
  foreign bodies, 322, 322f
  globe rupture, 321
  lens dislocation, 321, 322f
  periorbital trauma, 321
  vitreous hemorrhage, 321
Ovarian cysts
  blood loss from, 253
  pain due to, 254
  thrombus and free fluid, 253

P

Pacemaker therapy for AMI, 137–138
Pain control, 297
  epidural analgesia, 298
  lower extremity blocks, 300–301
  truncal blocks, 301–302
  upper extremity blocks, 298–299
PAPs, measurement of, 121–122
Paracentesis
  complications associated with, 288
  equipment and procedure tray for, 285
  indications and contraindications for, 285
  optimal site for, 285–286
  procedure
    abdominal cavity screening, 286
    free-hand technique, 287
    needle tip position, 287
Paranasal sinuses, ultrasound evaluation of
  anatomy of, 186
  technique for, 185–187
Parasternal long-axis focused echocardiography, 46f
Parasternal short-axis focused echocardiography, 46f
Parenchymal homogeneity, 235

Patient experience, critical care ultrasound, 6–7
PE and ACP, 122–123
Pediatric intensive care unit (PICU)
  equipments, 43
  portable notebook-type ultrasound system, 43
  problems encountered in, 43
Pediatric intensive care unit (PICU), bedside ultrasonography in
  airway ultrasound, 50
  benefits of CVLs, 44
  FAST examination, 50, 50f
  focused echocardiography, 45–47
  indications for, 44t
  novel uses of, 51–52
  procedural ultrasound, 51
  thoracic ultrasound
    for lung consolidation, 49–50
    for neonatal RDS, 50
    for pleural effusion, 47–48, 47f
    for pneumothorax assessment, 48–49
  vascular access, 43–45, 44f, 45f
Pelvic inflammatory disease (PID), 253
Pelvis
  anatomy of, 249
  infection source from, 253
  ultrasound examination of EV approach, 250–251
Penetrating cardiac injury, 176–177
Percutaneous cholecystostomy, 291
Percutaneous dilatational
  cannulation of trachea, 193
  examination of anterior neck prior to surgical, 192
  hypercarbia, 192
  malposition in, 192
  selection of insertion site, 193
  tracheostomy (PDT), 191–194
  ultrasound techniques for, 192–194
Pericardial effusion, 45f, 178–179, 178f
Pericardiocentesis, 133
  complication of, 278
  pitfall of, 283
Periorbital trauma, 321
Peripheral arterial hemodynamics, 263
Peripheral IV access, 316
Peripherally inserted central venous catheter (PICC), 303
  infection risk, 314
  insertion of, 315
  line kits, 314
  placement methods, 314
  thrombosis, 314
  tip malposition scanning, 304, 316
Peripheral vascular disease, baseline assessment of, 263
Perirenal hematoma, 243
Phased-array probes, 25–26
  echocardiographic image, 26f
Physician-sonographer, technical and interpretive skills of, 335

INDEX

Pleural effusion
  biopsy of, 278
  diagnostic sonography of, 274
  lung ultrasonography, 213
  patient positioning for, 273
  pleural ultrasound for, 198–204
  thoracic ultrasound for, 47–48, 47f
Pleural sliding, differential diagnosis for absence of, 49, 49f
Pleural ultrasound
  control for, 197
  ETT position, 189–191
  general considerations in, 197
  normal pleural examination, 198
  pleural effusion in, 198–204
Pneumonia with septic shock, GDE for, 62
Pneumoperitoneum, FAST identification, 222
Pneumothorax, 49f
  associated with thoracentesis, 274
  due to biopsy of lung lesions, 277
  due to ICB, 301–302
  lung ultrasonography for, 214–215
Pneumothorax assessment, thoracic ultrasound for, 48–49
Popliteal fossa block, 300
Population health, critical care ultrasound, 7
Portable ultrasonography machine
  for critical care, 298
  neuraxial blocks scanning by, 297
Postmyocardial infarction pericarditis, 140
Postrenal ARF, 239
Postural maneuvers, 186
Preload responsiveness identification, 124
Pretracheal soft tissue (PST) swelling, 189
Preventable medical errors (PME), 304
Procedural ultrasound, 51, 51t
Progressive hypotension, GDE for, 60
Prostatic urethra, catheter in, 246
Prosthetic valve function evaluation, 171
Providers and intensivists, tension between, 6
Pseudoaneurysm, 265
Pulmonary artery occlusion pressure (PAOP), 105, 106–107
Pulmonary ultrasonography, 4
Pulmonic valve (PV), evaluation of, 164–165, 165f
Pulsed Doppler transducer, 27
Pulse duration (PD), 16
Pulsed-wave Doppler (PWD), 18, 18f
  RVOT calculation with, 96
  stroke volume and cardiac output calculation with, 94–95
  VTI and LVOT calculation with, 95
Pulsed-wave parameters, 16, 16t
Pulse repetition period (PRP), 16
Pulse ultrasound, 16–17
Pyonephrosis, 243–244

Q
Quality assurance, 21

R
Radial artery catheterization, 312–313
Rapidly progressive glomerulonephritis (RPGN), 292
Receiver gain, 29, 29f
Receiver/processor, functions of, 29t
  signal amplification, 29, 29f
  signal compensation, 29, 30f
  signal compression, 29–31, 30f
  signal demodulation, 31, 31f
  signal rejection, 31
Recruitment maneuvers, 123
Refraction artifact, 36f
Relative hypovolemia, 105
Renal biopsy
  complications associated with, 295
  contraindications for, 293–294
  indications for, 292–293
  procedure
    laboratory testing, 294
    postbiopsy care, 295
    spinal needle movement, 294–295
  risk from, 293
  transvenous, 293
Renal collecting system, dilatation of, 239
Renal cysts, 239–241
Renal failure
  categorization of, 238
  end-stage, 241
  hydronephrosis, 238, 240
  renal cysts, 239–241
  ureteral obstruction, Doppler interrogation of, 239
Renal intraparenchymal abscess, 244
Renal obstruction, 239
Renal parenchymal damage, 238
Renal trauma, ultrasound of, 243
Restrictive CMP, 157f
  causes of, 157
  clinical features of, 156
  Doppler assessment of, 158, 158f
  two-dimensional and M-mode assessment of, 157, 157f
Retinal detachment, 323, 323f
Reverberation artifact, 35f
Right atrial pressure (RAP) estimation, 108–109, 109t
Right heart failure
  preload responsiveness identification in, 124
Right ventricle (RV), anatomy of, 115
Right ventricular (RV) dysfunction, 115
Right ventricular outflow tract (RVOT), 96
RV diasystolic overload
  echocardiographic features of
    reduced LV filling, 120
    RV diastolic volume, 120
    RV dilation, 118–119
    RV end-diastolic size, 119–120
RV infarction, 124
RV systolic overload
  echocardiographic features of
    eccentricity index, 116
    pulmonary artery and its bifurcation, 117–118, 117f, 118f
    pulmonary vascular impedance, 116
    septal dyskinesia, 116, 116f

S
Sciatic nerve
  blockade, 300
  subgluteal approach to, 301
Seashore sign, M-mode ultrasound image of, 210
Seldinger technique, 289, 292, 314
Septal and valvular injury, 176
Severe hypotension
  and respiratory distress, GDE for, 60
  and respiratory failure, GDE for, 59
Single-crystal imaging transducer, 27
Sinusogram, 186
Skin compression artifact, 282
Societe de Reanimation de Langue Francaise (SRLF), 38
Solid pleural abnormalities, 204–205
Solitary kidney, risk for, 293
Sonographically guided pleural biopsy, 278
Sound wave
  acoustic parameters
    amplitude, 10–11
    frequency and period, 9–10
    intensity, 12
    power, 11–12
    propagation speed, 12, 12f, 12t
    wavelength, 12–13
  definition of, 9
  interactions, 15
  nature of, 10
Spatial and temporal resolution of 2D image, factors determining, 27t
Spatial pulse length (SPL), 16
Splenic ultrasound, 227–228
Spontaneously breathing patients
  dynamic echocardiographic parameter estimation, 112–114
  respiratory cyclic variations of pulse pressure, 112
  response to PLR, 112–113
  SV, 114
  pneumothorax incidence in, 274
  vs. mechanically ventilated patient, 108–109
Standard transthoracic, transthoracic echocardiographic, 337f–338f
Static parameters
  static echocardiographic parameters, 107–108
  static pressure parameters, 106–107
Stroke volume, with pulsed-wave Doppler, 94–95

Subclavian vein, ultrasound-guided cannulation of, 310–311
Supraclavicular plexus, 299

T

Thoracentesis
  complications of, 274
  patient and operator positioning for, 274
  real-time visualization of, 275
Thoracic ultrasound
  convex-array/sector-scanning probes for, 273
  for lung consolidation, 49–50
  for neonatal RDS, 50
  patient positioning for, 273–274
  for pleural effusion, 47–48, 47f
  for pneumothorax assessment, 48–49
Time-gain compensation (TGC), 29
Tissue harmonic imaging (THI), 14
Tissue phantoms, 21, 22f
Transabdominal bladder, 236–237
Transabdominal (TAS) pelvic ultrasound examination
  for embryonic structures, 252
  using curved linear array, 249
Transcranial Doppler (TCD)
  acoustic windows of
    transforaminal and transorbital, 268
    transtemporal, 268–269
  applications of, 268
  circle of Willis, 269
  functionality of, 268
  middle cerebral artery (MCA) waveforms, 269
  parameters, 268
  vs. duplex vascular examination, 268
Transducer arrays
  longitudinal view of, 307
  orientation of, 307
  position of, 187
  problems with, 307–308
  selection, 304–305
  transverse view of, 306–307
  vein visualization and, 308
Transducers
  components of, 24f
    backing material, 23
    matching layer, 23
    PZT crystal, 23
    wire, 23
  definition of, 23
  display modes, 24, 25f
  manipulation, 66
  phased-array probes, 25–26
  single-crystal, 24
Transesophageal echocardiography (TEE), 163
  dynamic parameter estimation (See Dynamic echocardiographic parameter estimation)
  for fever, elevated white count, and hypotension, 82

GDE with, 57, 58
for hypotension, 81
  and severe LV failure, 82
  and urosepsis, 81
  and ventilatory support, 83
international training program for, 40
of LVEDA AND LVESA, 107, 107f
report, 338–339
for respiratory failure, 83
role in valve function evaluation, 171
for septic shock, 85, 86
for unexplained hypotension, 82, 84
vs. transthoracic echocardiography, 89–90
Transient LV apical ballooning syndrome, 160–161, 161f
Transthoracic biopsy procedures
  coaxial cutting needle technique, 277
  contraindications to, 277
  disadvantage of, 277
  ultrasound-guided needle biopsy, 276–278
Transthoracic echocardiography (TTE), 65, 163
  critical care (See Critical care TEE)
  dynamic parameter estimation (See Dynamic echocardiographic parameter estimation)
  examination, 66–67
  GDE with, 57, 58
  international training program for, 40
  limitations of, 180, 180f
  nomenclature, 66
  pediatric cardiac ICU, 45
  role in valve function evaluation, 171
  technical issues with, 65–66
  vs. transesophageal echocardiography, 89–90
Traumatic injuries
  causes of, 175
  indications for cardiac ultrasonography in, 176t
Traumatic vision, 321
Tricuspid valve (TV) evaluation, 164, 164f
Truncal blocks, 301–302
Tubo-ovarian abscess (TOA), 253
Tubo-ovarian complex (TOC), 253
Two-dimensional arrays, 27, 28t
Two-dimensional imaging, 26f
Two-dimensional imaging displays, 24

U

Ultrasound reports, abdominal and pelvic reports, 339t
Ultrasound artifacts, 33–36, 34t
Ultrasound equipment quality assurance, 21
Ultrasound examination of chest, report, 336
Ultrasound-guided cannulation
  of axillary vein, 312
  of femoral vein, 311–312

of internal jugular vein, 308–310
of subclavian vein, 310–311
Ultrasound-guided needle biopsy, 276–278
Ultrasound-guided paracentesis, 51f
Ultrasound-guided pericardiocentesis, 133
  equipment requirements for, 279
  pericardial effusion, 283
  site selection for, 279–281
  skin compression artifact in, 282
  sterile skin preparation for, 282
  vs. fluoroscopic guidance, 278
Ultrasound-guided procedures, classification of, 305–306
Ultrasound-guided tube thoracostomy, 275–276
Ultrasound image formation, 28
  signal amplification, 29, 29f
  signal compensation, 29, 30f
  signal compression, 29–31, 30f
  signal demodulation, 31, 31f
  signal rejection, 31
Ultrasound images
  bioeffects, 21–22
  factors affecting quality of, 14, 14t
Ultrasound imaging
  of abdomen, 339–340
  of axillary plexus, 300
  cannulation
    of neck/larynx, 335–336
    of pericardial effusion, 281
    of peripheral lung mass, 276
    of popliteal fossa, 301
  of chest, 336
  of femoral nerve, 300
Ultrasound imaging, basic assumptions for, 32t
Ultrasound in ICU. See Critical care ultrasound
Ultrasound machine
  components of, 27–28
  electrical pulses, 28
  receiver/processor, 29–31
  compression, 30f
  transducer output, 29
Ultrasound of neck/larynx, report, 335
Ultrasound reports by body region, 335–336
Ultrasound terminology, 33t
Ultrasound transducer, 23
Ultrasound waves, 10
  acoustic parameters
    amplitude, 10–11
    frequency and period, 9–10
    intensity, 12
    power, 11–12
    propagation speed, 12, 12f, 12t
    wavelength, 12–13
  continuous-wave, 16
  high- and low-frequency, 14t
  interactions, 15

Ultrasound waves, (Cont'd.)
  and medium, interactions of, 13–15
    acoustic impedance, 14
    attenuation, 13
    axial or longitudinal resolution, 14
    echo, 13
    reflection, 14
    reflective boundaries, 15
    refraction, 15, 15f
    tissue harmonics, 14
    ultrasound transmission, 14–15
  pulse waves, 15–16
Upper extremity
  arterial anatomy of, 263
  blockage, 298–299
  venous anatomy of, 258–260, 315
  venous examination, patient position for, 261
Upper extremity blocks, for pain control, 298–299
Ureteral obstruction, 239
Urinary bladder, color-flow Doppler of, 238
Urinary system, ultrasound evaluation of, 235
Urinary tract infection (UTI), 243–244, 293
Urosepsis, 243–244
  GDE for, 58
Uterus
  anatomy of, 249
  transabdominal longitudinal image of, 253
  ultrasound of, 250

V

Valsalva maneuver, 260
Vascular access procedures
  complications associated with, 303–304
  CVC placement, 303
  ultrasonography impact on, 304
Vascular occlusion, 267
Vein visualization, 308
Velocity–time integral (VTI), 95, 95f
Venous duplex examination of DVT
  equipment requirements for, 261–262
  flow characteristics, 261
  patient positioning, 261
  transverse compressions, 261–262
Venous duplex examination of extremities, 340–341
Venous systems
  of lower extremity, 258
  of upper extremity, 258
Viral pneumonia, 50f
Visceral-parietal pleural interface (VPPI), 188
Vitreous hemorrhage, 321
Volume responsiveness
  dynamic parameters of, 108
  vs. fluid challenge, 105–106

W

Wall-motion score index, 91–92
Wave interactions, 15

www.ingramcontent.com/pod-product-compliance
Lightning Source LLC
Chambersburg PA
CBHW051051300825
31884CB00012B/80